Essentials of Plastic Surgery

Q&A Companion

Essentials of
Plastic Surgery

Q&A Companion

ALEX P. JONES
FRCS (PLAST), MBCHB (HONS), BSC (HONS)
Consultant Plastic and Reconstructive Surgeon,
James Cook University Hospital,
Middlesbrough, Cleveland, United Kingdom

JEFFREY E. JANIS, MD, FACS
Professor of Plastic Surgery, Neurosurgery, Neurology, and Surgery;
Executive Vice Chairman, Department of Plastic Surgery,
Chief of Plastic Surgery, University Hospital,
Ohio State University Wexner Medical Center, Columbus, Ohio

With the Assistance of Dr. Anna R. Barnard

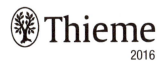

2016

Thieme Medical Publishers, Inc.
333 Seventh Ave.
New York, NY 10001

© 2016 by Thieme Medical Publishers, Inc.

No claim to original U.S. Government works

Printed in Germany

International Standard Book Number-13: 978-1-62623-659-2

This book contains information obtained from authentic and highly regarded sources. While all reasonable efforts have been made to publish reliable data and information, neither the author[s] nor the publisher can accept any legal responsibility or liability for any errors or omissions that may be made. The publishers wish to make clear that any views or opinions expressed in this book by individual editors, authors or contributors are personal to them and do not necessarily reflect the views/opinions of the publishers. The information or guidance contained in this book is intended for use by medical, scientific or health-care professionals and is provided strictly as a supplement to the medical or other professional's own judgement, their knowledge of the patient's medical history, relevant manufacturer's instructions and the appropriate best practice guidelines. Because of the rapid advances in medical science, any information or advice on dosages, procedures or diagnoses should be independently verified. The reader is strongly urged to consult the relevant national drug formulary and the drug companies' and device or material manufacturers' printed instructions, and their websites, before administering or utilizing any of the drugs, devices or materials mentioned in this book. This book does not indicate whether a particular treatment is appropriate or suitable for a particular individual. Ultimately it is the sole responsibility of the medical professional to make his or her own professional judgements, so as to advise and treat patients appropriately. The authors and publishers have also attempted to trace the copyright holders of all material reproduced in this publication and apologize to copyright holders if permission to publish in this form has not been obtained. If any copyright material has not been acknowledged please write and let us know so we may rectify in any future reprint.

Except as permitted under U.S. Copyright Law, no part of this book may be reprinted, reproduced, transmitted, or utilized in any form by any electronic, mechanical, or other means, now known or hereafter invented, including photocopying, microfilming, and recording, or in any information storage or retrieval system, without written permission from the publishers.

For permission to photocopy or use material electronically from this work, please access www.copyright.com (http://www.copyright.com/) or contact the Copyright Clearance Center, Inc. (CCC), 222 Rosewood Drive, Danvers, MA 01923, 978-750-8400. CCC is a not-for-profit organization that provides licenses and registration for a variety of users. For organizations that have been granted a photocopy license by the CCC, a separate system of payment has been arranged.

Trademark Notice: Product or corporate names may be trademarks or registered trademarks, and are used only for identification and explanation without intent to infringe.

Orders may be sent to: Thieme Publishers New York
333 Seventh Avenue, New York, NY 10001 USA
+1 800 782 3488, customerservice@thieme.com

Thieme Publishers Stuttgart
Rüdigerstrasse 14, 70469 Stuttgart, Germany
+49 [0]711 8931 421, customerservice@thieme.de

Thieme Publishers Delhi
A-12, Second Floor, Sector-2, Noida-201301
Uttar Pradesh, India
+91 120 45 566 00, customerservice@thieme.in

Thieme Publishers Rio de Janeiro, Thieme Publicações Ltda.
Edifício Rodolpho de Paoli, 25º andar
Av. Nilo Peçanha, 50 – Sala 2508,
Rio de Janeiro 20020-906 Brasil
+55 21 3172-2297 / +55 21 3172-1896

www.Thieme.com

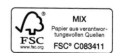

*To my family and friends for their love and support,
to my mentors for sharing their skills and knowledge,
and to my patients for making the art of plastic surgery so worthwhile*

A.P.J.

*To my family and source of strength,
Emily, Jackson, Brinkley, and Holden,
and to my source of inspiration,
my former, current, and future residents*

J.E.J.

EXECUTIVE EDITOR Sue Hodgson
SENIOR PROJECT EDITING MANAGER Carolyn Reich
GRAPHICS MANAGER Brett Stone
DIRECTOR OF ILLUSTRATION AND DESIGN Brenda Bunch
MANAGING EDITOR Suzanne Wakefield
EDITOR/PROJECT MANAGER Makalah Boyer
ILLUSTRATOR Sarah Taylor, Amanda Tomasikiewicz
PRODUCTION Debra Clark, Chris Lane
PROOFREADER Linda Maulin
INDEXER Matthew White

Foreword

This is a very valuable companion book to the second edition of *Essentials of Plastic Surgery*. It allows readers a chance to see whether they are retaining what they are reading. We all get lost from time to time in the journey to obtain knowledge through reading. Readers can "take a break" and refer to this book to see how they are progressing with objective help.

The questions are practical, useful, and reflect the style and content of questions frequently asked in examinations of all stripes. The contents of the question bank and the chapters in the text are an excellent mirror of the depth and breadth of the current state of knowledge in plastic surgery. If readers can answer all the questions in this book, they clearly have a handle on things! I would encourage all readers to challenge themselves to do just that.

Alex Jones and Jeff Janis are masters of plastic surgery. Their work in this book is of Herculean proportions. This labor of love is a gift to those who want to excel in the magic of our specialty.

Donald H. Lalonde, Hons BSc, MD, MSc, FRCSC
Professor of Surgery, Department of Plastic Surgery,
Dalhousie University, Saint John, New Brunswick, Canada

Foreword

It is a great privilege to be invited to write a foreword to this *Q&A Companion* of the very well established *Essentials of Plastic Surgery* by Dr. Jeffrey Janis. Dr. Janis has an enviable and international reputation in the field of surgical education. His collaboration with the young British plastic surgeon, Alex Jones, introduces a European perspective to the format.

The attention to detail that has gone into this *Q&A Companion* is obvious and will inculcate the lessons read in *Essentials of Plastic Surgery*.

I feel that it will be sought out not only by trainees but also by established surgeons in this era of revalidation and reaccreditation.

A.G.B. Perks, FRCS, FRCS (Plast), FRACS (Plast)
Consultant Plastic and Reconstructive Surgeon,
Head of Department of Plastic, Reconstructive & Burns Surgery,
Nottingham University Hospitals, Nottingham, United Kingdom;
President, 2013 and 2014, British Association of Plastic Reconstructive and Aesthetic Surgeons

Preface

Almost four years have passed since we first discussed producing a question and answer companion to the second edition of the popular *Essentials of Plastic Surgery*. We felt there was a paucity of texts available for self-assessment and that the market could benefit from a comprehensive, clinically oriented Q&A book to help readers cement the core principles covered within the *Essentials* text.

The second edition of *Essentials* has grown considerably from the first edition, now featuring 88 to 102 chapters, with approximately 35% additional content and nearly 1300 pages. The Q&A book closely reflects this content and contains nearly 1200 questions in 102 chapters, which are structured as both multiple choice questions (MCQ) and extended matching questions (EMQ) in single best answer format. The questions are designed to test the reader on the content of each *Essentials* chapter, with key emphasis on clinical application of this knowledge.

Each chapter mirrors the equivalent chapter from *Essentials,* with the same style and format and pertinent illustrations reproduced. Questions are repeated in the answer section to avoid the reader's having to page back and forth. The correct answer is fully explained, and incorrect answers are expanded to clarify them.

This learning resource is accompanied by an electronic version (e-book), which means that it can be readily accessed on smart phones and tablets. For those who prefer traditional books, the format is both compact and portable and is presented with high-quality production.

The book is intended to be used as a study aid, working through individual questions and answers in turn, or as a self-test in which multiple questions are undertaken, with a review at the end of the exercise.

We hope that readers find this to be a useful adjunct to the *Essentials* book on which it is based and that it acts as a comprehensive companion book that can be used to assess one's knowledge base of the spectrum of plastic surgery as presented in the parent book. We hope it will prove useful through your training and future life as a plastic surgeon.

Alex P. Jones
Jeffrey E. Janis

Acknowledgments

The creation of this book has required teamwork by a significant number of talented people, and I would like to express my gratitude for each person's part in developing this study tool. First, my appreciation to Dr. Jeff Janis for the comprehensive second edition of *Essentials of Plastic Surgery* as the source text for this *Q&A Companion* and for his insightful collaboration, commitment, and enthusiasm throughout the project. I would also like to thank all of the original contributors to the source text for providing such a wealth of information on which to base questions. A particular thank you is due to Karen Berger, who first expressed her belief in and support for this project. Michelle Berger invested a massive amount of time and energy as the book went through first and second layout versions.

Dr. Anna Barnard has been a significant contributor to this book, providing feedback and editing advice throughout the project. Furthermore, she provided specific expert input in the upper limb sections, for which she wrote the majority of questions.

Residents Terri Zomerlei and Ibrahim Khansa at Ohio State University Wexner Medical Center performed invaluable reviews of all content from a resident's perspective to ensure that the questions and answers were effectively presented and clinically relevant.

The manuscript and final pages took shape with the expert guidance of executive editor Sue Hodgson and the skilled hands of the St. Louis team of CRC Press/Taylor & Francis Group. With infinite patience and skill, editor/project manager Makalah Boyer spent endless hours shaping all stages of the book into a cohesive whole. Illustrators Sarah Taylor and Amanda Tomasikiewicz rendered excellent new drawings to augment the figures reproduced from the parent book, *Essentials of Plastic Surgery*. And my deep appreciation goes to the many members of the editing and production team, who represent the highest order of dedication to craftsmanship in book publishing.

Our goal was to produce a valuable resource for the plastic surgeons of today and tomorrow as they expand and refine their knowledge of our ever-growing field. The nature of plastic surgery demands innovators, and it is our hope that through *Essentials of Plastic Surgery* and this *Q&A Companion*, readers will reinforce their mastery of the fundamentals, which may prove necessary for the very next patient they see.

A.P.J.

Acknowledgments

A tremendous debt of gratitude is owed to a great number of people who put an incredible amount of time, energy, and effort into the creation, editing, and production of this Q&A Companion to the second edition of *Essentials of Plastic Surgery*.

It goes without saying that there could not be a companion book without a parent book, and to that end, I would like to thank the authors of the original chapters on whose work these questions were crafted and founded.

I also acknowledge with sincere appreciation Alex Jones, who literally poured his heart and soul into this book for years. As you will see from the quality of the book, these questions and answers were not written overnight, but rather were painstakingly written over a long period of time with many meticulous revisions and modifications. Alex's dedication, time, sweat, and passion come through in the final result, and it has been a distinct pleasure to work closely with him. His European perspective gives international flavor and relevance to the book and the types of questions it contains to make it applicable to plastic surgeons worldwide. Credit clearly is also due to Anna Barnard, who helped Alex on many of the chapters and whose work and effort absolutely need to be recognized.

The ultimate value of the book is truly in the eyes and hands of the end user, and to that end, I asked two of my current residents, Drs. Ibrahim Khansa and Terri Zomerlei, to review every one of the 102 chapters to make sure they were clinically relevant, useful, and clear. Their comments and input helped refine the book and raised the bar on its utility and practicality. I thank them for their insight, time, and willingness to take on such a task in the middle of their busy clinical responsibilities.

I would also like to recognize Karen Berger and Michelle Berger from Quality Medical Publishing, who originally welcomed the idea of this book and set the wheels in motion to its ultimate production. During the writing of this book, CRC Press/Taylor & Francis Group purchased the publication arm of Quality Medical Publishing, and therefore I had the distinct pleasure of working with an incredible team of experienced professionals, such as executive editor Sue Hodgson, project manager and editor Makalah Boyer, Suzanne Wakefield, managing editor, as well as Sarah Taylor, Brenda Bunch, Carolyn Reich, Brett Stone, Debra Clark, Chris Lane, Linda Maulin, and Matthew White. Without each of these individuals, this project simply could not have come to fruition. Their skill and expertise are clearly represented in every page.

Most of all, I would like to deeply and sincerely thank my wife, Emily, and our beautiful children, Jackson, Brinkley, and Holden. Their love, support, patience, and understanding is unequaled and unparalleled and is the only reason a book like this is possible in the first place. I owe them more than I could ever hope to repay, and I take nothing for granted.

J.E.J.

Contents

PART I ◆ FUNDAMENTALS AND BASICS

1. WOUND HEALING   3
2. GENERAL MANAGEMENT OF COMPLEX WOUNDS   13
3. SUTURES AND NEEDLES   19
4. BASICS OF FLAPS   26
5. FUNDAMENTALS OF PERFORATOR FLAPS   35
6. TISSUE EXPANSION   41
7. VASCULARIZED COMPOSITE ALLOGRAFTS AND TRANSPLANT IMMUNOLOGY   48
8. BASICS OF MICROSURGERY   55
9. BIOMATERIALS   62
10. NEGATIVE PRESSURE WOUND THERAPY   72
11. LASERS IN PLASTIC SURGERY   77
12. ANESTHESIA   85
13. PHOTOGRAPHY FOR THE PLASTIC SURGEON   94

PART II ◆ SKIN AND SOFT TISSUE

14. STRUCTURE AND FUNCTION OF SKIN   103
15. BASAL CELL CARCINOMA, SQUAMOUS CELL CARCINOMA, AND MELANOMA   110
16. BURNS   129
17. VASCULAR ANOMALIES   138
18. CONGENITAL NEVI   145

PART III ◆ HEAD AND NECK

19. HEAD AND NECK EMBRYOLOGY   153
20. SURGICAL TREATMENT OF MIGRAINE HEADACHES   159

Congenital Conditions

21	Craniosynostosis	167
22	Craniofacial Clefts	177
23	Distraction Osteogenesis	184
24	Cleft Lip	188
25	Cleft Palate	196
26	Velopharyngeal Dysfunction	206
27	Microtia	213
28	Prominent Ear	219

Traumatic Injuries

29	Facial Soft Tissue Trauma	226
30	Facial Skeletal Trauma	231
31	Mandibular Fractures	244
32	Basic Oral Surgery	250

Acquired Deformities

33	Principles of Head and Neck Cancer: Staging and Management	261
34	Scalp and Calvarial Reconstruction	272
35	Eyelid Reconstruction	279
36	Nasal Reconstruction	285
37	Cheek Reconstruction	296
38	Ear Reconstruction	304
39	Lip Reconstruction	312
40	Mandibular Reconstruction	319
41	Pharyngeal Reconstruction	326
42	Facial Reanimation	336
43	Face Transplantation	347

Part IV ♦ Breast

| 44 | Breast Anatomy and Embryology | 355 |
| 45 | Breast Augmentation | 362 |

46 Mastopexy 370
47 Augmentation-Mastopexy 378
48 Breast Reduction 383
49 Gynecomastia 392
50 Breast Cancer and Reconstruction 398
51 Nipple-Areolar Reconstruction 409

PART V ♦ TRUNK AND LOWER EXTREMITY

52 Chest Wall Reconstruction 419
53 Abdominal Wall Reconstruction 427
54 Genitourinary Reconstruction 435
55 Pressure Sores 443
56 Lower Extremity Reconstruction 451
57 Foot Ulcers 462
58 Lymphedema 471

PART VI ♦ HAND, WRIST, AND UPPER EXTREMITY

59 Hand Anatomy and Biomechanics 481
60 Basic Hand Examination 492
61 Congenital Hand Anomalies 498
62 Carpal Bone Fractures 509
63 Carpal Instability and Dislocations 514
64 Distal Radius Fractures 520
65 Metacarpal and Phalangeal Fractures 525
66 Phalangeal Dislocations 537
67 Fingertip Injuries 544
68 Nail Bed Injuries 553
69 Flexor Tendon Injuries 559
70 Extensor Tendon Injuries 568
71 Tendon Transfers 581
72 Hand and Finger Amputations 589

73	Replantation	594
74	Hand Transplantation	603
75	Thumb Reconstruction	610
76	Soft Tissue Coverage of the Hand and Upper Extremity	616
77	Compartment Syndrome	625
78	Upper Extremity Compression Syndromes	634
79	Brachial Plexus	644
80	Nerve Injuries	654
81	Hand Infections	664
82	Benign and Malignant Masses of the Hand	674
83	Dupuytren's Disease	681
84	Rheumatoid Arthritis	688
85	Osteoarthritis	697
86	Vascular Disorders of the Hand and Wrist	705

Part VII ♦ Aesthetic Surgery

87	Facial Analysis	715
88	Nonoperative Facial Rejuvenation	724
89	Fat Grafting	740
90	Hair Transplantation	748
91	Brow Lift	758
92	Blepharoplasty	768
93	Blepharoptosis	780
94	Face Lift	789
95	Neck Lift	804
96	Rhinoplasty	812
97	Genioplasty	825
98	Liposuction	831
99	Brachioplasty	841

100	ABDOMINOPLASTY	**850**
101	MEDIAL THIGH LIFT	**864**
102	BODY CONTOURING IN THE MASSIVE-WEIGHT-LOSS PATIENT	**872**

CREDITS **881**

INDEX **883**

Essentials of Plastic Surgery

Q&A Companion

Part I

Fundamentals and Basics

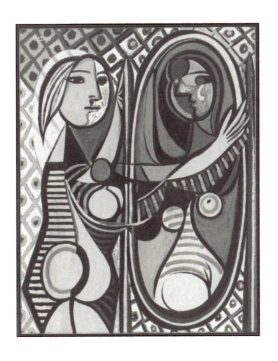

© 2015 Estate of Pablo Picasso / Artists Rights Society (ARS), New York.

1. Wound Healing

See *Essentials of Plastic Surgery,* second edition, pp. 3-9.

PHASES OF WOUND HEALING

1. **Which one of the following statements is true of the process of wound healing?**
   A. It is comprised of five key phases.
   B. Vasodilatation is the initial response after injury.
   C. Each of the key phases are distinct entities.
   D. Each of the phases are of similar duration.
   E. The wound healing process differs in fetal tissue.

2. **In the first 24 hours after a soft tissue injury, which one of the following represents the dominant cell type?**
   A. The neutrophil
   B. The macrophage
   C. The lymphocyte
   D. The fibroblast
   E. The myofibroblast

3. **Which one of the following collagen subtypes is most commonly found in the skin?**
   A. Type I
   B. Type II
   C. Type III
   D. Type IV
   E. Type V

4. **Which one of the following is true in a 6-week-old healing wound?**
   A. Net collagen production is positive.
   B. Net glycosaminoglycan production is positive.
   C. Net vasculogenesis is positive.
   D. Net glycosaminoglycan production is static.
   E. Net collagen production is static.

5. **Which one of the following collagen subtypes predominates in a 3-week-old healing wound?**
   A. Type I
   B. Type III
   C. Type V
   D. Type VII
   E. Type IX

6. **Ten weeks after direct closure of a wound to the forearm, what proportion of preinjury tensile strength can be expected across the scar?**
   A. 20%
   B. 40%
   C. 60%
   D. 80%
   E. 100%

GROWTH FACTORS

7. A patient sustains a wound to the right arm following trauma. After wash out in the emergency department, the wound is left to heal by secondary intention. *Which one of the following is correct regarding the effect of growth factors on this process?*
   A. FGF will decrease fibroblast proliferation.
   B. TGF-beta promotes fibroblast migration and proliferation.
   C. VEGF is produced by endothelial cells.
   D. EGF promotes endothelial proliferation.
   E. PDGF promotes keratinocyte proliferation.

CELL TYPES IN WOUND HEALING

8. *Which one of the following cell types is chiefly responsible for reducing the surface area of a granulating wound because of its contractile properties?*
   A. Fibroblast
   B. Keratinocyte
   C. Macrophage
   D. Lymphocyte
   E. Myofibroblast

CELLULAR PROCESS IN EPITHELIALIZATION

9. *Which one of the following is an important cellular process that facilitates mobilization of keratinocytes during healing of a split-thickness skin graft donor site?*
   A. Diapedesis
   B. Margination
   C. Loss of contact inhibition
   D. Differentiation
   E. Epithelialization

TYPES OF WOUND HEALING

10. *Which one of the following most accurately defines whether primary or secondary healing occurs within a cutaneous wound?*
    A. The mechanism of injury
    B. The amount of tissue damage
    C. The time healing takes to occur
    D. The method of wound closure
    E. How closely the wound edges are apposed

FACTORS AFFECTING WOUND HEALING

11. *In which one of the following conditions is normal wound healing expected after surgery?*
    A. Ehlers Danlos
    B. Progeria
    C. Werner syndrome
    D. Cutis laxa
    E. Smokers

12. *Which one of the following vitamins can be particularly useful to help wound healing in patients on long-term steroids?*
    A. Vitamin A
    B. Vitamin B
    C. Vitamin C
    D. Vitamin D
    E. Vitamin E

13. What is the single most important cause of a wound to fail to heal?
   A. Poor oxygen supply
   B. Denervation
   C. Radiation injury
   D. Poor nutrition
   E. Dry wound base

14. Debridement of a chronic wound can remove excess granulation tissue and expedite healing. **What else is thought to be responsible for impaired wound healing in chronic wounds that is removed during debridement?**
   A. Metalloproteases
   B. Lathyrogens
   C. Myofibroblasts
   D. TGF-beta
   E. Chondroitin sulfate

15. You see a patient who wishes to undergo a face lift. She has given up smoking after your advice and now uses only nicotine replacement medications. **Which one of the following represents a well-recognized effect of nicotine on tissues?**
   A. Reduced oxyhemoglobin concentrations
   B. Reduced platelet adhesion
   C. Reduced local inflammation
   D. Reduced local blood supply
   E. Toxic effects on keratinocytes

16. You have a patient with a large wound to the tibia after a fall and have closed this directly. He is due to start chemotherapy very soon. **When can the chemotherapy be started without detrimental effects on healing of this wound?**
   A. Immediately
   B. In 3 days
   C. In 14 days
   D. In 1 month
   E. There is no evidence to guide this decision

ABNORMAL SCARRING

17. **When examining a patient with an abnormally thickened scar, what is the key factor that will differentiate a keloid from a hypertrophic scar?**
   A. Elevation of the scar
   B. Erythema within the scar
   C. Growth beyond the original wound borders
   D. A biopsy of the scar tissue is the only way to differentiate
   E. The shape of the scar

TREATMENT FOR KELOID SCARS

18. A young female patient presents with a large keloid scar on her ear after a piercing. She has tried silicone gel and steroid injections with little improvement. **Which one of the following is correct?**
   A. No firm evidence supports pressure therapy and massage techniques to reduce scarring in such patients.
   B. Radiation therapy may be helpful for this patient, but the chance of recurrence is as high as 33%.
   C. The ongoing treatment plan would be the same if this patient had a hypertrophic scar.
   D. Silicone sheeting acts by increasing hydration while decreasing tissue temperature.
   E. Multimodality treatment is not advocated in this case.

Answers

PHASES OF WOUND HEALING

1. Which one of the following statements is true of the process of wound healing?
   E. The wound healing process differs in fetal tissue.
   Fetal wound healing during the first two trimesters differs from the normal wound healing process and is the subject of much research because of the perceived potential for scarless healing. The process is more of a regenerative process than a repair process often with the absence of an inflammatory phase.[1]
   Wound healing after birth represents a highly evolved and complex defense mechanism that helps to limit infection and further injury. The normal wound healing process is comprised of three (not five) phases. These are the inflammatory, the fibroproliferative, and the remodeling phases, respectively. The phases are not distinct entities and have overlap both in terms of timing and function. Each phase has a different duration and this can be quite variable. The inflammatory phase typically lasts for a week, the fibroproliferative phase lasts for two to three weeks, and the remodeling phase lasts for up to one year. Vasoconstriction is the initial response to injury in order to limit blood loss and lasts for 5 to 10 minutes after injury. Vasodilatation and increased tissue permeability follows this as part of the inflammatory phase to promote cellular access to the injured area. Knowledge of the key processes in wound healing is often tested in examinations and a solid understanding of these principles is important for clinical practice with respect to the management of different wound types.

2. In the first 24 hours after a soft tissue injury, which one of the following represents the dominant cell type?
   A. The neutrophil
   There are a number of key cell types involved in the wound healing process and they are generally specific to a particular phase of wound healing. For example, the neutrophil is the dominant cell type in the first 24 hours after injury. It serves to produce inflammatory mediators and undertake phagocytosis of damaged cells, but is not actually critical to wound healing. After 48 hours the macrophage becomes the dominant cell type. In contrast, this is critical to wound healing because it orchestrates growth factors such as TGF-beta, which promotes collagen production, remodeling, epithelialization, and chemotaxis. Lymphocytes are involved with the inflammatory phase, although their role is poorly defined. They are typically present towards the end of the first week after injury. The fibroblast is key to wound healing and moves into the wound after 48 hours. By the end of the first week, it represents the dominant cell type. Along with the myofibroblast, it has a key role in the fibroproliferative phase with the production of collagen.

3. Which one of the following collagen subtypes is most commonly found in the skin?
   A. Type I
   Collagen is a protein that forms the key building block for skin, bone, cartilage, and tendon. The basic structure consists of three left-handed polypeptide helices wound together to form a right-handed helix. It comprises two alpha-1 and one alpha-2 chains, each of these are formed by amino acid sequences; glycine-prolene-X and glycine-X-hydroxyprolene. There are more than

20 different collagen subtypes and type I is the most common in humans, representing 90% of all body collagen. It predominates in the skin, tendon, and bone. Type II is found in the cornea and articular cartilage. Type III is found in the vessel and bowel walls. Type IV is found in the basement membrane only.

4. **Which one of the following is true in a 6-week-old healing wound?**
   E. Net collagen production is static.
   At six weeks, the healing wound should be in the remodeling phase of wound healing. During this phase, net collagen production is static because an equilibrium is reached between collagen breakdown and collagen synthesis. Although there is no change in quantity, collagen continues to undergo remodeling with increased organization and formation of stronger cross-links. The ratio of different collagen subtypes also changes. Glycosaminoglycan production and vasculogenesis decrease as does the water content and cellular population.

5. **Which one of the following collagen subtypes predominates in a 3-week-old healing wound?**
   B. Type III
   As discussed in the explanation to question 3, there are more than twenty different types of collagen with type I representing 90% of all body collagen. The normal adult ratio of type I to type III within the skin is around 4:1. However, in the healing wound, type III collagen is made first and this subtype predominates in the proliferation and early remodeling phases until it is gradually replaced by type I collagen.

6. **Ten weeks after direct closure of a wound to the forearm, what proportion of preinjury tensile strength can be expected across the scar?**
   D. 80%
   In spite of the impressive ability of wounds to heal, tissues never regain 100% of their preinjury tensile strength. It is estimated that a healed wound will have, at best, around 80% of its preinjury tensile strength and this will be achieved between 60 days and one year after the injury. The evidence for this stems from a 1965 study by Levenson et al[2] where healing in rat skin wounds was assessed at various time intervals. Knowledge of skin strength at various time points following repair is clinically useful when considering suture selection, such that the suture is able to satisfactorily support the wound until adequate strength has been regained. For example, placement of buried dermal sutures in the face allows for external skin sutures to be removed at 5 days although the repair will still be weak at this stage. It also helps guide the clinician and patient with regard to resumption of normal activities following surgery. (See Chapter 3, *Essentials of Plastic Surgery*, second edition.)

GROWTH FACTORS

7. A patient sustains a wound to the right arm following trauma. After wash out in the emergency department, the wound is left to heal by secondary intention. **Which one of the following is correct regarding the effect of growth factors on this process?**
   B. TGF-beta promotes fibroblast migration and proliferation.
   Many growth factors are involved in the wound-healing process and most of these positively influence cell proliferation and migration. Accordingly, TGF-beta will promote fibroblast migration and proliferation. FGF will increase both fibroblast and keratinocyte proliferation. It also affects fibroblast chemotaxis. VEGF will promote endothelial cell proliferation and is produced by many

different cell types in response to hypoxia or injury. EGF promotes keratinocyte and fibroblast division rather than endothelial cell proliferation. PDGF promotes fibroblast, endothelial cell, and smooth muscle proliferation rather than keratinocyte proliferation.

CELL TYPES IN WOUND HEALING

8. Which one of the following cell types is chiefly responsible for reducing the surface area of a granulating wound because of its contractile properties?

E. Myofibroblast

Fibroblasts are the key cells responsible for forming extracellular matrix and collagen. They are present in both the early and late stages of wound healing and have a permanent presence in the dermis. Myofibroblasts are specialized fibroblasts that have contractile cytoplasmic microfilaments and distinct cellular adhesion structures. They are present in the early stages of wound healing and serve to collectively decrease the size of a wound. They usually remain within the wound for the first few weeks following injury. Keratinocytes are the major cells of the epidermis and are involved in wound healing and normal skin cell turnover. Macrophages and lymphocytes are both inflammatory cells that are involved in the orchestration of wound healing.

CELLULAR PROCESSES IN EPITHELIALIZATION

9. Which one of the following is an important cellular process that facilitates mobilization of keratinocytes during healing of a split-thickness skin graft donor site?

C. Loss of contact inhibition

The process of healing a split-thickness skin graft donor site is termed reepithelialization. This involves a series of cellular processes that enable keratinocytes from the wound edges to proliferate and move towards the center of the wound. Cells are usually held at the wound edge by contact inhibition and this must be lost to enable cells to mobilize. Following a loss of contact inhibition, cells move across the wound until they meet cells from the other side and contact inhibition is reestablished. While cells at the wound edge are migrating, basal cells further back from the wound edge proliferate to support the cell numbers required to bridge the wound. Differentiation of keratinocytes subsequently occurs to reestablish normal epithelial layers from basal layer to stratum corneum. Margination refers to the process of leukocytes moving from the axial zone (central higher flow zone) to the plasmatic zone (peripheral lower flow zone) within blood vessels and adhering to the vessel walls in order to exit the blood stream. Diapedesis refers to the process of cells passing through vessel walls once margination has taken place during the inflammatory phase of wound healing.

TYPES OF WOUND HEALING

10. Which one of the following most accurately defines whether primary or secondary healing occurs within a cutaneous wound?

E. How closely the wound edges are apposed

Healing is defined as primary, secondary, or tertiary (delayed primary). The key factor that differentiates whether primary or secondary healing occurs is how closely the wound edges are apposed. When the wound edges are reapproximated, such as when an incised wound is sutured, primary healing can occur. This results in the least amount of scar tissue production. In contrast, where there is a gap between the wound edges, such as when a finger pulp injury with tissue loss is left open, secondary wound healing will occur in order to fill in the missing tissue. More scar tissue is formed and the process involves a combination of contraction and epithelialization. Neither the mechanism of injury, the amount of tissue damage, nor the method of wound closure per se define whether primary or secondary intention occur, only the reapproximation of the wound edges. Even when tissue loss has occurred, primary healing is possible providing that the wound edges are debrided and well apposed. Complete healing is normally achieved most quickly in wounds that are closed primarily, but this is not a defining factor. Wound closure can be satisfactorily achieved with sutures, staples, or glue, and each of these techniques allow primary healing to take place. Tertiary healing or delayed primary healing are the same thing. They refer to wounds that are initially left open and then closed after debridement at a later stage. This is an approach commonly employed in infected wounds where closure is delayed until the infection has been satisfactorily treated.

FACTORS AFFECTING WOUND HEALING

11. In which one of the following conditions is normal wound healing expected after surgery?

D. Cutis laxa

Cutis laxa is a condition where there is a mutation in elastin fibers and this results in loose wrinkled skin and hypermobile joints. Some patients can benefit from resection of excess skin and this is safe as wound healing is normal.

The other conditions are all associated with abnormal wound healing. Ehlers Danlos syndrome is also known as cutis hyperelastica and is a genetic connective tissue disorder with abnormal collagen cross-linking. The condition is associated with thin friable skin, poor wound healing, hypertrophic scarring, and hypermobile joints. Progeria is also known as Hutchinson-Gilford syndrome and is also a genetic condition observed in children. Patients have premature aging with skin laxity and poor wound healing. Werner syndrome is adult progeria with similar features to Hutchinson-Gilford syndrome. In each of these conditions, surgery is best avoided where possible.

It is well accepted that there is an association between smoking and delayed wound healing, although the precise mechanism is not well understood. The constituents implicated within tobacco smoke include nicotine, carbon monoxide, and hydrogen cyanide. Sørensen undertook a systematic review in 2012[3] to consider the effects of smoking on wound healing and found that smoking temporarily decreases tissue oxygenation and aerobic metabolism, while it also attenuates both the inflammatory and proliferation phases of wound healing thereby decreasing collagen production. Cessation of smoking for four weeks before surgery appears to reverse some, but not all of the processes described.

12. Which one of the following vitamins can be particularly useful to help wound healing in patients on long-term steroids?

A. Vitamin A

Vitamins are vital to normal wound healing processes, but supplements typically help wound healing only when there is a deficiency present. Vitamin A is also known as retinol and has important functions in immunity, vision, and wound healing. It can help reverse delayed wound healing due to steroids and increase epithelialization in healing wounds. It is well accepted that steroids delay wound healing and animal and human studies have shown these negative effects to be reversed when vitamin A is used either topically or systemically. The mechanism is not well understood, and the benefit of using vitamin A is absent when steroids are not being given. Given this evidence, it may be particularly useful to prescribe vitamin A during the perioperative period in patients on long-term steroids such as for rheumatoid arthritis or ulcerative colitis.[4]

There are a number of different B vitamins including thiamine, folic acid, pyridoxine, and cobalamin which have important roles in metabolism and oxygen transport. Deficiencies of the B vitamins can therefore result in a broad range of conditions. Vitamin C is vital for hydroxylation reactions in collagen synthesis and a deficiency leads to scurvy, with immature fibroblasts, deficient collagen synthesis, capillary hemorrhage, and decreased tissue strength. Vitamin D is important for calcium regulation and a deficiency can lead to rickets in children or osteomalacia in adults. Vitamin E is an antioxidant that stabilizes membranes. Large doses inhibit healing and may cause dermatitis.

13. **What is the single most important cause of a wound to fail to heal?**
    A. **Poor oxygen supply**
    The single most common reason for a wound not to heal is tissue hypoxia. This can occur secondary to a number of causes such as poor vascularity, smoking, previous injury, or radiation therapy. The presence of infection with microorganisms greater than 10^5 per gram of tissue will decrease oxygen tension, lower the pH, and increase collagenase activity. Denervation of a wound will make it more susceptible to pressure damage and is a major factor in the development of sacral sores in paraplegic patients and foot ulcers in diabetic patients. A moist wound is thought to be beneficial to healing so wounds are often kept moist until reepithelialization is complete, but a dry wound is not the most significant factor in failure of a wound to heal. Radiation injury is a significant factor in wound healing and results from damage to blood vessels, which in turn causes poor oxygen supply to local tissues.

14. Debridement of a chronic wound can remove excess granulation tissue and expedite healing. **What else is thought to be responsible for impaired wound healing in chronic wounds that is removed during debridement?**
    A. **Metalloproteases**
    Matrix metalloproteases are enzymes involved in the normal healing process. They have multiple functions including removal of damaged extracellular matrix and bacteria, scar contraction and scar remodeling. They are often abundant in chronic wounds and in excess, have been implicated in slow wound healing and altered extracellular matrix turnover because they can result in degradation of normal proteins. Debridement of a chronic wound will reduce the content of metalloproteases and transform it back to an acute wound state. It can thereby improve healing in such cases. Lathyrogens such as betaaminoproprionitrile (BAPN) are amino acid derivatives found in food substances such as chickpeas. They can cause a decrease in collagen cross-linking and thereby affect wound healing when present in excess. Given their action on collagen, they may have a potential therapeutic effect on wound healing by decreasing scar tissue formation. Myofibroblasts were discussed in question 8 and represent a specialized subtype of fibroblasts. Their removal from the wound would only be beneficial if there was an excess number present. This is unlikely as they are usually only present in the early stages of wound healing. TGF-beta is an important growth factor in wound healing. It serves to promote fibroblast migration and proliferation. It is not present in fetal wounds and its absence may be one of the factors responsible for decreased scarring in utero. For this reason its manipulation may have a possible role in reducing scarring in adult wounds. Chondroitin sulfate is a component of glycosaminoglycans. Other components include hyaluronic acid, dermatan sulfate and heparin sulfate. Glycosaminoglycans form part of the extracellular matrix and are used clinically as fillers in cosmetic practice. They are not harmful to normal wound healing.

15. You see a patient who wishes to undergo a face lift. She has given up smoking after your advice and now uses only nicotine replacement medications. **Which one of the following represents a well-recognized effect of nicotine on tissues?**
    D. **Reduced local blood supply**
    Nicotine is a vasoconstrictor that reduces nutritional blood flow to the skin, resulting in tissue ischemia and the potential for impaired healing of injured tissues. Nicotine also increases platelet

adhesiveness (not decreases it), raising the risk of thrombotic microvascular occlusion and further tissue ischemia. In addition, it can reduce red blood cells, fibroblast and macrophage proliferation. Nicotine is therefore one of the components within cigarette smoke that may be responsible for the increased risk of wound complications associated with tobacco smoking.

There have been a number of studies to explore the precise role of nicotine in wound healing, both as a single agent and as part of cigarette smoking. However the mechanisms involved are complex and remain incompletely understood. At present, in spite of the effects of nicotine on wound healing, there is no clinical evidence to show that nicotine replacement therapy use in patients abstaining from smoking will significantly affect their wound healing. In high-risk procedures such as face lifting, it is still probably best to avoid both smoking and nicotine replacement therapy in order to minimize risk of wound complications. Other products in cigarette smoke such as carbon monoxide and hydrogen cyanide are responsible for reduced oxyhemoglobin concentrations, altered inflammation, and toxic cellular effects.[3,5,6]

16. You have a patient with a large wound to the tibia after a fall and have closed it directly. He is due to start chemotherapy very soon. **When can the chemotherapy be started without detrimental effects on healing of this wound?**
    C. In 14 days
    It is well accepted that antineoplastic agents affect wound healing. This evidence is based on both lab-based animal studies and clinical studies in humans. However there is unlikely to be any significant effect on wound healing, providing that chemotherapy treatment is delayed for 10-14 days after the wound has been closed. This makes sense given the anticipated healing time for a typical soft tissue wound.[7,8]

ABNORMAL SCARRING

17. **When examining a patient with an abnormally thickened scar, what is the key factor that will differentiate a keloid from a hypertrophic scar?**
    C. Growth beyond the original wound borders
    Keloid and hypertrophic scars each represent abnormal scarring processes and are differentiated clinically. The key defining feature of a keloid scar is that it grows beyond the original scar border, whereas a hypertrophic scar does not. Both keloid and hypertrophic scars are typically elevated and erythematous. The histological appearances are similar with high concentrations of type III collagen in each. Keloid scars are typically observed in patients 10 to 30 years of age and can occur spontaneously or secondary to injury. They tend to affect patients with darker skin tones most commonly. Females are more commonly affected than males. They commonly occur on the ear or anterior chest and rarely regress spontaneously. Hypertrophic scars have an equal sex ratio, are typically seen in younger age groups (less than 20 years of age), and appear soon after injury such as in children who have sustained a burn. All skin tones can be affected.

TREATMENT FOR KELOID SCARS

18. A young female patient presents with a large keloid scar on her ear after a piercing. She has tried silicone gel and steroid injections with little improvement. **Which one of the following is correct?**
    B. Radiation therapy may be helpful for this patient, but the chance of recurrence is as high as 33%.
    Treatment for keloids and hypertrophic scars involves topical silicone gel, compression garments, intralesional steroid injections (with or without debulking surgery), and radiation therapy (see Table 1-3, *Essentials of Plastic Surgery,* second edition). A key difference in management is that hypertrophic scars often improve with time and daily massage. Therefore they may not require

more involved interventions. Sometimes these scars soften with time but remain erythematous. In these circumstances, laser therapy with pulse dye can be beneficial.[9,10]

REFERENCES

1. Hu MS, Maan ZN, Wu JC, et al. Tissue engineering and regenerative repair in wound healing. Ann Biomed Eng 42:1494-1507, 2014.
2. Levenson SM, Geever EF, Crowley LV, et al. The healing of rat skin wounds. Ann Surg 161:293-308, 1965.
3. Sørensen LT. Wound healing and infection in surgery: the pathophysiological impact of smoking, smoking cessation, and nicotine replacement therapy: a systematic review. Ann Surg 255:1069-1079, 2012.
4. Hunt TK, Ehrlich HP, Garcia JA, et al. Effect of vitamin A on reversing the inhibitory effect of cortisone on healing of open wounds in animals and man. Ann Surg 170:633-641, 1969.
5. Silverstein P. Smoking and wound healing. Am J Med 93:22S-24S, 1992.
6. Warner DO. Perioperative abstinence from cigarettes: physiologic and clinical consequences. Anesthesiology 104:356-367, 2006.
7. Falcone RE, Nappi JF. Chemotherapy and wound healing. Surg Clin North Am 64:779-794, 1984.
8. Shamberger RC, Devereux DF, Brennan MF. The effect of chemotherapeutic agents on wound healing. Int Adv Surg Oncol 4:15-58, 1981.
9. Sidle DM, Kim H. Keloids: prevention and management. Facial Plast Surg Clin North Am 19:505-515, 2011.
10. Chike-Obi CJ, Cole PD, Brissett AE. Keloids: pathogenesis, clinical features, and management. Semin Plast Surg 23:178-184, 2009.

2. General Management of Complex Wounds

See *Essentials of Plastic Surgery,* second edition, pp. 10-16.

BLOOD GLUCOSE CONTROL
1. A diabetic patient is scheduled to undergo abdominal wall reconstruction. Preoperative hemoglobin A_1C is 12% and random blood glucose (RBG) level is 200 mg/dl. ***Which one of the following is correct?***
   A. A normal A_1C should be 8.5 when expressed as a percentage of glycosylated hemoglobin.
   B. The A_1C represents the patient's average glucose control over the previous 180 days.
   C. Postoperative infection risk is significantly increased for this patient, because the blood glucose level is higher than 180 mg/dl.
   D. Tight blood glucose control (<70 mg/dl) during the perioperative period will reduce the postoperative mortality risk.
   E. An elevated A_1C level linearly correlates with an increased risk of surgical site infections.

PREOPERATIVE ASSESSMENT OF NUTRITION
2. ***When assessing a patient's preoperative nutritional status before major surgery by monitoring blood albumin levels, which one of the following is correct?***
   A. The half-life of albumin is 3 days.
   B. A preoperative value of 4.3 g/dl is outside the normal range.
   C. Assessment is based on the rule of fives.
   D. Severe malnutrition would be suggested by preoperative values less than 3.0 g/dl.
   E. A low preoperative level is a strong predictor for postoperative mortality risk.

IMAGING IN COMPLEX WOUNDS
3. A 67-year-old smoker has exposed hardware after a wound breakdown over his fibular fracture. The hardware has been removed, but his wound is not progressing. His dorsalis pedis pulse is not palpable, and the posterior tibial pulse is weak. ***Which one of the following modalities is the most accurate and least harmful modality for imaging of this patient's peripheral arterial disease?***
   A. MRA
   B. Plain radiographs
   C. CTA
   D. Ultrasound
   E. Contrast angiography

VASCULAR ULCER MANAGEMENT
4. After assessing a patient who is malnourished and has a punched out ulcer on the lower leg, you decide to perform an ankle-brachial pressure test, which shows a value of 0.4. ***What does this result suggest?***
   A. Normal lower limb vasculature.
   B. Imminent ischemic gangrene is likely.
   C. Critical stenosis is present that warrants further intervention.
   D. Vessels are significantly calcified.
   E. Predominantly venous disease.

TISSUE RECONSTRUCTION AND WOUND CLOSURE

5. **What was the main limitation of the original reconstructive ladder concept?**
   A. That it did not include free tissue transfer.
   B. That the concept could only be practiced by plastic surgeons.
   C. That it did not include dermal matrices or negative pressure therapy.
   D. That the reconstructive process was performed in a stepwise manner.
   E. That primary closure was the first rung on the ladder.

NEGATIVE PRESSURE WOUND THERAPY

6. You are planning to temporize an abdominal wound with a negative pressure dressing after debridement. **Which one of the following is correct regarding negative pressure wound therapy?**
   A. It increases local blood flow and granulation tissue production.
   B. It reduces fluid exudate.
   C. It is contraindicated in recently debrided wounds.
   D. It can be useful for treating fistulas.
   E. It reduces mitotic activity in the wound.

SELECTION OF SKIN SUBSTITUTES

7. You are considering the use of a biologic skin substitute in a patient with an acute burn. Your patient is concerned about the use of tissues from animals and states that he would only consent to products that are purely synthetic or human derived. **Which one of the following is acceptable for use in this patient?**
   A. Biobrane
   B. Apligraf
   C. Transcyte
   D. SurgiMend
   E. AlloDerm

BIOLOGIC SKIN SUBSTITUTES

8. For each of the following descriptions, select the most likely skin substitute from the list. (Each option may be used once, more than once, or not at all.)
   A. *This contains cultured neonatal dermal fibroblasts on a silicone/collagen matrix using porcine collagen.*
   B. *This is a nylon mesh with silicone and chemically bound porcine collagen.*
   C. *This is a bilayer structure containing bovine collagen, human fibroblasts, and human keratinocytes.*

   Options:
   a. AlloDerm
   b. SurgiMend
   c. Integra
   d. Transcyte
   e. Apligraf
   f. Dermagraft
   g. Biobrane

Chapter 2 ▪ General Management of Complex Wounds

Answers

BLOOD GLUCOSE CONTROL

1. A diabetic patient is scheduled to undergo abdominal wall reconstruction. Preoperative hemoglobin A_1C is 12% and random blood glucose (RBG) level is 200 mg/dl. *Which one of the following is correct?*
   C. Postoperative infection risk is significantly increased for this patient, because the blood glucose level is higher than 180 mg/dl.
   In patients with or without diabetes, perioperative hyperglycemia (>180 mg/dl) carries a significantly increased risk of postoperative wound infection.[1]
   The hemoglobin A_1C is a blood test used to assess the long-term control of blood glucose. Because hemoglobin molecules remain in the blood for 3 months, it is possible to gauge glucose control over a 120-day period (not 180-day) by measuring glycosylated hemoglobin levels. A normal hemoglobin A_1C is around 6%. Tight blood glucose control with intensive insulin therapy and normoglycemia (<110 mg/dl) has shown a reduction in hospital deaths in some trials.[2] However, where glucose control is <7 mg/dl, there is an increased risk of death in critically ill patients.[3] Although postoperative hyperglycemia and undiagnosed diabetes increase the risk of surgical site infections, elevated hemoglobin A_1C does not linearly correlate.[4,5]

PREOPERATIVE ASSESSMENT OF NUTRITION

2. When assessing a patient's preoperative nutritional status before major surgery by monitoring blood albumin levels, which one of the following is correct?
   E. A low preoperative level is a strong predictor for postoperative mortality risk.
   Albumin can provide a useful indication of nutrition. Its half-life is 20 days, and a normal value is 3.6 to 5.4 g/dl. A value of 2.8 to 3.5 g/dl suggests mild malnutrition, 2.1 to 2.7 g/dl suggests moderate malnutrition, and less than 2.1 g/dl indicates severe malnutrition. A large study published in 1999 involving more than 50,000 patients showed that as preoperative albumin levels decreased, early postoperative mortality and morbidity increased exponentially.[6] The authors concluded that albumin was a useful predictor of outcome in major surgical procedures.
   Prealbumin, rather than albumin, has a half-life of 3 days and can be assessed by the rule of fives. A normal value is greater than 15 mg/dl, mild deficiency is less than 15 mg/dl, moderate is less than 10 mg/dl, and severe is less than 5 mg/dl.

IMAGING IN COMPLEX WOUNDS

3. A 67-year-old smoker has exposed hardware after a wound breakdown over his fibular fracture. The hardware has been removed, but his wound is not progressing. His dorsalis pedis is not palpable, and the posterior tibial pulse is weak. *Which one of the following is the most accurate and least harmful modality for imaging of this patient's peripheral arterial disease?*
   A. MRA
   A systemic review of imaging in the lower limb confirmed that peripheral arterial disease is best imaged using MRA, because this has an overall better diagnostic accuracy than CTA or ultrasonography. It also showed a patient preference of MRA over standard contrast angiography.[7] Plain radiographic films can demonstrate calcification of vessels and may be useful for assessment of fractures, foreign bodies, and osteomyelitis, rather than vascular imaging.

VASCULAR ULCER MANAGEMENT

4. After assessing a patient who is malnourished and has a punched out ulcer on the lower leg, you decide to perform an ankle-brachial pressure test, which shows a value of 0.4. **What does this result suggest?**
   C. Critical stenosis is present that warrants further intervention.
   The ankle-brachial pressure index is a noninvasive test used to investigate the lower limb vasculature. It compares a patient's lower limb arterial pressure with that of the upper limb and expresses it as a ratio. A normal ankle-brachial pressure index is between 0.9 and 1.2. A value greater than 1.2 suggests calcification as vessels become noncompressible. A value of 0.5 to 0.9 is associated with mixed arteriovenous disease. A value of less than 0.5 suggests critical arterial stenosis, and a value of less than 0.2 indicates that ischemic gangrene is likely. The clinical picture is consistent with the appearance of an arterial ischemic ulcer, and referral for a vascular opinion is recommended.

TISSUE RECONSTRUCTION AND WOUND CLOSURE

5. ***What was the main limitation of the original reconstructive ladder concept?***
   D. That the reconstructive process was performed in a stepwise manner.
   The reconstructive ladder was a concept described by Mathes and Nahai[8] used to categorize options for wound closure, progressing a stepwise manner of complexity from healing by secondary intention to free tissue transfer, with the simplest option being preferentially used first. The major conceptual understanding of the original concept was that each rung was mandatory to climb before hitting the next rung. This was corrected by Gottlieb and Krieger[9] who coined the term "reconstructive elevator," which they described in the Editorial section of *Plastic Reconstructive Surgery* in 1994 to emphasize that reconstruction is flexible and does not have to proceed in a stepwise fashion. Reconstruction should immediately proceed to the best option in any given scenario, taking into consideration the patient, the wound, and the resources available. The original reconstructive ladder did not include negative pressure dressings or dermal matrices; however this was not its major caveat. Janis et al[10] refined the reconstructive ladder to include dermal matrices and negative pressure wound therapy. Other models for reconstruction have included the reconstructive triangle[8] and the reconstructive matrix.[11] The reconstructive triangle includes tissue expansion, local flaps, and free tissue transfer. The reconstructive matrix contains three axes representing technological sophistication, surgical complexity, and patient-surgical risk. (See Figs. 2-1 and 2-2, *Essentials of Plastic Surgery,* second edition.)

NEGATIVE PRESSURE WOUND THERAPY

6. You are planning to temporize an abdominal wound with a negative pressure dressing after debridement. ***Which one of the following is correct regarding negative pressure wound therapy?***
   A. It increases local blood flow and granulation tissue production.
   Negative pressure wound therapy is commonly used to accelerate wound healing either as a sole means of wound closure or to prepare a wound for skin grafting. Argenta and Morykwas[12] first described the term in 1997 after their clinical experience. It is believed to cause deformation of cells that leads to an increase in their mitotic activity. Fluid exudate is removed during negative pressure therapy, but the production of fluid per se is not affected. Production of granulation tissue is increased. Use of negative pressure therapy should be avoided in wounds with exposed vessels, fistulas, active infection, or malignancy. It can safely be used after wound debridement providing that hemostasis is adequate and the points described above are addressed with respect to the other contraindications (see Chapter 10).

Chapter 2 ▪ General Management of Complex Wounds   17

SELECTION OF SKIN SUBSTITUTES

7. You are considering the use of a biologic skin substitute in a patient with an acute burn. Your patient is concerned about the use of tissues from animals and states that he will only consent to products that are purely synthetic or human derived. **Which one of the following is acceptable for use in this patient?**

E. AlloDerm

All of the products listed contain animal derivatives, with the exception of AlloDerm. This is a regenerative tissue matrix derived from cadaveric human dermis. It has been used successfully in burn patients to reduce joint contracture.[13] It is also used for breast and abdominal wall reconstruction. Biobrane contains porcine dermis and is used in partial thickness burns. Apligraf contains bovine collagen and is used in lower limb ulcers. Transcyte contains porcine collagen and is used in deeper burns. SurgiMend contains bovine dermis and is used in abdominal wall reconstruction. (See question 8 answer and Chapter 9, *Essentials of Plastic Surgery*, second edition.)

BIOLOGIC SKIN SUBSTITUTES

8. For the following scenarios, the best options are as follows:
   A. This contains cultured neonatal dermal fibroblasts on a silicone/collagen matrix using porcine collagen.
   d. Transcyte
   B. This is a nylon mesh with silicone and chemically bound porcine collagen.
   g. Biobrane
   C. This is a bilayer structure containing bovine collagen, human fibroblasts, and human keratinocytes.
   e. Apligraf

A number of biologic skin substitutes are available (see Chapter 9 and Table 2-1, *Essentials of Plastic Surgery*, second edition). They can be classified according to composition: human derived, animal derived, synthetic, or a combination of these. Human-derived substitutes include AlloDerm (LifeCell, Branchburg, NJ), which is cadaveric acellular dermis. Animal-derived products include Strattice (LifeCell), a porcine-derived acellular dermal matrix, and SurgiMend (TEI Biosciences, Boston, MA), a bovine-derived acellular matrix.

Combined animal/synthetic substitutes include Integra (Integra LifeSciences, Plainsboro, NJ), which comprises silicone and bovine collagen with shark glycosaminoglycans, and Biobrane (Smith & Nephew, London), which consists of nylon, silicone, and porcine collagen. Biobrane is used to dress superficial dermal burns, especially for children. It can accelerate healing, decrease pain, and reduce the number of dressing changes. Integra may be useful in deeper burns; the deep layer provides a scaffold for dermal regeneration, and the silicone layer supplies a temporary epidermis. After cellular and vascular ingrowth has occurred, the silicone layer can be removed and a split-thickness graft applied. Integra is sometimes preferred for late burn reconstruction because of potential problems with infection in the acute setting.

Apligraf (Organogenesis, Canton, MA), Dermagraft (Advanced Tissue Sciences, LaJolla, CA), and Transcyte (Smith & Nephew) all contain human fibroblasts and a synthetic component. Apligraf and Dermagraft are marketed for use in diabetic foot ulcers, whereas Transcyte is intended for use in burns. Transcyte includes newborn human fibroblast cells and a nylon mesh that is coated with porcine dermal collagen and bonded to a silicone membrane, similar to Biobrane. Apligraf also contains bovine type I collagen.

References

1. Kwon S, Thompson R, Dellinger P, et al. Importance of perioperative glycemic control in general surgery: a report from the Surgical Care and Outcomes Assessment program. Ann Surg 257:8-14, 2013.
2. Vanhorebeek I, Langouche L, Van den Berghe G. Tight blood glucose control: what is the evidence? Crit Care Med 35(9 Suppl):S496-S502, 2007.
3. Finfer S, Liu B, Chittock DR, et al. Hypoglycemia and risk of death in critically ill patients. New Engl J Med 367:1108-1118, 2012.
4. King JT Jr, Goulet JL, Perkal MF, et al. Glycemic control and infections in patients with diabetes undergoing noncardiac surgery. Ann Surg 253:158-165, 2011.
5. Latham R, Lancaster AD, Covington JF, et al. The association of diabetes and glucose control with surgical-site infections among cardiothoracic surgery patients. Infect Control Hosp Epidemiol 22:607-612, 2001.
6. Gibbs J, Cull W, Henderson W, et al. Preoperative serum albumin level as a predictor of operative mortality and morbidity: results from the National VA Surgical Risk Study. Arch Surg 134:36-42, 1999.
7. Collins R, Cranny G, Burch J, et al. A systematic review of duplex ultrasound, magnetic resonance angiography, and computed tomography angiography for the diagnosis and assessment of symptomatic, lower limb peripheral artery disease. Health Techol Assess 11:iii-iv, xi-xiii, 1-184, 2007.
8. Mathes SJ, Nahai F. Reconstructive Surgery: Principles, Anatomy, & Technique. St Louis: Quality Medical Publishing, 1997.
9. Gottlieb LJ, Krieger LM. From the reconstructive ladder to the reconstructive elevator. Plast Reconstr Surg 93:1503-1504, 1994.
10. Janis JE, Kwon RK, Attinger CE. The new reconstructive ladder: modifications to the traditional model. Plast Reconstr Surg 127(Suppl 1):S205-S212, 2011.
11. Erba P, Ogawa R, Vyas R, et al. The reconstructive matrix: a new paradigm in reconstructive plastic surgery. Plast Reconstr Surg 126:492-498, 2010.
12. Argenta LC, Morykwas MJ. Vacuum-assisted closure: a new method for wound control and treatment: clinical experience. Ann Plast Surg 38:563-576, 1997.
13. Yim H, Cho YS, Seo CH, et al. The use of AlloDerm on major burn patients: AlloDerm prevents post-burn joint contracture. Burns 36:322-328, 2010.

3. Sutures and Needles

See *Essentials of Plastic Surgery,* second edition, pp. 17-23.

SUTURE CHARACTERISTICS

1. **Following closure of an abdominoplasty with 2-0 Vicryl sutures, which one of the following is correct?**
   A. The sutures will lose half of their tensile strength within one week.
   B. The absorption process will occur through proteolysis.
   C. The rate of suture absorption will be unpredictable.
   D. The absorption process will be enzyme mediated.
   E. Inflammation will be less than if a natural suture was used.

2. **Which one of the following statements is correct regarding nonabsorbable sutures?**
   A. Suture materials with greater memory form more secure knots.
   B. Monofilament sutures display superior knot security compared with braided sutures.
   C. *Elasticity* is the tendency of a suture to return to its original length after stretching.
   D. Sutures with more memory are also more pliable and easier to handle.
   E. *Capillarity* refers to the tendency of a suture to absorb fluid and swell.

3. **What does the #-0 value refer to on a 3-0 nylon suture?**
   A. The suture diameter in Imperial measurement.
   B. The suture diameter in Metric measurement.
   C. The suture diameter in French measurement.
   D. The suture USP breaking strength.
   E. The relative breaking strength compared to stainless steel.

NEEDLE CONFIGURATIONS

4. The configuration of a needle varies according to its intended use. **Which one of the following statements is correct regarding needle selection?**
   A. A conventional cutting needle is ideal for suturing skin under tension.
   B. Taper needles are occasionally used for tendon repairs.
   C. The reverse cutting needle is more likely to result in *cheese wiring* of the dermis.
   D. Blunt tip needles are reserved for ophthalmic surgery.
   E. The point of a standard cutting needle is on the inner curve of the needle.

CURVED NEEDLE CHARACTERISTICS

5. Curved suture needles are commonly used in plastic surgery. **Which one of the following statements is correct regarding their needle characteristics?**
   A. Needle length is usually the same as chord length.
   B. Chord length is unaffected by needle curvature.
   C. Chord length is the direct distance between the needle point and swage.

D. Needle diameter is the same as chord length.
E. Curve radius can vary with five-eighths circle being most popular for plastic surgery applications.

SUTURE NAMES AND CHARACTERISTICS

6. Match the following suture descriptions to the most appropriate choice from the list. (Each option may be used once, more than once, or not at all.)
   A. This is a monofilament suture with hydrolytic absorption, medium memory, and a 7- to 10-day time to reach 50% original strength.
   B. This suture has low memory and hydrolytic absorption that loses 50% strength in 2 to 3 weeks. It is available as either a monofilament or braided suture and is known as polyglycolic acid.
   C. This braided, synthetic, nonabsorbable suture is available in coated or uncoated variants with moderate reactivity and good memory and handling.

   Options:
   a. Polyester
   b. Chromic gut
   c. Monocryl
   d. Biosyn
   e. Vicryl
   f. Dexon
   g. PDS
   h. Silk

WOUND CLOSURE

7. Which one of the following statements is true regarding wound closure?
   A. Braided sutures are popular for closure of animal bite wounds.
   B. Infection within a wound will slow the process of suture absorption and result in more suture granuloma problems.
   C. In the rat model, skin can be expected to regain 20% of its original strength after 1 week, and almost 95% by 6 weeks.
   D. Polydiaxone (PDS) is unlikely to adequately support a healing wound until 50% of original wound strength has been regained.
   E. Closure with stainless steel staples is rapid and causes a low amount of local tissue ischemia.

8. Why does the punctuate component of the railroad scar develop?
   A. Localized pressure necrosis
   B. Over tightening of sutures
   C. Localized wound infection
   D. Reepithelialization around the suture
   E. Premature suture removal

MICROSURGICAL SUTURES

9. When selecting appropriate sutures for microsurgical anastomoses, which one of the following statements is correct?
   A. A 10-0 nylon suture is the best choice for repair of a 100% divided radial artery.
   B. Different microsuture materials have broadly similar handling characteristics.
   C. An 8-0 suture is the best choice for repair of an adult proper digital artery.
   D. Sutures used for microsurgery are commonly nylon, polypropylene, or polyglytone.
   E. Microsuture needle characteristics decrease uniformly as suture material diameter decreases.

Chapter 3 ▪ Sutures and Needles   21

Answers

SUTURE CHARACTERISTICS

1. *Following closure of an abdominoplasty with 2-0 Vicryl sutures, which one of the following statements is correct?*
   E. Inflammation will be less than if a natural suture was used.

   Absorption of suture material can be either hydrolytic (which is more common and results in less tissue inflammation) or proteolytic. There is variation in the rate of suture absorption depending on material type (see Table 3-1, *Essentials of Plastic Surgery*, second edition) but Vicryl sutures will take 2 to 3 weeks for their strength to decrease to 50%. Most absorbable sutures lose half their strength within the first four weeks and will eventually be completely absorbed. The rate of absorption is proportional to the degree of polymerization and is quite predictable for any given suture. Some sutures such as Vicryl Rapide and Caprosyn (Polyglytone 6211) should be avoided in areas that require longer support as they lose half their strength in the first week. Proteolytic absorption is enzyme mediated and is associated with natural sutures such as those derived from beef or sheep intestine, which are often referred to as cat gut. Synthetic sutures such as polydiaxone (PDS) and polyglactin (Vicryl) absorb by the process of hydrolysis where water from tissues is absorbed into the suture material resulting in disruption of cross-links within the polymeric structure.

2. *Which one of the following statements is correct regarding nonabsorbable sutures?*
   C. Elasticity is the tendency of a suture to return to its original length after stretching.

   Elasticity is the tendency of a suture to return to its original length after stretching and can be helpful in wounds where postoperative swelling is anticipated; thereby ensuring that the suture retains sufficiently tight closure after the swelling reduces. Memory refers to the tendency of a suture to return to its original shape and sutures with more memory are usually less pliable, more difficult to handle, and have less knot security. For example, PDS has greater memory than Monocryl or Dexon. Knot security refers to the force required to cause a knot to slip and will be increased with braided sutures such as Vicryl or Ethibond, compared with monofilament sutures such as Monocryl. Fluid absorption is the amount of fluid retained by a suture and capillarity refers to the movement of fluid along the suture. Sutures with greater capillarity (for example, braided subtypes) are more likely to become colonized with bacteria, potentially leading to wound infection. The braided nature of these sutures also provides a greater surface area and recesses for organisms to adhere. For these reasons, sutures such as nylon are less likely to harbor infection when compared with a braided alternative such as Vicryl.

3. *What does the #-0 value refer to on a 3-0 nylon suture?*
   D. The suture USP breaking strength.

   It is a common misconception that the #-0 rating refers to the diameter of a suture. However, the rating for sutures refers to the United States pharmacopoenia (USP) breaking strength rating, rather than suture diameter. Therefore two different types of 3-0 suture can have different diameters but share the same breaking strength. As #-0 rating increases for any given suture, the diameter and breaking strength will both decrease.

NEEDLE CONFIGURATIONS

4. The configuration of a needle varies according to its intended use. **Which one of the following statements is correct regarding needle selection?**
   E. The point of a standard cutting needle is on the inner curve of the needle.

   There are five main types of needles: conventional cutting, reverse cutting, side cutting, taper point, and blunt tip. Each has a particular use/indication (see Fig. 3-1, *Essentials of Plastic Surgery,* second edition).

   A standard cutting needle has its cutting surface or point on the inner curve and is at risk of tearing through the tissues causing cheese wiring when closing wounds under tension. In contrast, a reverse cutting needle has its cutting edge on the outer curve and is therefore less likely to cause cheese wiring. Side cutting needles have two cutting surfaces or points and can be used in skin closure to reduce cheese wiring. Taper point or round bodied needles do not have a cutting surface on the needle beyond the sharp tip and are the standard choice for tendon repair to prevent cutting through the tendon fibers and previously placed suture passes/knots. Blunt tip needles are used for intraabdominal surgery and some high-risk patients.

CURVED NEEDLE CHARACTERISTICS

5. Curved suture needles are commonly used in plastic surgery. **Which one of the following statements is correct regarding their characteristics?**
   C. Chord length is the direct distance between the needle point and swage.

   Fig. 3-1 shows the key components of a curved needle. A needle has a point or tip at the leading edge and a swage at the other end where the thread is attached. Needle length is the distance from the swage to the needle point along the length of the needle body. Chord length is the direct or shortest distance between the swage and the needle point. It is therefore shorter than needle length in a curved needle. The curvature of a needle refers to the amount of a full circle involved and ranges from one fourth to five eighths, with three eighths being most common in plastic surgery applications. Chord length will differ according to needle curvature and will be greatest with the half-circle needle. Needle diameter refers to the thickness of the needle itself and is determined by the balance between providing sufficient material strength yet maintaining the smallest diameter possible for the required size suture

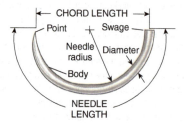

Fig. 3-1 Anatomy of a needle.

SUTURE NAMES AND CHARACTERISTICS
6. *For the following descriptions, the best options are as follows:*
   A. This is a monofilament suture with hydrolytic absorption, medium memory, and a 7- to 10-day time to reach 50% original strength.
   c. Monocryl
   This suture is also known as *poliglecaprone*. It is a popular choice for buried skin closure in plastic surgery as it handles well and has a low reactivity. Biosyn (Glycomer 631) is similar to Monocryl but retains its strength for 1 to 2 weeks longer.

   B. This suture has low memory and hydrolytic absorption that loses 50% strength in 2 to 3 weeks. It is available as either a monofilament or braided suture and is known as polyglycolic acid.
   f. Dexon
   This suture, known as *polyglycolic acid*, has very similar characteristics to Vicryl. The key difference is that Vicryl is always braided whereas Dexon may be either monofilament or braided. Vicryl Rapide is a similar braided suture to Vicryl but has a lower molecular weight and therefore loses its strength in just 5 days rather than 2 to 3 weeks. This is often used as an external skin suture in young children.

   C. This braided, synthetic, nonabsorbable suture is available in coated and uncoated variants with moderate reactivity and good memory and handling.
   a. Polyester
   Polyester sutures may be uncoated such as Mersilene (Ethicon), or coated such as Ethibond (Ethicon), Surgidac (U.S. Surgical Corporation), and Ticron (U.S. Surgical Corporation). Coating involves the process of adding a lubricant to improve suture passage and handling. Polyester sutures may be used for tendon or ligament repair and some surgeons use them for securing the SMAS during face lifts.

   PDS is polydiaxone and this is a monofilament suture that has low reactivity and maintains 50% strength until 4 weeks. For this reason it is often useful in closure of deep wounds such as closing Scarpa's fascia during abdominoplasty. Gut is an absorbable suture available in different subtypes. Plain gut loses half its strength in a week and chromic gut loses half its strength in two weeks. Silk is a nonabsorbable braided suture that will still lose its strength after one year and is often used for vessel ties and marker sutures (Tables 3-1 and 3-2).

Table 3-1 Qualities of Absorbable Sutures

Composition (proprietary name)	Time to 50% Strength	Configuration	Reactivity	Memory
Gut	Unpredictable			
Fast	5-7 days	Monofilament	High	Low
Plain	7-10 days	Monofilament	High	Low
Chromic	10-14 days	Monofilament	High	Low
Polyglytone 6211 (Caprosyn*)	5-7 days	Monofilament	Low	Medium
Poliglecaprone 25 (Monocryl†)	7-10 days	Monofilament	Low	Medium
Glycomer 631 (Biosyn†)	2-3 weeks	Monofilament	Low	Medium
Glycolide/lactide copolymer Low molecular weight (Vicryl Rapide*)	5 days	Braided	Low	Low
Regular (Polysorb†, Vicryl*)	2-3 weeks	Braided	Low	Low
Polyglycolic acid (Dexon S†)	2-3 weeks	Monofilament or braided	Low	Low
Polyglyconate (Maxon†)	4 weeks	Monofilament	Low	High
Polydioxanone (PDS II*)	4 weeks	Monofilament	Low	High

*Ethicon.
†U.S. Surgical Corporation.

Table 3-2 Qualities of Nonabsorbable Sutures

Composition (proprietary name)	Tensile Strength	Configuration	Reactivity	Memory/ Handling
Silk	Lost in 1 year	Braided	High	−−/Good
Nylon	81% at 1 year,			
Monofilament (Ethilon*, Monosof-Dermalon†)	72% at 2 years,	Monofilament	Low	+/Fair
Braided (Nurolon*, Surgilon†)	66% at 11 years	Braided	Low	−−/Good
Polypropylene (Prolene*, Surgipro†)	Indefinite	Monofilament	Low	++/Poor
Polybutester				
Uncoated (Novafil†)	Indefinite	Monofilament	Low	+/Fair
Coated (Vascufil†)	Indefinite	Monofilament	Low	−/Good
Polyester				
Uncoated (Mersilene*)	Indefinite	Braided	Moderate	−−/Good
Coated (Ethibond*, Surgidac†, Ticron†)	Indefinite	Braided	Moderate	−−/Good
Surgical steel	Indefinite	Monofilament or braided	Low	++/Poor

*Ethicon.
†Covidien.

Chapter 3 ▪ Sutures and Needles   25

WOUND CLOSURE

7. Which one of the following statements is true regarding wound closure?
E. Closure with stainless steel staples is rapid and causes a low amount of local tissue ischemia.

Stainless steel clips have a number of advantages over sutures for wound closure. Closure is faster and they cause less local tissue ischemia. Some surgeons feel that there is little or no difference in the cosmetic outcome when comparing skin staples to sutures and they certainly can be useful in certain situations such as closure of scalp wounds where they also have a useful hemostatic effect. When using staples on the trunk or limbs, it is important to ensure that a deep layer of sutures is still present if the staples are to be removed sufficiently early (5 to 7 days) in order to avoid permanent staple marks.

In general, monofilament sutures are a better choice than braided alternatives for closing wounds that have a high risk of developing postoperative infection (e.g., debrided bite wounds), because bacteria may be less adherent to them (as discussed in question 2). Infection in a wound will accelerate the process of suture absorption.

In the rat model, as described by Levenson et al,[1] skin strength can be expected to regain 5% of its original strength in 1 week, 50% by 4 weeks, and 80% by 6 weeks. In this model, wound strength at 1 year is thought to reach only 80% of original strength. PDS will have retained 50% of its original strength at 4 weeks and will remain in the wound for longer than 12 weeks. It will therefore support a wound until at least 60% to 70% of its original strength has been regained. (See Fig. 3-5, *Essentials of Plastic Surgery,* second edition.)

8. Why does the punctuate component of the railroad scar develop?
D. Reepithelialization around the suture

A railroad scar has two main components: punctuate scars and parallel rows of scar between them. The punctuate component occurs because of reepithelialization around the suture which causes a cylindrical cuff leading to a permanent suture tract. Early suture removal may help avoid this process. The parallel rows result from pressure necrosis on the skin and subcutaneous tissues and are exacerbated by over tightening of sutures and delayed suture removal. (See Fig. 3-5, *Essentials of Plastic Surgery,* second edition.)

MICROSURGICAL SUTURES

9. When selecting appropriate sutures for microsurgical anastomoses, which one of the following statements is correct?
B. Different microsuture materials have broadly similar handling characteristics.

Handling characteristics are largely similar between different microsuture materials, although differences can occur between needles depending on their size, shape, and needle point. The choice of suture size depends on the vessel or structure size. For example, repair of the radial artery is satisfactorily achieved with an 8-0 nylon (Ethilon). A 10-0 is usually unnecessarily small and is more appropriate for repair of an adult digital vessel. Suture materials in microsurgery are monofilament permanent materials like nylon and polypropylene (Prolene and Surgipro). As discussed in question 6, Polyglytone is an absorbable suture material used for wound closure (Caprosyn). Moving from a 9-0 to a 10-0 does not necessarily mean the needle will be smaller so needle size should always be confirmed before opening the suture material.

REFERENCE

1. Levenson SM, Geever EF, Crowley LV, et al. The healing of rat skin wounds. Ann Surg 161:293-308, 1965.

4. Basics of Flaps

See *Essentials of Plastic Surgery*, second edition, pp. 24-44.

BLOOD SUPPLY TO FLAPS

1. **Which one of the following is correct regarding blood supply to flaps?**
   A. Fasciocutaneous flaps rely most heavily on the subfascial vascular plexus.
   B. Axial pattern flaps are based on the subdermal plexus and are limited by set width to length ratios.
   C. An *angiosome* is defined as an area of skin only supplied by a named source artery.
   D. The parasympathetic system is most important in regulating blood flow to the skin.
   E. Neurocutaneous flaps are based on perforating arteries accompanying a cutaneous nerve.

PERFORATOR FLAPS

2. **For each of the following flaps, select the correct type of blood supply. (Each option may be used once, more than once, or not at all.)**
   A. Anterolateral thigh flap (ALT)
   B. Deep inferior epigastric artery perforator flap (DIEP)
   C. Groin flap
   D. Lateral arm flap

   Options:
   a. Indirect muscle perforator
   b. Indirect septal perforator
   c. Direct cutaneous perforator
   d. Variable indirect muscle or septal perforators

VENOUS FLAPS

3. **Which one of the following is correct regarding venous flaps?**
   A. They tend to have very predictable survival outcomes.
   B. They are traditionally classified into five groups according to vascular anatomy.
   C. They are commonly sensate given the proximity of cutaneous nerves.
   D. The mechanism of flap perfusion is poorly understood.
   E. Donor site morbidity is typically increased, compared to arterial flaps.

CLASSIFICATION OF MUSCLE FLAPS

4. Muscle flaps may be grouped according to their vascular anatomy. **Which one of the following is correct regarding the Mathes and Nahai classification of muscle flaps?**
   A. A gluteus maximus is a type II muscle flap.
   B. The tensor fascia lata flap represents a type I flap.
   C. Type IV muscle flaps have one dominant pedicle with secondary segmental pedicles.
   D. Flap types II and IV have the most reliable vascularity.
   E. The gracilis flap has two dominant pedicles but no secondary segmental pedicles.

Chapter 4 ■ Basics of Flaps   27

LOCAL FLAP TECHNIQUES

5. **Which one of the following statements regarding local flaps is correct?**
   A. Advancement flaps are traditionally single-pedicle rectangular flaps.
   B. Rotation flaps can be facilitated by the use of Burow's triangles or back-cuts.
   C. Transposition flaps are usually rotated laterally about a pivot point into a distant defect.
   D. A Z-plasty is a variation of an advancement flap.
   E. Limberg and Dufourmentel flaps have identical angles.

Z-PLASTY

6. You are selecting the internal angles for a Z-plasty procedure. **What angle should provide a theoretical 50% increase in central limb length?**
   A. Ten degrees
   B. Thirty degrees
   C. Forty-five degrees
   D. Sixty degrees
   E. Ninety degrees

7. **Which one of the following is correct regarding Z-plasty procedures?**
   A. A seventy-five degree Z-plasty provides the best compromise for central limb lengthening.
   B. Multiple Z-plasties in series are more effective for increasing skin length than a single, large Z-plasty.
   C. The double-opposing semicircular flap modification can effectively close circular defects.
   D. Actual gain in central limb length is very close to the theoretical predicted values.
   E. A Z-plasty with ninety-degree internal angles provides the least tension on closure.

FLAP PHYSIOLOGY

8. **Which one of the following acts as a vasoconstrictor on flap microcirculation?**
   A. Thromboxane A_2
   B. Bradykinin
   C. Acidosis
   D. Prostaglandin E_1
   E. Hypercapnia

FLAP DELAY

9. You are planning to delay a flap for reconstruction of a large skin defect to the head and neck. **Which one of the following is correct regarding flap delay?**
   A. It will require two surgical procedures spaced three to five days apart.
   B. It will specifically improve long-term survival of the entire flap.
   C. Delay preconditions the flap to ischemia but often results in early tissue necrosis.
   D. Flap tip viability is improved as a result of increased blood flow coupled with a decreased oxygen requirement.
   E. Of the five proposed mechanisms of flap delay, sympathetic stimulation is probably most important.

PHARMACOLOGIC INFLUENCES ON FREE FLAP SURVIVAL

10. **Based on reliable evidence, which one of the following is recommended for use in free tissue transfer to improve anastomotic patency during the first week?**
    A. Dextran
    B. Unfractionated heparin
    C. Low-molecular-weight heparin
    D. Calcium channel blockers
    E. Aspirin

PHARMACOLOGIC AGENTS IN FREE TISSUE TRANSFER

11. For each of the following descriptions, select the most appropriate answer from the list. (Each answer may be used once, more than once, or not at all.)
    A. This stimulates the conversion of plasminogen to plasmin and may be useful in early free flap salvage.
    B. This impairs endothelium-dependent skin vasodilation and may affect wound healing.
    C. This is an anticoagulant secreted by medicinal leeches that partly explains their benefit in venous compromised flaps.

Options:
a. Low-molecular-weight heparin
b. Hirudin
c. Nicotine
d. Aspirin
e. Streptokinase
f. Dextran
g. Nitroglycerin

FREE FLAP MONITORING

12. You are asked to assess a patient 24 hours after breast reconstruction with a DIEP flap. Which one of the following is the least helpful discriminator between arterial and venous occlusion in this flap?
    A. Capillary refill time
    B. Flap tissue turgor
    C. Flap skin color
    D. Flap surface temperature
    E. Flap dermal bleeding

13. Which one of the following is considered to be the most effective method for monitoring free flaps postoperatively?
    A. External Doppler ultrasound
    B. Transcutaneous oxygen tension
    C. Surface temperature
    D. Fluorescein injection
    E. Clinical observation

Answers

BLOOD SUPPLY TO FLAPS

1. *Which one of the following is correct regarding blood supply to flaps?*
   E. Neurocutaneous flaps are based upon perforating arteries accompanying a cutaneous nerve.

   Neurocutaneous flaps (such as the sural flap) receive their blood supply through the arteries accompanying the named nerve. Fasciocutaneous flaps are supplied by different levels of vascular plexus including the subfascial, intrafascial, and the intradermal layers, but the suprafascial and subdermal plexuses are considered to be the most important. *Axial pattern flaps* contain a specific direct cutaneous artery within the longitudinal axis of the flap. Examples include the pedicled groin and paramedian forehead flaps. This means they are not limited by specific set width to length ratios. An angiosome refers to a composite unit of skin and the underlying deep tissue supplied by a source artery, not just the skin area alone. The sympathetic (not parasympathetic) system is most important in regulating blood flow to the skin. Flaps based on the subdermal plexus that are limited to particular width to length ratios are described as *random pattern flaps;* for example, a transverse rectangular advancement flap on the forehead.

PERFORATOR FLAPS

2. *For the following flaps, the best options are as follows:*
   A. *Anterolateral thigh flap (ALT)*
      d. Variable indirect muscle or septal perforators
   B. *Deep inferior epigastric artery perforator flap (DIEP)*
      a. Indirect muscle perforator
   C. *Groin flap*
      c. Direct cutaneous perforator
   D. *Lateral arm flap*
      b. Indirect septal perforator

   The perforator vessels supplying flaps can be broadly classified as *direct* or *indirect*. Direct perforators pierce the deep fascia to supply skin, without having traversed deeper structures. Indirect perforators pass through deeper tissues, usually muscle or an intermuscular septum, before piercing the deep fascia. Blondeel et al[1] classified perforator flaps whose skin is supplied by an isolated perforating vessel or vessels into three categories: *myocutaneous perforator flaps* based on an indirect muscle perforator, *septocutaneous perforator flaps* based on an indirect septal perforator, and *direct cutaneous perforator flaps* based on direct cutaneous perforators. These are shown in Fig. 4-1.

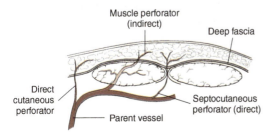

Fig. 4-1 Different types of direct and indirect perforator vessels with regard to their surgical importance: Direct perforator perforating the deep fascia only, indirect muscle perforator traveling through muscle before piercing the deep fascia, and indirect septal perforator traveling through the intermuscular septum before piercing the deep fascia.

VENOUS FLAPS

3. Which one of the following is correct regarding venous flaps?
D. The mechanism of flap perfusion is poorly understood.

The mechanism of flap perfusion is not well understood for venous flaps. Suggested mechanisms of venous flap perfusion include plasmatic imbibition, perfusion pressure, arteriovenous anastomoses, perivenous arterial networks, vein-to-vein interconnections, and circumvention of venous valves. Not only is their physiology poorly understood, survival can be unpredictable. Thatte and Thatte[2] have classified the following three types (not five) of venous flaps, according to their vascular anatomy:

Type I is an unipedicled venous flap with a single cephalad vein as the only vessel.
Type II is a bipedicled flow-through venous flap.
Type III is an arterialized venous flap in which one end of the vein is anastomosed to a feeding artery.

Venocutaneous flaps are not usually sensate, it is neurocutaneous flaps such as the sural flap that have this quality. Donor site morbidity is sometimes said to be reduced when compared to an arterial flap because no arterial sacrifice is required.

CLASSIFICATION OF MUSCLE FLAPS

4. Muscle flaps may be grouped according to their vascular anatomy. **Which one of the following is correct regarding the Mathes and Nahai classification of muscle flaps?**
B. The tensor fascia lata flap represents a type I flap.

The Mathes and Nahai classification[3] of muscle flap supply is as follows:

Type I: One vascular pedicle (e.g., tensor fascia lata)
Type II: One dominant and one or more minor pedicles (e.g., gracilis)
Type III: Two dominant pedicles (e.g., gluteus maximus)
Type IV: Segmental vascular pedicle (e.g., sartorius)
Type V: One dominant pedicle with secondary segmental pedicles (e.g., latissimus dorsi)

The TFL flap is a type I flap as it has one dominant pedicle arising from the lateral circumflex femoral artery. It may be harvested with an ALT flap: The gluteus maximus is a type III flap (not type II) as it has two dominant vascular pedicles: the superior and inferior gluteals. This means that the entire muscle can be based on either vessel. The gracilis is a type II flap according to the Mathes and Nahai classification as it has one proximal dominant pedicle and a more distal minor pedicle. The distant pedicle cannot support the entire muscle if raised on this vessel. Flap types I, III, and V have the most reliable vascularity.

LOCAL FLAP TECHNIQUES

5. Which one of the following statements regarding local flaps is correct?
B. Rotation flaps may be facilitated by the use of Burow's triangles or back-cuts.

Local flaps can be subclassified as *rotation, advancement, transposition,* or *interpolation* (see Figs. 4-9, and 4-12, *Essentials of Plastic Surgery,* second edition). Rotation flaps often have a semicircular design and rotate about a pivot point into an adjacent defect (Fig. 4-2). Direct closure of the donor site is usually possible. Use of a back-cut or Burow's triangle at the base will change the pivot point which can increase the reach of the flap tip.

Chapter 4 ■ Basics of Flaps

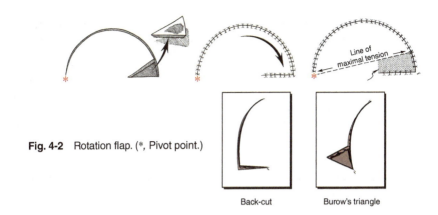

Fig. 4-2 Rotation flap. (*, Pivot point.)

Advancement flaps slide into an adjacent defect by stretching the skin or release of subcutaneous tissues without rotation or lateral movement. They can be rectangular or V-Y in design and small Burow's triangles at the base can also help advancement. Transposition flaps have elements of rotation and lateral advancement, and they rotate around a pivot point into an adjacent defect. Common examples include rhomboid flaps and Z-plasty flaps. Though Limberg and Dufourmentel flaps are both transposition flaps of a rhomboid design, they differ in the individual internal angles used. The Limberg flap is a rhomboid flap that uses two 60-degree angles and two 120-degree angles. The Dufourmentel flap is a narrower design with internal angles that are not fixed to specific numbers. The benefit of this flap is that it has a lesser arc of pivot and therefore reduces the likelihood of a dog-ear being created (see Figs. 4-9 through 4-12, *Essentials of Plastic Surgery,* second edition).

Z-PLASTY

6. You are selecting the internal angles for a Z-plasty procedure. **What angle should provide a theoretical 50% increase in central limb length?**
   C. Forty-five degrees
   A *Z-plasty* is a type of transposition flap with two adjacent triangular flaps that are reversed. Key factors in the design are that the three limbs should be of equal length, and the two internal angles should be equivalent (see Table 4-1, *Essentials of Plastic Surgery,* second edition). There is a consistent theoretical relationship between internal angle and percentage gain in central limb length. An angle of 30 degrees will allow an increase of 25%. Thereafter, for each increase in angle of 15 degrees, length increases by 25% (e.g., a 45-degree increase in angle gives a 50% increase in length, and a 60-degree increase in angle gives a 75% increase in length). In clinical practice actual gains in length may differ from the theoretical values because of skin laxity and adherence.

7. **Which one of the following is correct regarding Z-plasty procedures?**
   C. The double-opposing semicircular flap modification can effectively close circular defects.
   The double-opposing Z-plasty technique involves a curvilinear modification of the Z-plasty principle and is used to close circular defects (see Fig. 4-15, *Essentials of Plastic Surgery,* second edition). A 60-degree, rather than a 75-degree Z-plasty provides the best compromise for achieving increased central limb length without significant lateral tension (see Fig. 4-14, *Essentials of Plastic Surgery,* second edition).[4] Although combining multiple Z-plasties in series is a useful technique, more effective skin lengthening is achieved with a single, large Z-plasty.

A number of techniques involve Z-plasties, such as the jumping-man flap and four-flap Z-plasty. Both of these can be useful for correction of first-web-space tightness (see Fig. 61-7, *Essentials of Plastic Surgery*, second edition). The jumping-man flap or double-opposing Z, is created with a combination of Z-plasty flaps and a central V-Y advancement flap. The four flap Z-plasty moves flaps from an initial ABCD orientation to CABD orientation following transfer. For this reason it is sometimes referred to as the "Cadbury" flap. As discussed in question 6, the actual gain in the central limb length following a standard Z-plasty differs from the theoretical predicted value. This can range from 55% to 84%. Use of the 90-degree Z-plasty provides a large theoretical gain in length but results in high tension across the wound closure.[4]

FLAP PHYSIOLOGY

8. Which one of the following acts as a vasoconstrictor on flap microcirculation?
A. Thromboxane A_2

Blood flow to the skin is regulated by local and systemic factors. Systemic factors are neural through sympathetic adrenergic fibers and humeral through a number of chemical mediators. Thromboxane A_2 is a humoral vasoconstrictor, as are epinephrine, norepinephrine, serotonin, and prostaglandin $F_{2\alpha}$. Circulating vasodilators include bradykinin, histamine, and prostaglandin-E_1. Local control is affected by metabolic factors including hypercapnia, hypoxia, and acidosis. Each of these acts primarily as a vasodilator.

FLAP DELAY

9. You are planning to delay a flap for reconstruction of a large skin defect to the head and neck. **Which one of the following is correct regarding flap delay?**
D. Flap tip viability is improved as a result of increased blood flow coupled with a decreased oxygen requirement.

Flap delay involves surgical interruption of a portion of the blood supply to a flap prior to transfer. It may be useful to improve the viable length of a given flap (i.e., improve tip viability) but does not significantly affect more proximal areas such as the base which would have survived anyway. It requires two surgical procedures typically spaced ten to twenty-one days apart. Although in animal models, flaps have been successfully divided at three days, this time interval is not normally advised in clinical cases. Flap delay should not result in tissue necrosis as vascularity should not be compromised to such an extent. The process should cause a more mild degree of tissue ischemia.

There are two main theories regarding delay: that delay conditions tissues to ischemia allowing them to survive on less nutrient blood flow and that delay improves vascularity by opening up choke vessels between adjacent vascular territories. It is likely that a combination of these effects is responsible.

The five mechanisms believed to be involved in delay are sympathectomy, vascular reorganization, reactive hyperemia, acclimatization to hypoxia, and a nonspecific inflammatory reaction. Therefore loss of sympathetic stimulation, as opposed to an increase in sympathetic stimulation, is proposed to be a factor in delay.

PHARMACOLOGIC INFLUENCES ON FREE FLAP SURVIVAL

10. Based on reliable evidence, which one of the following is recommended for use in free tissue transfer to improve anastomotic patency during the first week?
C. Low-molecular-weight heparin

Of the medications listed, low-molecular-weight heparin has been shown to improve anastomotic patency while minimizing hemorrhage. Dextran was originally used as a volume expander and can decrease platelet adhesiveness and procoagulant activity. It also increases bleeding time and has been shown to improve short-term microvascular patency. However it is not routinely used because of its poor side effect profile including anaphylaxis, pulmonary edema, renal failure, and cardiac complications. Calcium channel blockers act on vascular smooth muscle and have been shown to improve flap survival in animal models. Aspirin acts on the cyclooxygenase pathway and decreases the synthesis of thromboxane A_2, a potent vasoconstrictor. Although some evidence suggests that anastomotic patency may be improved in the first twenty-four hours, beyond this time no further improvement is observed. There is currently no evidence to support the routine use of aspirin following free flap surgery.

PHARMACOLOGIC AGENTS IN FREE TISSUE TRANSFER

11. *For each of the following descriptions, select the most appropriate answer from the list. (Each answer can be used once, more than once, or not at all):*
  A. *This stimulates the conversion of plasminogen to plasmin and may be useful in early free flap salvage.*
  e. Streptokinase
  B. *This impairs endothelium-dependent skin vasodilation and may affect wound healing.*
  c. Nicotine
  C. *This is an anticoagulant secreted by medicinal leeches that partly explains their benefit in venous compromised flaps.*
  b. Hirudin

> The most common cause of free flap failure is venous insufficiency. This can secondarily compromise arterial inflow and lead to formation of a secondary thrombus. Antithrombolytic agents include streptokinase and urokinase, which are first-generation agents. Second-generation agents include tissue plasminogen activator and acylated plasminogen-streptokinase activator complex. These may be effective in flap salvage in the setting of microvascular thrombosis, because they convert plasminogen to plasmin, which acts to cleave fibrin at the thrombus site.
>
> Acute exposure of human skin vasculature to nicotine is associated with amplification of norepinephrine induced skin vasoconstriction and impaired endothelium-dependent skin vasodilation. Nicotine also increases platelet adhesiveness and increases the risk of wound breakdown following surgery (see Chapters 1 and 8).
>
> Medicinal leeches (Hirudo medicinalis) secrete a number of substances that affect coagulation. First, they inject hirudin (a naturally occurring anticoagulant) at the site of a bite. Second, they secrete hyalase which facilitates spread of hirudin through tissues and a vasodilatory substance that also contributes to bleeding. Leeches can be useful in flaps which have mild venous compromise.

FREE FLAP MONITORING

12. You are asked to assess a patient 24 hours after breast reconstruction with a DIEP flap. *Which one of the following is the least helpful discriminator between arterial and venous occlusion in this flap?*
  D. Flap surface temperature

> Cutaneous free flap monitoring is predominantly based on clinical assessment, although a number of adjuncts are available (Table 4-1). Common clinical features assessed are tissue color, capillary return, tissue turgor, flap temperature, and dermal bleeding characteristics. Of these features, all can usually be used to discriminate between venous and arterial insufficiency, with the exception of temperature, which is usually reduced in either case. A healthy flap should have a capillary refill time of 2 to 3 seconds. It should be a healthy pink color in pale skinned

individuals. Tissue turgor should be normal. Low turgor indicates underfilling of the flap (i.e., arterial compromise) and increased turgor indicates venous congestion. Needle testing of the dermis can be helpful as a healthy flap should bleed bright red blood. No blood or serous fluid indicates there is no inflow and dark red blood suggests there is inadequate venous outflow.

Table 4-1 *Signs of Arterial Occlusion and Venous Congestion*

	Arterial Occlusion	Venous Congestion
Skin color	Pale, mottled, bluish, or white	Cyanotic, bluish, or dusky
Capillary refill	Sluggish	Brisker than normal
Tissue turgor	Prunelike; turgor decreased	Tense, swollen; turgor increased
Dermal bleeding	Scant amount of dark blood or serum	Rapid bleeding of dark blood
Temperature	Cool	Cool

13. *Which one of the following is considered to be the most effective method for monitoring free flaps postoperatively?*
    E. Clinical observation
    Despite a number of technologically advanced tools for monitoring free flaps, clinical observation remains the most widely used and consistent method for monitoring a free flap. Of the clinical assessment modalities, bleeding from a dermal wound as described in question 12, is an accurate positive test, as the absence of bleeding indicates no arterial inflow and dark red blood indicates venous outflow insufficiency. A failed flap will leak serous straw colored fluid on dermal scratch testing. It is paramount to educate nursing and medical staff in accurate flap monitoring so that changes in flap appearance are identified and managed early. In buried flaps such as a bony fibula flap for reconstruction of the humerus, direct clinical observation of the flap is not possible so an internal Doppler placed on the artery or vein can be helpful. This involves securing a cuff around the vessel with ligaclips. The cuff is placed distal to the anastomosis and has a wire attached that connects to an external box providing audible confirmation of blood flow.

REFERENCES

1. Blondeel PN, Van Landuyt K, Hamdi M, et al. Perforator flap terminology: update 2002. Clin Plast Surg 30:343-346, 2003.
2. Thatte MR, Thatte RL. Venous flaps. Plast Reconstr Surg 91:747-751, 1993.
3. Mathes SJ, Nahai F. Classification of the vascular anatomy of muscles: experimental and clinical correlation. Plast Reconstr Surg 67:177-187, 1981.
4. McGregor AD, McGregor IA. Fundamental Techniques of Plastic Surgery and Their Surgical Applications, ed 10. Philadelphia: Churchill Livingstone, 2000.

5. Fundamentals of Perforator Flaps

See *Essentials of Plastic Surgery,* second edition, pp. 45-56.

ANATOMY OF PERFORATOR FLAPS
1. *Which one of the following statements is correct regarding perforator flaps?*
   A. An indirect perforator originates from the source artery and pierces the deep fascia without traversing any deeper structures.
   B. The terms *perforasome* and *angiosome* may be used interchangeably given they are the same thing.
   C. A direct perforator passes directly through an intermediary structure before crossing the deep fascia en route to the skin.
   D. Vessels that are septocutaneous perforators are considered to be direct perforators.
   E. Any given perforasome is composed of multiple angiosomes arising from the same source vessel.

CLASSIFICATION OF PERFORATOR FLAPS
2. *Which one of the following is correct regarding the classification of perforator flaps?*
   A. The Gent consensus recommends the use of suffixes to indicate the muscles involved.
   B. The Canadian classification system considers the anatomic region and muscle name.
   C. The only difference between the Canadian and Gent classification systems is the use of the word *artery* within the flap title.
   D. No single universally accepted classification system exists for perforator flaps.
   E. The Gent consensus names flaps according to the nutrient source vessel only.

ANTEROLATERAL THIGH FLAP
3. *Which one of the following statements is correct regarding the anterolateral thigh flap?*
   A. It is a fasciocutaneous flap which obtains its dominant supply from the transverse branch of the lateral circumflex femoral artery.
   B. The correct Canadian nomenclature is anterior lateral thigh perforator (ALTAP) flap.
   C. The correct Gent consensus nomenclature is lateral circumflex femoral artery perforator (LCFAP).
   D. LCFAP-*s* indicates that an anterolateral thigh flap is based on a septocutaneous perforator.
   E. It is normally a type A fasciocutaneous flap using the Mathes and Nahai classification.

4. You are planning to reconstruct a 12 by 8 cm defect on the dorsal foot and ankle of a woman following leiomyosarcoma resection. She has a BMI of 35 and is hypertensive, but is otherwise medically well. **Which one of the following is correct regarding the use of an anterolateral thigh flap (ALT) for this patient's reconstruction?**
   A. The ALT is ideal for reconstruction in this scenario.
   B. The ALT donor site will require skin grafting.
   C. Preoperative donor site angiography is mandatory in this setting.
   D. A radial forearm flap may be better for this woman.
   E. ALT pedicle length is unlikely to be sufficient for reconstruction.

TECHNIQUES FOR RAISING PERFORATOR FLAPS

5. While raising a deep inferior epigastric perforator (DIEP) flap for breast reconstruction, you are concerned regarding the size of the venae commitantes. The flap has been cut to size, preserving zones I through III. You have completed a satisfactory anastomosis and have inset the flap. The flap is running but capillary refill is very brisk and the flap is becoming blue. **Which one of the following is most likely to improve the flap viability?**
   A. Further reduction of flap volume
   B. Staged flap inset
   C. Postoperative use of leech therapy
   D. Anastomosis of the superficial inferior epigastric vein (SIEV)
   E. Administration of systemic heparin

6. You are planning to use a perforator flap to reconstruct a soft tissue defect and will be supervising your resident during the process. **Which one of the following should you tell them?**
   A. The minimal perforator diameter should be 2.0 mm.
   B. The inability to identify a visible perforator pulse does not matter.
   C. The plane of dissection should be close to the perforator.
   D. The perforator must be sited centrally in the skin flap.
   E. Including two perforators is required for optimal flap viability.

7. **When designing a freestyle perforator flap for reconstruction of a 9 cm diameter shoulder defect, which one of the following is the most useful preoperative investigation?**
   A. Handheld Doppler
   B. CT angiography
   C. Laser Doppler flowmetry
   D. Indocyanine green
   E. Tissue oximetry

LATERAL CIRCUMFLEX FEMORAL ARTERY PERFORATOR FLAP

8. You are planning to use a pedicled lateral circumflex femoral artery perforator (LCFAP) flap to reconstruct an abdominal wall defect. **Which muscle often requires dissection when raising this flap?**
   A. Vastus medialis
   B. Gracilis
   C. Gastrocnemius
   D. Biceps femoris
   E. Vastus lateralis

Chapter 5 ▪ Fundamentals of Perforator Flaps   37

Answers

ANATOMY OF PERFORATOR FLAPS
1. **Which one of the following statements is correct regarding perforator flaps?**
   D. Vessels that are septocutaneous perforators are considered to be direct perforators.
   Perforator flaps are vascularized areas of skin and subcutaneous tissue receiving blood supply from one or more perforators originating from a named source vessel. The perforating vessels can pass directly from the source vessel without traversing any deep structures or indirectly through muscle. This has clinical relevance with regard to the ease and speed with which flaps can be raised. Flaps with an intramuscular perforator path are more challenging and time consuming to raise. Angiosomes and perforasomes are not identical. Taylor and Palmer[1] described the 40 angiosomes in 1987, and Taylor[2] subsequently related them to perforator flaps in 2003. As discussed in Chapter 4, angiosomes represent a composite unit of skin and the underlying tissue supplied by a given source vessel. However, it was Saint-Cyr et al[3] who described the perforasome theory, representing a similar concept but the composite tissue is based on a single perforator from a given source vessel. This means that multiple perforasomes form each angiosome and in consequence there are around 300 perforasomes described.

CLASSIFICATION OF PERFORATOR FLAPS
2. **Which one of the following is correct regarding the classification of perforator flaps?**
   D. No single universally accepted classification system exists for perforator flaps.
   No single classification system for perforator flaps is universally accepted, but the two most commonly used are the Canadian classification system and the Gent consensus. With the Gent consensus, the flap is either named after the nutrient source vessel (e.g., deep inferior epigastric perforator [DIEP] flap) or the associated muscle or anatomic region in cases in which the source vessel supplies many other flaps (e.g., anterolateral thigh perforator [ALTP] or tensor fascia lata perforator [TFLP] flap).[4]
   The Canadian classification system also names the flap according to the source vessel, with the addition of the word *artery,* (e.g., deep inferior epigastric artery perforator [DIEAP] flap). In this system, when the source vessel supplies more than one flap, additional abbreviations are added. For example, a lateral circumflex femoral artery perforator flap involving the tensor fascia lata is named LCFAP-*tfl*[5] (see Fig. 5-6, *Essentials of Plastic Surgery,* second edition).

ANTEROLATERAL THIGH FLAP
3. **Which one of the following statements is correct regarding the anterolateral thigh flap?**
   D. LCFAP-*s* indicates that an anterolateral thigh flap is based on a septocutaneous perforator.
   The anterolateral thigh flap is a fasciocutaneous flap that may be based on the transverse branch of the lateral circumflex femoral artery, but the dominant supply is the descending branch. The correct Gent nomenclature for the anterolateral thigh flap is ALTP, whereas the Canadian classification system nomenclature is LCFAP. This becomes LCFAP-*vl* when the vastus lateralis is perforated (myocutaneous) and LCFAP-*s* when it is purely septocutaneous. The flap can be described using the Mathes and Nahai system according to the course of the perforator. This

classification contains three subtypes: A, B, and C. Type A is a direct cutaneous flap, type B is a septocutaneous flap, and type C is a musculocutaneous or myocutaneous flap.[6] The ALT can be a septocutaneous flap (i.e., type B) and this is most easy to raise as no intramuscular dissection is required. Often there are perforators passing through the vastus lateralis and in this case it would be a type C flap. This dissection is more time consuming and risks damage to the perforating vessels.

4. You are planning to reconstruct a 12 by 8 cm defect on the dorsal foot and ankle of a woman following leiomyosarcoma resection. She has a BMI of 35 and is hypertensive, but otherwise medically well. *Which one of the following is correct regarding the use of an anterolateral thigh flap (ALT) for this patient's reconstruction?*
   D. **A radial forearm flap may be better for this woman.**
   The ALT is a versatile flap that in many cases would be ideal for reconstructing the dorsum of the foot and ankle because it is often thin, pliable, and has a long pedicle enabling reach to the anterior or posterior tibial vessels. Furthermore, it can be raised as a chimeric flap with two separate skin paddles if there are separate defects involving medial and lateral malleoli, and it can limit surgery to a single limb. However, in obese individuals such as this patient, the ALT flap is often too thick and bulky and dissection may also be more challenging in these individuals. For this reason a radial forearm flap may be a better choice here.
   ALT skin paddle dimensions may be as large as 25 by 35 cm in some cases and flaps less than 10 cm width, such as in this case, can usually be closed directly. Those wider than 10 cm are likely to require a skin graft to the donor site, however this figure is still variable depending on individual patients' tissue characteristics. Preoperative angiography can be useful for evaluation of perforator flap vascularity, but is not essential. It is more likely to be useful to confirm leg vascularity and availability of recipient vessels, particularly in cases following lower limb trauma or in patients with peripheral vascular disease.

TECHNIQUES FOR RAISING PERFORATOR FLAPS

5. While raising a deep inferior epigastric perforator (DIEP) flap for breast reconstruction, you are concerned regarding the size of the venae commitantes. The flap has been cut to size preserving zones I through III. You have completed a satisfactory anastomosis and have inset the flap. The flap is running but capillary refill is very brisk and the flap is becoming blue. *Which one of the following is most likely to improve the flap viability?*
   D. **Anastomosis of the superficial inferior epigastric vein (SIEV)**
   The flap as described is showing signs of venous compromise. This can occur in DIEP flaps where there is inadequate connection between the superficial and deep inferior epigastric vascular systems. In cases such as this, where the venae commitantes are small, it is likely that the superficial system is large. When raising a DIEP flap the SIEV should be identified and preserved at the flap inferior margin and where compromise occurs, it can be anastomosed to a suitable vein. This is the most appropriate step in this scenario.
   In general, venous compromise can be due to a number of factors which must be systematically addressed. First the anastomotic patency must always be checked to ensure flow and that no external compression or twisting of the pedicle has occurred. In this case, the anastomoses are working satisfactorily. If one area of the flap (usually zone IV) is congested, this may be removed, but this has been done already. If the flap becomes brisk after inset it may be that compression is the cause and release of inset and staged closure may be helpful. Systemic heparin is not likely to

benefit this situation given the venous compromise. Use of leeches can help small flaps such as those on the digits that are venous congested but would not be the first choice in this scenario.

6. You are planning to use a perforator flap to reconstruct a soft tissue defect and will be supervising your resident during the process. **Which one of the following should you tell them?**
   C. The plane of dissection should be close to the perforator.
   When raising perforator flaps, dissection around the perforator must be meticulous with limited vessel manipulation such as twisting, stretching, and grasping. Dissection should be close to the vessel within the loose areolar plane as this facilitates good visibility of the vessel and minimizes risk of inadvertent damage. The minimal perforator diameter is 0.5 mm rather than 2.0 mm and the presence of a visible or palpable pulse is a strong indicator of a good perforator. Having the perforator centrally within the skin paddle is not required and in some propeller freestyle flaps the perforator is deliberately offset (see Fig. 5-7, *Essentials of Plastic Surgery,* second edition). The number of perforators that should be included in a flap is debated. DIEP flaps can be satisfactorily raised on single perforators, but some authors suggest that fat necrosis is reduced where more perforators are included.[7,8] Perforator quality is probably more important than perforator quantity for any given flap.[8]

7. ***When designing a freestyle perforator flap for reconstruction of a 9 cm diameter shoulder defect, which one of the following is the most useful preoperative investigation?***
   A. Handheld Doppler
   Preoperative methods for assessing perforator flaps include handheld Doppler, CT angiography, duplex ultrasonography and magnetic resonance angiography (MRA). Of these, the handheld Doppler will be ideal for most applications like this case where a freestyle flap is to be used because it is simple and reliable to help locate individual perforating vessels. CT angiography is more useful in flaps with variable anatomy such as the DIEP or superior gluteal artery perforator (SGAP) flap but is not essential when handheld methods can suffice. Indocyanine green is a useful *intraoperative* technique to help identify zones of adequate perfusion before committing to flap design. Laser Doppler flowmetry and tissue oximetry are methods used to monitor flaps postoperatively. They have high positive and negative predictive values but are expensive and not routinely used.

LATERAL CIRCUMFLEX FEMORAL ARTERY PERFORATOR FLAP

8. You are planning to use a pedicled lateral circumflex femoral artery perforator (LCFAP) flap to reconstruct an abdominal wall defect. **Which muscle often requires dissection when raising this flap?**
   E. Vastus lateralis
   As discussed in question 3, the LCFAP flap (also known as the ALT flap) is based on the lateral circumflex femoral artery and perforating vessels from this source vessel may pass through a portion of the vastus lateralis en route to the skin. In some cases, the perforators may be completely septal and in this situation intramuscular dissection is not required.
   Dissection of the gracilis muscle is required when raising an MCFAP flap which arises from the medial circumflex femoral vessels or the transverse upper gracillis (TUG) flap.[9,10] Intramuscular dissection of the medial head of gastrocnemius is required when raising a medial sural artery perforator flap (MSAP) flap.[11]

Perforator flaps have also been described based on the short head of biceps femoris and these may arise from either the popliteal or profunda femoris vessels.[12] In spite of a number of new perforator flaps having been described, the LCFAP or ALT remains one of the most popular workhorse flaps in reconstructive surgery.

REFERENCES

1. Taylor GI, Palmer JH. The vascular territories (angiosomes) of the body: experimental study and clinical applications. Br J Plast Surg 40:113-141, 1987.
2. Taylor GI. The angiosomes of the body and their supply to perforator flaps. Clin Plast Surg 30:331-342, 2003.
3. Saint-Cyr M, Wong C, Schaverien M, et al. The perforasome theory: vascular anatomy and clinical implications. Plast Reconstr Surg 124:1529-1544, 2009.
4. Blondeel PN, Van Landuyt KH, Monstrey SJ, et al. The "Gent" consensus on perforator flap terminology: preliminary definitions. Plast Reconstr Surg 112:1378-1382, 2003.
5. Geddes CR, Morris SF, Neligan PC. Perforator flaps: evolution, classification, and applications. Ann Plast Surg 50:90-99, 2003.
6. Mathes SJ, Nahai F. Reconstructive Surgery: Principles, Anatomy, and Technique. St Louis: Quality Medical Publishing, 1997.
7. Baumann DP, Lin HY, Chevray PM. Perforator number predicts fat necrosis in a prospective analysis of breast reconstruction with free TRAM, DIEP, and SIEA flaps. Plast Reconstr Surg 125:1335-1341, 2010.
8. Lindsey JT. Perforator number does not predict fat necrosis. Plast Reconstr Surg 127:1391-1392, 2011.
9. Hallock GG. The development of the medial circumflex femoral artery perforator flap. Semin Plast Surg 20:121-126, 2006.
10. Yousif NJ. The transverse gracilis musculocutaneous flap. Ann Plast Surg 31:382, 1993.
11. Cavadas PC, Sanz-Giménez-Rico JR, Gutierrez-de la Cámara A, et al. The medial sural artery perforator free flap. Plast Reconstr Surg 108:1609-1615; discussion 1616-1617, 2001.
12. Cavadas PC, Sanz-Jiménez-Rico JR, Landin L, et al. Biceps femoris perforator free flap for upper extremity reconstruction: anatomical study and clinical series. Plast Reconstr Surg 116:145-152, 2005.

6. Tissue Expansion

See *Essentials of Plastic Surgery,* second edition, pp. 57-66.

VISCOELASTIC PROPERTIES OF SKIN
1. **Which one of the following statements is correct regarding biologic tissue creep?**
   A. It forms the basis of intraoperative expansion.
   B. It involves displacement of water from ground substance.
   C. The elastic fibers become microfragmented.
   D. Collagen fibers undergo realignment.
   E. Cellular ingrowth and tissue regeneration are initiated.

SOFT TISSUE CHANGES DURING TISSUE EXPANSION
2. You have placed a submuscular tissue expander for immediate breast reconstruction following skin sparing mastectomy. **Which one of the following will occur in the soft tissues during tissue expansion?**
   A. The dermis will initially thicken but will normalize within 3 months.
   B. A capsule will form around the implant leading to improved skin flap viability.
   C. The pectoralis muscles will stretch and increase in bulk.
   D. The number and size of blood vessels within the overlying skin will decrease.
   E. The subcutaneous fat layer will thicken, thereby helping to provide additional implant cover.

EXPANDER SUBTYPES
3. **Which one of the following is a consistent feature of all internal tissue expanders?**
   A. Permanence
   B. Shape
   C. Filling portal
   D. Silicone elastomer shell
   E. Inflation method

TISSUE EXPANSION
4. **Which one of the following is correct regarding tissue expansion?**
   A. Expanders with remote ports require a magnet for accurate port location.
   B. Round expanders typically achieve 75% of their mathematically predicted tissue expansion.
   C. Expanders with differential expansion are useful in immediate breast reconstruction.
   D. Crescentic expanders achieve a greater percentage of their calculated expansion than any other implant shapes.
   E. Osmotic, self-inflating expanders are commonly used in clinical practice.

ADVANTAGES OF TISSUE EXPANSION

5. You are describing the risks and benefits of tissue expansion to a parent whose child requires excision of a giant cell nevus from the occipital scalp. *Which one of the following is the key advantage of tissue expansion for this child?*
   A. The number of general anesthetic procedures is minimized.
   B. The number of hospital clinic visits is reduced.
   C. The reconstruction can be completed more quickly.
   D. The defect is more likely to be closed directly using a hair-bearing skin flap.
   E. There is minimal functional and aesthetic impact during the expansion process.

TISSUE EXPANSION PLANNING

6. You are planning to expand tissue to resurface a scalp burn scar in an adult. *Which one of the following is correct regarding tissue expansion?*
   A. The base diameter of the expander should be 5 times the defect diameter.
   B. The expander should not be inflated beyond the listed volume.
   C. Selection of a crescenteric expander is a good choice in this scenario.
   D. The access incision is best placed parallel to the intended direction of expansion.
   E. The expander should be placed superficial to the galea.

THE EXPANSION PROCESS

7. You have placed an expander with an integrated port for delayed breast reconstruction. *Which one of the following is correct regarding the expansion process?*
   A. It should begin 6 weeks after implantation of the expander.
   B. It is best performed aseptically with a 14-gauge needle and sterile water.
   C. Expansion in the clinic should only be stopped once the patient feels discomfort.
   D. Skin blanching is a useful sign to guide expansion in a clinic setting.
   E. Risk of extrusion is reduced by early expansion.

ESTIMATION OF TISSUE AVAILABILITY AFTER EXPANSION

8. You are resurfacing a scalp defect using three expanders. *The amount of tissue available from each expander can be estimated by which of the following?*
   A. Base radius multiplied by circumference (dome length)
   B. Circumference (dome length) minus base radius
   C. Base radius divided by circumference (dome length)
   D. Circumference (dome length) minus base diameter
   E. Dome height minus base radius

CLINICAL APPLICATIONS

9. You see a 20-year-old girl in clinic with a large congenital nevus on the scalp measuring 10 by 10 cm. She would like it to be removed and you plan to use tissue expansion. *What is the maximum percentage of the scalp that can usually be reconstructed with tissue expansion without causing significant thinning of the remaining hair?*
   A. 15%
   B. 30%
   C. 50%
   D. 65%
   E. 75%

10. **Why is tissue expansion not generally advocated for standard nasal reconstruction with a forehead flap?**
   A. Forehead skin does not expand well.
   B. The donor site is fully closed directly without expansion.
   C. The risk of implant extrusion is high.
   D. The donor site heals well by secondary intention.
   E. A general anesthetic can be avoided.

COMPLICATIONS OF TISSUE EXPANSION

11. **When considering the anatomic location for tissue expansion, which one of the following has the highest complication rates?**
   A. Neck
   B. Scalp
   C. Chest
   D. Arm
   E. Leg

12. You see a patient following insertion of a submuscular breast expander for delayed breast reconstruction. She had 100 ml injected at the time of surgery and a small contour was created. She has had two further documented sessions of normal expansion with 80 ml on each occasion through the integrated port, but the chest wall now appears flat. *What is the most likely reason?*
   A. Insufficient volume injected at this stage
   B. Faulty valve on the integrated port
   C. Intraoperative damage to the implant
   D. Failure to inject the volumes directly into the expander
   E. Expander puncture during injection

Answers

VISCOELASTIC PROPERTIES OF SKIN
1. **Which one of the following statements is correct regarding biologic tissue creep?**
   E. Cellular ingrowth and tissue regeneration are initiated.
   Creep refers to a permanent elongation in tissues subjected to an external force. There are two types of creep: mechanical and biologic. Mechanical creep occurs where tissue is acutely stretched and results in collagen realignment, elastic fiber microfragmentation, water displacement, and recruitment of adjacent tissue. In contrast, biologic creep occurs where tissues are stretched for a prolonged period and cellular ingrowth is initiated. Changes include an increase in collagen production, angiogenesis, and epidermal proliferation.

SOFT TISSUE CHANGES DURING TISSUE EXPANSION
2. You have placed a submuscular tissue expander for immediate breast reconstruction following skin sparing mastectomy. **Which one of the following will occur in the soft tissues during tissue expansion?**
   B. A capsule will form around the implant leading to improved skin flap viability.
   There are a number of changes that occur in the skin and subcutaneous tissue during tissue expansion. A key factor is an increase in vascularity within expanded soft tissue because of an increased size and number of vessels secondary to angiogenesis. The highest vessel density is found at the junction of the capsule and host tissue and this was demonstrated by Pasyk et al[1] who analyzed the capsule, identifying four distinct layers. The outermost layer had a high density of collagen and blood vessels. This has clinical relevance in that the capsule itself can increase skin flap viability and should be left in situ following expansion where possible.
   The dermis thins, not thickens, fibroblasts and myofibroblasts increase in number, and sweat glands and hair follicles become less dense. Thickness does not return to normal until approximately 2 years after expansion. The epidermis thickens secondary to hyperkeratosis and normalizes after 6 months. Muscle tends to decrease in thickness and mass due to either compression or stretch from the expander (depending on which level the expander is placed). In this scenario muscle function is not usually significantly reduced by the expansion process itself, although the medial release and muscle undermining may do so. Fat is extremely sensitive to mechanical force and aggressive expansion is likely to cause fat necrosis. In general the subcutaneous layer thins and some permanent loss of fat occurs.

EXPANDER SUBTYPES
3. **Which one of the following is a consistent feature of all internal tissue expanders?**
   D. Silicone elastomer shell
   Internal tissue expanders are formed with a silicone elastomer shell surrounding an internal reservoir. They may be classified by shape, permanence, inflation mechanism, or filling portal type. Shapes include round, crescentic, and rectangular. Implants are commonly temporary but may be permanent such as some breast prostheses with a second inner compartment filled with silicone. Inflation is usually manual but can be self-filling as a result of osmosis when hypertonic expanders are used. The filling portal can be integrated or placed externally.

TISSUE EXPANSION

4. Which one of the following is correct regarding tissue expansion?
C. Expanders with differential expansion are useful in immediate breast reconstruction.

The use of permanent expanders is popular in breast reconstruction and they can be shaped with differential expansion of the upper/lower poles. This can help recreate a more natural breast contour with ptosis. They are comprised of a more highly projecting lower pole and a more modestly projecting upper pole. Expanders can have integrated or remote ports. Remote ports are either placed externally or subcutaneously and are palpable and therefore do not require a magnetic locator, which is reserved for integrated ports.

Expander geometry affects the amount of surface area gained. Expanders that are rectangular (not crescentic) achieve the greatest percentage of their calculated expansion at 38%. Crescentic expanders usually achieve values of approximately 32%, and round expanders typically achieve values of approximately 25%.

Osmotic, self-inflating expanders contain hypertonic sodium chloride crystals and fill by osmosis. The rate of expansion cannot be altered after insertion. Although commercially available, they are not commonly used in clinical practice. They tend to be occasionally used in pediatric patients with scalp or periorbital defects and are otherwise largely experimental.

ADVANTAGES OF TISSUE EXPANSION

5. You are describing the risks and benefits of tissue expansion to a parent whose child requires excision of a giant cell nevus from the occipital scalp. *Which one of the following is the key advantage of tissue expansion for this child?*
D. The defect is more likely to be closed directly using a hair-bearing skin flap.

Tissue expansion is useful, because it can facilitate closure of defects that otherwise require importation of distant tissue, but it has several disadvantages. It is staged and requires at least two surgical procedures; multiple surgical outpatient appointments are needed for expansion; completion of reconstruction is delayed; and appearance and function may be unacceptable for the patient and/or family during the expansion process. Placement of an expander also carries a risk of infection. Should this occur the expander would need to be removed.

TISSUE EXPANSION PLANNING

6. You are planning to expand tissue to resurface a scalp burn scar in an adult. *Which one of the following is correct regarding tissue expansion?*
C. Selection of a crescentic expander is a good choice in this scenario.

Shape selection of the expander depends on location and crescent shapes are often used in the scalp. These are normally placed subgaleally. Precise expander volume is not usually a concern because most can be safely overinflated beyond their recommended maximum volume. The base diameter of the expander should be 2 to 2.5 times the defect diameter (not 5 times).

The access incision for initial expander placement should ideally be perpendicular to the main axis of expansion (long axis of the expander) not parallel, to reduce tension across the scar. It should be placed at the edge of the defect so that it can be removed at the time of reconstruction.

THE EXPANSION PROCESS

7. You have placed an expander with an integrated port for delayed breast reconstruction. *Which one of the following is correct regarding the expansion process?*
D. Skin blanching is a useful sign to guide expansion in a clinic setting.

Expansion typically begins 2 to 3 weeks after surgery to allow time for the wound to heal sufficiently without tension. Expansion is best performed with a small needle (23-gauge or smaller). It is performed using sterile saline, which has a similar osmolarity to tissue fluids.

Patient discomfort and blanching are both indicators that expansion for that appointment is complete. Rapid expansion is associated with a greater risk of extrusion.

ESTIMATION OF TISSUE AVAILABILITY AFTER EXPANSION

8. You are resurfacing a scalp defect using three expanders. *The amount of tissue available from each expander can be estimated by which of the following?*
   D. Circumference (dome length) minus base diameter
   The amount of extra tissue available can be estimated by measuring the dome length and subtracting the base diameter (Fig. 6-1).

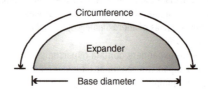

Circumference − Base diameter = Tissue available

Fig. 6-1 Amount of tissue available equals circumference minus base diameter.

CLINICAL APPLICATIONS

9. You see a twenty-year-old girl in clinic with a large congenital nevus on the scalp measuring 10 by 10 cm. She would like it to be removed and you plan to use tissue expansion. *What is the maximum percentage of the scalp that can usually be reconstructed with tissue expansion without causing significant thinning of the remaining hair?*
   C. 50%
   The scalp is well suited to reconstruction using tissue expansion providing patients are motivated and willing to tolerate a prolonged period with a deformed appearance of the head. Applications include tumor excision as in this case, burn alopecia, and other traumatic defects (as delayed procedures). Reconstruction outcomes will be specific to each individual patient and hair thinning will be dependent on both the site and size of the defect as well as the density of the patient's hair, however 50% is considered to be the maximum defect size that can be reconstructed in postburn patients without causing significant hair thinning.[2]

10. *Why is tissue expansion not generally advocated for standard nasal reconstruction with a forehead flap?*
    D. The donor site heals well by secondary intention.
    Forehead tissue expanders can be placed before raising a forehead flap with the intended benefit of facilitating direct closure of the donor defect. In practice this is not commonly performed because, in most cases, the caudal part of the donor site is closed directly and the residual defect on the scalp heals well by secondary intention. The forehead skin does expand well and has a relatively low rate of extrusion. A general anesthetic is standard practice for nasal reconstruction when using a forehead flap.[3]

Chapter 6 ■ Tissue Expansion   47

COMPLICATIONS OF TISSUE EXPANSION

11. When considering the anatomic location for tissue expansion, which one of the following has the highest complication rates?

E. Leg

In general, extremity tissue is associated with the highest complication rate when using tissue expansion techniques. The main complications are poor wound healing, implant extrusion, and infection. Of the extremities, the lower limb has the highest complication rate, especially when used below the knee. This does not mean tissue expansion cannot be used successfully in these locations, rather that patients and clinicians must be aware of the increased risks and these are taken into account. Other contributory risk factors such as diabetes, peripheral vascular disease, previous burn surgery, and previous radiation therapy must also be factored into the decision-making process.

12. You see a patient following insertion of a submuscular breast expander for delayed breast reconstruction. She had 100 ml injected at the time of surgery and a small contour was created. She has had two further documented sessions of normal expansion with 80 ml on each occasion through the integrated port, but the chest wall now appears flat. *What is the most likely reason?*

E. Expander puncture during injection

The most likely reason for an expander not to retain volume following injection of fluid is damage to the outer shell which allows fluid to leak out of the expander into the subcutaneous tissues. With modern implants, spontaneous volume loss is very unlikely to be due to faulty manufacture and is most likely due to the surgical team causing damage to the shell either during placement of the expander or during the expansion process itself.

A risk of using an expander with an integrated port is that the shell can fold over on itself when underfilled, so that when the injecting needle is passed into the valve it also passes through the shell. This is most likely to have occurred in this scenario. The expander is also at risk of damage during wound closure as the suture needle may inadvertently be passed through the silicone shell. If implants or expanders are returned to the manufacturer to assess deflation, the manufacturer is able to identify whether needle damage has occurred. Although in most cases, it is immediately obvious to see if the implant has been punctured, once it is removed.

It is unlikely that the fluid has not been injected into the expander providing that the magnetic finder has been used and the backing plate palpated during expansion, but this could potentially occur.

REFERENCES

1. Pasyk KA, Argenta LC, Austad ED. Histopathology of human expanded tissue. Clin Plast Surg 14:435-445, 1987.
2. MacLennan SE, Corcoran JF, Neale HW. Tissue expansion in head and neck burn reconstruction. Clin Plast Surg 27:121-132, 2000.
3. Burget GC. Axial paramedian forehead flap. In Strauch B, ed. Grabb's Encyclopedia of Flaps. Philadelphia: Lippincott, 1998.

7. Vascularized Composite Allografts and Transplant Immunology

See *Essentials of Plastic Surgery*, second edition, pp. 67-74.

TRANSPLANT TISSUE TYPES

1. **Which transplant type best describes the transfer of tissues between unrelated members of the same species?**
   A. Autograft
   B. Xenograft
   C. Allograft
   D. Isograft
   E. Vascularized graft

MAJOR HISTOCOMPATIBILITY COMPLEX ANTIGENS

2. **Which one of the following is correct regarding major histocompatibility complex (MHC) antigens?**
   A. There are three classes of MHC molecules.
   B. MHC molecules provide an immunologic fingerprint.
   C. Class I molecules display peptides from outside the cell.
   D. Class II molecules are present on all nucleated cells.
   E. HLA-DP, HLA-DR, and HLA-DQ are all class I molecules.

ACQUIRED IMMUNE SYSTEM

3. **Which one of the following is correct regarding the acquired immune system?**
   A. It plays a minor role in rejection of transplanted tissue.
   B. The sole primary mediators are the B lymphocytes.
   C. The acquired immune system is not capable of memory.
   D. It displays an enhanced secondary response.
   E. Activation of T cells requires a single stimulus.

ALLOGRAFT REJECTION

4. **Which one of the following is correct regarding allograft rejection?**
   A. Acute rejection occurs within the first few hours and is mediated by donor-specific antibodies.
   B. The direct pathway of donor organ recognition predominates in chronic rejection.
   C. Chronic rejection occurs over weeks to months and may be satisfactorily treated with steroids.
   D. Acute rejection is difficult to treat, and at present no reliable treatment exists.
   E. Accelerated rejection involves a secondary immune response mediated by sensitized T cells.

Chapter 7 ■ Vascularized Composite Allografts and Transplant Immunology 49

VASCULARIZED COMPOSITE ALLOGRAFT TRANSPLANTATION

5. You are part of the team preparing a patient for a full-face transplant. Tissue components to be included are skin, muscle, nerve, vessels, mucosa, and bone. An immunosuppressive regimen needs to be selected. **Which one of the following is the most antigenic tissue?**
   A. Fat
   B. Muscle
   C. Nerve
   D. Bone
   E. Skin

BANFF GRADING FOR ACUTE REJECTION

6. A patient presents with diffuse erythema of the skin after facial transplantation and frank epidermal necrosis is confirmed histologically. **Which one of the following grades best describes the problem according to the Banff criteria?**
   A. Grade 0
   B. Grade I
   C. Grade II
   D. Grade III
   E. Grade IV

IMMUNOSUPPRESSION

7. From the list, select the immunosuppressive agent that is most likely described in each of the following statements. (Each answer may be used once, more than once, or not at all.)
   A. *This agent works through inhibition of calcineurin, leading to inhibition of gene expression and T-cell activation. It has similar side effects to cyclosporin but displays increased neurotoxicity.*
   B. *This agent inhibits NF-kB, thereby inhibiting gene expression and activation of T cells. Side effects include hypertension, hyperlipidemia, hyperglycemia, and osteoporosis.*
   C. *This agent is a humanized monoclonal antiinterleukin (IL-2R) CD25 antibody that prevents interleukin-2–mediated activation. Side effects include hypersensitivity reactions.*

   Options:
   a. Sirolimus (Rapamune)
   b. Daclizumab (Zenapax)
   c. Azathioprine (Imuran)
   d. Mycophenolate mofetil (Cellcept)
   e. Muromonab-CD3 (Orthoclone OKT3)
   f. Prednisolone (Prednisone)
   g. Tacrolimus (Prograf)

IMMUNOSUPPRESSION THERAPY

8. A patient attends their weekly review 3 months after hand transplant surgery. On examination they have developed erythema and papules to the skin. **Which one of the following represents part of the first-line management of this patient, assuming that their tacrolimus levels are therapeutic?**
   A. Add sirolimus
   B. Add monoclonal antibodies
   C. Add polyclonal antithymocyte globulin
   D. Increase prednisolone
   E. Increase mycophenolate mofetil

COMPLICATIONS OF IMMUNE SUPPRESSION

9. *Following VCA, what would be the most likely presentation of malignancy secondary to immunotherapy?*
A. Hemoptysis
B. Keratotic skin lesion
C. Pathologic fracture
D. Lymphadenopathy
E. Change in bowel habit

THE PANEL REACTIVE ANTIBODY TEST

10. A patient awaiting face transplant surgery undergoes a panel reactive antibody test and receives a high score of 80%. ***What impact does this have on the patient's potential for transplantation surgery and why might the transfer team be disappointed?***
A. The patient is more likely to find a suitable donor.
B. The patient is less likely to find a suitable donor.
C. The patient will require less immunologic medical treatment.
D. The patient will have an increased risk of infection after surgery.
E. The transplant will never be able to proceed.

Chapter 7 ▪ Vascularized Composite Allografts and Transplant Immunology   51

Answers

TRANSPLANT TISSUE TYPES

1. **Which transplant type best describes the transfer of tissues between unrelated members of the same species?**
   C. Allograft
   An *allograft* is transplanted from an unrelated member of the same species (e.g., a cadaveric split-thickness skin graft or donor kidney transplant). An *isograft* is tissue that is transferred from one individual to another who is genetically identical. An *autograft* is tissue that is transplanted within the same individual (e.g., a split-thickness skin graft or free deep inferior epigastric artery perforator [DIEP] flap). A *xenograft* is tissue that is transplanted from one species to another, such as a porcine heart valve when implanted in a human. Grafts can be vascularized such as a hand transplant, or nonvascularized such as a split-thickness graft and can be transferred between individuals or within the same individual depending on the graft in question.

MAJOR HISTOCOMPATIBILITY COMPLEX ANTIGENS

2. **Which one of the following is correct regarding major histocompatibility complex (MHC) antigens?**
   B. MHC molecules provide an immunologic fingerprint.
   The MHC antigens are part of the cell-mediated immune response and in humans they are referred to as *human leukocyte antigen* (HLA) *molecules*. They are relevant to allograft rejection and provide an immunological fingerprint. There are two classes of molecules (not three) and they differ in a number of ways. Class I (HLA-A, HLA-B, and HLA-C) molecules are present on all nucleated cells, whereas class II (HLA-DP, HLA-DQ, and HLA-DR) are only found on antigen-presenting cells such as monocytes, macrophages, and B cells. Class I molecules present target peptides generated from within the cell, whereas class II molecules target peptides acquired from outside the cell following processes such as phagocytosis.

ACQUIRED IMMUNE SYSTEM

3. **Which one of the following is correct regarding the acquired immune system?**
   D. It displays an enhanced secondary response.
   The acquired immune system plays an important role in rejection of transplanted tissue, and both B and T lymphocytes are involved in the process. A key factor in the acquired immune system is that it is capable of memory, and its response to a second exposure can be more vigorous with a more rapid onset. Activation of T cells requires three (not one) signals/stimuli: (1) recognition of the foreign antigen, (2) a costimulatory signal, and (3) release of cytokines.

ALLOGRAFT REJECTION

4. **Which one of the following is correct regarding allograft rejection?**
   E. Accelerated rejection involves a secondary immune response mediated by sensitized T cells.
   Types of allograft rejection may be categorized as *hyperacute, accelerated, acute,* or *chronic.* Hyperacute rejection occurs within minutes to hours and is mediated by donor-specific antibodies that circulate before transplantation. These antibodies are acquired by prior exposure to an alloantigen after pregnancy, blood transfusion, or previous transplants. Accelerated rejection occurs within the first few days after a transplant. It represents a secondary immune response that is mediated by sensitized T cells. Treatment involves steroids and lymphocyte-depleting agents. Acute rejection occurs in the weeks or months following a transplant and may be cell mediated (T-cell–mediated response) or humoral (B-cell/antibody–mediated response). However, the only type of acute rejection reported in vascularized composite allografts is cell mediated. Treatment for cell-mediated acute rejection involves pulse steroids, optimization of maintenance therapy, and lymphocyte-depleting agents. Chronic rejection occurs over months to years via the indirect pathway of donor organ recognition. Treatment is very challenging, with no successful treatment available.

VASCULARIZED COMPOSITE ALLOGRAFT TRANSPLANTATION

5. You are part of the team preparing a patient for a full-face transplant. Tissue components to be included are skin, muscle, nerve, vessels, mucosa, and bone. An immunosuppressive regimen needs to be selected. **Which one of the following is the most antigenic tissue?**
   E. Skin
   Vascularized composite allografts (VCAs) contain numerous tissue types within a single graft such as skin, bone, muscle, and nerve. Of these tissue components, skin is the most antigenic, and as a result, direct inspection is important to identify acute rejection. This may manifest as erythematous macules, diffuse redness, or asymptomatic papules.

BANFF GRADING FOR ACUTE REJECTION

6. A patient presents with diffuse erythema of the skin after facial transplantation and frank epidermal necrosis is confirmed histologically. **Which one of the following grades best describes the problem according to the Banff criteria?**
   E. Grade IV
   The Banff 2007 grading system (Box 7-1) for acute rejection has five categories ranging from 0 to IV.[1] Grade 0 represents no rejection. Grade IV is the most severe rejection, and these patients present with frank necrosis of the epidermis or other skin structures. In face allografts, the transplanted mucosal surfaces may be similarly affected.

Chapter 7 ■ Vascularized Composite Allografts and Transplant Immunology

Box 7-1 *BANFF 2007 GRADING SYSTEM FOR ACUTE REJECTION*[1]

Grade 0 (no rejection)
- No or rare inflammatory infiltrates

Grade I (mild rejection)
- Mild perivascular infiltration
- No involvement of the overlying epidermis

Grade II (moderate rejection)
- Moderate to severe perivascular inflammation with or without mild epidermal and/or adnexal involvement (limited to spongiosis and exocytosis)
- No epidermal dyskeratosis or apoptosis

Grade III (severe rejection)
- Dense inflammation and epidermal involvement, with epithelial apoptosis, dyskeratosis, and/or keratinolysis

Grade IV (necrotizing acute rejection)
- Frank necrosis of the epidermis or other skin structures

IMMUNOSUPPRESSION

7. **For the following scenarios, the best options are as follows:**
   A. **This agent works through inhibition of calcineurin, leading to inhibition of gene expression and T-cell activation. It has similar side effects to cyclosporin but displays increased neurotoxicity.**
      g. Tacrolimus
   B. **This agent inhibits NF-kB, thereby inhibiting gene expression and activation of T cells. Side effects include hypertension, hyperlipidemia, hyperglycemia, and osteoporosis.**
      f. Prednisolone
   C. **This agent is a humanized monoclonal antiinterleukin (IL-2R) CD25 antibody that prevents interleukin-2–mediated activation. Side effects include hypersensitivity reactions.**
      b. Daclizumab

   A number of immunosuppressants are available, involving a variety of pathways (see Table 7-1, *Essentials of Plastic Surgery*, second edition). Common examples include the monoclonal antibodies, steroids, and calcineurin inhibitors. Although Tacrolimus can cause neurotoxicity, it has been found to enhance nerve recovery after coaptation.[2]

IMMUNOSUPPRESSION THERAPY

8. A patient attends their weekly review 3 months after hand transplant surgery. On examination they have developed erythema and papules to the skin. **Which one of the following represents part of the first-line management of this patient assuming that their tacrolimus levels are therapeutic?**
   D. Increase prednisolone

   This patient displays signs of acute rejection. This is managed with rescue therapy and involves systemic corticosteroids often alongside topical immunosuppressants such as clobetasol and protopic. It is important to confirm that calcineurin inhibitors such as tacrolimus are at therapeutic levels and if not, this must be addressed. Second-line agents include induction therapy agents, sirolimus and high-dose tacrolimus. Monoclonal antibodies and polyclonal antithymocyte globulin are part of a standard induction therapy regimen.

COMPLICATIONS OF IMMUNE SUPPRESSION

9. *Following VCA, what would be the most likely presentation of malignancy secondary to immunotherapy?*
   B. Keratotic skin lesion
   The most common malignancy after transplant surgery is skin cancer. The most likely subtype is squamous cell carcinoma (SCC) and this would first present as a keratotic skin lesion. The reason for the increased risk is immune suppression therapy. This is one of a number of reasons why close follow-up by a plastic surgery team is required.

   Hemoptysis is a sign of lung cancer, pathologic fractures are signs of bone metastases, lymphadenopathy may represent metastatic spread of an SCC or other tumor. Alternatively, posttransplant lymphoproliferative disease may occur. This is a B-cell proliferation due to neutropenic immune suppression. Symptoms range from infectious mononucleosis-like lesions to frank lymphoma. Change in bowel habit is associated with benign and malignant processes in the GI tract but not specifically to immune suppression therapy.

THE PANEL REACTIVE ANTIBODY TEST

10. A patient awaiting face transplant surgery undergoes a panel reactive antibody test and receives a high score of 80%. *What impact does this have on the patient's potential for transplantation surgery and why might the transfer team be disappointed?*
    B. The patient is less likely to find a suitable donor.
    Panel reactive antibodies are used to determine whether a patient has specific human leukocyte antigen antibodies.[3] A sample of a patient's blood is tested against the lymphocytes of 100 blood donors. The number of donors to which the patient has a reaction is expressed as a percentage (0% to 100%). A high percentage indicates that a patient has a high risk of acute rejection and may have to wait an extended time for a suitable donor. Medical treatment would not differ based on this result and although the chances of being able to proceed with transplant are reduced, the result does not mean that transplant is excluded for this patient. The infection rate posttransplant is unaffected by this result.

REFERENCES

1. Cendales LC, Kanitakis J, Schneeberger S, et al. The Banff 2007 working classification of skin-containing composite tissue allograft pathology. Am J Transplant 8:1396-1400, 2008.
2. Konofaos P, Terzis JK. FK506 and nerve regeneration: past, present and future. J Reconstr Microsurg 29:141-148, 2013.
3. U.S. Department of Health and Human Services. Organ Procurement and Transplantation Network. Available at http://optn.transplant.hrsa.gov/resources/allocationcalculators.asp?index75.

8. Basics of Microsurgery

See *Essentials of Plastic Surgery,* second edition, pp. 75-86.

CONTRAINDICATIONS TO FREE TISSUE TRANSFER

1. You are giving a lecture to residents which includes patient selection for free tissue transfer and microsurgery. **Which one of the following should you tell them to help guide their clinical practice?**
   A. Free tissue transfer is contraindicated in certain age groups.
   B. Free tissue transfer in smokers is associated with increased flap loss.
   C. Preoperative irradiation is a contraindication to free tissue transfer.
   D. Smoking after digital replantation significantly increases failure rates.
   E. Patients with a history of multiple VTE should not undergo free tissue transfer.

EQUIPMENT AND INSTRUMENTATION

2. When performing a microvascular anastomosis for free tissue transfer, which one of the following is correct?
   A. Heparinized saline is used in concentrations of 10,000 U/ml.
   B. Topical papaverine is a sodium channel blocker used to reduce vasospasm.
   C. Microvascular clamps should have a closing pressure of less than 30 g/mm^2.
   D. Operating loupes should not be routinely used for vascular anastomoses.
   E. Coupler devices should be reserved for end-to-end venous anastomoses.

TECHNICAL CONSIDERATIONS

3. Which one of the following is correct regarding microvascular surgery?
   A. Vessel inflow should be checked with the strip test before the anastomosis is performed.
   B. The adventitia should be trimmed flush to the vessel end.
   C. It is advisable to start with the simplest and most accessible anastomosis.
   D. Vessels are best manipulated by holding the adventitia.
   E. A set number of sutures will be required depending on vessel diameter.

4. You have just completed a microsurgical anastomosis and released the clamps. Flow seems to be partially impaired, the vessel is not completely tubular, and there is a significant single-point leak in the anterior vessel wall. **What is the next step in management of this situation?**
   A. Place an additional suture to close the leak.
   B. Clamp the vessels and cut out the anastomosis.
   C. Flush the anastomosis with heparinized saline.
   D. Apply lidocaine to reduce vessel spasm.
   E. Clamp the vessel and carefully inspect suture placement.

SIZE DISCREPANCY IN MICROVASCULAR ANASTOMOSES

5. During anastomosis of a lower-limb free flap, a size discrepancy of 2 mm between the donor artery and the recipient artery is found. *How is this challenge best addressed?*
   A. Spatulation of the larger vessels
   B. Triangular wedge excision from the smaller vessels
   C. Use of a coupler device
   D. Perform an end-to-side technique
   E. Cut the larger vessels obliquely

END-TO-SIDE ANASTOMOSES

6. *When reconstructing an open Gustilo IIIB tibial fracture with a free latissimus dorsi (LD) muscle, what is the major advantage of using an end-to-side arterial anastomosis to the posterior tibial artery?*
   A. Operating time should be reduced.
   B. Anastomotic patency will be improved.
   C. Fewer sutures would be required.
   D. The anastomosis is technically easier.
   E. In-line flow to the foot can be maintained.

FREE FLAP MONITORING

7. You see a patient on the first evening after a free transverse rectus abdominis (TRAM) flap breast reconstruction. *Which one of the following is correct regarding monitoring of this flap?*
   A. Arterial insufficiency presents with a purple, swollen flap.
   B. Doppler monitoring is consistently reliable.
   C. Thermography is most reliable for intraoral flaps.
   D. Venous insufficiency presents with slow egress of bright red blood to pinprick.
   E. A relative drop in flap surface temperature versus reference surface temperature indicates vascular compromise.

8. *Following circumferential reconstruction of a pharynx with a jejunal free flap, which one of the following represents the best modality for postoperative monitoring?*
   A. Clinical examination
   B. Laser Doppler flowmetry
   C. Tissue oximetry
   D. Implantable Doppler device
   E. Handheld Doppler device

FREE FLAP FAILURE

9. *Which one of the following is correct regarding failure of free flaps?*
   A. Success rates for free flaps are between 70% and 80% in experienced hands.
   B. The no-reflow phenomenon is the most common cause of flap failure.
   C. The no-reflow phenomenon is due to the absence of a patent anastomosis.
   D. Time from recognition of a failing flap to restoration of flow is most critical to successful salvage.
   E. The no-reflow phenomenon is usually reversible in the first 48 hours after surgery.

ANTICOAGULANTS IN MICROSURGERY

10. *Which one of the following is correct regarding heparin use in free flap surgery?*
    A. Heparin inhibits platelet aggregation via cyclooxygenase.
    B. Heparin binds to antithrombin and activates factor Xa.
    C. Heparin may be indicated when an anastomosis clots intraoperatively.
    D. Microvascular anastomotic patency is improved with systemic heparin.
    E. Systemic anticoagulation with heparin has minimal effect on hematoma rates.

MICRONEURAL REPAIR

11. After a laceration to the arm, a patient requires repair to the ulnar nerve. *Which one of the following is correct regarding repair of the transected nerve?*
    A. Direct repair under tension is preferable to interpositional grafting.
    B. Perineural repair is more difficult but has superior outcomes.
    C. Outcomes with sural nerve grafts are superior to those with vein grafts and synthetic tubes.
    D. Epineural repair with 10-0 sutures has the best overall outcomes.
    E. Accurate fascicular alignment with trimming where necessary will optimize outcomes.

Answers

CONTRAINDICATIONS TO FREE TISSUE TRANSFER
1. You are giving a lecture to residents which includes patient selection for free tissue transfer and microsurgery. **Which one of the following should you tell them to help guide their clinical practice?**
    D. Smoking after digital replantation significantly increases failure rates.
    Smoking can have significant detrimental effects on wound healing and success in digital replantation, but it does not appear to lead to an increase in free flap loss. Free tissue transfer has been performed on young and old patients with good outcomes, and age per se is not a major concern. Rather, it is the overall general health of a patient that is important. A patient must be able to tolerate the potentially long general anesthetic and insult of major surgery and be compliant with postoperative therapy. A natural concern with regard to free tissue transfer in children is vessel size but often the vessels are of good caliber and will also be free of atherosclerotic disease, making the procedure more straightforward. In elderly patients vessels may be more friable or stiff and have atherosclerosis which makes free tissue transfer more challenging. Preoperative radiation can also make vessel dissection and anastomosis more difficult, but it does not represent a contraindication to surgery. Many breast reconstructions are performed after radiation therapy, as are salvage cases in head and neck cancer. Additional care must, however, be taken with vessel handling as the vessels tend to be more fragile and are more prone to intimal damage. If patients have a history of multiple venous thromboembolism (VTE) then a hypercoagulable disorder should be excluded, however VTE per se is not a contraindication to free tissue transfer. Adequate prophylaxis with calf compression garments/hose/stocking and low-molecular-weight heparin will of course be required. Additional intraoperative heparin may be given. The risk of VTE can be assessed using the Caprini score.[1]

EQUIPMENT AND INSTRUMENTATION
2. When performing a microvascular anastomosis for free tissue transfer, which one of the following is correct?
    C. Microvascular clamps should have a closing pressure of less than 30 g/mm^2.
    It is important to use the correct microvascular equipment in order to avoid damage to vessels and anastomoses. Microvascular clamps are specifically designed to prevent trauma to the endothelium and should have a closing pressure of less than 30 g/mm^2. Heparinized saline is used in concentrations of 100 U/ml (not 10,000 U/ml). Topical papaverine works by blocking calcium (not sodium) channels and is useful to reduce vasospasm. Alternatively 1% to 2% lidocaine or verapamil can be used. Ideally a microscope with at least 10× magnification should be used for vascular anastomoses; however it is acceptable to use higher magnification loupes such as 3 to 4.5× for larger vessels. The coupler device is ideally suited to venous anastomoses, and can be used in both end-to-end and end-to-side connections. Although originally intended for venous anastomoses, it has been adopted by many surgeons for arterial anastomoses too. Spector et al[2] used them routinely in the artery for breast reconstruction in TRAM and DIEP flaps with good results when the thoracodorsal pedicle was the arterial source vessel.

Chapter 8 ■ Basics of Microsurgery   59

TECHNICAL CONSIDERATIONS

3. Which one of the following is correct regarding microvascular surgery?
   D. Vessels are best manipulated by holding the adventitia.

   During microvascular surgery, it is vital that vessel trauma, desiccation, and tension across the anastomosis are minimized. Carefully grasping the adventia is preferred to stabilize the vessel during dissection. The strip test is sometimes called an *Acland test* and is performed *after* the anastomosis has been completed. It involves carefully grasping the vessel distal to the anastomosis with two forceps and then gently milking blood distally so the vessel is empty between the two forceps. On release of the proximal forceps, the vessel should fill if the anastomosis is working correctly. The *spurt test* is used to check inflow *before* anastomosis is performed. This involves releasing all clamps from the input vessel, flushing with heparinized saline solution, and testing blood flow. Most surgeons advocate trimming of the adventitia to preserve 2 to 5 mm of exposed vessel end. The needle should enter the vessel at 90 degrees, not 45 degrees. The most difficult anastomosis should be done first as should the most difficult sutures within a given anastomosis.

4. You have just completed a microsurgical anastomosis and released the clamps. Flow seems to be partially impaired, the vessel is not completely tubular, and there is a significant single-point leak in the anterior vessel wall. **What is the next step in management of this situation?**
   E. Clamp the vessel and carefully inspect suture placement.

   This scenario describes the appearance of having backwalled the anastomosis. This is evidenced by the reduced flow and misshapen vessel appearance with high pressure causing a leak at the anterior wall. In this situation, reapplication of the clamps is necessary and careful progressive suture removal is advocated so that the suture causing the backwalling can be identified and replaced. In some situations it may be better to cut out the anastomosis and start again but in the first instance careful inspection is a better choice. Placing an additional suture would be appropriate if flow was good and no backwalling was suspected. Flushing the vessel may be helpful if the occlusion was secondary to a small amount of debris or thrombotic material. Application of lidocaine is useful to reduce spasm but not required in this case. The number of sutures required for an anastomosis will depend on the diameter of the vessel and the suture used. It is best to use the least number of sutures that will achieve a satisfactory seal.

SIZE DISCREPANCY IN MICROVASCULAR ANASTOMOSES

5. During anastomosis of a lower-limb free flap, a size discrepancy of 2 mm between the donor artery is found. **How is this challenge best addressed?**
   D. Perform an end-to-side technique

   A number of techniques are available to overcome size discrepancies between vessels. These include methods to increase the smaller vessel (spatulation) or to reduce the larger vessel (triangular wedge). Cutting the smaller vessel obliquely can also be helpful. Alternatively, an end-to-side anastomosis may be most appropriate for large discrepancies. This is an approach often taken for head and neck cases where the flap vein is anastomosed into the internal jugular vein. It is less commonly performed for arteries but is an acceptable technique for this scenario (see Fig. 8-12, *Essentials of Plastic Surgery,* second edition). The coupler device can be very useful for managing a size discrepancy between donor and recipient veins and may also be useful in some arterial anastomoses, as discussed in question 2. However, in the lower limb the vessels are likely to be too thick or stiff walled to work well with a coupler and they are not routinely used in this setting.

END-TO-SIDE ANASTOMOSES

6. When reconstructing an open Gustilo IIIB tibial fracture with a free latissimus dorsi (LD) muscle, what is the major advantage of using an end-to-side arterial anastomosis to the posterior tibial artery?

E. In-line flow to the foot can be maintained.

The main benefit of using an end-to-side anastomosis in this situation is the preservation of distal flow through the posterior tibial artery. This is particularly relevant given the history of trauma. An alternative is to use a flow-through flap (e.g. ALT) with two in-line anastomoses. End-to-side and end-to-end anastomoses both have equivalent patency and generally require a similar amount of sutures and operating time. Surgeons often find end-to-end anastomoses easier to perform than end-to-side, but it will depend on personal preference.

FREE FLAP MONITORING

7. You see a patient on the first evening after a free transverse rectus abdominis (TRAM) flap breast reconstruction. *Which one of the following is correct regarding monitoring of this flap?*

E. A relative drop in flap surface temperature versus reference surface temperature indicates vascular compromise.

The usual appearance of arterial insufficiency is a pale, cool flap with no capillary return and no bleeding to pinprick. A purple, swollen appearance with egress of dark blood (not bright red) to pinprick is characteristic of a congested flap secondary to venous outflow obstruction. Doppler imaging is a useful adjunct to flap monitoring, but it can be unreliable because of transmission of signals from adjacent vessels. Thermography measures skin surface temperature using a thermocouple device. Both venous and arterial occlusion can cause flap surface temperature to drop. Khouri and Shaw[3] reported that a relative difference in flap surface temperature versus reference surface temperature of more than 1.8° C had a 98% sensitivity for vascular compromise and a 75% predictive value; however, accuracy was considered to be poor in intraoral flaps. Absolute flap temperature changes, without a reference nonflap temperature, are less reliable, because they are affected by changes in ambient or body temperature.

8. *Following circumferential reconstruction of a pharynx with a jejunal free flap, which one of the following represents the best modality for postoperative monitoring?*

D. Implantable Doppler device

In the situation of a buried free flap, the most reliable monitoring method is to use an implantable Doppler device. This can be placed directly on either the anastomosed artery or vein and secured with a small ligaclip. Rates of salvage are reported to be very high using this device but sometimes the signal can be lost when in fact the vessel is still running. Clinical examination is difficult with buried flaps other than systemic parameters such as blood pressure and urine output. A handheld Doppler can be useful for some buried flaps but transmission from other vessels can compromise reliability. Laser Doppler and tissue oximetry each require the presence of a skin paddle for monitoring.

FREE FLAP FAILURE

9. Which one of the following is correct regarding failure of free flaps?

D. Time from recognition of a failing flap to restoration of flow is most critical to successful salvage.

Early recognition and surgical reexploration of a failing flap are critical to optimization of outcomes in free flap surgery. Most flaps can be salvaged if surgery is performed within the first two hours following recognition of the problem. Accurate postoperative free flap monitoring is therefore key to free flap success. It is tailored to specific flaps but in general a combined approach of clinical examination to assess color, capillary refill, turgor, and temperature, along with Doppler assessment, is advised for free flap monitoring. The most common cause of flap failure is an anastomotic problem, leading to venous or arterial insufficiency. The no-reflow phenomenon is believed to be caused by endothelial swelling, platelet aggregation, and leaky capillaries in the presence of a patent anastomosis. It is less commonly seen as a cause of flap failure and although it may be reversible at approximately 4 to 8 hours, this is unlikely after 12 hours.

ANTICOAGULANTS IN MICROSURGERY

10. *Which one of the following is correct regarding heparin use in free flap surgery?*
    C. Heparin may be indicated when an anastomosis clots intraoperatively.
    Some surgeons give a dose of intravenous heparin just before disconnecting or just after reconnecting the flap, with the intention of reducing thrombosis at the anastomotic site. Others will reserve this for when the first anastomosis has clotted and the anastomosis must be redone. Aspirin inhibits platelet aggregation via cyclooxygenase. Heparin binds antithrombin III and results in inhibition of both antithrombin and factor Xa. No evidence suggests that systemic heparin will improve anastomotic patency, except perhaps in cases in which intraoperative clotting has occurred or the anastomosis requires revision. The use of systemic heparin increases the risk of postoperative bleeding, but its action is short-lived compared with low molecular heparin.

MICRONEURAL REPAIR

11. After a laceration to the arm, a patient requires repair to the ulnar nerve. *Which one of the following is correct regarding repair of the transected nerve?*
    E. Accurate fascicular alignment with trimming where necessary will optimize outcomes.
    Different techniques exist to repair transected nerves. They include epineural, perineural, or grouped fascicular. Outcomes are similar with all techniques, but perineural techniques may be technically more difficult. Grouped fascicular techniques can be helpful for larger nerves such as the ulnar nerve at the wrist, where specific branches can be identified. It is vital that neither excessive tension nor buckling of fascicles occurs at the repair site. For this reason, accurate trimming and use of interpositional grafts are advocated where necessary. The choice of graft in short defects in sensory nerves may be less important, because vein grafts and polyglycolic acid tubes can have comparable outcomes to donor nerves such as the sural and antebrachial cutaneous nerves. Processed allograft conduits provide a further option, with results superior to those obtained with polyglycolic acid tubes. However, in larger defects autologous sural nerve grafts are the benchmark.

REFERENCES

1. Pannucci CJ, Bailey SH, Dreszer G, et al. Validation of the Caprini risk assessment model in plastic and reconstructive surgery patients. J Am Coll Surg 212:105-112, 2011.
2. Spector JA, Draper LB, Levine JP, et al. Routine use of microvascular coupling device for arterial anastomosis in breast reconstruction. Ann Plast Surg 46:365-368, 2006.
3. Khouri RK, Shaw WW. Monitoring of free flaps with surface temperature recordings: Is it reliable? Plast Reconstr Surg 89:495-499, 1992.

9. Biomaterials

See *Essentials of Plastic Surgery,* second edition, pp. 87-106.

GENERAL PRINCIPLES OF BIOMATERIALS

1. Biomaterials are commonly used in plastic surgery for a variety of different applications. ***Which one of the following statements is correct regarding biomaterials?***
   A. Biomaterials are by definition, synthetic materials.
   B. *Permanence* refers to the long-term durability of a biomaterial.
   C. Implants derived from synthetic material are termed *alloplasts*.
   D. *Allografts* represent living tissue derived from the host.
   E. *Xenografts* are derived from the same species animal donor.

GRAFT SUBTYPES

2. ***Which one of the following statements is correct regarding graft substitutes?***
   A. Allografts represent the benchmark for biomaterials.
   B. Autografts must be processed to reduce their antigenicity.
   C. The use of alloplastic materials prevents donor site morbidity and host reaction.
   D. The use of allogenic materials prevents the risk of disease transmission.
   E. Xenografts have more antigenic potential than homografts.

AUTOGRAFTS IN GENERAL

3. ***Which one of the following is an advantage of using an autograft?***
   A. Reduced duration of surgery
   B. Good tolerance and incorporation
   C. Avoidance of a donor site
   D. Limitless tissue quantity
   E. Reduced early morbidity

AUTOLOGOUS SKIN GRAFTS

4. You are planning a staged resurfacing of a 70% total body surface area burn. ***Which one of the following is correct?***
   A. Split-thickness grafts initially obtain their nutrients through the process of inosculation.
   B. Immune rejection is not a risk associated with cultured epidermal autografts.
   C. Split-thickness grafts range in thickness from 5 to 30/10,000 of an inch.
   D. Cultured epidermal autografts require 3 weeks to achieve a satisfactory cell expansion.
   E. Split-thickness grafts have less secondary contraction than full-thickness grafts.

ACELLULAR DERMAL MATRIX

5. You see a patient 14 days after mastectomy and immediate implant reconstruction with an acellular dermal matrix (ADM) sling. A large patch of erythema has developed over the lower pole of the reconstruction. The patient remains systemically well and afebrile. *Which one of the following is correct?*
   A. This is unusual and the patient must be closely monitored.
   B. A course of oral antibiotics should be prescribed.
   C. This is unrelated to the surgical technique.
   D. The patient is likely to need surgery to remove the implant.
   E. The patient requires reassurance only at this stage.

6. You are considering the use of Permacol to augment an abdominal wall repair and read that it is a crosslinked porcine dermal matrix. *Which one of the following is the main advantage of cross-linking in an ADM?*
   A. Improved tissue incorporation
   B. Increased material strength
   C. Reduced local tissue inflammation
   D. Fewer bowel wall adhesions
   E. Lesser chance of infection

ALLOGRAFT MATERIALS

7. You see a patient who has undergone breast reconstruction with AlloDerm and an implant. *Which one of the following is true of this ADM?*
   A. It is manufactured from bovine dermis.
   B. Its use results in a moderate host response.
   C. Incorporation into the host tissue is rare.
   D. It contains no cellular elements.
   E. Resorption rates are very consistent.

8. A patient has a 10 by 10 cm defect over the posterior ankle, exposing the Achilles tendon. A 2 by 2 cm area of tendon lacks paratenon cover centrally. You are planning to use Integra. *Which one of the following is correct regarding Integra?*
   A. It has a trilaminar structure.
   B. It contains collagen and glycosaminoglycans only.
   C. A key benefit is the relatively low cost.
   D. It will avoid the need for a skin graft.
   E. It can be used successfully in areas of exposed tendon.

SKIN AND SOFT TISSUE SUBSTITUTES

9. A patient with 20% superficial partial-thickness burns undergoes wound debridement in the OR. *Which one of the following dressings is indicated in this case?*
   A. Apligraf
   B. Orcel
   C. Transcyte
   D. Dermagraft
   E. Biobrane

10. When working in a major burn unit on fellowship you are advised to use Transcyte as a temporary dressing for a patient with mid-depth burns. **How does Transcyte differ from Biobrane?**
    A. A nylon mesh
    B. Porcine collagen
    C. A silicone coating
    D. Neonatal fibroblasts
    E. Bovine collagen

11. **For each of the following descriptions, select the most likely option. (Each option may be used once, more than once, or not at all.)**
    A. This noncrosslinked, bovine pericardium ADM can be used to smooth facial wrinkles.
    B. This bilaminar structure contains bovine collagen and silicone and is used in deep burns in conjunction with skin grafting at 2 to 4 weeks.
    C. This product has a 10-day shelf life and is used in venous and diabetic foot ulcers. It is made from neonatal fibroblasts and bovine collagen.

    Options:
    a. Transcyte
    b. Dermagraft
    c. Integra
    d. Veritas
    e. Apligraf
    f. Tutopatch

BONE AUTOGRAFTS

12. During mandibular reconstruction a 1 cm bone graft is required. **What is the main benefit of using a cortical bone graft over a cancellous bone graft?**
    A. Healing is primarily by osteogenesis
    B. Revascularization is more rapid
    C. Maintenance of volume is better
    D. Donor site morbidity is less
    E. It will be less prone to infection

SYNTHETIC BONE SUBSTITUTES

13. You are using methylmethacrylate to reconstruct the calvarium. **What is the main problem with using this biomaterial?**
    A. High cost
    B. Difficulty conforming
    C. Poor biocompatibility
    D. Lack of strength
    E. Risk of adjacent tissue damage

CARTILAGE AUTOGRAFTS

14. You are planning to use autologous cartilage to reconstruct a major nasal defect. **Which one of the following represents a caveat with cartilage grafting?**
    A. It commonly becomes infected.
    B. It has a high chance of resorption.
    C. It is difficult to precisely sculpt.
    D. It has a tendency to warp.
    E. Donor site morbidity is high.

ALLOPLASTIC MATERIALS

15. You are considering the use of alloplastic facial implants in your aesthetic practice. **Which one of the following materials represents a nonresorbable alloplastic material made with high-density polyethylene?**
    A. Mersiline
    B. Medpor
    C. Gore-Tex
    D. Marlex
    E. Prolene

RECONSTRUCTION WITH COMPOSITE MESH

16. **What is the main clinical indication for using composite materials such as Proceed, Sepramesh, and TiMesh?**
    A. Breast reconstruction
    B. Scalp reconstruction
    C. Abdominal wall reconstruction
    D. Chest wall reconstruction
    E. Lower limb reconstruction

SILICONE

17. **Which one of the following is a consistent finding with silicone as a biomaterial?**
    A. Fibrous encapsulation
    B. Resorption
    C. Incorporation
    D. Rejection
    E. Degradation

Answers

GENERAL PRINCIPLES OF BIOMATERIALS

1. Biomaterials are commonly used in plastic surgery for a variety of different applications. *Which one of the following statements is correct regarding biomaterials?*

   C. Implants derived from synthetic material are termed alloplasts.

   Biomaterials can be either naturally occurring (autograft, allograft, or xenograft) or synthetic (alloplastic). Permanence is arguably the most important clinical aspect of an implanted material and is achieved when harmony exists between host and implant. It therefore refers to the long-term biocompatibility between host and implant rather than durability of the implant. Allografts are either living or nonliving tissue derived from the same species donor, (e.g., cadaveric skin grafts), whereas autografts are derived from the host, (e.g., traditional skin grafts). Xenografts are derived from a different species donor, (e.g. bovine/porcine) and include skin substitutes and acellular dermal matrices.

GRAFT SUBTYPES

2. *Which one of the following statements is correct regarding graft substitutes?*

   E. Xenografts have more antigenic potential than homografts.

   Xenografts must be acellular to prevent a strong immunogenic host response. Homografts such as vascular composite grafts are cellular but still require antirejection therapy (see Chapter 7). Autografts, not allografts, represent the benchmark to which biomaterials are compared. They do not require processing to reduce their antigenicity, because they originate from the host. Although donor site morbidity is not a problem with alloplastic materials, they cause a host reaction such as capsule formation around a breast implant. Allogenic materials include allografts and homografts. Each carries a risk of infectious disease transmission.

AUTOGRAFTS IN GENERAL

3. *Which one of the following is an advantage of using an autograft?*

   B. Good tolerance and incorporation

   Autografts are the benchmark for reconstruction, because they are well tolerated by the host and become incorporated into adjacent tissue to provide lifelong reconstruction. However, the disadvantages include the need for a donor site, potential for donor site morbidity, increased surgical time for harvest, and a finite amount of available tissue.

   An example is the use of alveolar bone graft in cleft lip and palate patients. This can provide permanent bone stock in the alveolus at the expense of temporary donor site morbidity at the hip, which results in a prolonged surgical time and lengthened hospital stay. Hydroxyapatite synthetic material is an alternative substitute that could be used in this setting.

AUTOLOGOUS SKIN GRAFTS

4. You are planning a staged resurfacing of a 70% total body surface area burn. *Which one of the following is correct?*

   D. Cultured epidermal autografts take 3 weeks to achieve a satisfactory cell expansion.

   Cultured epidermal autografts (CEA) use murine (mouse) fibroblasts and calf serum, which may cause immune reactions that lead to rejection. They are expensive and time consuming, requiring

3 weeks to obtain a 10,000-fold expansion of keratinocytes. Epicel (Genzyme, Cambridge, MA) is FDA approved for use in patients with deep or full-thickness burns that are more than 30% total body surface area (TBSA).[1]

Split-thickness grafts initially adhere to the wound with formation of a fibrin layer. During the next 24 to 48 hours, the graft swells and obtains nutrients from the wound bed by diffusion. This process is called *serum imbibition*. During the following days, recipient and donor site vessel ends align. This process is known as *inosculation* and occurs in nature when tree branches join together. The final process is called *revascularization*, which involves full ingrowth of host capillaries into the graft. Split-thickness grafts are harvested at measures of 1000th of an inch not 10,000ths of an inch and have more (not less) secondary contraction than full-thickness grafts.

ACELLULAR DERMAL MATRIX

5. You see a patient 14 days after mastectomy and immediate implant reconstruction with an acellular dermal matrix (ADM) sling. A large patch of erythema has developed over the lower pole of the reconstruction. The patient remains systemically well and afebrile. **Which one of the following is correct?**
   E. **The patient requires reassurance only at this stage.**

   ADMs are immunologically inert, but they can mimic cellulitis when used in conjunction with implants or expanders in breast reconstruction. This is termed *red breast syndrome*. It does not indicate active infection and therefore does not warrant antibiotic therapy. The manufacturers suggest thorough washing of the product before use, because the chemicals and/or preservatives within the ADM are likely responsible for this phenomenon. It is unlikely the patient will need further treatment and will just require reassurance at this time. If she was febrile with a red, hot breast this would be a different matter and would support the presence of an infectious process.

6. You are considering the use of Permacol to augment an abdominal wall repair and read that it is a crosslinked porcine dermal matrix. **Which one of the following is the main advantage of cross-linking in an ADM?**
   B. **Increased material strength**

   Acellular dermal matrices are nonliving dermal components from an allogenic or xenogenic donor comprised of collagen, elastin, laminin, and glycosaminoglycans. They have a broad range of uses in plastic surgery. A limited number of ADMs are cross-linked and this serves to strengthen the material, prolong its lifespan, and reduce antigenicity. However this comes at the expense of delayed incorporation, prolonged inflammation, increased infection rate, and bowel adhesion formation. In essence cross-linking tends to make biologic material behave more like a synthetic material.

ALLOGRAFT MATERIALS

7. You see a patient who has undergone breast reconstruction with AlloDerm and an implant. **Which one of the following is true of this ADM?**
   D. **It contains no cellular elements.**

   AlloDerm is an acellular dermal matrix manufactured from human cadaveric tissue, not a bovine source. It has a minimal host response, because it no longer contains antigenic cells. It is well incorporated into tissues, but it can have variable resorption rates. AlloDerm is the most extensively used ADM in the U.S. for breast surgery and has the largest body of evidence in this setting. However, it is not licensed for use in the European marketplace and a porcine alternative is offered instead (Strattice).

68   Part I ■ Fundamentals and Basics

8. A patient has a 10 by 10 cm defect over the posterior ankle, exposing the Achilles tendon. A 2 by 2 cm area of tendon lacks paratenon cover centrally. You are planning to use Integra. **Which one of the following is correct regarding Integra?**
   E. **It can be used successfully in areas of exposed tendon.**
   Integra is a bilaminar dermal regeneration template used for skin replacement. It consists of a collagen and glycosaminoglycan base with a silicone upper layer that acts as a temporary epidermis. The silicone layer is removed after 3 to 4 weeks and is replaced with a skin graft. Integra is expensive but can be very useful over exposed tendon without paratenon or bone without periosteum, as it helps convert a nongraftable wound bed to a graftable one.

SKIN AND SOFT TISSUE SUBSTITUTES

9. A patient with 20% superficial partial-thickness burns undergoes wound debridement in the OR. **Which one of the following dressings is indicated in this case?**
   E. **Biobrane**
   Biobrane is useful as a temporary dressing for the management of superficial partial-thickness burns. It is a composite dressing made with porcine collagen embedded in nylon mesh. It also has a semipermeable silicone outer layer. It can be placed directly onto a clean burn wound but must be removed 7 to 14 days after application. The recipient site will then either need skin grafting or may have reepithelialized depending on burn depth. It is particularly useful for children following scald burns when the precise burn depth is uncertain because it decreases pain, reduces the number of dressing changes, and allows for reepithelialization of superficial areas thereby helping to differentiate between deep and more superficial areas of burn injury and avoid unnecessary skin grafting. Transcyte and Orcel may be indicated in deeper burns, while Apligraf and Dermagraft are indicated for the management of lower limb venous or diabetic ulcers.[2]

10. When working in a major burn unit on fellowship you are advised to use Transcyte as a temporary dressing for a patient with mid-depth burns. **How does Transcyte differ from Biobrane?**
    D. **Neonatal fibroblasts**
    Transcyte is a product manufactured with the same core components as Biobrane (nylon mesh, silicone, and porcine dermis) with the addition of neonatal fibroblasts seeded into the mesh. Various studies have shown its use to be effective in the management of partial-thickness burns. Healing rates have been shown to be superior, with reduction of pain and length of hospital stay. One study that compared Biobrane with Transcyte showed faster burn healing with Transcyte and this may be attributed to the neonatal cells and the associated growth factors. Although much emphasis has been placed on the development of cellular bilayered matrices such as Transcyte, they are expensive and consideration should still be given as to the benefits over more traditional therapy before embarking on their use. Neither Transcyte nor Biobrane contain bovine collagen.[3-6]

11. **For each of the following descriptions, select the most likely option. (Each option may be used once, more than once, or not at all).**
    A. *This noncrosslinked, bovine pericardium ADM can be used to smooth facial wrinkles.*
       f. **Tutopatch**
          Both Tutopatch and Veritas are derived from noncrosslinked bovine pericardium and may be used in abdominal wall reconstruction. However, only Tutopatch is used in smoothing of facial wrinkles.
    B. *This bilaminar structure contains bovine collagen and silicone and is used in deep burns in conjunction with skin grafting at 2 to 4 weeks.*
       c. **Integra**
          Integra is the only option listed that has a bilaminar construct containing silicone and bovine collagen. It is recommended for use in deep burns where sufficient autograft is not available. It is also indicated for areas where there is a nongraftable bed (see question 8) and for use in the management of burn scar contracture.
    C. *This product has a 10-day shelf life and is used in venous and diabetic foot ulcers. It is made from neonatal fibroblasts and bovine collagen.*
       e. **Apligraf**
          Apligraf is formed with neonatal fibroblasts and keratinocytes onto a bovine matrix. It has a short half-life of 10 days and is indicated for noninfected venous and diabetic lower limb ulcers (see Chapter 57).

          Transcyte (as discussed in question 10) contains porcine dermis and silicone with neonatal fibroblasts and is used as a temporary cover for deep burn injuries. Dermagraft also contains neonatal fibroblasts but these are seeded onto a biodegradable mesh (polyglactin). It is indicated for use in diabetic and venous ulcers of the lower limb.

BONE AUTOGRAFTS

12. During mandibular reconstruction a 1 cm bone graft is required. **What is the main benefit of using a cortical bone graft over a cancellous bone graft?**
    C. **Maintenance of volume is better**
       Autologous bone grafts may be either cortical or cancellous. Autologous bone sources include calvarium, iliac crest, rib, fibula, and radius. The advantages of using either cortical or cancellous autologous bone are a relative resistance to infection and a lack of host response to the graft. Disadvantages include variable graft resorption rates and donor site morbidity. Cortical bone grafts provide immediate structural support to the recipient site and maintain significantly more volume than cancellous bone grafts over time.[7] The healing is primarily by osteoconduction whereas in cancellous grafts healing is primarily by osteogenesis. Osteoconduction means that the graft serves as a nonviable scaffold for new bony ingrowth, whereas osteogenesis means that osteoblasts within the graft directly produce bone. Osteoinduction means that growth factors within the graft directly produce bone. Osteoinduction means that growth factors within the graft stimulate osteogenesis in host tissue. To an extent, all bone autografts have components of these healing processes but the relative importance differs. Revascularization is slower for cortical bone grafts and donor site morbidity may also be increased compared with cancellous graft harvest.

SYNTHETIC BONE SUBSTITUTES

13. You are using methylmethacrylate to reconstruct the calvarium. *What is the main problem with using this biomaterial?*
    ### E. Risk of adjacent tissue damage
    Methylmethacrylate is a nonresorbable high-density porous polymer used as a bone cement that also has clinical application in cranial reconstruction, forehead augmentation, and filling gaps in fractures. It is inexpensive, easily molded, inert, biocompatible, and has a high compression strength. However, it involves an exothermic reaction when mixed and can lead to local tissue damage unless adequate tissue cooling is achieved.

CARTILAGE AUTOGRAFTS

14. You are planning to use autologous cartilage to reconstruct a major nasal defect. *Which one of the following represents a caveat with cartilage grafting?*
    ### D. It has a tendency to warp.
    Autologous cartilage grafts are commonly used to reconstruct the nose, eyelid, and ear. Infection and resorption are rare. It is generally quite easy to sculpt but does have a tendency to warp. Donor sites include the ear, nasal septum, and ribs. Donor site morbidity is low, especially when harvested from the conchal bowl or nasal septum.

ALLOPLASTIC MATERIALS

15. You are considering the use of alloplastic facial implants in your aesthetic practice. *Which one of the following materials represents a nonresorbable alloplastic material made with high-density polyethylene?*
    ### B. Medpor
    Medpor is a high-density polyethylene material available as mesh and various implants, including chin, nasal, malar, and temporal prostheses. Gore-Tex is expanded polytetrafluoroethylene (ePTFE) that is available as mesh, tubes, and blocks. In mesh form it is used for chest and abdominal wall reconstruction; as a solid it is used for facial augmentation. Marlex is a heavyweight polypropylene mesh that is used in chest and abdominal wall reconstruction. Mersilene is a polyethylene terephthalate (PET) mesh with microporous components that is used in abdominal hernia repair.

RECONSTRUCTION WITH COMPOSITE MESH

16. *What is the main clinical indication for using composite materials such as Proceed, Sepramesh, and TiMesh?*
    ### C. Abdominal wall reconstruction
    The new breed of composite mesh materials include Proceed, Sepramesh, Parietex, C-Qur, and TiMesh. These products are mostly used in ventral hernia repairs of the abdominal wall. They can be subdivided into two groups: (1) tissue separating meshes–Proceed, Sepramesh, and Parietex; (2) coated meshes–C-Qur and TiMesh.
    The tissue separating meshes include a nonresorbable polymer on one surface and a biologic or resorbable material on the other side. The porous synthetic is placed against the abdominal wall to encourage host tissue incorporation, while the bioresorbable surface is placed against the viscera to limit bowel adhesions. The polymer is commonly polypropylene and the resorbable material commonly contains cellulose. Coated meshes comprise of a synthetic mesh such as polypropylene coated on both sides with a low inflammatory material such as titanium or omega fatty acids.

SILICONE

17. Which one of the following is a consistent finding with silicone as a biomaterial?
A. Fibrous encapsulation

Silicone is a nonresorbable polymer based on the element silicon. It has FDA approval as a solid and is most commonly used in breast implant prostheses. Fibrous encapsulation is a consistent finding with silicone implants and this is the basis of capsule formation and subsequent capsular contraction. Fibrous encapsulation can be a useful feature in the context of tissue expansion as the capsule develops a reliable blood supply that can be left in situ under local skin flaps.

Silicone is nonporous so it does not facilitate tissue ingrowth in the form of incorporation. However, it is inert so it is not rejected by tissues and is resistant to degradation thereby having a long lifespan following implantation.

REFERENCES

1. US Food and Drug Administration. Epicel® cultured epidermal autograft (CEA)-H990002.Available at http://www.fda.gov/MedicalDevices/ProductsandMedicalProcedures/DeviceApprovalsandClearances/Recently-ApprovedDevices/ucm074878.htm.
2. Whitaker IS, Worthington S, Jivan S, et al. The use of Biobrane by burn units in the United Kingdom: a national study. Burns 33:1015-1020, 2007.
3. Noordenbos J, Dore C, Hansbrough JF. Safety and efficacy of transcyte for the treatment of partial-thickness burns. J Burn Care Rehabil 20:275-281, 1999.
4. Lukish JR, Eichelberger MR, Newman KD, et al. The use of bioactive skin substitute decreases length of stay for pediatric burn patients. J Pediatr Surg 36:1118-1121, 2001.
5. Amani H, Dougherty WR, Blome-Eberwein S. Use of Transcyte and dermabrasion to treat burns reduces length of stay in burns of all size and etiology. Burns 32:828-832, 2006.
6. Kumar RJ, Kimble RM, Boots R, et al. Treatment of partial-thickness burns: a prospective, randomized trial using Transcyte. ANZ J Surg 74:622-626, 2004.
7. Ozaki W, Buchman SR. Volume maintenance of onlay bone grafts in the craniofacial skeleton: microarchitecture versus embryologic origin. Plast Reconstr Surg 102:291-299, 1998.

10. Negative Pressure Wound Therapy

See *Essentials of Plastic Surgery,* second edition, pp. 107-114.

THEORIES OF NEGATIVE PRESSURE WOUND THERAPY

1. **Which one of the following is not thought to be a mechanism of action of negative pressure wound therapy (NPWT)?**
   A. Removal of excess tissue fluid and improved oxygenation
   B. Removal of matrix metalloproteases and acute phase proteins
   C. An increase in cellular proliferation
   D. Reduction in bacterial load and contraction of wound edges
   E. Increased ratios of collagen type III to I production

MECHANICAL MECHANISMS

2. **Which one of the following is thought to be largely responsible for wound edges drawing closer together during NPWT?**
   A. Microstrain
   B. Macrostrain
   C. Nanostrain
   D. Equilibration of stresses
   E. Strain neutralization

CONTACT LAYERS IN NEGATIVE PRESSURE WOUND THERAPY

3. Different foam dressings can be used with negative pressure dressing systems. **What is the main theoretical clinical benefit of using foam with a larger pore size?**
   A. Reduced infection
   B. Increased tissue production
   C. Increased fluid removal
   D. Reduced pain
   E. Lower financial cost

4. **Which one of the following base layers has the largest volume of evidence supporting its use in NPWT?**
   A. Polyvinyl foam
   B. Polypropylene foam
   C. Polyurethane foam
   D. Silver-coated sponge
   E. Honeycomb gauze

5. A number of different base layers can be used in conjunction with NPWT and selection can affect outcome. **Which one of the following is correct regarding base layer selection?**
   A. Silver-coated sponge dressings are beneficial to decrease wound odor.
   B. PVA white foam should be used when rapid granulation is required.
   C. Use of gauze as a base layer tends to increase pain compared with foam dressings.
   D. Healing times are reduced when using foam rather than gauze.
   E. NPWT avoids the need for a nonadherent base layer on skin grafts.

Chapter 10 ▪ Negative Pressure Wound Therapy

PRESSURES USED IN NEGATIVE PRESSURE WOUND THERAPY

6. You are choosing a setting for a negative pressure dressing. *Which one of the following represents the pressure at which the maximum increase in blood flow is observed?*
   A. 25 mm Hg
   B. 50 mm Hg
   C. 75 mm Hg
   D. 100 mm Hg
   E. 125 mm Hg

FACTORS TO OPTIMIZE NEGATIVE PRESSURE WOUND THERAPY

7. *Which one of the following is most likely to accelerate granulation tissue production during NPWT?*
   A. Adjunctive fluid instillation
   B. A continuous pressure of 150 mm Hg
   C. Intermittent pressure mode
   D. A polyvinyl alcohol foam base layer
   E. Dressing changes every other day

CLINICAL USE OF NEGATIVE PRESSURE WOUND THERAPY

8. *In which one of the following scenarios can NPWT be indicated?*
   A. After sentinel node biopsy of the axilla
   B. Over a directly closed ankle wound
   C. On a cellulitic wound to the hand after a dog bite debridement
   D. Over a chronic wound to the elbow with eschar present
   E. Over a latissimus dorsi reconstruction of an open tibial fracture

9. You are setting up a new wound multidisciplinary team in your hospital and will be working alongside specialists from vascular, general, orthopedics, and cardiothoracic surgery to develop the use of NPWT across departments. *Which one of the following is correct and should be taken into account when planning the service?*
   A. There is no strong evidence to support the use of NPWT in diabetic foot disease.
   B. The incidence of limb amputation in diabetic foot disease is unaffected by NPWT.
   C. The evidence supporting NPWT as a primary treatment in venous ulcers is weak.
   D. NPWT on large abdominal or chest wall defects has no beneficial effect on respiratory function.
   E. NPWT with split-thickness skin grafts can improve their appearance but is not cost effective.

Answers

THEORIES OF NEGATIVE PRESSURE WOUND THERAPY

1. **Which one of the following is not thought to be a mechanism of action of negative pressure wound therapy (NPWT)?**
   E. Increased ratios of collagen type III to I production
   The precise mechanism of action of negative pressure therapy is largely unknown, but three common theories prevail. The fluid-based theory proposes that interstitial fluid, which may otherwise compromise the microcirculation and oxygen delivery, and contain substances that negatively impact wound healing, is removed from the wound.[1] The second is a mechanically driven process in which cell proliferation is increased in response to mechanical tissue stress. This stimulates angiogenesis and cellular growth and helps to draw in the wound edges. The third mechanism is a reduction in bacterial load.[2,3] However, it is not proven that negative pressure therapy will specifically alter collagen ratios.[4]

MECHANICAL MECHANISMS

2. **Which one of the following is thought to be largely responsible for wound edges drawing closer together during NPWT?**
   B. Macrostrain
   Macrostrain refers to the process whereby negative pressure will cause the contact wound dressing to collapse. Negative pressure becomes equally distributed across the wound and force is transferred to the wound edges, bringing them closer together. *Microstrain* refers to the microdeformation that occurs across a foam dressing in a negative pressure system. This leads to induction of mechanical stress and stimulation of angiogenesis. The other terms are not used to describe processes in NPWT.

CONTACT LAYERS IN NEGATIVE PRESSURE WOUND THERAPY

3. Different foam dressings can be used with negative pressure dressing systems.[2,3] **What is the theoretical clinical benefit of using foam with a larger pore size?**
   B. Increased tissue production
   Black polyurethane foam is hydrophobic and has pore sizes of 400 to 600 μm compared with a pore size between 60 and 270 μm in polyvinyl alcohol white foam. The theoretical benefit is that tissue growth is maximized. However, there is no clear evidence to show that pore size makes a significant difference in the clinical setting.

4. **Which one of the following base layers has the largest volume of evidence supporting its use in NPWT?**
   C. Polyurethane foam
   Polyurethane foam was used as the original contact dressing for NPWT and most published evidence relates to this dressing. As discussed in question 3, polyurethane foam has a pore size designed to maximize tissue growth and is typically a black-colored synthetic. More recently different foam types and gauze alternatives have become available as other manufacturers have entered into the market for NPWT devices (see question 5).

5. A number of different base layers can be used in conjunction with NPWT and selection can affect outcome. *Which one of the following is correct regarding base layer selection?*
   A. **Silver-coated sponge dressings are beneficial to decrease wound odor.**
   Silver-coated dressings can be useful to decrease malodor in certain wounds. This probably occurs secondary to decreasing bacterial cell counts. PVA white foam should be used in areas where rapid rates of granulation are less desirable, not more. Gauze may decrease pain during dressing changes compared with foam but no differences have been observed between the two dressings in terms of decreasing wound size, healing time, or time to prepare for grafting. When using NPWT with skin grafts, it is recommended to use an nonadherent base layer underneath the foam or gauze dressing.

PRESSURES USED IN NEGATIVE PRESSURE WOUND THERAPY

6. You are choosing a setting for a negative pressure dressing. *Which one of the following represents the pressure at which the maximum increase in blood flow is observed?*
   E. **125 mm Hg**
   Subatmospheric pressure is used in NPWT. This may be continuous or intermittent. The pressures commonly used range from 50 to 125 mm Hg, and the maximum increase in blood flow is seen at 125 mm Hg.[5]

FACTORS TO OPTIMIZE NEGATIVE PRESSURE WOUND THERAPY

7. *Which one of the following is most likely to accelerate granulation tissue production during NPWT?*
   C. **Intermittent pressure mode**
   The use of intermittent pressure (5 minutes on, 2 minutes off) has been shown to produce more rapid granulation tissue deposition. Polyvinyl alcohol foam is less likely to produce rapid granulation. No evidence supports changing a dressing every other day to accelerate granulation and it is common to change NPWT dressings twice weekly providing the wound is clean. Fluid instillation can be used with either continuous or intermittent pressures. This technique involves instillation of isotonic solution containing antibiotic or antibacterial products and may contribute to improved infection control.

CLINICAL USE OF NEGATIVE PRESSURE WOUND THERAPY

8. *In which one of the following scenarios can NPWT be indicated?*
   B. **Over a directly closed ankle wound**
   Although it may seem counterintuitive to use negative pressure therapy on a directly closed wound, incisional NPWT has been used in wounds with early signs of inadequate healing or those located on anatomic sites at high risk of poor healing. Examples include following internal fixation of lower limb fractures. The benefits are believed to result from a continuous evacuation of excessive drainage fluid, which prevents skin irritation, bacterial colonization, and edema. NPWT should not be used in the following scenarios: exposed vessels and nerves, malignancy in the wound, untreated osteomyelitis, fresh anastomotic site, or in a site with necrotic tissue with eschar still present.

9. You are setting up a new wound multidisciplinary team in your hospital and will be working alongside specialists from vascular, general, orthopedics, and cardiothoracic surgery to develop the use of NPWT across departments. **Which one of the following is correct and should be taken into account when planning the service?**
   C. **The evidence supporting NPWT as a primary treatment in venous ulcers is weak.**

   Evidence is currently lacking for the use of NPWT as a primary treatment in venous ulcers, although its use as an adjunct to skin grafting in these cases is supported. In contrast there is Level I evidence to support the use of NPWT in the primary management of diabetic foot ulcers both in terms of time to wound closure and decreased incidence of limb amputation.[6,7] In large abdominal wall and chest defects, NPWT can be beneficial to respiratory function with decreased ventilator support requirement and shorter duration in high dependency care.[8,9] The use of NPWT on split-skin grafts has Level I evidence to support its use and is especially useful in areas such as the perineum and axilla.[10] It not only improves graft appearance, but it also improves graft take in some situations and has been shown to reduce subsequent hospital stay. This would have a major impact on cost savings that would potentially outweigh the NPWT costs.[11-13]

REFERENCES

1. Argenta LC, Morykwas MJ. Vacuum-assisted closure: a new method for wound control and treatment: clinical experience. Ann Plast Surg 38:563-576, 1997.
2. Urschel JD, Scott PG, Williams HTG. The effect of mechanical stress of soft and hard tissue repair: a review. BR J Plast Surg 42:182-186, 1988.
3. Plikaitis CM, Molnar JA. Subatmospheric pressure wound therapy and the vacuum-assisted closure device: basic science and current clinical successes. Expert Rev Med Devices 3:175-184, 2006.
4. Morykwas MJ, Argenta LC, Shelton Brown EI, et al. Vacuum-assisted closure: a new method for wound control and treatment: animal studies and basic foundation. Ann Plast Surg 38:553-562, 1997.
5. Morykwas MJ, Faler BJ, Pearce DJ, et al. Effects of varying levels of subatmospheric pressure on the rate of granulation tissue formation in experimental wounds in swine. Ann Plast Surg 47:547-551, 2001.
6. Korber A, Franckson T, Grabbe S, et al. Vacuum assisted closure device improves the take of mesh grafts in chronic leg ulcer patients. Dermatology 216:250-256, 2008.
7. Vuerstaek JD, Vainas T, Wuite J, et al. State-of-the-art treatment of chronic leg ulcers: a randomized controlled trial comparing vacuum-assisted closure (VAC) with modern wound dressings. J Vasc Surg 44:1029-1037, 2006.
8. Armstrong DG, Lavery LA. Negative pressure wound therapy after partial diabetic foot amputation: a multicenter, randomized controlled trial. Lancet 366:1704-1710, 2005.
9. Blume PA, Walters J, Payne W, et al. Comparison of negative pressure wound therapy using vacuum-assisted closure with advanced moist wound therapy in the treatment of diabetic foot ulcers: a multicenter randomized controlled trial. Diabetes Care 31:631-636, 2008.
10. Raja SG, Berg GA. Should vacuum-assisted closure therapy be routinely used for management of deep sternal wound infection after cardiac surgery? Interact Cardiovasc Thorac Surg 6:523-528, 2007.
11. Llanos S, Danilla S, Barraza C, et al. Effectiveness of negative pressure closure in the integration of split thickness skin grafts: a randomized, double-masked, controlled trial. Ann Surg 244:700-705, 2006.
12. Moisidis E, Heath T, Boorer C, et al. A prospective, blinded, randomized, controlled clinical trial of topical negative pressure use in skin grafting. Plast Reconstr Surg 14:917-922, 2004.
13. Braakenburg A, Obdeijn MC, Feitz R, et al. The clinical efficacy and cost effectiveness of the vacuum-assisted closure technique in the management of acute and chronic wounds: a randomized controlled trial. Plast Reconstr Surg 118:390-397, 2006.

11. Lasers in Plastic Surgery

See *Essentials of Plastic Surgery,* second edition, pp. 115-124.

TARGET CHROMOPHORES

1. Laser therapy relies on the process of photothermolysis which targets specific tissue chromophores according to laser characteristics. For each of the following laser procedures, select the correct target chromophore. (Each answer may be used once, more than once, or not at all.)
   A. The chromophore in hair removal
   B. The chromophore in ablative resurfacing
   C. The chromophore in vascular lesions

   Options:
   a. Oxyhemoglobin
   b. Melanin
   c. Elastin
   d. Water
   e. CO_2
   f. Collagen

LASER SELECTION

2. A 30-year-old woman is referred to clinic with a bright red spot on her cheek. It measures 2 mm in diameter with radiating telangiectasia. It disappears on digital pressure and rapidly reappears. *How can this best be treated with laser therapy?*
   A. Q-switched potassium titanyl phosphate (KTP)
   B. Green dye
   C. Er:YAG
   D. CO_2
   E. Fraxel

3. Match each of the following descriptions to the most appropriate option. (Each option may be used once, more than once, or not at all.)
   A. This laser is commonly used to treat very superficial rosacea and telangiectasia.
   B. This laser is in the near-infrared spectrum and is useful for treating deeper vascular lesions.
   C. This laser is a good choice for removal of a black tattoo.

   Options:
   a. Ruby
   b. Q-switched potassium titanyl phosphate (KTP)
   c. Nd:YAG
   d. Er:YAG
   e. Diode
   f. Q-switched Nd:YAG
   g. KTP

VASCULAR LESIONS

4. A patient presents with a purple discolored patch to the left side of her face. It has been present since birth and has always grown in proportion to the patient's overall growth. It currently measures 6 cm by 8 cm. A plan is made for treatment with a pulsed dye laser. **When treating these lesions, when is treatment most likely to be effective?**
   A. In darker skinned individuals
   B. In young adult patients
   C. When the lesion is in the trigeminal nerve V_2 distribution
   D. When the lesion is lightly pigmented
   E. When the lesion is on the hands or feet

HAIR REMOVAL

5. You see a young blonde patient in your office who wishes to have hair removal treatment. **Which one of the following would be the most suitable treatment modality for her?**
   A. Fraxel
   B. Diode
   C. Nd:YAG
   D. IPL
   E. Pulsed dye

TATTOO REMOVAL

6. You see a patient in your office following treatment to remove a multicolored tattoo. The initial treatment has been partly successful but there remains residual green pigment. **Which laser would be best to target these areas in subsequent treatment?**
   A. Q-switched Nd:YAG
   B. Q-switched alexandrite
   C. Nd:YAG
   D. Er:YAG
   E. Pulsed dye

7. You see a patient in clinic with a tattoo of a multicolored cartoon bear character. She wishes to have this removed with laser treatment. **Which color ink is most likely to be resistant to laser treatment?**
   A. Black
   B. Green
   C. Red
   D. Yellow
   E. Brown

LASERS IN HYPERTROPHIC SCARS

8. You are asked to see a young girl in clinic following a 10% TBSA superficial dermal burn that was treated conservatively one year ago. Most areas healed well but some areas remained thickened and were treated with steroids. The scars have now flattened but remain erythematous. **What laser treatment is most appropriate to reduce the residual hyperpigmentation of her scar?**
   A. Ruby
   B. Alexandrite
   C. Diode
   D. Pulsed dye
   E. Er:YAG

FACIAL REJUVENATION

9. You consult with a 70-year-old white female in clinic who has deep rhytids and has requested ablative resurfacing. **Which one of the following is best for this patient?**
   A. Er:YAG
   B. Alexandrite
   C. IPL
   D. Fraxel
   E. Nd:YAG

LASER RESURFACING

10. A patient is seen in clinic requesting laser skin resurfacing. **Which one of the following medications should be discontinued prior to treatment to reduce the risk of scarring?**
    A. SPF 50 sunblock
    B. Hydroquinone
    C. Tretinoin
    D. Metronidazole
    E. Isotretinoin

WAVELENGTHS FOR COMMON LASERS

11. For each of the following wavelengths, select the corresponding laser type. *(Each answer may be used once, more than once, or not at all.)*
    A. Wavelength 1064 nm
    B. Wavelength 2940 nm
    C. Wavelength 585 nm

    Options:
    a. KTP
    b. Alexandrite
    c. Nd:YAG
    d. CO_2
    e. Er:YAG
    f. Diode
    g. Pulsed dye
    h. Ruby

LASER SAFETY

12. When using the CO_2 laser to treat an intraoral malignancy, which one of the following statements is correct?
    A. The operating site must be free of wet towels and drapes as they represent a fire hazard.
    B. The operating room staff does not need eye protection unless directly involved in the procedure.
    C. Masks and plume evacuation must be used to prevent particle transmission.
    D. A standard endotracheal tube must be used instead of a laryngeal mask.
    E. The lead surgeon does not require formal training and accreditation in laser safety.

Answers

TARGET CHROMOPHORES
1. **For each of the following laser procedures, select the correct target chromophore. (Each answer may be used once, more than once, or not at all.)**
   A. **The chromophore in hair removal**
      b. **Melanin**
   B. **The chromophore in ablative resurfacing**
      d. **Water**
   C. **The chromophore in vascular lesions**
      a. **Oxyhemoglobin**

   The term *selective photothermolysis* is derived from three terms. *Photo* referring to "light," *thermo* relating to "heat," and *lysis* referring to damage or destruction of cells. Lasers work by using a light source to create energy and heat specific targets within tissue, called *chromophores*. Common chromophores are as follows:
       Vascular lesions—hemoglobin and oxyhemoglobin
       Pigmented skin lesions—melanin
       Hair removal—melanin
       Tattoo pigment—tattoo pigment
       Ablative resurfacing—water
       Laser liposuction—water and fat

   Hair removal works best on dark hairs as the chromophore target is melanin within the hair. Water is the chromophore for ablative lasers such as CO_2 and Er:Yag. The target chromophores for vascular lesions are hemoglobin and oxyhemoglobin. Collagen and elastin are not chromophores but may be affected by laser treatment. For example, use of a resurfacing laser, such as CO_2 will target water in the dermis and stimulate the regeneration of collagen and elastin which can tighten the skin.

   The amount of tissue damage during laser treatment depends upon the wavelength, power, spot size, and exposure time (pulse width). The term thermal relaxation time is the time for target chromophores to dissipate 51% of the energy they have absorbed, into the surrounding tissue. If this time is exceeded collateral damage occurs due to excessive heat production. The ideal pulse time must be shorter than thermal relaxation time (usually one half). It represents the time for target chromophores to selectively absorb energies while protecting surrounding tissues.

LASER SELECTION
2. **A 30-year-old woman is referred to clinic with a bright red spot on her cheek. It measures 2 mm in diameter with radiating telangiectasia. It disappears on digital pressure and rapidly reappears.** *How can this best be treated with laser therapy?*
   A. **KTP**

   KTP is a popular choice for laser treatment of spider nevi. A spider nevus is an enlarged artery with radiating vessels supplied by it. This gives the appearance of a spider body with legs. The cause is not known but they can be associated with liver or thyroid disease. Most commonly, they present as an isolated condition and can often resolve spontaneously. Laser therapy can be useful for the treatment of persistent spider nevi in a single visit. Other vascular lasers may also be considered such as yellow pulsed dye, ruby, alexandrite, and diode as they all target hemoglobin and cause local coagulation to the main source vessel.[1] Green dye is used for café au lait macules. Er:Yag, fraxel, and CO_2 are all used for resurfacing.

3. *Match each of the following descriptions to the most appropriate option. (Each option may be used once, more than once, or not at all.)*
   A. *This laser is commonly used to treat very superficial rosacea and telangiectasia.*
      g. **KTP**
   B. *This laser is in the near-infrared spectrum and is useful for treating deeper vascular lesions.*
      c. **Nd:YAG**
   C. *This laser is a good choice for removal of a black tattoo.*
      f. **Q-switched Nd:YAG**

   Vascular lasers are KTP, pulsed dye, and Nd:YAG. All of these can be used for rosacea, port-wine stains, and telangiectasia. KTP has a penetration depth up to 1 mm at 532 nm. Pulsed dye laser has a penetration depth of around 0.5 mm to 1.0 mm at 585 nm. Both KTP and pulsed dye are within the visible spectrum, but Nd:YAG is in the infrared range. Nd:YAG can penetrate more deeply (up to 8 mm) and is ideal for deeper vascular lesions.

   Tattoo removal is best achieved using Q-switched lasers. These penetrate to the upper papillary dermis and selectively target ink particles by color depending on laser type. Dark inks such as black and blue are best treated with the Nd:YAG laser at 1064 nm although many Q-switched lasers also work well.

VASCULAR LESIONS

4. *A patient presents with a purple discolored patch to the left side of her face. It has been present since birth and has always grown in proportion to the patient's overall growth. It currently measures 6 cm by 8 cm. A plan is made for treatment with a pulsed dye laser.* **When treating these lesions, when is treatment most likely to be effective?**
   D. **When the lesion is lightly pigmented**

   The patient described, has a port-wine stain or capillary malformation. Port-wine stains represent a collection of abnormally formed capillaries within the skin, resulting in a red or purple colored mark. Most port-wine stains are present at birth, as in this case, but they can also be acquired. They are relatively common and occur in 1:300 infants with an equal sex distribution.

   The pulsed dye laser is commonly used to improve the appearance of port-wine stains as it targets oxyhemoglobin within the abnormal vessels using a 585 nm wavelength. Cases generally require a series of treatments at regular intervals. These often require general anesthesia in children. Treatment outcomes can be quite successful although most lesions never fully disappear. In general the outcome following treatment with pulsed dye laser is best in lighter colored lesions, in children and patients with lighter skin tones (Fitzpatrick I-III). Treatment can be started from the age of 6 months. Better responses are observed in the head and neck region with the exception of the trigeminal nerve V_2 distribution. The anatomic area associated with the poorest response is the extremities. Long-term follow-up shows that these lesions darken again over time once treatment has finished. In most cases the port-wine stain at ten years after treatment has an appearance midway between the before and after injury color. For this reason patients must be informed of the risk of darkening over time.[2]

HAIR REMOVAL

5. You see a young blonde patient in your office who wishes to have hair removal treatment. *Which one of the following would be the most suitable treatment modality for her?*

D. IPL

In general, laser hair removal is less effective in blonde patients but can be fairly successful using IPL. Lasers used for dark hair removal target the melanin and include diode, alexandrite and Nd:YAG. Alexandrite is commonly used for lighter skin tones. Nd:YAG is safest for darker skin tones to reduce risks of hypopigmentation.

TATTOO REMOVAL

6. You see a patient in your office following treatment to remove a multicolored tattoo. The initial treatment has been partly successful but there remains residual green pigment. *Which laser would be best to target these areas in subsequent treatment?*

B. Q-switched alexandrite

Green tattoo inks are best treated with a laser of wavelength 650 nm. Suitable choices include alexandrite (755 nm) and ruby (694 nm). Q-switched lasers are preferable over pulsed for tattoo removal. They use high bursts of energy in short time intervals and create acoustic waves that result in mechanical pigment disruption. The pigments that are fragmented can then be phagocytized by macrophages.

7. You see a patient in clinic with a tattoo of a multicolored cartoon bear character. She wishes to have this removed with laser treatment. *Which color ink is most likely to be resistant to laser treatment?*

D. Yellow

Multicolored tattoos are very difficult to treat and will require multiple therapies with different lasers. Of the colors listed, yellow will be most difficult to treat as this and orange are highly resistant to treatment. These colors best absorb light in the UV range which is absorbed by, and damages, melanocytes. This affects the ability of light to penetrate the dermis.

LASERS IN HYPERTROPHIC SCARS

8. You are asked to see a young girl in clinic following a 10% TBSA superficial dermal burn that was treated conservatively one year ago. Most areas healed well but some areas remain thickened and were treated with steroids. The scars have now flattened but remain erythematous. *What laser treatment is most appropriate to reduce the residual hyperpigmentation of her scar?*

D. Pulsed dye

Scars that remain erythematous due to increased vascularity may be treated with either pulsed dye, Nd:YAG or KTP lasers. They target oxyhemoglobin and decrease the number and proliferation of fibroblasts and subsequent type III collagen deposition.

FACIAL REJUENATION

9. You consult with a 70-year-old white female in clinic who has deep rhytids and has requested ablative resurfacing. *Which one of the following is best for this patient?*

A. Er:YAG

Water is the target chromophore for ablative resurfacing. Options include CO_2 (10,600 nm) or Er:YAG (2940 nm). Energy absorption by water is significantly more efficient with Er:YAG than

Chapter 11 ■ Lasers in Plastic Surgery   83

with CO_2 lasers. There is also less thermal diffusion. For these reasons, Er:YAG may provide a more consistent result (see Chapter 88, *Essentials of Plastic Surgery,* second edition). Nd:YAG is a nonablative resurfacing laser. Fraxel and IPL are also nonablative techniques that may be used for less aggressive resurfacing.

LASER RESURFACING

10. A patient is seen in clinic requesting laser skin resurfacing. **Which one of the following medications should be discontinued prior to treatment to reduce the risk of scarring?**

E. Isotretinoin

Isotretinoin is related to vitamin A and is taken orally to treat acne. The precise mechanism of action is not known but it works by suppressing activity in the sebaceous glands of the skin and by decreasing the amount of oil produced. It can make the skin fragile and cause delayed wound healing and scarring. This may be a direct result of damage to the epithelial cells of the adnexal structures which usually provide cells that repopulate the resurfaced skin wound. It can also increase the risk of wound infection and sensitivity to UV light. Therefore isotretinoin should be stopped six to twelve months before resurfacing treatment to minimize the risk of scarring, poor wound healing, and hyperpigmentation.[3,4]

Using tretinoin and hydroquinone for 4 to 6 weeks pretreatment will stimulate rapid healing and help prevent posttreatment hyperpigmentation. Antivirals should be given 48 hours before and 7 to 10 days after ablative laser resurfacing. Use of sunblock before and after treatment is normally advised. Metronidazole is a treatment for use in acne and does not specifically need to be stopped for laser surgery. However laser therapy should not be given during a bout of active acne as it will likely result in poor scarring.

WAVELENGTHS FOR COMMON LASERS

11. For each of the following wavelengths, select the corresponding laser type (Box 11-1). (Each answer may be used once, more than once, or not at all.)
   A. Wavelength 1064 nm
      c. Nd:YAG
   B. Wavelength 2940 nm
      e. Er:YAG
   C. Wavelength 585 nm
      g. Pulsed dye

Box 11-1   *WAVELENGTHS OF COMMON LASERS*

Vascular	**Melanin Target (hair removal, solar lentigines, or tattoo removal)**
KTP: 532 nm	Alexandrite: 755 nm
Pulsed dye: 585 nm	Ruby: 694 nm
Nd:YAG: 1064 nm	Diode: 810 nm
Ablative Resurfacing	
CO_2: 10,600 nm	
Er:YAG: 2940 nm	

KTP, Potassium titanyl phosphate.

The electromagnetic spectrum relevant to lasers in plastic surgery includes the UV (200 to 400 nm), visible (400 to 750 nm), near-infrared (750 to 1400 nm) and mid-infrared (1400 to 20,000 nm). Most vascular lasers are within the visible range (as this corresponds to the wavelength of hemoglobin), and most that target melanin are in the near-infrared spectrum. Those that target water are within the mid-infrared spectrum.

LASER SAFETY

12. When using the CO_2 laser to treat an intraoral malignancy, which one of the following statements is correct?

C. Masks and plume evacuation must be used to prevent particle transmission.

When using a laser for therapeutic interventions, it is vital that strict safety measures are in place.[5] The responsibility of this falls on both the surgeon and OR lead to ensure the safety measures are maintained. It is important to have formal training and accreditation in laser prior to using it in clinical practice. Eye protection with laser specific goggles/glasses is mandatory for all personnel and masks should be worn, particularly in cases with malignancy or risk of viral transmission. Plume evaluation is required when using CO_2 or erbium lasers. Wet swabs should be placed around the operative site to reduce the chance of local burns and ignition risks when using the CO_2 laser. In this case a reinforced endotracheal tube must also be used with low FiO_2 flows (less than 30%) to reduce the risk of flash burn or inhalation.

REFERENCES

1. Erceg A, Greebe RJ, Bovenschen HJ, et al. A comparative study of pulsed 532-nm potassium titanyl phosphate laser and electrocoagulation in the treatment of spider nevi. Dermatol Surg 36:630-635, 2010.
2. Huikeshoven M, Koster PH, de Borgie CA, et al. Redarkening of port-wine stains 10 years after pulsed-dye-laser treatment. N Engl J Med 356:1235-1240, 2007.
3. Layton A. The use of isotretinoin in acne. Dermato-endocrinology 1:162-169, 2009.
4. Tanna N, Meyers AD. Skin resurfacing laser surgery. Available at *http://emedicine.medscape.com/article/838501-overview#a05*.
5. Public Health England: Non-Ionising Radiation Service. Overview of the optical radiation course. Available at *https://www.phe-protectionservices.org.uk/nir/courses/overview/*.

12. Anesthesia

See *Essentials of Plastic Surgery,* second edition, pp. 125-139.

AMERICAN SOCIETY OF ANESTHESIOLOGISTS STATUS

1. You are planning surgery on a patient who will require a general anesthetic. Their medical history includes well-controlled diabetes mellitus and hypertension. These conditions do not presently limit the patient's functional status. **According to the American Society of Anesthesiologists (ASA) classification, what is the ASA status of this patient?**
   A. ASA 1
   B. ASA 2
   C. ASA 3
   D. ASA 4
   E. ASA 5

LOCAL ANESTHETIC ACTION

2. You have injected a local anesthetic agent as a digital ring block prior to digital nerve repair. **Which one of the following statements is true regarding how the anesthetic agent will take effect?**
   A. The first clinical effect will be a loss of proprioception.
   B. Nerve blockade will occur secondary to an effect on calcium channels.
   C. The resting potential of nerves will be affected.
   D. Propagation of action potentials within axons is impaired.
   E. The action will differ significantly depending on which anesthetic agent is used.

LOCAL ANESTHETICS

3. **Which one of the following statements regarding lidocaine as an injectable local anesthetic agent is correct?**
   A. The maximum safe dose of plain lidocaine is 7 mg/kg.
   B. Metabolism is predominantly renal.
   C. It is an amide local anesthetic compound.
   D. True allergies occur secondary to paraaminobenzoic acid (PABA) production.
   E. Onset of action usually takes five or six minutes.

SAFE DOSE SELECTION OF LOCAL ANESTHETICS

4. A woman weighing 55 kg (121 pounds) is having several basal cell carcinomas excised from her face. Lidocaine with epinephrine is given. **What is the commonly accepted maximum safe dose of anesthetic agent she can receive?**
   A. 11 ml of 1% lidocaine with epinephrine
   B. 16 ml of 1% lidocaine with epinephrine
   C. 38 ml of 1% lidocaine with epinephrine
   D. 16 ml of 0.5% lidocaine with epinephrine
   E. 76 ml of 2% lidocaine with epinephrine

5. A patient weighing 60 kg (132 pounds) is under general anesthesia and has a 25 cm by 15 cm split-thickness skin graft donor site on the thigh. Postoperative pain relief is needed. *Based on a maximum safe dose of 2 mg/kg, how much bupivacaine (Marcaine) can she receive?*
   A. 12 ml of 2%
   B. 16 ml of 0.5%
   C. 24 ml of 0.75%
   D. 48 ml of 0.25%
   E. 96 ml of 1%

LOCAL ANESTHETIC ADDITIVES

6. *What is the main effect of adding sodium bicarbonate to a local anesthetic solution?*
   A. It prolongs the duration of the anesthetic.
   B. It reduces localized bleeding.
   C. It allows a higher dose of anesthetic agent to be administered.
   D. It speeds the onset of anesthetic blockade.
   E. It helps stop precipitation of the anesthetic.

7. *When using local anesthetic to inject into a split-skin graft donor site, which one of the following agents can be added to improve local tissue distribution?*
   A. Sodium bicarbonate
   B. Clonidine
   C. Hyaluronidase
   D. Morphine
   E. Hyaluronic acid

LOCAL ANESTHETICS CONTAINING EPINEPHRINE

8. You are planning an excisional biopsy and local flap reconstruction of a large basal cell carcinoma on the face. *Which one of the following is the main disadvantage of adding epinephrine to the anesthetic solution?*
   A. The effect on duration of anesthesia
   B. The effect on anesthetic absorption rate
   C. The effect on patient discomfort
   D. The effect on anesthetic dosage allowance
   E. The effect on localized bleeding

9. *Which one of the following is only a relative contraindication to giving epinephrine with a local anesthetic?*
   A. Anesthesia of the penis
   B. A skin flap with limited perfusion
   C. Digital vessels compromised by infection or trauma
   D. Diabetic patients
   E. Dilutions of less than 1:60,000 to block a digit

CARDIOTOXICITY IN LOCAL ANESTHESIA

10. *Which one of the following is the most cardiotoxic local anesthetic agent?*
    A. Lidocaine
    B. Bupivacaine
    C. Lidocaine with epinephrine
    D. Cocaine
    E. Ropivacaine

TOXICITY WITH LOCAL ANESTHETIC AGENTS

11. You are operating on a patient and have just completed an injection of local anesthetic. The patient becomes unwell. **Which one of the following is most commonly the first sign of systemic toxicity?**
    A. Perioral numbness and a metallic taste in the mouth.
    B. Cardiac or respiratory arrest.
    C. Muscle twitching or convulsion.
    D. Visual disturbances.
    E. Disorientation and hallucinations.

TOPICAL LOCAL ANESTHETIC AGENTS

12. Topical local anesthetics are useful preoperatively, especially in the pediatric population. **Which one of the following is a topical anesthetic that contains lidocaine and prilocaine in equal concentrations?**
    A. EMLA
    B. LMX-4
    C. Betacaine
    D. Topicaine
    E. Tetracaine

ANESTHETIC TECHNIQUES

13. Match each of the following descriptions to the most appropriate option. (Each option may be used once, more than once, or not at all.)
    A. This type of block is useful for upper limb surgery and is usually performed under ultrasound guidance.
    B. This is a type of regional anesthesia that involves two tourniquets and intravenous injection.
    C. This technique involves injection of anesthetic agent into the subarachnoid space to provide central nerve blockade affecting motor and sensory function.

    Options:
    a. Peripheral nerve block
    b. Regional nerve block
    c. Spinal block
    d. Field block
    e. Bier block
    f. Epidural block

Answers

AMERICAN SOCIETY OF ANESTHESIOLOGISTS STATUS

1. You are planning surgery on a patient who will require a general anesthetic. Their medical history includes well-controlled diabetes mellitus and hypertension. These conditions do not presently limit the patient's functional status. *According to the American Society of Anesthesiologists (ASA) classification, what is the ASA status of this patient?*
   B. ASA 2
   The ASA physical status grade has six classes (1-6) ranging from a normal healthy patient (1) to one that is brain dead (6). The full categories are shown below:
   Class 1: A normal healthy patient
   Class 2: Mild systemic disease with no functional limitation
   Class 3: Severe systemic disease with functional limitation
   Class 4: Severe systemic disease that is a constant threat to life
   Class 5: Moribund and not expected to survive without surgery
   Class 6: Brain dead patient for organ retrieval
   This has clinical relevance for assessing the risk of surgery for individual patients and can help to guide which procedures can safely be offered and the appropriate level of care a patient will require (e.g. day case versus overnight admission and postoperative ward care versus high dependency). The ASA status also forms part of the WHO surgical checklist and facilitates communication between the surgeon and the anesthetist about a patient's general fitness for surgery. A patient's ASA status will also impact the billing costs for medical care in most medical systems.[1]

LOCAL ANESTHETIC ACTION

2. You have injected a local anesthetic agent as a digital ring block prior to digital nerve repair. *Which one of the following statements is true regarding how the anesthetic agent will take effect?*
   D. Propagation of action potentials within axons is impaired.
   Local anesthetic agents work in a broadly similar manner by interfering with sodium channels, thereby preventing an influx of sodium within the neuronal membrane. This does not affect the resting membrane potential but does impair propagation of the action potential. There is a differential sensitivity of nerve fibers that results in smaller fibers and those that are myelinated being blocked more quickly. (See Table 12-3 and Fig. 12-1, *Essentials of Plastic Surgery,* second edition.) The clinical sequence is as follows:
   1. Vasodilatation
   2. Loss of pain and temperature
   3. Loss of proprioception
   4. Loss of pressure sensation
   5. Loss of motor function

Chapter 12 ▪ Anesthesia   89

LOCAL ANESTHETICS

3. Which one of the following statements regarding lidocaine as an injectable local anesthetic agent is correct?

C. It is an amide local anesthetic compound.

Local anesthetic agents are classified as either amides or esters depending on their chemical composition. Amides are more commonly used in clinical practice and may be identified by the presence of the letter *i* in their prefix. For example, lidocaine, bupivacaine, mepivacaine, and prilocaine. The maximum safe dose for lidocaine with epinephrine is 7 mg/kg, but without epinephrine it is only 3 to 5 mg/kg. Absolute maximum safe dose is 300 mg. (See Table 12-4, *Essentials of Plastic Surgery,* second edition.) Lidocaine is metabolized in the liver (not the kidney) and its onset of action is rapid (usually within two minutes). The elimination half-life is 90 minutes to 120 minutes and the duration of action is up to one hour without and six hours with epinephrine. True allergies are rare for amide anesthetic agents such as lidocaine. PABA is a by-product of metabolism of esters (such as procaine and tetracaine) not amides and is often responsible for hypersensitivity reactions following administration of these compounds. Methylparaben is a preservative found in some ester and amide local anesthetics that resembles PABA and may cause an allergic reaction.

SAFE DOSE SELECTION OF LOCAL ANESTHETICS

4. A woman weighing 55 kg (121 pounds) is having several basal cell carcinomas excised from her face. Lidocaine with epinephrine is given. *What is the commonly accepted maximum safe dose of anesthetic agent she can receive?*

C. 38 ml of 1% lidocaine with epinephrine

Lidocaine is a short-acting local anesthetic commonly used in plastic surgery. It is an amide that has a rapid onset of action and is often combined with epinephrine. The safe dose of lidocaine with epinephrine is 7 mg/kg. The safe dose without is 3 to 5 mg/kg. This lady can therefore safely have 38 ml of 1% lidocaine with epinephrine.[2] The calculation is shown below:

7 mg × 55 kg = 384 mg
A 1% solution contains 10 mg in 1 ml
Therefore she can have 384/10 = 38.4 ml

Option A is based on a calculation of 2 mg/kg which is a maximum safe dose for Chirocaine. Option B is based on a calculation of 3 mg/kg which is a maximum safe dose for lidocaine with epinephrine. Option D refers to a safe maximum volume for 2% lidocaine with epinephrine, not 0.5%. Option E refers to a safe volume for 0.5% lidocaine with epinephrine, but would exceed the maximum safe dose for 2% lidocaine with epinephrine by four times. In the clinical setting it is vital to have a good understanding of safe dosing for commonly used local anesthetic agents.

5. A patient weighing 60 kg (132 pounds) is under general anesthesia and has a 25 cm by 15 cm split-thickness skin graft donor site on the thigh. Postoperative pain relief is needed. *Based on a maximum safe dose of 2 mg/kg, how much bupivacaine (Marcaine) can she receive?*
   D. 48 ml of 0.25%
   The safe dose of bupivacaine is 2 mg to 2.5 mg per kg and is not significantly altered by the addition of epinephrine.[2] This lady can therefore safely have 48 ml of 0.25% bupivacaine or levobupivacaine. The calculation is shown below:

   $$2 \text{ mg} \times 60 \text{ kg} = 120 \text{ mg}$$
   A 0.25% solution contains 2.5 mg in 1 ml
   Therefore she can have $120/2.5 = 48$ ml

   Option A is the maximum safe volume of 1% not 2% bupivacaine. Option B is the maximum safe volume of 1% bupivacaine. Option C is the maximum safe volume of 0.5% bupivacaine. Option E is the maximum safe volume of 0.125% bupivacaine. Levobupivacaine (Chirocaine) and ropivacaine (Naropin) are both isomers of bupivacaine developed to reduce the cardiotoxicity of bupivacaine. They have become popular alternatives to bupivacaine as a result. Safe doses are 2 to 3 mg/kg for levobupivacaine and 3 to 4 mg/kg for ropivacaine, with maximum recommended doses of 150 mg and 200 mg, respectively. Use of local anesthetic in patients who have skin grafts taken under general anesthetic is very useful and should be routinely performed. This has the benefit of reducing intraoperative and postoperative pain. Often patients who have split-graft harvest state that the donor site is the most painful part of the procedure so anything that can be performed to minimize this is recommended.

LOCAL ANESTHETIC ADDITIVES

6. *What is the main effect of adding sodium bicarbonate to a local anesthetic solution?*
   D. It speeds the onset of anesthetic blockade.
   Sodium bicarbonate can be added to local anesthetic solutions to speed the onset of blockade. This works by reducing the acidity of the anesthetic and releasing unionized anesthetic agent. The dose should be 8.4% $NaHCO_3$ added in a ratio of 1:9 with lidocaine. Care should be taken with agents such as bupivacaine as bicarbonate can lead to precipitation. An additional benefit of using bicarbonate is that it can decrease pain during injection, presumably as a result of the decreased acidity and perhaps in part to a more rapid onset of anesthesia.[3,4]

7. *When using local anesthetic to inject into a split-skin graft donor site, which one of the following agents can be added to improve local tissue distribution?*
   C. Hyaluronidase
   Hyaluronidase can be useful to help improve local anesthetic distribution within subcutaneous tissues and may be most useful in large split-skin graft donor sites. One prospective randomized double-blind study showed that the area of anesthesia is significantly increased by adding hyaluronidase to 1% lidocaine, while decreasing tissue distortion. However, the addition of hyaluronidase may increase pain on injection. As discussed in question 5, bicarbonate can reduce pain on injection of a local anesthetic but does not have any significant effect on its distribution. Morphine does not directly affect the anesthetic distribution but can provide improved pain relief. Clonidine is an alpha 2 adrenergic agonist that has analgesic effects. It can intensify and prolong anesthesia by reducing acidity.[5]

LOCAL ANESTHETICS CONTAINING EPINEPHRINE

8. You are planning an excisional biopsy and local flap reconstruction of a large basal cell carcinoma on the face. *Which one of the following is the main disadvantage of adding epinephrine to the anesthetic solution?*
C. The effect on patient discomfort.

Using epinephrine with a local anesthetic serves a number of useful purposes but it may increase pain on injection as it requires the solution to be more acidic. This is because epinephrine is unstable in solution at physiological pH.[3,4]

Other potential disadvantages to utilizing epinephrine include increased myocardial irritability leading to tachycardia, hypertension, or arrhythmias. For this reason, particular caution should be exercised when using epinephrine in patients with cardiac disease.

There are multiple beneficial effects of adding epinephrine to a local anesthetic solution. It causes local vasoconstriction and therefore maintains the anesthetic agent at the required site. It reduces bleeding and increases the duration of action. It also enables higher doses to be given safely. For example, lidocaine can be administered at doses of 3 to 5 mg/kg without epinephrine and up to 7 mg/kg when epinephrine is added. In addition, it will shorten the time to onset of anesthesia.

Factors to reduce pain during injection of a local anesthetic include slow infiltration, the addition of bicarbonate (see question 5) and ensuring the product is not cold (particularly relevant in products that are stored in the refrigerator).

9. *Which one of the following is only a relative contraindication to giving epinephrine with a local anesthetic?*
D. Diabetic patients

Contraindications to using epinephrine in local anesthetics can be classified as absolute or relative.

Absolute contraindications include use in the penis, skin flaps with limited perfusion, and when the digital vessels are already compromised. The use of epinephrine in healthy digits is considered safe but dilutions greater than 1:200,000 are recommended. Most of the time a digital tourniquet can be used to reduce bleeding in a digit, negating the need for epinephrine. Relative contraindications for epinephrine use include hypertension, diabetes, cardiac disease, thyrotoxicosis, and certain drug interactions such as with the monoamine oxidase inhibitors (MAO). These can cause a hypertensive crisis when epinephrine is used, secondary to formation of a pool of available endogenous catecholamines.

CARDIOTOXICITY IN LOCAL ANESTHESIA

10. *Which one of the following is the most cardiotoxic local anesthetic agent?*
B. Bupivacaine

Bupivacaine is known to have the greatest cardiac toxicity, especially after inadvertent intravascular injection. Ropivacaine was developed to provide a long duration of action with less cardiac toxicity. Symptoms of cardiovascular toxicity include hypotension, arrhythmias, and cardiovascular collapse.

The use of epinephrine can also cause cardiac problems and should be carefully monitored.

TOXICITY WITH LOCAL ANESTHETIC AGENTS

11. You are operating on a patient and have just completed an injection of local anesthetic. The patient becomes unwell. *Which one of the following is most commonly the first sign of systemic toxicity?*
    A. Perioral numbness and a metallic taste in the mouth.

    Toxicity due to local anesthetics can be unpredictable but generally parallels increasing plasma concentration and tongue numbness or a metallic taste are early signs (see Fig. 12-3, *Essentials of Plastic Surgery,* second edition). Toxicity can be subclassified into CNS, cardiovascular, or idiosyncratic effects. CNS effects include dizziness, metallic taste in the mouth, perioral numbness, tinnitus, and seizures. Cardiovascular effects include hypotension and arrhythmias. Idiosyncratic effects include anaphylaxis in patients with hypersensitivity to esters, increased relative toxicity associated with liver disease and the effects of epinephrine.

TOPICAL LOCAL ANESTHETIC AGENTS

12. Topical local anesthetics are useful preoperatively, especially in the pediatric population. *Which one of the following is a topical anesthetic that contains lidocaine and prilocaine in equal concentrations?*
    A. EMLA

    There are a number of topical local anesthetic agents in common use, the vast majority of which contain lidocaine in varying concentrations between 2.5% and 5%. EMLA contains 2.5% prilocaine and 2.5% lidocaine. EMLA stands for **E**utectic **M**ixture of **L**ocal **A**nesthetic which refers to the situation where two chemical compounds solidify at a lower temperature when mixed together than they do separately. In practical terms, this means that EMLA is a convenient consistency at room temperature for topical use.

    Key points to remember when using EMLA are that it takes one hour to provide an anesthetic effect which then lasts for a further two hours, and that it requires placement of an occlusive dressing over the cream once it has been applied.

    Topical local anesthetics with just lidocaine include LMX-4 and LMX-5 (the number refers to the percentage of lidocaine), Betacaine, and topicaine. Tetracaine contains 4% tetracaine only without lidocaine.

ANESTHETIC TECHNIQUES

13. Match each of the following descriptions to the most appropriate option. (Each option may be used once, more than once, or not at all.)
    A. This type of block is useful for upper limb surgery and is usually performed under ultrasound guidance.
    b. Regional nerve block
    B. This is a type of regional anesthesia that involves two tourniquets and intravenous injection.
    e. Bier block
    C. This technique involves injection of anesthetic agent into the subarachnoid space to provide central nerve blockade affecting motor and sensory function.
    c. Spinal block

    Nerve blocks may be local, regional, or central. Local blocks are useful for performing surgery on small areas such as individual digits and removal of skin lesions in most areas. Regional blocks allow more complex procedures to be undertaken and are particularly useful for upper limb procedures such as cubital tunnel release and flexor tendon repair. They involve injection of local anesthetic around a group of nerves under ultrasound guidance such as the brachial plexus. Intravenous regional blocks include the Bier block which was traditionally used to manipulate distal radial fractures. It involves intravenous injection of anesthetic under double tourniquet control.

Central blocks include spinal and epidural anesthesia. Epidural anesthesia is used in obstetrics and blocks sensory function but not usually motor. It is performed as a continuous technique and requires larger total volumes of anesthetic. Spinal anesthesia involves injection into the subarachnoid space and usually blocks both motor and sensory functions.

REFERENCES

1. Dripps RD. New classification of physical status. Anesthesiology 24:111, 1963.
2. British National Formulary. Available at *www.bnf.org*.
3. Mutalik S. How to make local anaesthesia less painful. J Cutan Anesthet Surg 1:37-38, 2008.
4. Brandis K. Alkalinisation of local anaesthetic solutions. Aust Prescr 34:173-175, 2011.
5. Nevarre DR, Tzarnas CD. The effects of hyaluronidase on the efficacy and on the pain of administration of 1%. Plast Reconstr Surg 101:365-369, 1998.

13. Photography for the Plastic Surgeon

See *Essentials of Plastic Surgery*, second edition, pp. 140-164.

BENEFITS OF PHOTOGRAPHY IN PLASTIC SURGERY

1. **Which function of photographs is probably the most useful from a patient's perspective?**
   A. Medicolegal protection
   B. Education and research
   C. Measurement of outcomes and enhanced communication
   D. Marketing
   E. Optimization of clinical care

STANDARDIZED PHOTOGRAPHY

2. **When taking photographs of patients before and after surgery, which one of the following is correct?**
   A. Digital zoom gives superior image quality to optical zoom.
   B. A change in background can be corrected for by white balancing the camera.
   C. Saving the image as a JPEG file preserves image quality better than TIFF format.
   D. A straight on flash angle is best for facial views.
   E. The same focal length should be used for comparative images.

STANDARDIZED FACE AND NECK VIEWS

3. **When taking photographs before a face lift, which one of the following statements is correct?**
   A. The Frankfort plane will give the most accurate image of the submental tissue.
   B. All images should be taken as closeups.
   C. A true lateral image can be ensured by viewing across the oral commissures.
   D. The oblique view must show the tip of the nose touching the far cheek.
   E. It is important to include worm's-eye (basal) and bird's-eye (cephalic) views.

STANDARDIZED RHINOPLASTY VIEWS

4. **When taking preoperative images for a patient seeking a rhinoplasty, which one of the following might conceal an underlying dynamic problem?**
   A. Taking a standardized oblique view
   B. Keeping the patient's face relaxed throughout
   C. Aligning the nasal tip with the eyebrows in full basal view
   D. Using a cephalic view to record deviation
   E. Taking closeups in a landscape (horizontal) format

Chapter 13 ■ Photography for the Plastic Surgeon   95

STANDARD BODY VIEWS

5. **Which one of the following statements is correct when taking photographs of the trunk before an abdominoplasty?**
   A. The patient should stand with their feet together.
   B. The patient should raise their arms above the head.
   C. The patient should wear their own choice of underwear.
   D. The camera should be level with the xiphisternum.
   E. The diver's view should be taken in the oblique plane.

STANDARD BREAST SERIES

6. **Which one of the following statements is correct regarding the standard breast series?**
   A. The patient's hands should be on their hips.
   B. Photographs should be taken vertically (portrait).
   C. The camera should be placed at the level of the clavicle fold.
   D. Reductions, mastopexies, and reconstructions should be photographed with the patient's arms positioned behind the body.
   E. After latissimus dorsi reconstruction, lateral views are taken with the patient's arms elevated above the head.

PHOTOGRAPHIC CONSENT

7. **Which one of the following statements is correct regarding consent for photographs?**
   A. Written patient authorization for photographs is always required.
   B. Standards of care should comply with those published by the Health Insurance Portability and Accountability Act (HIPAA).
   C. Key elements of protected health information are limited to name, date of birth, address, and social security number.
   D. Even when photographs are taken for treatment purposes, written patient consent is required.
   E. Satisfactory anonymity on facial views is achieved by blacking out the eyes.

Answers

BENEFITS OF PHOTOGRAPHY IN PLASTIC SURGERY

1. **Which function of photographs is probably the most useful from a patient's perspective?**

   C. Measurement of outcomes and enhanced communication

   All of these options are useful reasons for photography before and after treatment in plastic surgery. The most useful function from a patient's perspective is probably to help measure outcomes and improve communication. For example, patients can be shown photographs of other patients to help them better understand likely outcomes, including scarring and cosmesis. They can also review their own preoperative and postoperative photographs with their surgeon to see positive and negative aspects of their outcome. When reviewing photographs with patients postoperatively, it is interesting how they often forget how they looked preoperatively and having photographs for discussion helps to reestablish this.

   Clinical photography in plastic surgery is very important for education and research among clinicians. This should help to improve clinical care. Medicolegal protection may apply to both surgeon and patient. The use of patient photographs in marketing carries a high risk and is not advisable. Courts have imposed liability in cases in which the provider has exploited the patient for commercial benefit.

STANDARDIZED PHOTOGRAPHY

2. **When taking photographs of patients before and after surgery, which one of the following is correct?**

   E. The same focal length should be used for comparative images.

   It is important to use the same focal length for comparative images (e.g., before and after rhinoplasty). A change in focal length can have dramatic distorting effects (Fig. 13-1). This can be achieved by using the same lens on a camera with interchangeable lenses, or by fixing the focal distance on a single lens camera and physically moving the camera to achieve focus.

   Optical zoom gives a superior image as digital zoom simply mimics a greater zoom without gaining image detail. A consistent background and white balancing should be used but one cannot compensate for errors in the other. Saving an image in JPEG format uses lossy compression (i.e., image data is reduced each time it is saved), whereas TIFF format preserves image data but can be less practical for file storage. A separate bounce flash angled 45 degrees upwards is recommended for consistent lighting and less flattening than a straight on flash in facial views.

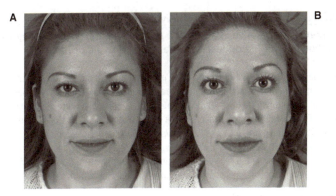

Fig. 13-1 Image **A** was created using a 105 mm lens 1:10. Image **B** was created with a 50 mm lens 1:10, which shows the lens distortion called a *barrel distortion*.

STANDARDIZED FACE AND NECK VIEWS

3. **When taking photographs before a face lift, which one of the following statements is correct?**
   C. A true lateral image can be ensured by viewing across the oral commissures.

   A true lateral image can be ensured by viewing across the oral commissures (Fig. 13-2). This can be achieved by asking the patient to open their mouth to check alignment. It is important as underrotation and overrotation may markedly distort the appearance. A face-lift series should include anterior, lateral, and oblique views. Images should be taken from both a distance and close up to aid with scale, perspective, and proportion. The oblique view can either show the nasal tip touching the far cheek, or the nasal dorsum touching the medial canthus according to surgeon preference.

   The Frankfort plane tends to exaggerate submental fullness compared to the natural horizontal facial plane. Therefore this natural plane is generally preferred for face and neck images. To exaggerate the submental tissues, a reading view is used, which flexes the neck. Additional views with the teeth gritted will demonstrate platysmal banding (see Fig. 13-9, *A* and *B*, *Essentials of Plastic Surgery*, second edition). Bird's-eye and worm's-eye views are more typical of a rhinoplasty or midface/facial fracture series (see Fig. 13-13, *Essentials of Plastic Surgery*, second edition).

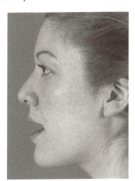

Fig. 13-2 A true lateral image may be obtained by viewing straight across the two oral commissures to verify correct rotation.

STANDARDIZED RHINOPLASTY VIEWS

4. When taking preoperative images for a patient seeking a rhinoplasty, which one of the following might conceal an underlying dynamic problem?

B. Keeping the patient's face relaxed throughout

The rhinoplasty series is difficult and often needs minor adjustment. Keeping the patient's face relaxed throughout may misrepresent preoperative problems when release of depressor septi is required. To demonstrate this, additional anterior and lateral views are required with the patient smiling. The oblique view may either have the nasal tip touching the cheek or the dorsum touching the medial canthus (see Fig. 13-5, *Essentials of Plastic Surgery,* second edition). Also see Figs. 13-13 through 13-15, *Essentials of Plastic Surgery,* second edition for additional rhinoplasty views and note that while the full-face views are portrait (see Fig. 13-8, *Essentials of Plastic Surgery,* second edition) closeup images are better taken as landscape (horizontal) views.

STANDARD BODY VIEWS

5. Which one of the following statements is correct when taking photographs of the trunk before an abdominoplasty?

E. The diver's view should be taken in the oblique plane.

The diver's view is taken in the oblique plane and demonstrates abdominal skin laxity by asking the patient to lean forward with the abdomen relaxed (Fig. 13-3). The standard body series is described in Box 13-6 and Figs. 13-16 and 13-17, *Essentials of Plastic Surgery,* second edition and should include the patient standing with the feet parallel at hip width. The patient should wear standardized undergarments, the camera should be level with the umbilicus and the patient's arms should be no higher than breast level.

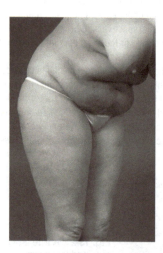

Fig. 13-3 The diver's view is an oblique view with the patient folded over while relaxing the abdomen.

Chapter 13 ▪ Photography for the Plastic Surgeon   99

STANDARD BREAST SERIES

6. *Which one of the following statements is correct regarding the standard breast series?*
   E. After latissimus dorsi reconstruction, lateral views are taken with the patient's arms elevated above the head.
   Images obtained after latissimus dorsi breast reconstruction include a posterior view with the arms down and a lateral view with the arms placed above the head. These views allow assessment of the donor site. In the standard breast series, the patient's arms are relaxed by their side with one additional anterior view with the hands pushed on the hips to view the pectoralis major. The breast is best photographed with a 50 mm lens at 1 m. Horizontal (landscape) photographs are taken for this series. They should extend from above the shoulders to below the umbilicus for correct proportion. The camera is ideally placed at the level of the areola, not the clavicle fold.

PHOTOGRAPHIC CONSENT

7. *Which one of the following statements is correct regarding consent for photographs?*
   B. Standards of care should comply with those published by the Health Insurance Portability and Accountability Act (HIPAA).
   The U.S. Department of Health and Human Services has published standards to protect the privacy of patients' identifiable health information. This comprises many elements, ranging from telephone number and IP address to credit card number and fingerprints or voiceprints. The standards are documented as the Health Insurance Portability and Accountability Act (HIPAA). According to these guidelines, patient authorization is not always required for photographs to be taken. However the purpose of obtaining photographs is categorized into two groups: treatment or nontreatment and the need for consent differs between the two groups. Nontreatment purposes include education, research, or patient education. Treatment purposes do not technically require patient authorization; however, nontreatment purposes do. According to HIPAA, a situation in which all identifiable information is removed from the photograph is an exception. It is important to recognize that all identifiable information cannot be removed from a face, and merely blacking out the eyes is not acceptable. Facial views therefore will always require formal consent specific to the required use.

Part II

Skin and Soft Tissue

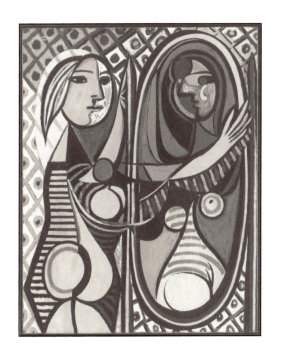

© 2015 Estate of Pablo Picasso / Artists Rights Society (ARS), New York.

14. Structure and Function of Skin

See *Essentials of Plastic Surgery,* second edition, pp. 167-175.

CELLULAR CONTENT OF THE SKIN

1. Match each of the following descriptions to the most appropriate skin cell. (Each option may be used once, more than once, or not at all.)
   A. An epidermal cell involved in the immune response
   B. A neural crest derivative of the epidermis involved in touch
   C. An epidermal cell responsible for increased skin uptake of melanin following sun exposure

Options:
a. Merkel cell
b. Fibroblast
c. Langerhans cell
d. Mast cell
e. Keratinocyte
f. Melanocyte

SENSORY RECEPTORS OF THE SKIN

2. Which one of the following is found in the dermis and is tested by assessing light touch and dynamic two-point discrimination?
   A. Naked nerve fiber
   B. Meissner's corpuscle
   C. Merkel cell
   D. Pacinian corpuscle
   E. Ruffini ending

APPENDAGES OF THE DERMIS

3. Match each of the following descriptions to the most appropriate skin appendage. (Each option may be used once, more than once, or not at all.)
   A. A dermal appendage involved in thermoregulation
   B. A dermal appendage involved in vibration pressure sensation
   C. A dermal appendage involved in sustained pressure and hot temperature sensation

Options:
a. Ruffini ending
b. Bulb of Krause
c. Apocrine sweat gland
d. Pacinian corpuscle
e. Naked nerve fiber
f. Eccrine sweat gland

LAYERS OF THE EPIDERMIS

4. Which one of the following statements is correct regarding the epidermis?
   A. The stratum corneum and stratum lucidum contain viable keratinocytes.
   B. The stratum granulosum is the only layer containing both viable and nonviable cells.
   C. The stratum basale is multilayered and has mitotically active keratinocytes.
   D. The stratum spinosum contains melanocytes, tactile cells, and granular dendrocytes.
   E. The stratum lucidum is translucent and tends to be thicker in the axilla and scalp.

5. **Which one of the following epidermal layers is only found in the hands and feet?**
   A. Stratum basale
   B. Stratum spinosum
   C. Stratum granulosum
   D. Stratum lucidum
   E. Stratum corneum

STRUCTURE AND FUNCTION OF THE DERMIS

6. **Which one of the following statements is correct regarding the dermis?**
   A. The ratio of collagen types I to III is uniform throughout the dermis.
   B. The dermis has a consistent thickness throughout the body.
   C. The papillary dermis represents 30% of total dermal thickness.
   D. Mature elastic fibers are present throughout the entire dermis.
   E. Ground substance facilitates diffusion of metabolites within the dermis.

COLLAGEN SUBTYPES

7. **In which anatomic location is collagen subtype II most likely to be found?**
   A. Bone
   B. Tendon
   C. Hyaline cartilage
   D. Ligament
   E. Blood vessels

SKIN DISORDERS AND WOUND HEALING

8. **For which one of the following patients is it generally acceptable to proceed with elective surgery?**
   A. Iron deficiency
   B. Cutis laxa
   C. Cutis hyperelastica
   D. Hutchinson-Gilford syndrome
   E. Werner's syndrome

CLINICAL SCENARIOS

9. **Match each of the following descriptions to the most likely diagnosis. (Each option may be used once, more than once, or not at all.)**
   A. A 12-year-old girl presents with joint hypermobility; thin, fragile tissue; and subcutaneous hemorrhages.
   B. A 20-year-old patient presents with skin laxity, yellow plaques, and cardiopulmonary problems but has normal wound healing.
   C. A 17-year-old micrognathic patient displays growth retardation, alopecia, and prominent ears.

   Options:
   a. Cutis laxa
   b. Parkes-Weber syndrome
   c. Ehlers-Danlos syndrome
   d. Progeria
   e. Osler-Weber-Rendu disease
   f. Werner's syndrome
   g. Pseudoxanthoma elasticum

Answers

CELLULAR CONTENT OF THE SKIN

1. *For the following descriptions, the best options are as follows:*
   A. *An epidermal cell involved in the immune response*
      c. **Langerhans cell**
   B. *A neural crest derivative of the epidermis involved in touch*
      a. **Merkel cell**
   C. *An epidermal cell responsible for increased skin uptake of melanin following sun exposure*
      e. **Keratinocyte**

   A number of different cells are found within the skin, with functions ranging from provision of structure through sensation, protection, and immunity. Langerhans cells are part of the macrophage/monocyte cell lineage and are antigen-presenting cells involved in immunity. Merkel cells are found in the epidermis, and provide constant touch and pressure sensation. They are thought to be of neuroendocrine origin and are clinically relevant in that they can undergo malignant change resulting in an aggressive form of skin cancer (see Chapter 15).

   The keratinocyte is the predominant cell of the epidermis and provides a protective physical barrier and UV protection by the uptake of melanin produced by melanocytes. A common misunderstanding is that melanocytes retain the melanin pigment and are solely responsible for the increased skin pigmentation with tanning. However it is the increased uptake by keratinocytes, following increased production by the melanocytes, that provides the increased skin pigmentation. Fibroblasts are the building blocks of the dermis and are responsible for collagen production. Mast cells are found within the dermis and are involved in the allergic response (see Table 14-1, *Essentials of Plastic Surgery*, second edition).

SENSORY RECEPTORS OF THE SKIN

2. *Which one of the following is found in the dermis and is responsible for light touch and dynamic two-point discrimination?*
   B. **Meissner's corpuscle**

   All of the answer selections are involved in skin sensation.
   The Meissner's corpuscle is involved in light touch and dynamic two-point discrimination (Fig. 14-1). It represents a type of unmyelinated nerve ending most commonly found in the fingertips and lips. A reduction in the number of Meissner's corpuscles is observed with increasing age and may be partly responsible for age related changes in manual dexterity (see Table 14-1, *Essentials of Plastic Surgery*, second edition).[1]

   Naked nerve fibers or free nerve endings are the simplest sensory receptor and are located along the dermoepidermal junction. They consist of multiple small terminal branches of afferent nerves and provide a primitive function for temperature, touch, and pain sensation. Merkel cells are associated with free nerve endings, particularly in thicker skin. They are also involved with touch and pressure sensation. Pacinian corpuscles are large sensory receptors involved in pressure, coarse touch, vibrations, and tension. They are located in the deeper layers of the skin as well as in ligaments and joint capsules and have the appearance of an onion on microscopy.

Pacinian corpuscles can be recognized when operating around nerve fibers and can be useful to guide dissection when trying to identify damaged or divided nerves, particularly in the palm. Ruffini corpuscles are spindle shaped structures on microscopy found most often in the foot soles. They are associated with pressure and touch sensation.[2]

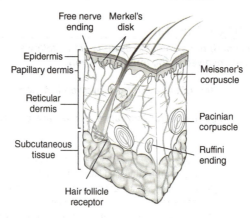

Fig. 14-1 Sensory receptors of the integument.

APPENDAGES OF THE DERMIS

3. *For the following descriptions, the best options are as follows:*
   A. *A dermal appendage involved in thermoregulation*
      f. **Eccrine sweat gland**
   B. *A dermal appendage involved in vibration pressure sensation*
      d. **Pacinian corpuscle**
   C. *A dermal appendage involved in sustained pressure and hot temperature sensation*
      a. **Ruffini ending**

   Eccrine sweat glands are found within the skin throughout the body and are involved in thermoregulation by the production of watery hypotonic fluid, whereas apocrine glands produce thickened secretions in the axilla and groin. These are involved in conditions such as hidradenitis suppurativa where patients have recurrent infective episodes affecting the axilla or groin. Pacinian corpuscles have been described in question 2 and are found within the dermis. They are involved in vibration and deep pressure sensation. Ruffini endings are slow adapting mechanoreceptors found in the skin and are high in density in the nail bed region and foot sole (see Table 14-1, *Essentials of Plastic Surgery,* second edition).

   Krause end bulbs are delicate receptors located in the oropharynx and eye. Naked nerve fibers are the simplest form of sensory receptor with slow rates of conduction. They are located in many supporting structures throughout the body, including the skin.[2]

   Other dermal appendages include the hair follicles, sebaceous glands, and erector pili. An important function of the epithelial lined appendages is in wound healing as they provide a source of epithelial cells to facilitate reepithelialization of partial-thickness injuries (see Chapters 1 and 2).

LAYERS OF THE EPIDERMIS

4. Which one of the following statements is correct regarding the epidermis?
   B. The stratum granulosum is the only layer containing both viable and nonviable cells.
   The epidermis consists of four or five layers, depending on the anatomic location. The layers from superficial to deep may be remembered using the mnemonic, "come let's get some beer." The layers are as follows: stratum corneum, stratum lucidum, stratum granulosum, stratum spinosum, and stratum basale. The upper two layers contain nonviable keratinocytes, while the deepest two layers consist only of viable keratinocytes. The stratum granulosum is the transition zone and is three to four layers thick. It contains both viable and nonviable cells. It has clinical relevance in melanomas as the Breslow thickness is measured from this layer to the deepest part of the tumor. The stratum corneum and stratum lucidum do not contain viable cells. The stratum basale is a single layer and contains melanocytes, tactile cells, granular dendrocytes, and mitotically active keratinocytes. The stratum spinosum contains only viable keratinocytes. The stratum lucidum is translucent but is not present in the axilla or face.

5. Which one of the following epidermal layers is only found in the hands and feet?
   E. Stratum corneum
   The stratum corneum or cornified layer of the skin is only found in glabrous areas which are the sole of the foot and palm. These areas represent the thickest areas of skin and provide excellent protective function (see Table 14-2, *Essentials of Plastic Surgery,* second edition).
   Sometimes these areas are used as skin graft donor sites when palm or foot sole defects are being reconstructed. Two passes are required with the dermatome. The first pass removes the superficial layer of keratinocytes and the second removes a deeper layer used as a graft. The original layer is then replaced on the donor site.

STRUCTURE AND FUNCTION OF THE DERMIS

6. Which one of the following statements is correct regarding the dermis?
   E. Ground substance facilitates diffusion of metabolites in the dermis.
   Ground substance is an amorphous transparent material with a semifluid gel consistency. It allows metabolite diffusion and comprises glycosaminoglycans in the form of hyaluronic acid and proteoglycans. Hyaluronic acid is an important component of ground substance and is used as an injectable filler to plump out the dermis for management of rhytids (see Chapter 88). The dermis comprises two layers: the more superficial papillary dermis and the deeper reticular dermis. The ratio of collagen types I to III differs according to dermal layer, with the papillary dermis having a higher concentration of type III collagen. Dermal thickness has significant variability according to the anatomic location. The scalp, back, palms, and foot soles are generally thickest and the eyelids are thinnest. The papillary dermis is much thinner than the reticular dermis (approximately 1/20th) and has a thickness more similar to the epidermis. Mature elastic fibers are only present in the reticular dermis. Understanding of the different skin layers and being able to recognize them clinically is useful when managing trauma injuries such as burns. Burns are classified according to depth and can be first degree, second degree, and third degree. First degree burns do not involve the dermis and heal quickly. Third degree burns involve the entire dermis and adnexal structures and have a prolonged healing time that means they are usually excised and skin grafted. Second degree burns can be either superficial or deep and will involve different levels of the dermis. In general the more superficial dermal burns can heal within a few weeks because the dermal appendages are present and facilitate reepithelialization. In deeper dermal burns this will not be possible and they are generally treated the same as full-thickness burns.

COLLAGEN SUBTYPES

7. In which anatomic location is collagen subtype II most likely to be found?
  C. Hyaline cartilage
    There are more than 20 types of collagen and of these, type I represents 90% of the body total. Type II is found in the cornea and hyaline cartilage. Other important subtypes are III and IV. Type III predominates in immature wounds, vessel, and bowel walls. Type IV is found in the basement membrane (see Chapter 1 in *Question and Answer* and Table 14-3, *Essentials of Plastic Surgery*, second edition).

SKIN DISORDERS AND WOUND HEALING

8. For which one of the following patients is it generally acceptable to proceed with elective surgery?
  B. Cutis laxa
    Cutis laxa is a very rare condition associated with degeneration of elastic fibers in the dermis. The name is derived from Latin meaning "loose skin" and it therefore results in hyperextensible skin with the appearance of premature aging. It can be autosomal dominant, recessive, or crosslinked and in general recessive inheritance results in the most severe form. It is often most noticeable on the face, neck, axilla, and groin. It can also affect connective tissues of the lungs, heart, vessels, and joints. In spite of this, wound healing is normal and it is considered safe to proceed with surgery.
    In contrast, the other options are all associated with abnormal wound healing. Deficiencies in iron, copper, and vitamin C all interfere with collagen production. Cutis hyperelastica is also known as Ehlers-Danlos syndrome and is a connective tissue disorder with abnormal collagen cross-linking resulting in poor wound healing and thin friable skin. Hutchinson-Gilford and Werner's syndromes are both types of progeria (premature aging conditions) and wound healing is impaired.[3,4]

CLINICAL SCENARIOS

9. For the following scenarios, the best options are as follows:
  A. A 12-year-old patient presents with joint hypermobility; thin, fragile tissue; and subcutaneous hemorrhages.
    c. Ehlers-Danlos syndrome
  B. A 20-year-old patient presents with skin laxity, yellow plaques, and cardiopulmonary problems but has normal wound healing.
    g. Pseudoxanthoma elasticum
  C. A 17-year-old micrognathic patient displays growth retardation, alopecia, and prominent ears.
    d. Progeria

    Ehlers-Danlos syndrome is also known as *Cutis hyperelastica*. It has an incidence of 1:400,000, with variable inheritance patterns. It is a connective tissue disorder with an abnormality of collagen cross-linking. This results in hypermobile joints and thin, friable, and hyperextensive skin. Patients have poor wound healing and a tendency for hypertrophic scarring. Surgery should be avoided when possible.
    Pseudoxanthoma elasticum is a condition with cutaneous, ocular, and cardiac manifestations. The cutaneous manifestations include yellow plaques that typically involve the neck and first appear in adolescence.
    Progeria is also known as *Hutchinson-Gilford syndrome* and is an autosomal recessive condition. It is very rare with an incidence of 1:1,000,000 that has features of premature aging in children. Patients first present with signs such as failure to thrive, retarded growth,

craniosynostoses, micrognathia, baldness, and prominent ears. They display abnormal skin laxity and loss of subcutaneous fat associated with poor wound healing. Werner's syndrome (also known as *adult progeria*) is a rare autosomal recessive condition with features of premature aging. Other associated features include altered skin pigmentation, microangiopathy, diabetes, and a high-pitched voice.

As discussed in question 8 and Chapter 1, cutis laxa is a rare connective tissue disorder in which the skin becomes inelastic and hangs loosely due to degeneration of elastic fibers, but healing is normal. Parkes-Weber syndrome is characterized by an extremity port-wine stain with a deeper venous and lymphatic malformation and an arteriovenous fistula. Osler-Weber-Rendu disease is also known as *hereditary hemorrhagic telangiectasia* and involves multiple malformed ectatic vessels in the skin, mucous membranes, and viscera.

REFERENCES

1. Cauna N, Ross LL. The fine structure of Meissner's touch corpuscles of human fingers. Biophys Biochem Cytol 8:467-482, 1960.
2. Burkitt HG, Young B, Heath JW. Wheater's Functional Histology: A Text and Colour Atlas. London: Churchill Livingstone, 2003.
3. Arnold M, Barbul A. Nutrition and wound healing. Plast Reconstr Surg 117(7 Suppl):42S-58S, 2006.
4. Campos AC, Groth AK, Branco AB. Assessment and nutritional aspects of wound healing. Curr Opin Clin Nutr Metab Care 11:281-288, 2008.

15. Basal Cell Carcinoma, Squamous Cell Carcinoma, and Melanoma

See *Essentials of Plastic Surgery*, second edition, pp. 176-194.

Basal Cell Carcinoma

DEMOGRAPHICS OF BASAL CELL CARCINOMA

1. *Which one of the following statements is correct regarding basal cell carcinoma (BCC)?*
   A. Incidence has recently plateaued.
   B. It more commonly affects females.
   C. It usually affects the trunk and limbs.
   D. The most commonly affected single site is the upper lip.
   E. It is the most common eyelid malignancy.

RISK FACTORS FOR BASAL CELL CARCINOMA

2. *Which one of the following is a risk factor more typical of SCC rather than BCC?*
   A. Immune suppression
   B. Human papilloma virus
   C. Fitzpatrick skin types I and II
   D. Sun exposure
   E. Advancing age

GORLIN'S SYNDROME

3. You are referred a patient with a diagnosis of Gorlin's syndrome. *Which one of the following is a typical feature of this condition?*
   A. Recurrent dental abscesses
   B. Posterior plagiocephaly
   C. Yellowish plaques on the scalp
   D. Multiple small red pits on the palm
   E. Coffee-colored patches in the axilla

BASAL CELL CARCINOMA SUBTYPES

4. *For each of the following descriptions, select the most likely BCC subtype. (Each option may be used once, more than once, or not at all.)*
   A. This is the most common type of BCC.
   B. This is the most aggressive type of BCC.
   C. This type of BCC is often mistaken for psoriasis, fungal infection, or eczema.

   Options:
   a. Superficial spreading
   b. Micronodular
   c. Mixed pattern
   d. Nodular
   e. Infiltrative
   f. Morpheaform

Chapter 15 ▪ Basal Cell and Squamous Cell Carcinoma and Melanoma

RISK STRATIFICATION FOR BASAL CELL CARCINOMA
5. *Which one of the following represents a low-risk BCC?*
   A. A 10 mm diameter BCC on the genitals
   B. A 7 mm diameter BCC on the nasal tip
   C. A 4 mm diameter BCC on the hand with lymphovascular invasion
   D. An 18 mm diameter BCC on the trunk
   E. A 9 mm diameter micronodular BCC on the thigh

NONSURGICAL MANAGEMENT OF BASAL CELL CARCINOMA
6. *Which one of the following is correct?*
   A. Photodynamic therapy (PDT) uses 5-aminolevulinic acid to create free radicals that destroy target cells but its use should be limited to treating superficial BCCs.
   B. Radiation therapy can be used for most types of BCC, is administered as a single treatment dose, and avoids surgery.
   C. Topical treatment of BCCs with Imiquimod or 5-fluorouracil (5-FU) is uniformly effective, because these agents are able to penetrate deep into the reticular dermis.
   D. Standard cryotherapy involves cooling cells to –40° and is indicated for tumors up to 54 mm deep.
   E. Vismodegib has received FDA approval as a first-line BCC treatment as an alternative to surgery or radiation therapy.

SURGICAL MANAGEMENT OF BASAL CELL CARCINOMA
7. You have a patient in the OR with a 5 mm diameter pearly nodular lesion on the forehead which you suspect to be a BCC. It has well-defined borders and visible telangiectasia. *What peripheral excision margin should you use?*
   A. 2 mm
   B. 4 mm
   C. 6 mm
   D. 8 mm
   E. 10 mm

8. *What is the major advantage of Mohs surgery for BCC management?*
   A. The intraoperative time is reduced.
   B. Complex reconstruction is avoided.
   C. Completeness of excision is confirmed intraoperatively.
   D. Cure rates are 100%.
   E. Excision and reconstruction are completed in a single stage.

Cutaneous Squamous Cell Carcinoma

RISK FACTORS FOR SQUAMOUS CELL CARCINOMA
9. *Which one of the following factors most increases the risk of developing an SCC?*
   A. Fitzpatrick skin types I and II
   B. Sun exposure
   C. Arsenic and hydrocarbons
   D. Human papilloma virus
   E. Immune suppression after transplant surgery

SQUAMOUS CELL CARCINOMA–RELATED DEATHS

10. *An SCC on which one of the following sites will most commonly result in death?*
    A. Ear
    B. Lip
    C. Trunk
    D. Limb
    E. Scalp

RISK FACTORS FOR RECURRENCE OF SQUAMOUS CELL CARCINOMA

11. Which one of the following describes a low-risk SCC?
    A. A tumor with depth of invasion of 4 mm
    B. A recurrent tumor
    C. A 2.5 cm diameter tumor
    D. A tumor on the upper lip
    E. A verrucous tumor subtype

TREATMENT OF CUTANEOUS SQUAMOUS CELL CARCINOMA

12. You see an 85-year-old otherwise healthy patient with a thick, necrotic 2 cm diameter SCC involving the left cheek and preauricular region. There is no obvious palpable lymphadenopathy present and the lesion remains mobile over deeper tissues. **Which one of the following is correct regarding management of this patient?**
    A. The lesion should be excised with a 4 mm margin and closed directly.
    B. Radiotherapy is the best modality for management in this case.
    C. The patient is unlikely to benefit from elective nodal dissection.
    D. The lesion must be treated with Mohs micrographic surgery.
    E. Posttreatment follow-up will be every 3 months for 5 years.

Melanoma

MELANOMA SUBTYPES

13. *Which one of the following is the most common melanoma subtype?*
    A. Superficial spreading
    B. Nodular
    C. Lentigo maligna
    D. Acral-lentiginous
    E. Desmoplastic

14. You see a 45-year-old white patient in your office who has evidence of new-onset, single-digit linear pigmented nail streak. You are concerned that this may be melanoma, and you perform a biopsy. **With which melanoma subtype may this presentation be associated?**
    A. Desmoplastic
    B. Amelanotic
    C. Ocular
    D. Superficial spreading
    E. Acral-lentiginous

15. **When assessing a patient in clinic with a suspected melanoma, which one of the following would be most in keeping with development of a nodular subtype?**
    A. Development within a long-standing mole
    B. Development de novo
    C. Development from a Hutchinson freckle
    D. Development within a sun-protected site
    E. Development from a Spitz nevus

MELANOMA PROGNOSIS

16. When reviewing the histopathology report of a melanoma specimen, what is the single most important histologic prognostic factor for the patient?
   A. Mitotic count
   B. Ulceration
   C. Perineural invasion
   D. Breslow thickness
   E. Clark's level

AMERICAN JOINT COMMITTEE ON CANCER MELANOMA STAGING CLASSIFICATION

17. For each of the following scenarios, select the correct melanoma staging classification of the American Joint Committee on Cancer (AJCC). (Each option may be used once, more than once, or not at all.)
   A. A patient has a melanoma of Breslow thickness (BT) 2.5 mm, three nodes, and metastases involving the skin.
   B. A patient has a 0.9 mm BT MM with no nodal or metastatic involvement and a mitotic rate of two per mm^2.
   C. A patient has a melanoma of BT 4.2 mm with micrometastases diagnosed after sentinel node lymph biopsy and no further metastatic spread.

Options:
a. T3N1M1a
b. T3N2M1a
c. T3N2M1b
d. T1aN0M0
e. T1bN0M0
f. T1cN0M0
g. T4N2aM0
h. T4N2bM0
i. T4N3M0

SURGICAL MANAGEMENT OF MELANOMA

18. Which one of the following is correct regarding the surgical management of melanoma?
   A. A full-thickness excision biopsy is required for all suspected melanomas.
   B. Long-term survival is improved by excision of the deep fascial layer during a wide local excision.
   C. Amputation proximal to the proximal interphalangeal joint is recommended for subungual melanomas of the digit.
   D. Sentinel lymph node biopsy is only indicated in stage II and III patients.
   E. A positive Cloquet's node is not the only indication for pelvic dissection.

NONSURGICAL MANAGEMENT OF MELANOMA

19. Which one of the following is correct regarding nonsurgical management of melanoma?
   A. Sentinel lymph node biopsy is a useful therapeutic treatment for melanoma.
   B. Elective lymph node dissection shows a survival benefit only with melanomas greater than 4 mm.
   C. The use of dacarbazine or cisplatin may help to reduce the tumor burden.
   D. Radiation therapy is often indicated as a primary treatment for cutaneous melanoma.
   E. Interferon alpha-2 can give a disease-free survival benefit in early disease.

EXCISION MARGINS IN MELANOMA

20. For each of the following scenarios, select the most appropriate peripheral surgical excision margin based on current evidence. (Each option may be used once, more than once, or not at all.)
    A. A primary melanoma with a BT of 3.2 mm
    B. An in situ melanoma
    C. A primary melanoma with a BT of 0.9 mm

    Options:
    a. 1 mm
    b. 5 mm
    c. 1 cm
    d. 2 cm
    e. 3 cm
    f. 4 cm

TREATMENT IN ADVANCED-STAGE MELANOMA

21. In a patient with stage IV melanoma who has tested positive for BRAF, which one of the following treatment modalities is specifically indicated?
    A. Radiotherapy
    B. Dacarbazine
    C. Cisplatin
    D. Vemurafenib
    E. Vinblastin

22. Which one of the following is a monoclonal antibody directed to the receptor CTLA-4, approved by the FDA for patients with unresectable melanoma?
    A. Ipilimumab
    B. MAGE-A3
    C. Imatinib
    D. Interleukin-2
    E. Canvaxin

MELANOMA FOLLOW-UP

23. Following complete resection of a 2.5 mm Breslow thickness melanoma from the calf, for how long should a patient be followed, assuming they have no palpable lymph nodes?
    A. One year
    B. Two years
    C. Five years
    D. Ten years
    E. Lifelong

Chapter 15 ▪ Basal Cell and Squamous Cell Carcinoma and Melanoma

General Topics in Skin Cancer

CLINICAL SCENARIOS IN SKIN CANCER

24. Match each of the following descriptions to the most appropriate clinical diagnosis. (Each option may be used once, more than once, or not at all.)
   A. A 65-year-old patient presents with multiple raised verrucous papules with varied deep pigmentation affecting the back.
   B. A teenage patient presents with a single yellowish verrucous plaque on the neck.
   C. A young adult presents with multiple BCCs and opacity of the mandible on panorex or radiograph.

Options:
   a. Pyogenic granuloma
   b. Amelanotic melanoma
   c. Becker nevus
   d. Gorlin's syndrome
   e. Seborrheic keratosis
   f. Pigmented BCC
   g. Nevus of Jadassohn
   h. Xeroderma pigmentosum

25. Match each of the following descriptions to the most appropriate clinical diagnosis. (Each option may be used once, more than once, or not at all.)
   A. A patient has a dome-shaped keratotic lesion that displayed initial rapid growth followed by spontaneous regression after 7 weeks.
   B. A patient has red plaques involving the penis, and the histology shows cytologic atypia and normal basal cells.
   C. This is the most common premalignant lesion of the oral mucosa, with a 15% risk of malignant transformation.

Options:
   a. Marjolin's ulcer
   b. SCC
   c. BCC
   d. Erythroplasia of Queyrat
   e. Actinic keratosis
   f. Merkel cell tumor
   g. Erythroplakia
   h. Leukoplakia
   i. Keratoacanthoma

Answers

Basal Cell Carcinoma

DEMOGRAPHICS OF BASAL CELL CARCINOMA

1. *Which one of the following statements is correct regarding basal cell carcinoma (BCC)?*
   E. It is the most common eyelid malignancy.
   BCC is a malignant tumor of the skin arising from the basal cells of the epidermis and it represents the most common type of eyelid malignancy. It is the most common type of skin cancer with more than 2 million cases reported annually in the U.S. It has rapidly rising incidence which is probably due to a combination of increasing population age, increased sun exposure, and better detection. Males are affected more commonly than females. At least 80% of BCCs occur in the head and neck region with the most common sites being the nose, eyelid, and ear. Other sites that are often affected include the cheek, lip, neck, and brow.

RISK FACTORS FOR BASAL CELL CARCINOMA

2. *Which one of the following is a risk factor more typically of SCC rather than BCC?*
   B. Human papilloma virus
   Human papilloma virus (HPV) is not associated with development of BCCs. It is however associated with SCC of the skin and mucous membranes such as the oropharynx and oral cavity. It also is implicated in cervical cancer. Risk factors for BCC include skin type and color, increasing age, male sex, sun exposure, immune compromise, genetic predisposition, and carcinogen exposure.

GORLIN'S SYNDROME

3. You are referred a patient with a diagnosis of Gorlin's syndrome. *Which one of the following is a typical feature of this condition?*
   D. Multiple small red pits on the palm
   A common finding in patients with Gorlin's syndrome is the presence of multiple small red pits on the palm or foot sole. They appear as small depressions and are caused by partial or complete absence of the stratum corneum. They are typically 2 to 3 mm diameter with a similar depth. They are present in up to one third of patients by the start of the second decade, and almost all patients by age 20.[1] Although the presence of three or more palmar pits constitutes a major diagnostic criterion in Gorlin syndrome, pits may also be seen in patients with other conditions, such as psoriasis.[2]

   Gorlin's syndrome (nevoid basal cell syndrome) is an autosomal dominant condition affecting chromosome 9 that is characterized by multiple BCCs at an early age. These patients will require lifelong review and multiple procedures for tumor excision. Another common feature associated with Gorlin's is development of odontogenic keratocysts, which show as radiolucent areas on panore. Recurrent dental abscesses are not a specific finding. There are often cranial abnormalities which include absence of the falx cerebri, hypertelorism, and a broad nasal root. Neither posterior plagiocephaly or recurrent dental abscesses are typical findings. A yellowish plaque on the skin may represent a sebaceous nevus which itself is benign but has the potential for transformation to BCC in around 10% of cases. Coffee-colored patches are typical of neurofibromatosis.

BASAL CELL CARCINOMA SUBTYPES

4. *For the following scenarios, the best options are as follows:*
   A. *This is the most common type of BCC.*
      d. Nodular
   B. *This the most aggressive type of BCC.*
      f. Morpheaform
   C. *This type of BCC is often mistaken for psoriasis, fungal infection, or eczema.*
      a. Superficial spreading

   More than 20 subtypes of BCC have been described. The most common subtype is nodular (50% to 60%) and other common subtypes are micronodular (15%), and superficial spreading (9% to 15%) (see Fig. 15-1, *Essentials of Plastic Surgery*, second edition).

   Subtypes differ in their behavior and the most aggressive is morpheaform which have a high incidence of positive margins following excision. These tend to present as an "enlarging scar" without history of trauma and have a flat or slightly elevated scarlike appearance. Infiltrative subtypes are also quite aggressive, whereas nodular subtypes are fairly low risk.

   The classic appearance of a BCC is a raised lesion with a rolled edge, visible telangiectasia and central ulceration. This appearance is most in keeping with a nodular subtype. Superficial spreading BCCs are located in the epidermis with no dermal invasion. They are pink, flat scaly patches with ulceration and crusting rather than the classic nodular appearances described above. Accordingly, they can be confused with fungal infections or eczema.

RISK STRATIFICATION FOR BASAL CELL CARCINOMA

5. *Which one of the following represents a low-risk BCC?*
   D. An 18 mm diameter BCC on the trunk

   BCCs less than 2 cm diameter on the trunk or proximal limbs are considered low-risk lesions. Low-risk subtypes are nodular and superficial. High-risk subtypes are morpheaform, sclerosing, and micronodular. Risk factors for the recurrence of BCCs depend on many factors including the subtype, diameter, depth, anatomic site, clarity of borders, rate of growth, and histopathologic findings (see Table 15-2, *Essentials of Plastic Surgery,* second edition). High-risk lesions based on size (diameter) are larger than 2 cm on the trunk or proximal limbs; larger than 1 cm on the cheek, forehead, or scalp; and larger than 6 mm on the central face, genitalia, hands, or feet. Other factors suggestive of high risk include poor differentiation, perineural/lymphovascular invasion, rapid growth, and recurrent tumors. In a standard histopathological report key features should be detailed such as subtype, diameter, depth, completeness of excision (mm), perineural or perivascular involvement, and tumor growth/regression in order to determine further treatment and the risk of recurrence.

NONSURGICAL MANAGEMENT OF BASAL CELL CARCINOMA

6. *Which one of the following is correct?*
   A. Photodynamic therapy (PDT) uses 5-aminolevulinic acid to create free radicals that destroy target cells but its use should be limited to treating superficial BCCs.

   PDT uses the light-activated photosensitizing drug 5-aminolevulinic acid to create oxygen free radicals that selectively destroy target cells. It can be used in premalignant or superficial lesions, but should not be used in deeper or high-risk lesions. Radiation therapy provides an alternative to surgery and can be effective for most BCCs. It tends to be reserved for older patients (age 60 and older) and has cure rates >90%. One of the caveats of radiation therapy is that multiple treatments are required over a four- to six-week period and it requires a diagnostic biopsy to be obtained before treatment. Furthermore, completeness of excision cannot be confirmed and subsequent surgery to the area is more challenging. Topical treatments with either Imiquimod or 5-FU can be effective in low-risk superficial lesions, because they can destroy the surface cells. They should not be used in deeper lesions because they cannot destroy deeper cells and risk growth recurrence due to residual tumor cell presence. Standard cryotherapy involves cooling the tissues to −40° during repeated freeze-thaw cycles, but it is not indicated for tumors deeper than 3 mm. It has a more useful role in management of early actinic keratosis. Vismodegib is a hedgehog inhibitor with FDA approval for use in locally advanced BCC when other treatment forms have been exhausted, and therefore is not a first line treatment. Adverse effects include muscle spasm, alopecia, ageusia, and fatigue.

SURGICAL MANAGEMENT OF BASAL CELL CARCINOMA

7. You have a patient in the OR with a 5 mm diameter pearly nodular lesion on the forehead which you suspect to be a BCC. It has well-defined borders and visible telangiectasia. *What peripheral excision margin should you use?*

   B. 4 mm

   Excision margins required for well-defined BCCs are commonly 4 mm, while those for infiltrative subtypes are significantly greater. Studies have been undertaken using Mohs techniques to assess completeness of excision in BCCs with increasing margins. These studies have shown that excision of small (<20 mm) well-defined lesions using a 3 mm peripheral margin will result in complete removal in 85% of cases. Increasing this margin to 4 mm will increase complete excision rates to around 95%. This suggests that around 5% of well-defined BCCs will have tumor extension beyond 4 mm that cannot be identified clinically. Morpheaform and large BCCs will require peripheral margins of 13 to 15 mm to achieve 95% complete excision. Margins of 3 mm and 5 mm provide clearance in only 66% and 82% of these cases, respectively. Depth of excision is less well guided but in general taking a cuff of subcutaneous fat with the specimen is believed to be sufficient. In cases where completeness of excision is uncertain at the time of surgery, a further deeper specimen should be taken and carefully labeled. If excision is still uncertain then the wound should be temporized with a dressing and histological confirmation of completeness should be obtained before proceeding with reconstruction.[3-5]

   Mohs micrographic surgery involves sequential horizontal excision using a topographic map of the lesion and repeated excision until all positive tumor margins are clear. Reported cure rates are higher than standard excision at 99%. In addition, tissue conservation is increased. For this reason, Mohs is indicated not only in recurrent tumors but also in primary tumors in cosmetically sensitive areas, aggressive tumor subtypes such as morpheaform and sclerosing variants and those with poorly delineated peripheral margins.

8. *What is the major advantage of Mohs surgery for BCC management?*

   C. Completeness of excision is confirmed intraoperatively.

   Mohs micrographic surgery involves sequential horizontal excision using a topographic map of the lesion with repeated excision until all positive tumor margins are clear. The main benefits are that completeness can be confirmed because tissue is assessed at every margin and this is confirmed at the time of surgery. In contrast, standard histological analysis does not sample every margin so completeness cannot be guaranteed. Furthermore, the procedure would need to be staged if confirmation of excision is required before reconstruction. Reported cure rates

are higher than standard excision at 99%, but 100% cure is still not achieved. A further benefit is that tissue conservation is increased because only involved margins are reexcised in contrast to a standard surgical approach where an arbitrary margin is taken. For this reason, Mohs is indicated in both primary and recurrent tumors, particularly those in cosmetically sensitive areas. It is also useful in treating aggressive tumor subtypes such as morpheaform and sclerosing variants and those with poorly delineated peripheral margins. The problem with Mohs is that it takes significantly longer to treat each patient and the patients must wait for the analysis to be performed at each excision stage. Patients still require complex reconstruction in many cases with flaps or grafts. Some Mohs surgeons can and do reconstruct the defects created, but many will return the patient back to the reconstructive plastic surgeon once excision is complete. Therefore many patients still have a staged procedure with regard to reconstruction.

Cutaneous Squamous Cell Carcinoma

RISK FACTORS FOR SQUAMOUS CELL CARCINOMA

9. **Which one of the following factors most increases the risk of developing an SCC?**
   E. **Immune suppression after transplant surgery**
   All of the options represent risk factors for SCC. However, the risk of developing an SCC after immunosuppression for renal transplant is increased by 253 times, making this the most significant single-risk factor. Immunosuppression after transplant usually involves combination therapy with steroids (prednisolone) and immunomodulators such as mycophenolate mofetil (MMF) and tacrolimus.
   Patients with lighter skin tones (Fitzpatrick I to II) have an increased risk. Overall lifetime sun exposure, episodes of sunburn, and the use of tanning beds can further increase the risk. Carcinogens implicated include pesticides, arsenic, and organic hydrocarbons. Viruses such as HPV and herpes are also implicated. This emphasizes the importance of assessing these areas during history in patients with suspected SCCs and providing prevention advice.

SQUAMOUS CELL CARCINOMA–RELATED DEATHS

10. **An SCC on which one of the following sites will most commonly result in death?**
    A. **Ear**
    SCCs arising on the external ear are particularly high-risk lesions that can spread through the lymphatics to the parotid gland and neck. Of all the head and neck skin SCC sites, the pinna is considered to be the most likely site to result in death. Other high-risk sites include the temple, forehead, scalp, and lower lip. In each of these sites, metastatic spread can occur in the neck or parotid nodes. For this reason elective nodal dissection may be considered in some cases. Other high-risk factors for metastases should also be considered such as tumor diameter (>2 cm), depth (>4 mm), poor differentiation, incomplete margins, and perineural invasion as a tumor spread can proceed along nerves.[6-9]

RISK FACTORS FOR RECURRENCE OF SQUAMOUS CELL CARCINOMA

11. **Which one of the following describes a low-risk SCC?**
    E. **A verrucous tumor subtype**
    Many factors are used to classify SCCs as low-risk or high-risk.[10] Factors that characterize low-risk lesions include the following: sun-exposed sites, excluding the lip and the ear, diameter less than 2 cm, depth less than 4 mm, tumor confined to the dermis, well-differentiated or verrucous subtypes, and no evidence of host immune suppression. Factors that characterize

high-risk lesions are the following: involvement of the ear or lip, diameter greater than 2 cm, depth greater than 4 mm, moderate or poor differentiation, host immune suppression, recurrence, and non-sun-exposed sites such as the perineum (see Table 15-1, *Essentials of Plastic Surgery*, second edition).

TREATMENT OF CUTANEOUS SQUAMOUS CELL CARCINOMA

12. You see an 85-year-old otherwise healthy patient with a thick, necrotic 2 cm diameter SCC involving the left cheek and preauricular region. There is no obvious palpable lymphadenopathy present and the lesion remains mobile over deeper tissues. **Which one of the following is correct regarding management of this patient?**
    C. The patient is unlikely to benefit from elective nodal dissection.
    Wide local excision is the most suitable management for this patient and a peripheral margin greater than 6 mm is required. Many surgeons would opt for a 1 cm margin in this case given the size and thickness of the tumor and its anatomic location. Cure rates for primary surgery are around 95%. Wound closure in patients of this age group is usually achieved with local flap techniques given the skin laxity in the cheek and neck at this age. Primary radiotherapy has a cure rate of 90% and is reserved for patients in whom surgery is not advisable, or as adjuvant therapy in high-stage large or recurrent tumors.

    Elective lymph node dissection is not advocated for cutaneous SCC, in contrast to an equivalently sized intraoral tumor. The technique is, however, indicated in cases where there is evidence of tumor spread to the parotid capsule or contiguous nodal basin drainage as may be suggested by adherence of the tumor to underlying deep structures. SLNB is sometimes indicated for node-negative patients with high-risk tumors. Mohs surgery is not required in this case given the high cure rates with standard surgical techniques. Following surgical excision, the patient should be followed up in clinic for an extended period. This should be on a 3- to 6-month basis for 2 years, then every 6 to 12 months for 3 years, then annually thereafter.

Melanoma

MELANOMA SUBTYPES

13. **Which one of the following is the most common melanoma subtype?**
    A. Superficial spreading
    There are a number of different melanoma subtypes and the most common cutaneous variant is superficial spreading, representing more than half of all melanomas (50% to 70%). Nodular subtypes are the next most common, representing between 15% to 30% of all cases. Lentigo maligna and acral-lentiginous usually each represent less than 10% of all melanomas, and desmoplastic subtypes are least common, representing around 1% of all cases.

14. You see a 45-year-old white patient in your office who has evidence of new-onset, single-digit linear pigmented nail streak. You are concerned that this may be melanoma, and you perform a biopsy. **With which melanoma subtype may this presentation be associated?**
    E. Acral-lentiginous
    Acral-lentiginous melanoma can occur on the palms and foot soles, subungually, or in other sun-protected sites. Melanonychia is often a benign finding, but if it involves a single digit, it should raise concerns. Melanonychia represents a linear pigmented streak within the nail and is associated with this melanoma subtype.

Chapter 15 ▪ Basal Cell and Squamous Cell Carcinoma and Melanoma   121

15. **When assessing a patient in clinic with a suspected melanoma, which one of the following would be most in keeping with development of a nodular subtype?**
   B. Development de novo
   Development of melanoma commonly differs between subtypes. For example, nodular melanoma typically arises de novo in normal skin. It appears as a dome-shaped pigmented lesion that may resemble a blood blister. It displays a lack of horizontal growth so keeps sharp demarcation. Nodular melanomas are aggressive and more commonly affect men. Superficial spreading subtypes tend to arise from long-standing junctional or compound nevi, and patients may have noticed a change in the color, size, or borders of the lesion. These tumors tend to have a prolonged horizontal growth before vertical growth commences. A Hutchinson freckle is also known as a senile freckle or lentigo maligna and this is an in situ melanoma. It can progress to form lentigo maligna melanoma, which is the least aggressive subtype and is related to sun exposure. The Hutchinson freckle represents the horizontal growth phase and the vertical growth phase represents the transition to melanoma. Melanomas in sun-protected sites tend to be acral-lentiginous and are seen on the soles or palms. They have a long radial growth phase followed by transition to a vertical growth phase. A spitz nevus is a smooth dome-shaped benign lesion seen in children or young adults that represents a proliferation of enlarged spindle melanocytes. It does not represent a precursor to melanoma, although there is a melanoma subtype call spitzoid melanoma that has a similar histologic appearance to a spitz nevus.

MELANOMA PROGNOSIS

16. **When reviewing the histopathology report of a melanoma specimen, what is the single most important histologic prognostic factor for the patient?**
   D. Breslow thickness
   All of the options are important factors in melanoma, but Breslow thickness (BT) is the single most important factor. It represents the measurement of tumor depth from the granular layer of the epidermis to the deepest extension of the tumor. BT is used to stage the disease using the TNM classification system and to plan subsequent treatment. A number of key features will be displayed on a histological report for melanoma including those listed in answer options A, B, C, and E. For example, the mitotic rate (especially relevant to tumors less than 1 mm deep) and ulceration (relevant to all tumors), perineural or perivascular invasion, and Clark's level which relates to the anatomic depth of the tumor. Completeness of excision is also critical to plan further management, and subtype and growth phase are both important to provide information on prognosis.

AMERICAN JOINT COMMITTEE ON CANCER MELANOMA STAGING CLASSIFICATION

17. **For the following scenarios, the best options are as follows (see Table 15-3, Essentials of Plastic Surgery, second edition):**
   A. *A patient has a melanoma of Breslow thickness (BT) 2.5 mm, three nodes, and metastases involving the skin.*
      b. T3N2M1a
   B. *A patient has a 0.9 mm BT MM with no nodal or metastatic involvement and a mitotic rate of two per mm^2.*
      e. T1bN0M0
   C. *A patient has a melanoma of BT 4.2 mm with micrometastases diagnosed after sentinel node lymph biopsy and no further metastatic spread.*
      g. T4N2aM0

The American Joint Committee on Cancer (AJCC) has produced guidelines for melanoma staging based on the TNM (tumor, node, metastasis) system. In this classification, tumors are initially classified by their Breslow depth as T1 to T4 lesions, with lesions less than 1 mm graded as T1, those between 1.01 mm and 2.0 mm as T2, those between 2.01 mm and 4.0 mm as T3, and those greater than 4 mm as T4. The presence of ulceration or mitotic rate greater than 1 will upgrade a T1a lesion to T1b. For T2, 3, and 4 tumors the presence of ulceration will upgrade them to T2b, 3b, and, 4b, respectively. The mitotic rate does not alter the T classification for these tumors.[11]

Nodal status is N0 (no spread), N1 (spread to one nearby lymph node), N2 (spread to 2 or 3 nearby lymph nodes) and N3 (spread to 4 or more lymph nodes). Again this is further altered by pathological information on micrometastases, in transit satellites, and macrometastases which may be obtained following SNLB or excisional surgery.

Metastatic spread is subclassified as M1a, b, or c, depending on the extent and type of metastases present.

Once the T, N, and M groups have been determined, they are combined to give an overall stage called stage grouping. This provides prognostic information which is also used to guide treatment (Tables 15-1 and 15-2).

Table 15-1 *AJCC TNM Melanoma Staging Classification, 2010*

Tumor Classification	Depth of Invasion
TX	Primary tumor cannot be assessed
Tis	Melanoma in situ
T1	<1.0 mm
T2	1.01-2.0 mm
T3	2.01-4.0 mm
T4	>4.0 mm

NOTE: a and b subcategories of T: a, without ulceration and mitosis <1/mm^2; b, with ulceration or mitoses >1/mm^2.

Node Classification	
NX	Cannot be assessed
N1	One node
N2	Two to three nodes
N3	Four or more nodes, matted, or in transit satellites with metastatic nodes

NOTE: a, b, and c subcategories of N: a, micrometastasis (diagnosed after sentinel lymph node biopsy); b, macrometastasis (clinically positive nodes); c, in transit satellites without nodes (N2 only).

Metastatic Classification	
M1a	Metastases to skin, subcutaneous, distant nodes
M1b	Metastases to lung
M1c	Metastases to other viscera or any distant site combined with elevated serum LDH

Chapter 15 ▪ Basal Cell and Squamous Cell Carcinoma and Melanoma

Table 15-2 *Pathologic Staging*

Stage	Tumor	Node	Metastasis
Stage 0	Tis	N0	M0
Stage IA	T1a	N0	M0
Stage IB	T1b	N0	M0
	T2a	N0	M0
Stage IIA	T2b	N0	M0
	T3a	N0	M0
Stage IIB	T3b	N0	M0
	T4a	N0	M0
Stage IIC	T4b	N0	M0
Stage IIIA	T(1-4)a	N1a	M0
	T(1-4)a	N2a	M0
Stage IIIB	T(1-4)b	N1a or N2a	M0
	T(1-4)a	N1b, N2b, or N2c	M0
Stage IIIC	T(1-4)b	N1b, N2b, or N2c	M0
	Any T	N3	M0
Stage IV	Any T	Any N	M1

SURGICAL MANAGEMENT OF MELANOMA

18. **Which one of the following is correct regarding the surgical management of melanoma?**

   E. **A positive Cloquet's node is not the only indication for pelvic dissection.**

   In patients with positive nodal disease or positive sentinel lymph nodes, therapeutic lymph node dissection is advocated. In patients with positive groin disease an extended procedure to include dissection of pelvic nodes is required in some cases. The indications include where multiple groin nodes are clinically palpable, where there is CT or ultrasound evidence of multiple groin nodes involved, where multiple groin nodes are found to be positive during sentinel lymph node biopsy (SLNB), and where there is a conglomerate of groin nodes.

   Full-thickness excision biopsies (1 to 3 mm margins) are required for the vast majority of suspected melanomas in order to confirm diagnosis, completely remove the lesion and fully assess their histological features including Breslow thickness. However, full-thickness biopsies are not required for subungual melanoma as this offers no prognostic information. Incisional biopsies may be considered for low-suspicion lesions or cosmetically sensitive regions. Shave biopsies are not recommended.

   Long-term survival is not improved by excising the deep fascial layer and recommendations are to perform the wide local excision down to the fascial layer only. Removal of the fascia may increase metastatic spread. Recommendations for subungual melanoma are that amputation is performed proximal to the distal interphalangeal joint, not the proximal interphalangeal joint. Sentinel lymph node biopsy is a staging procedure and is indicated in both stage Ib and stage II disease but not stage III, as by definition nodal spread must have already taken place.

NONSURGICAL MANAGEMENT OF MELANOMA

19. **Which one of the following is correct regarding nonsurgical management of melanoma?**

   C. **The use of dacarbazine or cisplatin may help to reduce the tumor burden.**

   As discussed in question 18, dacarbazine and cisplatin are chemotherapy agents that may be considered in melanoma to reduce tumor burden, but they are generally only palliative. Sentinel lymph node biopsy is a staging procedure, not a therapeutic procedure, that is used in patients with intermediate depth melanomas in order to identify whether the tumor has spread to the sentinel lymph node. If SNLB is positive, then progression to completion lymphadenectomy should proceed. There remains debate about the clinical benefits of SNLB as overall life expectancy does not appear to be improved, but local tumor recurrence may be; further evidence is awaited. Elective lymph node dissection appears to have a survival benefit only in intermediate melanoma (1 to 2 mm) and is not routinely performed because of the comorbidity involved unless the SLNB or clinical examination is positive for lymph node involvement. Radiation therapy is rarely indicated as a primary treatment of melanoma except for lentigo maligna or desmoplastic lesions. Interferon can be useful in patients with regional nodal disease or deep primary tumors.

EXCISION MARGINS IN MELANOMA

20. For the following scenarios, the best options are as follows:
    A. A primary melanoma with a BT of 3.2 mm
       d. 2 cm
    B. An in situ melanoma
       b. 5 mm
    C. A primary melanoma with a BT of 0.9 mm
       c. 1 cm

    Evidence for the selection of excision margins in melanoma is provided by six key papers considering five major studies.[12-18]

    Recommended peripheral margins for melanoma excision vary between different guidelines and this reflects the available evidence and differences in its interpretation (Table 15-3).

    In situ disease is commonly excised with a 5 mm margin. Melanomas less than 1 mm in depth are commonly excised with a 1 cm margin. Thicker melanomas are excised with a 2 cm margin.

    Most evidence for peripheral margin selection relates to melanoma on the trunk and excludes the head, neck, and distal limbs. In clinical practice, margins should be tailored to patients on an individual basis depending on site, size, and tumor biology, ideally in a multidisciplinary team setting.

Table 15-3 United States Excision Margin Guidelines for Melanoma Excision

Primary Tumor Type	Recommended Peripheral Excision Margin	Commonly Recommended Deep Excision Margin
In situ disease	5 mm	Cuff of subcutaneous tissue
Less than 1 mm Breslow depth	1 cm	To next fascial plane
1.01 mm to 2 mm Breslow depth	1 to 2 cm (wider is preferable if possible, depending on tumor site, patient, and surgeon preference)	To next fascial plane
2.01 mm to 4 mm Breslow depth	1 to 2 cm (wider is preferable if possible, depending on tumor site, patient, and surgeon preference)	To next fascial plane
Greater than 4.01 mm Breslow depth	2 cm	To next fascial plane

Chapter 15 ▪ Basal Cell and Squamous Cell Carcinoma and Melanoma 125

TREATMENT IN ADVANCED-STAGE MELANOMA

21. In a patient with stage IV melanoma who has tested positive for BRAF, which one of the following treatment modalities is specifically indicated?

D. Vemurafenib

Vemurafenib is a BRAF inhibitor with FDA approval that is used for advanced-stage melanoma. It is indicated in patients who are BRAF-positive (i.e., those who have a mutation of the intracellular signaling kinase BRAF). Mutations in the BRAF gene are present in 40% to 70% of melanomas, leading to uncontrolled cell proliferation. Vemurafenib has been shown to increase overall survival and progression-free survival when compared with dacarbazine (a standard monochemotherapeutic agent).[19] Although the survival improvements have been statistically significant, the real benefits have been modest as lifespan was extended by just a few months in most cases. A further problem with BRAF inhibitors such as vemurafenib is that resistance can occur. For this reason, combination therapy is also being studied. Also, patients have an increased risk of developing SCC while taking this treatment. Furthermore the financial implications of using this drug are significant with a course of treatment costing many thousands of dollars. Radiotherapy may be indicated as adjuvant treatment following lymphadenectomy with more significant disease and can be used in palliation for metastatic disease. Dacarbazine, cisplatin, and vinblastin are standard chemotherapy agents used in combination rather than individually that are generally palliative only with modest response rates.[20]

22. Which one of the following is a monoclonal antibody directed to the receptor CTLA-4, approved by the FDA for patients with unresectable melanoma?

A. Ipilimumab

Immune-based treatment options for patients with advanced-stage melanoma can be subclassified as immune agents such as interleukin-2, checkpoint inhibitors such as ipilimumab, or signal transduction inhibitors such as vemurafenib (described in question 21) and trametinib.

Ipilimumab is a monoclonal antibody that blocks the CTLA-4 receptor (a downregulator of T-cells). The resultant stimulation of T-cells may present a risk for immune-related reactions. It received FDA approval in 2011 for patients with advanced-stage melanoma. Imatinib (also known as *Glivec*) is a tyrosine kinase inhibitor that works by blocking growth pathways within a variety of tumors. Canvaxin and MAGE-A3 have been trialed as vaccines against melanoma in advanced disease, but results have not been particularly successful.

MELANOMA FOLLOW-UP

23. Following complete resection of a 2.5 mm Breslow thickness melanoma from the calf, how long should a patient be followed, assuming they have no palpable lymph nodes?

E. Lifelong

Standard follow-up for melanoma patients varies according to country but in the U.S. lifelong surveillance is currently advised by the National Comprehensive Cancer Network (NCCN) and American Academy of Dermatology (AAD). The German Cancer Society and German Dermatologic Society recommend ten-year follow-up for most stages as do the Swiss, while the British Association of dermatologists advise follow-up according to stage and this varies from five to ten years. The Australian and New Zealand guidelines also vary according to stage with five-year follow-up advised for stage I and lifelong for stages II and III.

Typical follow-up will involve clinical assessment with review of the primary site and nodal basins as well as review of other skin sites for new or changing pigmented lesions. Local recurrence usually occurs within 5 cm of the original lesion within the first 3 to 5 years. In the first five years patients are typically seen at 3- to 6-monthly intervals. Beyond five years patients are seen on an annual basis. Routine imaging beyond five years is not recommended.[21]

General Topics in Skin Cancer

CLINICAL SCENARIOS IN SKIN CANCER

24. For the following scenarios, the best options are as follows:
   A. A 65-year-old patient presents with multiple raised verrucous papules with varied deep pigmentation affecting the back.
      e. Seborrheic keratosis
   B. A teenage patient with a single yellowish verrucous plaque on the neck.
      g. Nevus of Jadassohn
   C. A young adult with multiple BCCs and opacity of the mandible on panorex or radiograph.
      d. Gorlin's syndrome

   Seborrheic keratoses are benign lesions commonly found on the trunk of older patients. They are slow growing and have a raised verrucous appearance with varying degrees of pigmentation. They may often be mistaken for melanomas but do not usually require excision unless patients are catching them leading to traumatic bleeding episodes.

   A sebaceous nevus of Jadassohn is a yellowish plaque that is present at birth and often changes during puberty. It has a 10% to 15% chance of malignant transformation to a BCC and is therefore excised on a preventative basis. Gorlin's syndrome is an autosomal dominant inherited condition, discussed in question 3, associated with multiple BCCs, odontogenic keratocysts, palmar and plantar pits, calcification of the falx cerebri, and bifid ribs.

   A pyogenic granuloma represents an unstable benign lesion that appears following trauma. It appears as a raised lesion that frequently bleeds. It is excised and sent for histological analysis. Amelanotic melanoma can be difficult to diagnose as by its nature it is nonpigmented. Diagnosis is by excision and histological analysis. Pigmented BCCs may mimic melanomas and can sometimes be confused with seborrheic keratosis. Where there is doubt regarding the diagnosis, excision and histological analysis is justified. Xeroderma pigmentosum is an autosomal recessive inherited condition of impaired DNA synthesis that results in multiple epithelial malignancies.

25. For the following scenarios, the best options are as follows:
   A. A patient has a dome-shaped keratotic lesion that displayed initial rapid growth followed by spontaneous regression after 7 weeks.
      i. Keratoacanthoma
   B. A patient has red plaques involving the penis, and the histology shows cytologic atypia and normal basal cells.
      d. Erythroplasia of Queyrat
   C. This is the most common premalignant lesion of the oral mucosa, with a 15% risk of malignant transformation.
      h. Leukoplakia

   Keratoacanthomas are premalignant skin lesions with a typical domed-shaped appearance and a keratin plug. Their clinical and histologic appearance closely resembles a well-differentiated SCC. They usually progress rapidly over a number of weeks before spontaneous regression begins. They are frequently excised to exclude an SCC diagnosis. Bowen's disease is an in situ condition displaying an erythematous plaque with sharp borders and slight scaling. When found on the penis, vulva, or oral mucosa, they are known as *erythroplasia of Queyrat*.

Leukoplakia is the most commonly seen premalignant lesion of the oral mucosa and appears as a white patch. Erythroplakia is less common but has a higher risk of malignant change. Actinic keratosis is commonly seen in elderly white patients with a significant lifetime sun exposure. The lesions appear as scaly, keratotic macules, or papules and often respond well to treatment with 5-FU or cryotherapy. They have a risk of transformation to SCC. Merkel cell tumors can have a similar clinical appearance to BCC or SCC or nodular melanoma and should be promptly excised with a generous margin. They tend to be locally aggressive even with complete excision and patients should be followed closely.

REFERENCES

1. Lo Muzio L. Nevoid basal cell carcinoma syndrome (Gorlin syndrome). Orphanet J Rare Dis 3:32, 2008.
2. Kimonis VE, Goldstein AM, Pastakia B, et al. Clinical manifestations in 105 persons with nevoid basal cell carcinoma syndrome. Am J Med Genet 69:299-308, 1997.
3. Breuninger H, Dietz K. Prediction of subclinical tumor infiltration in basal cell carcinoma. J Dermatol Surg Oncol 17:574-578, 1991.
4. Wolf DJ, Zitelli JA. Surgical margins for basal cell carcinoma. Arch Dermatol 123:340-344, 1987.
5. Kimyai-Asadi A, Goldberg LH, Peterson SR, et al. Efficacy of narrow-margin excision of well-demarcated primary facial basal cell carcinomas. J Am Acad Dermatol 53:464-468, 2005.
6. Veness MJ. High-risk cutaneous squamous cell carcinoma of the head and neck. J Biomed Biotechnol 8:572, 2007.
7. Habif TP, ed. Clinical Dermatology: A Color Guide to Diagnosis and Therapy, ed 4. St Louis: Elsevier, 2004.
8. Miller S, Alam M, Anderson J, et al. NCCN Guidelines. Clinical practice guidelines in oncology: basal cell and squamous cell skin cancers version 2, 2012. Available at *http://www.nccn.org/professionals/physician_gls/f_guidelines.asp#nmsc*.
9. Immerman SC, Scanlon EF, Christ M, et al. Recurrent squamous cell carcinoma of the skin. Cancer 51:1537, 1983.
10. Motley RJ, Preston PW, Lawrence CM. Multi-professional Guidelines for the Management of the Patient with Primary Cutaneous Squamous Cell Carcinoma. London, United Kingdom: British Association of Dermatology, 2009.
11. Available at *https://cancerstaging.org/references-tools/quickreferences/Documents/MelanomaSmall.pdf*.
12. Veronesi U, Cascinelli N, Adamus J, et al. Thin stage I primary cutaneous malignant melanoma. Comparison of excisions with margins of 1 or 3 cm. N Engl J Med 318:1159-1162, 1988.
13. Balch CM, Urist MM, Karakousis CP, et al. Efficacy of 2-cm surgical margins for intermediate-thickness melanomas (1 to 4 mm): results of a multi-institutional randomized surgical trial. Ann Surg 218:262-267, 1993.
14. Cohn-Cedermark G, Rutqvist LE, Andersson R, et al. Long term results of a randomized study by the Swedish Melanoma Study Group on 2-cm versus 5-cm resection margins for patients with cutaneous melanoma with a tumor thickness of 0.8-2.0 mm. Cancer 89:1495-1501, 2000.
15. Khayat D, Rixe O, Martin G, et al; French Group of Research on Malignant Melanoma. Surgical margins in cutaneous melanoma (2 cm versus 5 cm for lesions measuring less than 2.1-mm thick). Cancer 97:1941-1946, 2003.

16. Balch C, Soong SJ, Smith T, et al. Long-term results of a prospective surgical trial comparing 2 cm vs 4 cm excision margins for 740 patients with 1-4 mm melanomas. Ann Surg Oncol 8:101-108, 2001.
17. Thomas JM, Newton-Bishop J, A'Hern R, et al; United Kingdom Melanoma Study Group; British Association of Plastic Surgeons; Scottish Cancer Therapy Network. Excision margins in high-risk malignant melanoma. N Engl J Med 350:757-766, 2004.
18. Marsden JR, Newton-Bishop JA, Burrows L, et al; British Association of Dermatologists (BAD) Clinical Standards Unit. Revised UK guidelines for the management of cutaneous melanoma 2010. J Plast Reconstr Aesthet Surg 63:1401-1419, 2010.
19. Chapman P, Hauschild A, Robert C, et al. Improved survival with vemurafenib in melanoma with BRAF V600E mutation. N Engl J Med 364:2507-2516, 2011.
20. Maverakis E, Cornelius LA, Bowen GM, et al. Metastatic melanoma–a review of current and future treatment options. Acta Derm Venereol 95:516-524, 2015.
21. Trotter SC, Sroa N, Winkelmann RR, et al. A Global Review of Melanoma Follow-up Guidelines. J Clin Aesthet Dermatol 6:18-26, 2013.

16. Burns

See *Essentials of Plastic Surgery*, second edition, pp. 195-202.

PROGNOSIS AFTER SEVERE BURN INJURY

1. **Which one of the following factors is a major predictor of survival used when calculating the Baux score in a patient with a severe, acute burn injury?**
   A. The depth of the burn
   B. The burn subtype
   C. The age of the patient
   D. The first aid treatment provided
   E. The patient's past medical history

PATHOPHYSIOLOGY

2. A 22-year-old patient with a thermal injury is referred to you. The referring unit described the injury as a second-degree burn. **Which one of the following is correct regarding second-degree burns?**
   A. Blistering is usually present.
   B. Sensation is usually absent.
   C. Capillary refill is rarely present.
   D. The entire dermis is normally involved.
   E. The skin appendages are completely destroyed.

BURN TISSUE HISTOLOGY

3. The early management of burn injuries is based on Jackson's burn model. **Which area of the burn is most likely to benefit from early aggressive resuscitation according to this model?**
   A. Zone of necrosis
   B. Zone of stasis
   C. Zone of infiltration
   D. Zone of coagulation
   E. Zone of hyperemia

TRANSFER TO A BURN CENTER

4. **Which one of the following adult burns should be managed locally by a well-equipped plastic surgery department without referral to a burn center?**
   A. A 4% third-degree burn involving the upper forearm and hand.
   B. A 15% first-degree burn involving the trunk and upper limbs.
   C. A 12% second-degree burn involving the lower limbs.
   D. A 1% hydrofluoric acid burn to the hand.
   E. A 4% second-degree flash burn to the face and neck in an enclosed space.

MANAGEMENT OF ELECTRICAL BURNS

5. A 70 kg patient has sustained a high-voltage electrical burn to the left lower limb and is admitted acutely to the burn center. A normal EKG was obtained on admission. Clinical observations are normal, but the involved limb is tense and painful, with intracompartmental pressures measured at 20 mm Hg. Urine output is 30 ml per hour but is colored dark brown. **Which one of the following is correct?**
    A. Urine output should be maintained above 75 ml per hour.
    B. Bicarbonate and mannitol are contraindicated.
    C. Fasciotomy is not indicated at present.
    D. No further cardiac monitoring is required.
    E. The urine discoloration indicates renal failure.

ACUTE MANAGEMENT OF BURNS

6. *For each of the following clinical scenarios, select the most appropriate initial investigation or approach. (Each option may be used once, more than once, or not at all.)*
    A. *A 14-year-old youth has an isolated flash burn injury to the upper face and eyes after throwing an aerosol can onto a bonfire. His speech and breathing are not compromised. He is otherwise well.*
    B. *A 47-year-old man sustains an inhalation burn while working on underground gas pipes when an explosion occurred. He has second-degree burns to his face, neck, and forearms. The Glasgow Coma Scale (GCS) score is 15, but he has a hoarse voice.*
    C. *A 25-year-old man sustains a high-voltage electrical injury while climbing close to a railway.*

Options:
   a. Basic airway assessment and bronchoscopy
   b. Arterial blood gas
   c. Chest radiograph
   d. Ophthalmology referral
   e. EKG
   f. Early prophylactic intubation
   g. Full advanced trauma life support (ATLS) approach

MANAGEMENT OF CHEMICAL BURNS

7. Which one of the following is the most appropriate treatment for a patient after a chemical injury with phenol?
    A. Application of calcium gluconate gel
    B. Copious irrigation and neutralization with a weak acid
    C. Copious irrigation alone
    D. Irrigation followed by application of polyethylene glycol
    E. Application of copper sulfate

BURN RESUSCITATION

8. Which one of the following is the correct resuscitation volume for a 95 kg patient with 42% TBSA burns (using the modified Parkland formula)? The patient had 3 L before arrival at the burn unit, and the burn occurred 4 hours ago.
    A. 1250 ml per hour for 4 hours, then 500 ml per hour for 16 hours
    B. 1000 ml per hour for 8 hours, then 400 ml per hour for 16 hours
    C. 1000 ml per hour for 4 hours, then 500 ml per hour for 16 hours
    D. 1500 ml per hour for 4 hours, then 500 ml per hour for 16 hours
    E. 750 ml per hour for 12 hours, then 580 ml per hour for 12 hours

ESTIMATION OF BURN EXTENT

9. You are asked to see an adult patient in the emergency room. On examination, the patient has a large burn to the left arm and thorax that involves almost all of the left upper limb and half of the anterior trunk. *What is your estimate of burn extent?*
- A. 12%
- B. 18%
- C. 24%
- D. 28%
- E. 32%

OPERATIVE MANAGEMENT

10. *When considering the operative management of a major burn–injured patient, which one of the following is correct?*
- A. Fascial excision increases blood loss.
- B. Tangential excision creates a more severe deformity.
- C. Volume of excision is purely dependent on availability of blood for transfusion.
- D. Typical blood loss for burn excision can be estimated as 0.5 ml per cm^2 burn.
- E. Allograft material is usually required for early wound cover.

POSTOPERATIVE MANAGEMENT

11. *Which one of the following statements is true regarding early postoperative management of acute burns?*
- A. Systemic antibiotics should be routinely prescribed for patients.
- B. The Curreri formula must be used to calculate precise caloric requirements.
- C. Total parenteral nutrition is preferred over enteral feeding to rest the gut.
- D. Metabolic demands are increased by 300% so nutritional intake should be tripled.
- E. A calorie/nitrogen ratio of 100:1 is recommended for optimal nutritional support.

NUTRITIONAL REQUIREMENTS

12. *Which one of the following represents the Curreri formula?*
- A. 20 kcal/kg/day + 40 kcal/%TBSA/day
- B. 25 kcal/kg/day + 40 kcal/%TBSA/day
- C. 25 kcal/kg/day + 60 kcal/%TBSA/day
- D. 20 kcal/kg/day + 60 kcal/%TBSA/day
- E. 25 kcal/kg/day + 25 kcal/%TBSA/day

TOPICAL ANTIMICROBIALS IN BURN WOUNDS

13. A patient with a large burn treated with a topical antibacterial agent for *Pseudomonas* infection develops a metabolic acidosis and compensatory hyperventilation. *Which one of the following agents may be responsible for this clinical picture?*
- A. Silver sulfadiazine
- B. Mafenide acetate
- C. Sodium hypochlorite
- D. Silver nitrate
- E. Manuka honey

SIGNS OF SEPSIS

14. You see a 30-year-old lady on the burn unit as staff are concerned she is becoming septic. She has a 20% TBSA second-degree burn that has been debrided and grafted. She weighs 45 kg and was previously fit and well. *Which one of the following observations would best support a diagnosis of sepsis?*
- A. A respiratory rate of 12 breaths per minute
- B. A core temperature of 35 degrees Celsius
- C. A random blood glucose of 85 mg/dl
- D. A systolic blood pressure of 90 mm Hg
- E. A urine output of 20 ml per hour

Answers

PROGNOSIS AFTER SEVERE BURN INJURY
1. **Which one of the following factors is a major predictor of survival used when calculating the Baux score in a patient with a severe, acute burn injury?**
   C. The age of the patient
   The Baux score is a predictor of mortality after a burn injury. It takes into account a patient's age, the % TBSA burn, and the presence or absence of inhalation injury. A Baux score is calculated by adding age and % TBSA burn. A score greater than 100 in the presence of an inhalation injury or 110 without an inhalation injury is associated with a 50% mortality. The other factors are also relevant to the prognosis—in particular the patient's preinjury status, the burn subtype and burn depth, but do not form part of the Baux scoring system.

PATHOPHYSIOLOGY
2. A 22-year-old patient with a thermal injury is referred to you. The referring unit described the injury as a second-degree burn. **Which one of the following is correct regarding second-degree burns?**
   A. Blistering is usually present.
   A characteristic finding in most second-degree burns is that blistering is present. Burn depth is classified as first-degree, second-degree, or third-degree. First-degree burns involve the epidermis only, and third-degree burns involve the entire dermis and adnexal structures. Second-degree burns can be superficial or deep, involving variable amounts of dermis and both types usually have blistering. Deeper second-degree and third-degree burns can be insensate, but superficial second-degree burns are characteristically painful. The clinical relevance of the adnexal structures being preserved in partial-thickness burns is that the ability for reepithelialization is maintained as these epithelial-lined structures are able to provide a source of keratinocytes in the center of the wound. Burn appearance can guide clinical estimation of injury depth. More superficial second-degree burns will be pink and blanch with pressure. Deep second-degree burns may display fixed staining or pallor similar to a full-thickness injury.

BURN TISSUE HISTOLOGY
3. The early management of burn injuries is based on Jackson's burn model. **Which area of the burn is most likely to benefit from early aggressive resuscitation according to this model?**
   B. Zone of stasis
   The model for burn histology involves three areas. The central zone of coagulation is sometimes called the *zone of necrosis* and is nonviable. This is treated by excision and grafting. The surrounding zone of stasis is initially viable. High-quality, timely treatment can prevent necrosis in this zone and avoid the need for excision and grafting. The zone of hyperemia is sometimes called the *zone of inflammation* and is viable. No zone of infiltration is present (see Table 16-1, *Essentials of Plastic Surgery,* second edition).[1]

TRANSFER TO A BURN CENTER

4. **Which one of the following adult burns should be managed locally by a well-equipped plastic surgery department without referral to a burn center?**
   B. A 15% first-degree burn involving the trunk and upper limbs
   First-degree burns involve the epidermis only and display erythema without blistering. They are commonly a result of sunburn. It is unusual to have to admit or refer a patient with a first-degree burn to the hospital or burn center, even at 15% TBSA unless pain control is not being achieved. This may be more likely in the pediatric population. Criteria for transfer of patients to a burn center include partial-thickness burns greater than 10% TBSA, third-degree burns, and burns involving the hands, feet, genitalia, or major joints. Additional criteria include electrical burns, inhalation injury, burns in the context of associated trauma, burn–injured patients with significant preexisting medical disorders, and children, when the hospital does not have the facilities to care for them. Patients with chemical burns should also be referred to a burn center and in particular hydrofluoric acid burns even as small as 1% can be life threatening so require immediate referral.

MANAGEMENT OF ELECTRICAL BURNS

5. A 70 kg patient has sustained a high-voltage electrical burn to the left lower limb and is admitted acutely to the burn center. A normal EKG was obtained on admission. Clinical observations are normal, but the involved limb is tense and painful, with intracompartmental pressures measured at 20 mm Hg. Urine output is 30 ml per hour but is colored dark brown. **Which one of the following is correct?**
   A. Urine output should be maintained above 75 ml per hour.
   In this case the patient shows signs of myoglobinuria secondary to extensive muscle damage, but not renal dysfunction. This must be carefully treated with fluid therapy to ensure that urine output is maintained between 75 ml and 100 ml per hour. This aims to minimize myoglobin precipitation and subsequent renal damage. Bicarbonate and mannitol are not contraindicated and, in fact, may be useful in cases of myoglobinuria. The involved limb is at risk of compartment syndrome and a painful, tense limb in the setting of a high-voltage electrical injury should be considered for early fasciotomy. The threshold for fasciotomy is usually an intracompartmental pressure of greater than 30 mm Hg, but a decision to operate is made on clinical factors and would be warranted in this case given the clinical presentation. Following a high voltage injury, there is a significant risk of cardiac arrhythmia and in spite of a normal admission EKG, continued cardiac monitoring is required in the acute phase.

ACUTE MANAGEMENT OF BURNS

6. **For the following scenarios, the best options are as follows:**
   A. A 14-year-old youth has an isolated flash burn injury to the upper face and eyes after throwing an aerosol can onto a bonfire. His speech and breathing are not compromised. He is otherwise well.
      d. Ophthalmology referral
   B. A 47-year-old man sustains an inhalation burn while working on underground gas pipes when an explosion occurred. He has second-degree burns to his face, neck, and forearms. The Glasgow Coma Scale (GCS) score is 15, but he has a hoarse voice.
      g. Full ATLS approach

C. *A 25-year-old man sustains a high-voltage electrical injury while climbing close to a railway.*
  g. **Full ATLS approach**
     Patients with facial burns are at high risk of airway and ocular injury. The airway and eyes should be assessed in all of these patients. However, the 14-year-old youth shows no evidence of airway injury and the event occurred in an open space. This patient will have a high risk of corneal damage and should receive an early ophthalmology consult. In the absence of a local ophthalmology service, assessment of the cornea can be made using fluorescein. The 47-year-old man is at high risk of immediate airway compromise and needs to be managed accordingly using an ATLS approach. He may require intubation given the mechanism of injury and this will be part of the ATLS approach. The 25-year-old man is at a high risk of other associated injuries and requires an ATLS approach. He too may require early intubation although may not do so given the injury mechanism. In this case, continued EKG monitoring is required specifically for the electrical injury, but again this will form part of the ATLS approach.

MANAGEMENT OF CHEMICAL BURNS

7. *Which one of the following is the most appropriate treatment for a patient after a chemical injury with phenol?*
   D. **Irrigation followed by application of polyethylene glycol**
      In general, chemical burns should initially be managed with copious irrigation. Some chemicals such as phenol require specific treatments such as topical application of polyethylene glycol. Phenol burns have severe local and systemic toxic effects that can result in death with relatively small volumes.

      Hydrofluoric acid burns release fluoride ions that bind with calcium, leading to profound hypocalcemia. These burns should be treated with calcium gluconate to chelate the fluoride ions. Alkalines should be treated with copious irrigation, but neutralization with weak acids should be avoided. Phosphorus should be stained with copper sulfate solution and surgically removed.

BURN RESUSCITATION

8. *Which one of the following is the correct resuscitation volume for a 95 kg patient with 42% TBSA burns (using the modified Parkland formula)? The patient had 3 L before arrival at the burn unit, and the burn occurred 4 hours ago (Box 16-1).*
   A. **1250 ml per hour for 4 hours, then 500 ml per hour for 16 hours**

Box 16-1 *The Modified Parkland Formula*

4 ml/kg/%TBSA burn = Total fluid volume for the first 24 hours from the time of injury
Half of this volume is given in the first 8 hours, and the rest is given over the last 16 hours.
4 ml × 95 (kg) × 42 (%TBSA) = (15960 ml) or 16 L total fluid volume
Therefore 8 L are given in the first 8 hours, and 8 L are given over the next 16 hours.
The burn occurred 4 hours ago and 3 L were already given. Therefore the remaining fluid
   requirement in the next 4 hours is 5 L (1250 ml/hour), followed by 500 ml/hour for 16 hours.

ESTIMATION OF BURN EXTENT

9. You are asked to see an adult patient in the emergency room. On examination, the patient has a large burn to the left arm and thorax that involves almost all of the left upper limb and half of the anterior trunk. **What is your estimate of burn extent?**
   B. 18%
   Assessment of burn extent is commonly performed using Lund and Browder charts (Fig. 16-1). The approximate areas are as follows:
   - Head and neck 9%
   - Anterior and posterior trunk 18% (each)
   - Lower limbs 18% (each)
   - Upper limbs 9% (each)
   - Perineum 1%

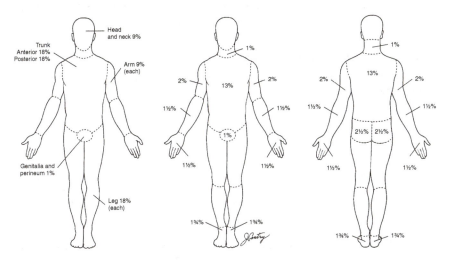

Fig. 16-1 Calculation of total body surface area.

Alternative ways to assess burn extent include the 1% rule and serial halving. The 1% rule is based on the assumption that the palm and fingers represent 1% of the total TBSA. For smaller burns this is a useful approach. Serial halving is useful for a rapid estimation of a large burn and involves making repeated assessments of the burn area stating whether more than half or less than half is involved.[2]

OPERATIVE MANAGEMENT

10. When considering the operative management of a major burn–injured patient, which one of the following is correct?
    D. Typical blood loss for burn excision can be estimated as 0.5 ml per cm^2 burn.
    Blood loss during burn excision can be estimated at 0.5 ml loss for each cm^2 burn injury debrided. Potential blood loss and the amount of blood available for transfusion both need to be considered when deciding how much excision can be performed in one sitting. The volume of excision achievable will also, however, depend on many other factors and the amount of blood available

is only one component. For example, the patient's premorbid status, the area and depth of burn, the timing in relation to the burn injury, and the tissue availability to cover the wound.

A benefit of fascial excision with respect to bleeding is that blood loss is reduced. However it does leave a more severe contour deformity and may result in unnecessary removal of healthy tissue.

Tangential excision provides a better contour and depth control as tissue is excised until bleeding tissue is identified. However, blood loss is more difficult to control. When excising large burn areas, it is vital to keep the patient warm and volume repleted from a cardiovascular perspective. Systematic staged excision of individual areas can help to minimize heat and fluid loss intraoperatively.

The benchmark for grafting is to use the patient's own skin (autograft) rather than use cadaveric (allograft). This is because cadaveric grafts are only temporary and the graft is rejected 3 to 4 weeks after reconstruction. Autograft STSG is then required at this stage. Other options for temporary burn cover include semisynthetic and synthetic materials such as Biobrane, Transcyte, and Integra (see Chapter 9).

POSTOPERATIVE MANAGEMENT

11. *Which one of the following statements is true regarding early postoperative management of acute burns?*
   E. A calorie/nitrogen ratio of 100:1 is recommended for optimal nutritional support.
   After a major burn injury, nutritional support is vital to help wound healing. Due to the catabolic state, a caloric to nitrogen ratio of 100:1 is recommended. A patient's metabolic demands significantly increase after a major burn, but only by 120% to 150%, not by 300%. Enteral feeding is preferred over total parenteral feeds, and prophylactic proton pump inhibitors are recommended to protect the gut which is at risk of stress ulcer formation. Total parenteral feeding may be indicated if there is a sustained period of ileus or some other reason for absorption to be impaired. The Curreri formula is one method of calculating daily caloric needs, but it does not have to be used (see question 12).

   Systemic antibiotics are required in the presence of active infection and the choice should be guided by culture sensitivities. Prophylactic antibiotics are not routinely required. Early debridement and topical antimicrobials are probably more appropriate. Minimizing antibiotics where possible is best in order to avoid resistance.

NUTRITIONAL REQUIREMENTS

12. *Which one of the following represents the Curreri formula?*
   B. 25 kcal/kg/day + 40 kcal/%TBSA/day
   The Curreri formula is one method of calculating the required caloric intake after a major burn injury.[3,4] Although formulas like this are useful tools to guide treatment, care should be taken when they are used, because overestimation of caloric requirements is possible.

TOPICAL ANTIMICROBIALS IN BURN WOUNDS

13. A patient with a large burn treated with a topical antibacterial agent for *Pseudomonas* infection develops a metabolic acidosis and compensatory hyperventilation. **Which one of the following agents may be responsible for this clinical picture?**
   B. Mafenide acetate
   Mafenide acetate is available in 5% and 8.5% forms and has a large amount of data to support its use as an effective topical antibacterial agent. It is particularly useful for treating wounds that are infected with pseudomas. Mafenide is a potent carbonic anhydrase inhibitor that can cause

hyperchloremic metabolic acidosis and compensatory hyperventilation. In some cases this can be fatal. Other caveats are that prolonged use of mafenide can promote growth of candida in the wound and it is painful for the patient on application.

Silver-containing agents are popular in burn dressings as they have a broad spectrum of cover for both gram-positive and gram-negative organisms. They include silver nitrate and silver sulfadiazine. Sodium hypochlorite also has a broad spectrum of cover and at concentrations of 0.025% is bactericidal without inhibiting fibroblasts. Manuka honey is popular as a topical antibacterial agent in many wounds including burns. The antibacterial qualities derive in part from generation of bactericidal hydrogen peroxide. Honey has a low pH, creating an environment that also limits bacterial growth and its high sugar content interferes with bacterial cell division and the development of biofilms. Low toxicity of human keratinocytes and dermal fibroblasts has been demonstrated.[5,6]

SIGNS OF SEPSIS

14. You see a 30-year-old lady on the burn unit as staff are concerned she is becoming septic. She has a 20% TBSA second-degree burn that has been debrided and grafted. She weighs 45 kg and was previously fit and well. *Which one of the following observations would best support a diagnosis of sepsis?*

B. A core temperature of 35 degrees Celsius

Patients with large burns are at high risk of developing sepsis and it is key to identify this early so that appropriate treatment can be instigated. The key signs include hyperventilation, hypothermia or hyperthermia, hyperglycemia, obtundation, ileus, hypotension, and oliguria. Core temperature should normally be around 37 degrees Celsius but can vary according to activity level, site of measurement and time of day. The normal range for respiratory rate in an adult is 12 to 16 breaths per minute. A normal random blood glucose should be between 80 and 110 mg/dl (4.3 to 6.1 mmol/l). A systolic blood pressure of 90 mm Hg is normal in many young females, but this is patient specific and can represent a sign of sepsis in many patients. A urine output of approximately 0.5 ml per hour would be normal in this patient.

A retrospective review of more than 5000 pediatric patients with a burn injury showed that of the 144 patients who died and underwent autopsy, 47% had sepsis confirmed as the primary cause of death. A further 29% had respiratory compromise as the primary cause of death. Many patients subsequently developed multiorgan system failure as a result. This highlights the importance of recognizing and treating sepsis early following a burn injury.[7]

REFERENCES

1. Jackson DM. The diagnosis of the depth of burning. Br J Surg 40:588-596, 1953.
2. Jones AP, Barnard AR, Allison KP. Trauma: burns. In Nutbeam T, Boylan M, eds. ABC of Prehospital Emergency Medicine. Oxford, UK: BMJ Books, 2013.
3. Turner WW Jr, Ireton CS, Hunt JL, et al. Predicting energy expenditures in burned patients. J Trauma 25:11-16, 1985.
4. Mendonça Machado N, Gragnani A, Masako Ferreira L. Burns, metabolism and nutritional requirements. Nutr Hosp 26:692-700, 2011.
5. Herndon DN. Total Burn Care, ed 3. Philadelphia: Elsevier, 2012.
6. Lee DS, Sinno S, Khachemoune A. Honey and wound healing: an overview. Am J Clin Dermatol 12:181, 2011.
7. Williams FN, Herndon DN, Hawkins HK, et al. The leading causes of death after burn injury in a single pediatric burn center. Crit Care 13:R183, 2009.

17. Vascular Anomalies

See *Essentials of Plastic Surgery*, second edition, pp. 203-210.

EPIDEMIOLOGY OF HEMANGIOMAS

1. **Which one of the following statements regarding hemangiomas is correct?**
   A. They represent the most common tumor in infancy.
   B. They occur twice as often in males, compared with females.
   C. Twenty percent of hemangiomas occur in the head and neck region.
   D. All subtypes typically develop a few weeks after birth.
   E. Most patients have two or more concurrent lesions.

MANAGEMENT OF HEMANGIOMAS

2. A 3-month-old infant is seen in clinic with an enlarging vascular lesion to the buttock. It began as a small spot shortly after birth and has grown to measure 1.5 cm diameter. There had been some episodes of bleeding following minor trauma, but it has been stable for the past three weeks. **How best can this patient be managed?**
   A. Propanolol
   B. Steroids
   C. Laser
   D. Surgery
   E. Observation

CLINICAL COURSE OF HEMANGIOMAS

3. You are discussing long-term outcomes with the family of a 6-week-old infant with a 1 cm infantile hemangioma to the cheek. **Which one of the following should you tell them?**
   A. Involution is most likely to complete within a year.
   B. Involution is unlikely to occur without treatment.
   C. Further growth is unlikely.
   D. Involution occurs in 75% of cases by age 5.
   E. Involution may be incomplete, and the infant may require surgery.

HEMANGIOMA CLINICAL SCENARIOS

4. For each of the following descriptions, select the most appropriate option. (Each option may be used once, more than once, or not at all.)
   A. This is the most common complication of a hemangioma.
   B. This occurs when there is profound thrombocytopenia in conjunction with a hemangioma.
   C. A patient has retinal hemangiomas and hemangioblastomas of the cerebellum in conjunction with pancreatic cysts.

   Options:
   a. Maffucci's syndrome
   b. PHACE syndrome
   c. von Hippel-Lindau disease
   d. Kasabach-Merritt syndrome
   e. Congestive cardiac failure
   f. Visual obstruction
   g. Ulceration
   h. Bleeding
   i. Infection

VASCULAR MALFORMATIONS

5. Which one of the following statements is correct regarding vascular malformations?
   A. They are not usually present at birth.
   B. They grow proportionally with the child and often regress.
   C. The autonomic nervous system has little influence on their development.
   D. They represent structural anomalies because of faulty embryonic morphogenesis.
   E. During embryonic development, capillaries develop from arterial and venous precursors.

PORT-WINE STAINS (CAPILLARY MALFORMATIONS)

6. Which one of the following statements regarding port-wine stains is correct?
   A. They affect 3 in 100 newborn babies.
   B. The neck is the most common anatomic location.
   C. They often correspond to the distribution of the facial nerve.
   D. They are more commonly observed in males.
   E. If left untreated, 70% will progress to a cobblestone ectasia.

SYNDROMES INVOLVING VASCULAR ANOMALIES

7. Match each of the following descriptions of vascular anomaly to the most appropriate option. (Each option may be used once, more than once, or not at all.)
   A. This syndrome is characterized by microcephaly, multiple lipomas, and vascular malformations.
   B. This syndrome includes an arteriovenous fistula, port-wine stain, and venous/lymphatic malformation in an extremity with associated skeletal hypertrophy.
   C. This syndrome is characterized by multiple malformed ectatic vessels in skin, mucous membranes, and viscera.

   Options:
   a. Riley-Smith syndrome
   b. Bannayan-Zonana syndrome
   c. Osler-Weber-Rendu disease
   d. Sturge-Weber syndrome
   e. Klippel-Trenaunay syndrome
   f. Parkes-Weber syndrome

8. Match each of the following descriptions to the most appropriate option. (Each option may be used once, more than once, or not at all.)
   A. This condition is associated with a patchy port-wine stain on an extremity and deeper venous and lymphatic malformation.
   B. This condition is characterized by a large, facial port-wine stain with V_1 and V_2 involvement and venous malformation of the pia mater and arachnoid mater.
   C. This condition is associated with pseudopapilledema, microcephaly, and vascular malformations.

   Options:
   a. Riley-Smith syndrome
   b. Blue rubber bleb nevus syndrome
   c. Osler-Weber-Rendu disease
   d. Sturge-Weber syndrome
   e. Klippel-Trenaunay syndrome
   f. Parkes-Weber syndrome

VENOUS MALFORMATIONS

9. Which one of the following statements is correct regarding venous malformations?
   A. They increase in size when elevated.
   B. They are treated successfully with the Er:YAG laser.
   C. They are usually painless.
   D. They tend to enlarge in puberty and pregnancy.
   E. They are no longer treated with sclerotherapy.

LYMPHATIC MALFORMATIONS

10. Which one of the following statements is correct regarding lymphatic malformations?
    A. They have little effect on adjacent bone growth.
    B. They rarely occur in combination with venous abnormalities.
    C. They are commonly associated with clear cutaneous vesicles.
    D. They rarely become infected.
    E. Morbidity is low after surgical excision.

ARTERIOVENOUS MALFORMATIONS

11. When managing arteriovenous malformations, which one of the following is correct?
    A. Although pulsatile, they are generally low-flow lesions.
    B. Their vascular anatomy is best imaged using MRI.
    C. Embolization is indicated before surgical excision.
    D. Rates are low following complete excision.
    E. Consumptive coagulopathy is generally managed intraoperatively.

Chapter 17 ▪ Vascular Anomalies 141

Answers

EPIDEMIOLOGY OF HEMANGIOMAS

1. *Which one of the following statements regarding hemangiomas is correct?*
   A. They represent the most common tumor in infancy.
   Hemangiomas are the most common tumor in infancy. They are abnormal endothelial proliferations and are considered to be true tumors. They are found more commonly in females, with a female/male ratio of 3:1. They are usually seen in the head and neck region (60%, not 20%) but may occur on the trunk, limbs, or intracranially. Hemangiomas can be divided into infantile and congenital subtypes. Most are infantile and these develop shortly after birth appearing as a small red spot. Congenital hemangiomas however are fully grown at birth and are classified as two forms, rapidly involuting (RICH) or noninvoluting (NICH). Most patients with hemangiomas have a single lesion, although some do have more than one. Presentation with multiple hemangiomas is most often as part of a syndrome such as Maffuci's or PHACE syndrome.

MANAGEMENT OF HEMANGIOMAS

2. A 3-month-old infant is seen in clinic with an enlarging vascular lesion to the buttock. It began as a small spot shortly after birth and has grown to measure 1.5 cm diameter. There had been some episodes of bleeding following minor trauma, but it has been stable for the past three weeks. ***How best can this patient be managed?***
   E. Observation
   The mainstay of treatment for hemangiomas is conservative management given that the vast majority are self-limiting and resolve over time. This infant is at risk of further bleeding episodes and should be seen again in clinic, but does not require further intervention as present. Hemangiomas may be treated with surgery, laser therapy, steroids, or other injectable agents if they are causing visual or airway obstruction, or bleeding and ulceration that is difficult to control with conservative measures. There has been recent interest in the use of beta blocker medication in the form of propranolol for treatment of ulcerated hemangiomas and results so far appear promising. Starkey and Shahidullah[1] published a comprehensive review of evidence on this topic in 2011. Propranolol is thought to restrict growth in hemangiomas by causing vasoconstriction, inhibition of VEGF, and induction of apoptosis. Typical doses are 1 to 3 mg/kg/day for up to 12 months. Potential side effects include bradycardia, bronchoconstriction, and hypotension.
   Bleomycin is a chemotherapeutic agent that has also shown promising results in the management of ulcerated hemangiomas and other vascular malformations.[2] Steroids may be injected locally or given systemically to arrest growth of hemangiomas but do not cause regression. Laser therapy can be used for hemangiomas in the acute setting to help with ulceration, or in the later stages of regression to remove residual color from the area.

CLINICAL COURSE OF HEMANGIOMAS

3. You are discussing long-term outcomes with the family of a 6-week-old infant with a 1 cm infantile hemangioma to the cheek. ***Which one of the following should you tell them?***
   E. Involution may be incomplete, and the infant may require surgery.
   The vast majority of infantile hemangiomas will involute spontaneously and parents and other family members should be reassured about this. However, a number of patients will have residual

fullness at the site of the hemangioma that may require surgical excision. Others may have residual discoloration that may benefit from laser therapy. Infantile hemangiomas appear shortly after birth and have an initial phase of rapid growth. This often lasts for 6 to 18 months before involution begins. Therefore this child is likely to have further growth of the hemangioma before involution. Involution has usually occurred in 50% of patients by the age of five, 70% by the age of seven, and 90% by the age of nine. Congenital hemangiomas differ in their ability to spontaneously involute. They are of two types: RICH and NICH. Both are present at birth but only RICH involute spontaneously. They do so within the first year of life. NICH lesions do not respond well to pharmacotherapy and may need surgery if problematic.

HEMANGIOMA CLINICAL SCENARIOS

4. *For the following descriptions, the best options are as follows:*
   A. *This is the most common complication of a hemangioma.*
      g. **Ulceration**
         Ulceration is the most common complication of hemangiomas. Other common complications include bleeding, infection, and emotional/psychological issues. Hemangiomas located close to the periorbital region risk visual obstruction that if untreated can lead to anisometropia. Hemangiomas located around the oral or nasal cavities can affect feeding and risk airway obstruction. Hemangiomas in the perineum can cause problems with toileting and hygiene, with subsequent sores and infection.
   B. *This occurs when there is profound thrombocytopenia in conjunction with a hemangioma.*
      d. **Kasabach-Merritt syndrome**
         Kasabach-Merritt syndrome is a combination of hemangioma, thrombocytopenia, and coagulopathy. Although infrequent, it is potentially fatal in infants with rapidly growing vascular lesions, and early recognition with prompt management is essential. This topic is often tested in plastic surgery exams.
   C. *A patient has retinal hemangiomas and hemangioblastomas of the cerebellum in conjunction with pancreatic cysts.*
      c. **von Hippel-Lindau disease**
         von Hippel-Lindau disease is a rare inherited condition that involves hemangiomas of the retina, hemangioblastomas of the cerebellum, and pancreatic, liver, and adrenal gland cysts. Seizures and mental retardation can also occur. It is inherited in an autosomal dominant fashion and results from a mutation in the von Hippel-Lindau tumor suppressor gene. It occurs in around 1 in 30,000 births and patients are at risk of developing various different malignant tumors as well as benign proliferations. PHACE syndrome involves large facial hemangiomas associated with posterior fossa malformations, arterial abnormalities, coarctation of the aorta, and eye abnormalities.
         Maffucci's syndrome involves enchondromas with multiple cutaneous hemangiomas.

VASCULAR MALFORMATIONS

5. *Which one of the following statements is correct regarding vascular malformations?*
   D. **They represent structural anomalies because of faulty embryonic morphogenesis.**
      Vascular malformations can be subdivided into **capillary, venous, arteriovenous,** and **lymphatic** subtypes. They occur because of faulty embryonic morphogenesis. They are present at birth and grow with the child, but they do not regress. The autonomic nervous system influences vascular development. This explains why some abnormalities such as port-wine stains occur in specific

Chapter 17 ▪ Vascular Anomalies   143

nerve distributions. During embryonic development, venous and arterial channels appear after the initial capillary network has been formed.

PORT-WINE STAINS (CAPILLARY MALFORMATIONS)

6. *Which one of the following statements regarding port-wine stains is correct?*
   E. **If left untreated, 70% will progress to a cobblestone ectasia.**
   Port-wine stains affect 0.3% of newborn babies and most commonly occur on the face (80%). One of the main reasons for treating them early in life is to avoid development of a cobblestone appearance which can occur in adulthood if left untreated. They can correspond to the trigeminal nerve distribution, but not the facial nerve and are sometimes accompanied by ocular and central nervous system disorders. Females are affected three times as often as males. Treatment modalities include pulsed dye or Nd:YAG laser.

SYNDROMES INVOLVING VASCULAR ANOMALIES

7. *For the following scenarios, the best options are as follows:*
   A. *This syndrome is characterized by microcephaly, multiple lipomas, and vascular malformations.*
      b. **Bannayan-Zonana syndrome**
   B. *This syndrome includes an arteriovenous fistula, port-wine stain, and venous/lymphatic malformation in an extremity with associated skeletal hypertrophy.*
      f. **Parkes-Weber syndrome**
   C. *This syndrome is characterized by multiple malformed ectatic vessels in skin, mucous membranes, and viscera.*
      c. **Osler-Weber-Rendu disease (hereditary, hemorrhagic telangiectasia)**
      There are a number of conditions associated with vascular anomalies. These are shown in Tables 17-3 and 17-4, *Essentials of Plastic Surgery,* second edition. Those that are associated with port-wine stains include Sturge-Weber, Klippel-Trenaunay, and Parkes-Weber.
      Syndromes with other vascular malformations include Bannayan-Zonana, Riley-Smith, Blue rubber bleb and Osler-Weber-Rendu. Syndromes associated with hemangiomas include Maffucci's, von Hippel-Lindau, and PHACE, which are shown in Table 17-1, *Essentials of Plastic Surgery,* second edition.

8. *For the following scenarios, the best options are as follows:*
   A. *This condition is associated with a patchy port-wine stain on an extremity and deeper venous and lymphatic malformation.*
      e. **Klippel-Trenaunay syndrome**
   B. *This condition is characterized by a large, facial port-wine stain with V_1 and V_2 involvement and venous malformation of the pia mater and arachnoid mater.*
      d. **Sturge-Weber syndrome**
   C. *This condition is associated with pseudopapilledema, microcephaly, and vascular malformations.*
      a. **Riley-Smith syndrome**
      See Tables 17-1, 17-3, and 17-4, *Essentials of Plastic Surgery,* second edition.

VENOUS MALFORMATIONS

9. Which one of the following statements is correct regarding venous malformations?

D. They tend to enlarge in puberty and pregnancy.

Venous malformations are present at birth and can grow significantly during pregnancy or puberty if they are hormone sensitive. They decrease in size when elevated and swell in a dependent position. Demonstrating this is a key part of the clinical examination of these lesions. They commonly cause aching, especially in the extremities such as where varicose veins are present. Sclerotherapy is a popular treatment modality, with a variety of different injectables, and laser therapy is successful with Nd:YAG rather than Er:YAG laser.

LYMPHATIC MALFORMATIONS

10. Which one of the following statements is correct regarding lymphatic malformations?

C. They are commonly associated with clear cutaneous vesicles.

Clear cutaneous vesicles signify a dermal lymphatic component in a vascular malformation. Bony overgrowth and simultaneous venous anomalies are common associations. Lymphatic malformations frequently become infected and require aggressive antibiotic therapy. Surgery to lymphatic malformations is associated with many complications, including delayed wound healing, infection, and prolonged drainage. Success treating these with intralesional bleomycin has shown promising results.[2]

ARTERIOVENOUS MALFORMATIONS

11. When managing arteriovenous malformations, which one of the following is correct?

C. Embolization is indicated before surgical excision.

Arteriovenous malformations (AVMs) are high-flow pulsatile lesions that are difficult to treat surgically and require preoperative embolization to minimize risk of bleeding during resection. It is usual to embolize AVMs 24 to 72 hours before surgery. The main risk for patients undergoing resection of AVMs is bleeding due to the high flow and consumptive coagulopathy. The latter must be addressed preoperatively with correction of any clotting dysfunction. Preoperative imaging consists of an MRI to determine the extent of the lesion and surrounding soft tissue involvement. Angiography is required to indentify the feeding vessels and vascular anatomy. Recurrence rates are high after surgical excision and for this reason generous margins should be taken where possible. Patients may need not only hypotensive anesthesia but also cardiopulmonary bypass in some situations. Management of these malformations is a multidisciplinary task, given the complexity and high risks of morbidity and mortality.

REFERENCES

1. Starkey E, Shahidullah H. Propranolol for infantile haemangiomas: a review. Arch Dis Child 96:890-893, 2011.
2. Sainsbury DC, Kessell G, Fall AJ, et al. Intralesional bleomycin injection treatment for vascular birthmarks: a 5-year experience at a single United Kingdom unit. Plast Reconstr Surg 127:2031-2044, 2001.

18. Congenital Nevi

See *Essentials of Plastic Surgery*, second edition, pp. 211-214.

GIANT CONGENITAL NEVOCYTIC NEVI

1. **When examining a patient with a giant congenital nevocytic nevus, which one of the following features is a consistent finding?**
   A. A bathing suit distribution
   B. Multiple satellite lesions
   C. Leptomeningeal involvement
   D. A verrucous surface texture to the nevus
   E. Spina bifida with meningomyelocele

HISTOLOGY OF CONGENITAL AND ACQUIRED NEVI

2. **Which one of the following statements is correct regarding congenital and acquired nevi?**
   A. Congenital nevi tend to be located more superficially within the dermis compared with acquired nevi.
   B. Small, medium, and large congenital nevi each have very different histological features.
   C. Congenital nevi differ from acquired nevi in their involvement with skin appendages.
   D. Growth of congenital nevi is often disproportionate to overall patient growth.
   E. All types of congenital and acquired nevi can have extension into muscle and bone.

RISK OF MALIGNANT TRANSFORMATION

3. **Which one of the following statements regarding malignant transformation of CNN is correct?**
   A. Management with respect to the potential for malignant transformation remains controversial.
   B. There is minimal lifetime risk of malignant transformation in smaller CNN.
   C. The most common age range for malignant transformation of giant CNN is 10 to 20 years.
   D. Transformation of giant CNN to melanoma occurs in more than a third of cases.
   E. Malignant transformation carries a better prognosis compared with other melanoma subtypes.

MANAGEMENT OF GIANT CONGENITAL NEVOCYTIC NEVI

4. **Which one of the following is probably the most important indication to treat a giant CNN?**
   A. Cosmetic appearance
   B. Parental request
   C. Psychological effects
   D. Risk of malignant change
   E. Site and size of lesion

MANAGEMENT OF CONGENITAL NEVOCYTIC NEVI

5. *When planning management of CNN, which one of the following statements is correct?*
   A. Nongiant cell congenital nevi should be assessed three times per year.
   B. Early excision is not warranted in lesions just because they are difficult to monitor.
   C. Any atypical congenital nevi should be excised regardless of size.
   D. Reconstruction of giant CNN will require tissue expansion to achieve primary closure.
   E. Laser or curettage are recommended for smaller lesions and have low recurrence rates.

DIAGNOSIS OF PIGMENTED SKIN LESIONS

6. A baby is found to have a 3 cm diameter, steel-blue macule in the lumbosacral region soon after birth. *Which one of the following is the most likely diagnosis?*
   A. Mongolian spot
   B. Blue nevus
   C. Spitz nevus
   D. Café au lait spot
   E. Halo nevus

CLINICAL SCENARIOS INVOLVING PIGMENTED SKIN LESIONS

7. *For each of the following clinical scenarios, select the most likely diagnosis. (Each option may be used once, more than once, or not at all.)*
   A. A white baby girl presents with a yellowish waxy plaque on the scalp. She is otherwise fit and well.
   B. An Asian newborn baby has a right-sided, blue-brown periocular macule with a 2 cm diameter.
   C. An adolescent male presents with a 10 cm diameter, tan-colored, hairy lesion on the right shoulder. It has been present for 6 months.

Options:
   a. Nevus spilus
   b. Epidermal nevus
   c. Becker's nevus
   d. Nevus of Ota
   e. Nevus of Ito
   f. Dysplastic nevus
   g. Sebaceous nevus

Answers

GIANT CONGENITAL NEVOCYTIC NEVI
1. When examining a patient with a giant CNN, which one of the following features is a consistent finding?
D. A verrucous surface texture to the nevus

Giant cell nevi have a verrucous appearance, but satellite lesions are commonly seen.[1] Neurocutaneous manifestations include leptomeningeal extension, meningomyelocele, and spina bifida. Leptomeningeal melanosis is considered to be more likely in the presence of scalp or dorsal spinal cutaneous lesions. Suspicion of these warrants further investigation with MRI. Giant cell nevi vary in their anatomic location and accordingly can be *bathing suit, stocking,* or *coat sleeve* (see Table 18-1, *Essentials of Plastic Surgery,* second edition).

HISTOLOGY OF CONGENITAL AND ACQUIRED NEVI
2. Which one of the following statements is correct regarding congenital and acquired nevi?
C. Congenital nevi differ from acquired nevi in their involvement with skin appendages.

Congenital nevi consist of nevus cells located in the deeper dermis and can invade skin appendages, vessels, and nerves. In contrast, acquired nevi tend to consist of nevus cells that are limited to the papillary and upper reticular dermis and do not involve skin appendages. The histologic appearance of all congenital nevi is largely similar but giant cell nevi differ in that they may have extension into muscle, bone, and dura. After birth, CNN grow in proportion to body size.

RISK OF MALIGNANT TRANSFORMATION
3. Which one of the following statements regarding malignant transformation of CNN is correct?
A. Management with respect to the potential for malignant transformation remains controversial.

The risk of malignant transformation in congenital nevi and their preemptive management is a controversial topic for which there are many opinions. This is because many factors remain uncertain, such as the true lifetime risk of malignant change for any given lesion, and the impact of prophylactic excision in reducing development of subsequent cutaneous or noncutaneous malignancy.

The lifetime risk of malignant change is probably 1% to 5% for small congenital nevi. The risk in medium CNN is uncertain, and neither small- nor medium-sized CNN are likely to change before puberty. In contrast, giant CNN have a 5% to 10% risk of malignant transformation, and half of these will occur between ages 3 and 5 years. The size and site of a giant CNN as well as the number of satellite lesions appears to impact the risk of malignant transformation. Trunk lesions have a higher risk of malignant transformation as do those greater than 40 cm in diameter. When malignant transformation occurs in giant nevi, the prognosis is poor.[2,3]

MANAGEMENT OF GIANT CONGENITAL NEVOCYTIC NEVI

4. **Which one of the following is probably the most important indication to treat a giant CNN?**
   D. Risk of malignant change
   All of the above may need to be considered for selection of treatment. Cosmesis will often be very important to parents and patients. It is particularly important to patients as they begin to develop social awareness. The site, size, and location of the lesion and availability of tissue for reconstruction play a significant role in decision-making. Both scarring from surgery and the original nevus can carry significant potential psychological effects. However, the most important reason for treating a nevus is the potential risk of malignant change.

MANAGEMENT OF CONGENITAL NEVOCYTIC NEVI

5. **When planning management of CNN, which one of the following statements is correct?**
   C. Any atypical congenital nevi should be excised regardless of size.
   Early excision of small and medium congenital nevi is warranted if they are difficult to monitor (e.g., on the back or scalp) or if they have atypical features such as color variegation, abnormal borders, or growth. Nongiant nevi can be observed on an annual basis (not every 4 months) unless suspicious, in which case a diagnostic biopsy is performed instead. Giant CNN should be excised completely as soon as possible after appropriate imaging. Reconstruction often requires a combination of tissue expansion, grafts, and flaps but is dependent on size and anatomic location. For example, giant CNN representing 1% TBSA located on the trunk may be closed directly without expansion techniques. Laser and curettage are not recommended for managing CNN as they are associated with high recurrence rates.

DIAGNOSIS OF PIGMENTED SKIN LESIONS

6. **A baby is found to have a 3 cm diameter, steel-blue macule in the lumbosacral region soon after birth. *Which one of the following is the most likely diagnosis?***
   A. Mongolian spot
   Mongolian spots are more common in races with darkly pigmented skin and can vary from a couple of centimeters to 20 cm. They are present at birth and usually disappear during childhood. In contrast, blue nevi usually appear in late adolescence and are small (less than 1 cm). They are typically blue or black and can be located on the hands, feet, head, or neck. A Spitz nevus is a red or pigmented dome-shaped papule that usually appears at birth and is commonly found on the head or neck. Excision is normally recommended. Café au lait spots are well circumscribed homogeneous macular coffee-colored lesions often seen with neurofibromatosis. A halo nevus has a white halo around the nevus due to a lymphocytic reaction and most commonly is found on the back during puberty.

CLINICAL SCENARIOS INVOLVING PIGMENTED SKIN LESIONS

7. *For the following scenarios, the best options are as follows:*
   A. A white baby girl presents with a yellowish waxy plaque to the scalp. She is otherwise fit and well.
   g. Sebaceous nevus
   A number of lesions can sometimes be confused with CNN. A sebaceous nevus is a solitary yellowish waxy plaque usually found on the scalp. It has a risk of malignant transformation to BCC in the region of 10% or 15%.
   B. An Asian newborn baby has a right-sided, blue-brown periocular macule with a 2 cm diameter.
   d. Nevus of Ota
   The nevus of Ota has an onset at birth or within the first year of life and during puberty. It is especially common in Asians and blacks. It appears as a blue-brown unilateral periocular macule varying in size from a few centimeters to one which affects half of the face.
   C. An adolescent male presents with a 10 cm diameter, tan-colored, hairy lesion on the right shoulder. It has been present for 6 months.
   c. Becker's nevus
   A Becker's nevus has an onset in adolescence and lesions are commonly unilateral affecting the shoulder. Their color varies from tan to brown with irregular margins.

   A nevus spilus is usually an acquired lesion that is a tan macular spot 1 to 4 cm diameter speckled with dark brown papules or macules. An epidermal nevus is present at birth or develops shortly after, and is a tan or brown warty macule or papule with or without plaques or hair and it is often located on the extremities.

   The nevus of Ito usually appears at birth and is typically seen in Asians and blacks. It appears as a large blue-brown lesion on the posterior shoulder innervated by the supraclavicular and lateral cutaneous brachial nerves. A dysplastic nevus often occurs during or after puberty and has different areas of pigmentation. They are usually larger than 6 mm and commonly found on the trunk.

REFERENCES

1. Foster RD, Williams ML, Barkovich AJ, et al. Giant congenital melanocytic nevi: the significance of neurocutaneous melanosis in neurologically asymptomatic children. Plast Reconstr Surg 107:933-941, 2001.
2. Krengel S, Marghoob AA. Current management approaches for congenital melanocytic nevi. Dermatol Clin 30:377-387, 2012.
3. Marghoob AA, Borrego JP, Halpern AC. Congenital melanocytic nevi: treatment modalities and management options. Semin Cutan Med Surg 26:231-240, 2007.

Part III

Head and Neck

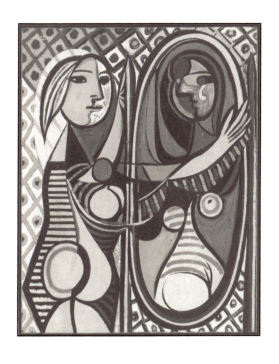

© 2015 Estate of Pablo Picasso / Artists Rights Society (ARS), New York.

19. Head and Neck Embryology

See *Essentials of Plastic Surgery*, second edition, pp. 217-222.

HUMAN EMBRYOLOGY
1. *Which one of the following statements is correct?*
   A. The nervous system derives from the mesodermal layer.
   B. The endoderm forms the gastrointestinal and genitourinary tracts.
   C. The heart and great vessels derive from both ectoderm and mesoderm.
   D. Bone, cartilage, muscle, dermis, and epidermis derive from mesoderm.
   E. Hair follicles, sebaceous glands, and eccrine sweat glands derive from ectoderm.

PHARYNGEAL (BRANCHIAL) ARCHES
2. *Which one of the following statements is correct?*
   A. The muscles of mastication are derived from the second arch.
   B. The digastric muscle develops from two separate arches.
   C. The facial nerve and facial musculature derive from different arches.
   D. Levator veli palatini and tensor veli palatini arise from the same arch.
   E. The ossicles derive from a single pharyngeal arch.

PHARYNGEAL (BRANCHIAL) GROOVES
3. *Which one of the following statements is correct?*
   A. Groove I develops into the internal auditory meatus and tympanic membrane.
   B. The most common branchial groove sinus derives from cleft IV and runs from the sternocleidomastoid muscle to the tongue base.
   C. Branchial cleft abnormalities are most often detected in the fourth decade of life as discharging sinuses.
   D. The cervical sinus is formed from grooves II through IV, and incomplete obliteration is the cause of branchial sinus tracts.
   E. Branchial clefts from cleft II differ from cleft III by their relationship to the internal jugular vein.

PHARYNGEAL (BRANCHIAL) POUCHES
4. *Which one of the following statements is correct?*
   A. The first pouch gives rise to the external auditory canal.
   B. The second pouch gives rise to the lingual tonsil.
   C. The third pouch gives rise to the superior parathyroid and thymus.
   D. The fourth pouch gives rise to the ultimobranchial body and T-cells.
   E. The fourth pouch migrates above the third pouch.

HEAD AND NECK DEVELOPMENT

5. **Which one of the following statements is correct?**
   A. The tongue is formed from two different arches.
   B. The thyroid gland develops from the tongue.
   C. The external ear receives contribution from all arches.
   D. The facial skeleton forms by endochondral ossification.
   E. The face develops from paired frontonasal prominences.

EMBRYOLOGIC ORIGINS OF ADULT STRUCTURES

6. **Match each of the following adult anatomic structures to its specific embryologic origin. (Each option may be used once, more than once, or not at all.)**
   A. Philtrum
   B. Lower lip
   C. Secondary palate

   Options:
   a. Frontonasal prominence
   b. Maxillary prominence
   c. Medial nasal prominence
   d. Lateral nasal prominence
   e. Ophthalmic prominence
   f. Mandibular prominence

7. **Match each of the following adult anatomic structures to its specific embryologic origin. (Each option may be used once, more than once, or not at all.)**
   A. Primary palate
   B. Nasal alae
   C. Nasal septum

   Options:
   a. Frontonasal prominence
   b. Maxillary prominence
   c. Medial nasal prominence
   d. Mandibular prominence
   e. Lateral nasal prominence
   f. Ophthalmic prominence

Answers

HUMAN EMBRYOLOGY

1. *Which one of the following statements is correct?*
   E. Hair follicles, sebaceous glands, and eccrine sweat glands derive from ectoderm.
   The ectoderm forms the epidermis and the epidermal appendages. This has clinical relevance to the healing process in partial-thickness wounds as the ectodermally derived skin appendages such as hair follicles, eccrine and apocrine sweat glands, and sebaceous glands are epithelial lined and provide a source of keratinocytes for reepithelialization. This knowledge also helps to understand how certain conditions present. For example, the fact that skin and neural tissue share embryologic origin explains why patients with neurofibromatosis develop both skin and nerve tissue tumors. The mesodermal derivatives are also clinically relevant to plastic surgery as this embryologic layer forms bone, cartilage, muscle, connective tissue, and blood vessels. The endoderm has less applicability to plastic surgery as it forms the lining of the gastrointestinal and respiratory tracts and the digestive organ parenchyma.

PHARYNGEAL (BRANCHIAL) ARCHES

2. *Which one of the following statements is correct?*
   B. The digastric muscle develops from two separate arches.
   There are six pharyngeal arches and each comprises a mixture of endoderm, mesoderm, and ectoderm such that all layers of the head and neck can be formed (Table 19-1). Knowledge of the embryologic origins of the head and neck has clinical relevance to plastic surgery. For example, each of the digastric muscles has an anterior and a posterior belly, which have different embryologic origins. The anterior belly develops from the first arch along with the muscles of mastication and tensor veli palatini. The main nerve derived from this arch is the trigeminal and this supplies these structures. The posterior belly develops from the second arch which also forms the muscles of facial expression and the stapes. The main nerve derived from this arch is the facial nerve and this supplies these structures (Fig. 19-1).

   When the facial nerve is damaged, the muscles of facial expression become paralyzed but the trigeminally supplied muscles of mastication and anterior belly of digastric remain functional. Therefore the digastric muscle can be transferred to the lower lip to compensate for marginal nerve branch weakness and the temporalis muscle can be transferred to compensate for buccal and zygomatic nerve branch weakness. Of further interest is that facial nerve paralysis also results in a loss of sound dampening and again this can be explained by embryologic development because the nerve to the stapedius, the stapedius itself, and the stapes are all derived from the second arch. The other two ossicles (incus and malleus) are derived from the first arch.

   A common exam question relates to the innervation of the palatal musculature. All but one are innervated by the pharyngeal plexus as they are derived from arches four to six. The tensor veli palatini opens the Eustachian tube and is derived from the first arch and so has trigeminal innervation (see Chapters 25 and 42).

Table 19-1 *Pharyngeal Arch Derivatives*

Arch	Nerve	Artery	Bone	Muscle
I	**CN V**	Maxillary	Greater wing of sphenoid, incus, malleus, **maxilla**, zygomatic, temporal (squamous), **mandible**	**Muscles of mastication,** anterior digastric, mylohyoid, tensor tympani, **tensor veli palatini**
II	**CN VII**	Stapedial (corticotympanic)	Stapes, styloid process, stylohyoid ligament, lesser horn and upper body of hyoid	**Muscles of facial expression,** posterior digastric, stylohoid, stapedius
III	**CN IX**	Common carotid, proximal internal carotid	Greater horns and lower body of hyoid	Stylopharyngeus
IV/VI	**CN X**	Aortic arch, right subclavian, origin of pulmonary arteries, ductus arteriosus	Laryngeal cartilages	**Pharyngeal constrictors, levator veli palatini,** palatoglossus, striated upper esophageal muscles, **laryngeal** muscles

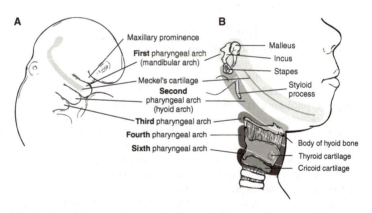

Fig. 19-1 A, Lateral view of pharyngeal arches. **B,** Cartilaginous and bony structures.

PHARYNGEAL (BRANCHIAL) GROOVES

3. *Which one of the following statements is correct?*
   D. **The cervical sinus is formed from grooves II through IV, and incomplete obliteration is the cause of branchial sinus tracts.**

   There are five pharyngeal grooves (also known as clefts), and the cervical sinus is formed from grooves II through IV. Failure of the sinus to obliterate leads to the formation of a branchial sinus tract, cyst, or fistula. These are often detected in the second (not fourth) decade of life as neck swellings and those formed from groove II are most common. Groove I forms the **external** auditory meatus and tympanic membrane, not the **internal** auditory meatus, which is formed by the first pharyngeal pouch (see question 4). Grooves II and III differ in their relationship to the internal and external **carotids** (not the **internal jugular vein**). A groove II anomaly runs **between** the external and internal carotid arteries toward the tonsillar fossa, and a groove III anomaly passes **under** the internal carotid. Knowledge of this anatomy can be useful intraoperatively when excising branchial sinuses.

PHARYNGEAL (BRANCHIAL) POUCHES

4. *Which one of the following statements is correct?*
   E. The fourth pouch migrates above the third pouch.
   There are five pharyngeal pouches which grow inward between the pharyngeal arches. The fourth pouch migrates above the third pouch during embryonic development. This explains why the third pouch forms the inferior parathyroid, and the fourth pouch forms the superior parathyroid. The first pouch forms the internal auditory canal (the first groove forms the external auditory canal), and the second pouch forms the palatine (not the lingual) tonsil. The ultimobranchial body forms from the fifth pouch and produces the thyroid C cells.

HEAD AND NECK DEVELOPMENT

5. *Which one of the following statements is correct?*
   B. The thyroid gland develops from the tongue.
   The clinical relevance of the thyroid developing from the foramen caecum of the tongue is that during embryologic development, the thyroid moves caudally to its final destination in the neck just below the cricoid cartilage. If a persistent connection is retained between these two structures then a thyroglossal duct cyst may form and this presents as a painless midline neck swelling in the region of the hyoid bone. A cyst can develop anywhere along the path of the descending thyroid between the tongue base and thyroid, but cysts close to the tongue and floor of the mouth are uncommon. Clinical examination of a patient with a thyroglossal cyst will display swelling elevation on protrusion of the tongue. Treatment is by complete surgical excision under general anesthesia. Recurrence is likely to occur if excision is incomplete.
   The tongue is formed from three arches (I, III, and IV), not just two. The anterior two thirds originates from the first arch and receives sensory innervation from the lingual nerve (trigeminal nerve branch) and taste sensation from the facial nerve through the chordae tympani. The posterior third originates from arches III and IV, with sensory and taste innervation from the glossopharyngeal and vagus nerves. The hypoglossal nerve supplies motor innervation to the tongue. The external ear is formed from arches I and II and develops in the neck region before passing cranially during the first trimester. This explains why microtia usually results in an inferiorly placed ear remnant.
   The bones of the facial skeleton including the maxilla, mandible, frontal, squamous, and parietal bones are formed by the process of intramembranous ossification. In contrast, the bones of the skull base including the sphenoid, ethmoid, mastoid, and petrous temporal bone are formed by endochondral ossification from cartilage precursors. Meckels cartilage is an exception to the rule as this forms the malleus and mandibular condyle via endochondral ossification.
   The face develops from five prominences; the paired mandibular and maxillary prominences and the single frontonasal prominence. This has clinical relevance to the development of Tessier clefts and cleft lip/palate (see Chapters 22, 24, and 25).

EMBRYOLOGIC ORIGINS OF ADULT STRUCTURES

6. *For the following anatomic structures, the best options are as follows:*
   A. Philtrum
       c. Medial nasal prominence
   B. Lower lip
       f. Mandibular prominence
   C. Secondary palate
       b. Maxillary prominence
           As discussed in question 5, the face develops from the paired maxillary and mandibular prominences along with the frontonasal prominence, which comprises the medial and lateral

nasal prominences. The medial nasal prominence forms the primary palate, the midmaxilla, midlip, philtrum, central nose, and nasal septum. The lateral nasal prominence forms the nasal alae. The mandibular prominences form the mandible, lower lip, and face. The maxillary prominences form the secondary palate, lateral maxilla, and lateral lip. Knowledge of the embryologic development and fusion of these prominences provides the basis for understanding the concepts of cleft lip, cleft palate, and Tessier clefts (see Chapters 22, 24, and 25).

7. **For the following anatomic structures, the best options are as follows:**
   A. Primary palate
      c. Medial nasal prominence
   B. Nasal alae
      e. Lateral nasal prominence
   C. Nasal septum
      c. Medial nasal prominence

   As discussed in question 5, the face develops from the paired maxillary and mandibular prominences along with the frontonasal prominence, which comprises the medial and lateral nasal prominences. The medial nasal prominence forms the primary palate, the midmaxilla, midlip, philtrum, central nose, and nasal septum. The lateral nasal prominence forms the nasal alae. The mandibular prominences form the mandible, lower lip, and face. The maxillary prominences form the secondary palate, lateral maxilla, and lateral lip. Knowledge of the embryologic development and fusion of these prominences provides the basis for understanding the concepts of cleft lip, cleft palate, and Tessier clefts (see Chapters 22, 24, and 25) (Fig. 19-2).

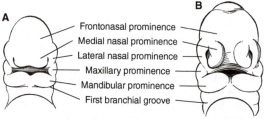

Fig. 19-2 Embryonic development of the human face. **A,** Week 5. **B,** Week 6. **C,** Week 7.

20. Surgical Treatment of Migraine Headaches

See *Essentials of Plastic Surgery*, second edition, pp. 223-233.

MEDICAL THERAPY FOR MIGRAINES
1. *Which one of the following medications is used to stop a migraine attack once it has started?*
   A. Propranolol
   B. Gabapentin
   C. Diphenhydramine
   D. Sumatriptan
   E. Verapamil

TRIGGER ANATOMY
2. *Peripheral compression of which one of the following cranial nerves may be indicated in development of migraine headaches?*
   A. Facial
   B. Trigeminal
   C. Olfactory
   D. Vagus
   E. Glossopharyngeal

3. *Which one of the following tissue types is not implicated as a source contributing to migraine headaches?*
   A. Muscle
   B. Fascia
   C. Tendon
   D. Bone
   E. Blood vessel

4. *During surgical exploration of the supraorbital nerve, what is the most likely anatomic arrangement causing compression at the supraorbital notch?*
   A. A bony spicule
   B. A fascial band
   C. A muscular band
   D. A narrow foramen
   E. A double septum

5. You are undertaking nerve decompression of the greater occipital nerve. *Which muscle does the greater occipital nerve pass through just before it enters the trapezius?*
   A. Splenius capitis
   B. Semispinalis capitis
   C. Rectus capitis
   D. Obliquus capitis inferior
   E. Medialis capitis superiori

SYMPTOMS RELATED TO DIFFERENT MIGRAINE HEADACHES

6. A patient who is generally fit and well presents with a history of morning migraine headaches. The patient was recently advised by a dentist to use a night mouthguard. **Which type of migraine is most likely?**
   A. Rhinogenic
   B. Occipital
   C. Temporal
   D. Frontal
   E. Parietal

7. A 30-year-old surgeon presents with a history of migraines that occur most often after she works out at the gym. The attacks can be particularly bad after a full day of operating. **Which type of migraine is most likely?**
   A. Rhinogenic
   B. Temporal
   C. Occipital
   D. Frontal
   E. Parietal

MANAGEMENT OF PATIENTS WITH MIGRAINE HEADACHES

8. A 40-year-old patient has severe migraine headaches two or three times each week, with pain originating above the eyebrows, radiating into the forehead and scalp. Attacks are helped, but not arrested, by manual pressure on the brow. She has been prescribed Sumatriptan and propanolol and also uses NSAIDs. **What is the next best step in management of this patient?**
   A. Record a migraine journal for one month
   B. Add in zolmitriptan and elitriptan
   C. Inject local anesthetic into the brow
   D. Inject botulinum toxin A into the brow
   E. Surgically decompress the supraorbital nerve

9. *In which anatomic area is local nerve block with lidocaine or bupivacaine particularly useful for assessment of nerve irritation trigger points in migraine patients?*
   A. Brow
   B. Temple
   C. Occiput
   D. Neck
   E. Nose

10. When botulinum toxin A is given as migraine therapy, what percentage reduction in intensity or frequency of migraines is generally required to define significant improvement?
    A. 10%
    B. 20%
    C. 40%
    D. 50%
    E. 70%

11. **Which one of the following sensory nerves is most likely to be intentionally sacrificed in migraine surgery, resulting in an area of residual paresthesia?**
    A. Greater occipital nerve
    B. Lesser occipital nerve
    C. Supraorbital nerve
    D. Supratrochlear nerve
    E. Zygomaticotemporal nerve

12. **Which one of the following is correct regarding the surgical management of migraines?**
   A. Supraorbital nerve decompression requires an endoscopic approach.
   B. Greater occipital nerve decompression may involve elevation of a fat flap.
   C. Surgery should be considered the mainstay of treatment for most migraine patients.
   D. Most surgical approaches involve resection of bone or osteotomies.
   E. Correction of a deviated septum is first-line treatment for most cases.

OUTCOMES AFTER MIGRAINE SURGERY

13. **Which one of the following patients is most likely to have a good result after migraine surgery?**
   A. A patient with a high number of migraines each month
   B. A patient with a history of previous whiplash injury
   C. A patient with migraines first starting in their twenties
   D. A patient who has multiple trigger sites decompressed
   E. A patient who undergoes surgery at a younger age

Answers

MEDICAL THERAPY FOR MIGRAINES

1. Which one of the following medications is used to stop a migraine attack once it has started?

D. Sumatriptan

Having baseline knowledge of medications used to treat a migraine is important when assessing patients for migraine surgery. There are three main types of medication used to manage migraines; prophylactic agents, abortive agents, and acute analgesics. The triptans, including sumatriptan, represent an abortive type of therapy and are given to prevent a suspected early migraine or stop an attack once it has begun. They act on serotonin 5-HT receptors and inhibit release of neuropeptides. The frequency of triptan use is a useful guide to both the frequency and severity of migraine attacks. Recording a journal of triptan use is also helpful for comparison before and after intervention with botox injections or surgery.

Prophylactic agents have the goal of reducing severity and frequency of migraine attacks. They are subclassified as beta blockers (e.g., propranolol), calcium channel blockers (e.g., verapamil), antidepressants (e.g., amitriptyline), anticonvulsants (e.g., gabapentin or valproate), or antihistamines (e.g., diphenhydramine).

Acute analgesics have the goal of relieving mild-to-moderate symptoms of migraine during an episode. These comprise NSAIDs such as ibuprofen, aspirin, or diclofenac. Another popular agent is acetaminophen.

TRIGGER ANATOMY

2. Peripheral compression of which one of the following cranial nerves may be indicated in development of migraine headaches?

B. Trigeminal

Migraine headaches have traditionally been treated with medications as described in question 1. However, migraines persist in many patients, in spite of these medical treatments and as a result, new surgical approaches to their management have been developed. These are based on the theory that extracranial sensory branches of the trigeminal and cervical spinal nerves can be irritated, entrapped, or compressed at points throughout their anatomic course. Surgical treatments are aimed at addressing the compression sites in order to reduce compression and ultimately the frequency and severity of migraine attacks.[1]

Specific compression of the facial, vagus, or glossopharyngeal nerves is not thought to be responsible for the development of migraines although patients can experience visual disturbances and abnormal smells or tastes before or during an attack. Nasal abnormalities such as a deviated septum may be implicated in migraines via irritation of the anterior and posterior ethmoid and nasopalatine nerves, which are branches of the trigeminal nerve, but the olfactory nerve which is responsible for the sense of smell is not involved.

3. Which of the following tissue types is not implicated as a source contributing to migraine headaches?

C. Tendon

A number of different anatomic trigger points of the trigeminal nerve and cervical plexus have been implicated in the development of migraine headaches. A variety of tissue types have been attributed to the compression or irritation, but tendon is not one of them.

Tissues implicated in causing compression and/or irritation of the nerves include muscle, fascia, bone, and vessel. For example, supraorbital nerve triggers may be caused by the corrugators or procerus muscles, bone, and fascia at the supraorbital foramen, or by the adjacent supraorbital artery (see Figs. 20-1 and 20-3, *Essentials of Plastic Surgery,* second edition). In addition, cartilage may be implicated in intranasal compression by the effects of septal deviation on paranasal branches of the trigeminal nerve (branches of the sphenopalatine ganglion).

4. **During surgical exploration of the supraorbital nerve, what is the most likely anatomic arrangement causing compression at the supraorbital notch?**
   B. A fascial band
   Compression of the supraorbital nerve is implicated in migraine headaches and can occur at a number of sites. In approximately 86% of cases there is a fascial band across the supraorbital notch that may be the cause of compression in this area. The anatomy of fascial compression is subclassified into the subgroups type I, type II, and type III, depending on the anatomic arrangement of fascia and bone.

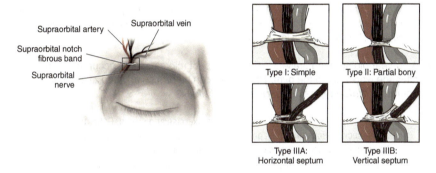

Fig. 20-1 Bony, fascial, and vascular compression of the supraorbital nerve.

Type I represents a single fascia band over a single foramen and is the most common type. Type II bands have partial bony spicules that extend to the neurovascular bundle. Type III bands contain a horizontal *(A)* or vertical *(B)* septum that encases the nerve (Fig. 20-1). Muscular sites of compression beyond the supraorbital foramen include the corrugator and procerus muscles.

5. **Which muscle does the greater occipital nerve pass through just before it enters the trapezius?**
   B. Semispinalis capitis
   The greater occipital nerve is the medial branch of the dorsal primary ramus of C2 (Fig. 20-2).

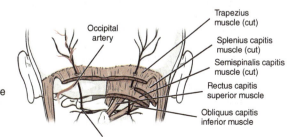

Fig. 20-2 Greater occipital nerve anatomy.

The trunk exits approximately 3 cm below and 1.5 cm lateral to the occipital protuberance. It passes around the obliquus capitis inferior and then the rectus capitis superior before piercing the semispinalis capitis medially. It finally passes through the trapezius, where it is closely associated with the occipital artery. Surgical access to this nerve is through a 5 cm long midline incision a few centimeters below the occipital protuberance.

SYMPTOMS RELATED TO DIFFERENT MIGRAINE HEADACHES

6. A patient who is generally fit and well presents with a history of morning migraine headaches. The patient was recently advised by a dentist to use a night mouthguard. *Which type of migraine is most likely?*
   C. Temporal
   Temporal migraine often occurs in the morning and is associated with bruxism (grinding of the teeth) overnight. Pain is often associated with the temporalis or masseter muscles and originates just lateral and cephalad to the lateral canthus. Patients with temporal headaches may describe improvement with manual pressure applied to the area of the superficial temporal artery during a migraine attack.[2] It is postulated that pulsation of the superficial temporal artery causes irritation to local sensory nerve fibers.[3] For this reason, some surgical treatments involve tying off the superficial temporal artery for such patients.

7. A 30-year-old surgeon presents with a history of migraines that occur most often after she works out at the gym. The attacks can be particularly bad after a full day of operating. *Which type of migraine is most likely?*
   C. Occipital
   Occipital migraines can be triggered by heavy exercise and stress. Patients often have tight posterior neck musculature. Pain originates just lateral to the midline, a few centimeters caudal to the occipital tuberosity and there is often a tender site on manual palpation close to the origin of trapezius. Irritation of the greater occipital nerve, which is a branch of C2 (see question 5 and Fig. 20-2), is thought to be implicated in this type of migraine and may be due to muscle or fascial compressions, or irritation from the occipital artery.

MANAGEMENT OF PATIENTS WITH MIGRAINE HEADACHES

8. A 40-year-old patient has severe migraine headaches two or three times each week, with pain originating above the eyebrows, radiating into the forehead and scalp. Attacks are helped, but not arrested, by manual pressure on the brow. She has been prescribed sumatriptan and propanolol and also uses NSAIDs. *What is the next best step in management of this patient?*
   D. Inject botulinum toxin A into the brow
   This patient has reached a stage where a trial of Botox injection is warranted. The main aim of using Botox is to test the effectiveness of providing temporary decompression of the trigeminal or cervical nerves at specific migraine trigger sites (see Fig. 20-9, *Essentials of Plastic Surgery*, second edition).

   Before the Botox injection a patient should record a journal of migraine headaches and medication use, but this patient has already done so and has provided a clear history. She is already taking a triptan so there is no benefit in adding in other triptans in this case. Furthermore, manipulation of medications is best left to the treating neurologist. Injection of local anesthetic will provide immediate short-term relief by anesthetizing the target nerve but will not reliably predict outcome or appropriateness of surgery for most trigger sites including the brow. Moving to surgical decompression is only indicated for this patient, once a positive result of trigger site anatomy from Botox has been demonstrated.

9. **In which anatomic area is local nerve block with lidocaine or bupivacaine particularly useful for assessment of nerve irritation trigger points in migraine patients?**
   B. Temple
   Local nerve block (as discussed in question 8), may be undertaken using lidocaine or bupivacaine to identify triggers that Botox misses, such as the auriculotemporal nerve in temporal headaches. The auriculotemporal nerve is a branch of V_3 and extends through the parotid gland, then travels over the temporomandibular joint (TMJ) before dividing over the zygomatic arch and within the layers of the temporaparietal fascia. It provides sensation to the tragus, the anterior portion of the ear, and posterior temple. Compression may be caused by soft tissues of the temple or the superficial temporal artery. Muscular compression is not typical so Botox is not useful here. The other sites are more likely to benefit from Botox injection for trigger point assessment. However all sites can be targeted with local anesthetic block as acute treatment of active migraines.

10. **When botulinum toxin A is given as migraine therapy, what percentage reduction in intensity or frequency of migraines is generally required to define significant improvement?**
    D. 50%
    Botulinum toxin A has been approved for use in the prophylactic management of chronic migraine headaches. As discussed in question 8, it is primarily used as an effective test to confirm suspected trigger sites. Its efficacy should be measured and recorded in a journal. *Improvement* is defined as a 50% reduction in the intensity or frequency of migraines over a 4-week period. Patients who improve may then be considered for surgery. It is sometimes also used as repeated long-term treatment for patients with chronic migraines who prefer not to proceed with surgery, but have displayed a significant response to therapy.

11. **Which one of the following sensory nerves is most likely to be intentionally sacrificed in migraine surgery, resulting in an area of residual paresthesia?**
    E. Zygomaticotemporal nerve
    Temporal migraines can be triggered by compression of the zygomaticotemporal or auriculotemporal nerves which are branches of the trigeminal nerve. The zygomaticotemporal nerve arises from the maxillary division (V_2), and the auriculotemporal nerve arises from the mandibular division (V_3). The zygomaticotemporal nerve supplies a small patch of skin on the parietal scalp and is a nerve that is avulsed rather than decompressed in order to improve symptoms of migraine. The other nerves listed are all regularly preserved and sources of irritation or compression are removed.

12. **Which one of the following is correct regarding the surgical management of migraines?**
    B. Greater occipital nerve decompression may involve elevation of a fat flap.
    Greater occipital nerve release may be combined with elevation of a fat flap in order to protect the nerve and reduce the chance of compression recurrence. Supraorbital nerve decompression may be achieved through endoscopic, open brow, or transpalpebral approaches. Surgery should

not be the mainstay of treatment for most migraine patients. It is used for patients who have an established diagnosis of migraine by a neurologist and have a failure of traditional medication. Most surgical approaches involve decompression of muscle, fascial bands, and ablation of blood vessels as the primary aim and do not require osteotomies or foraminotomies except on rare occasion.

OUTCOMES AFTER MIGRAINE SURGERY

13. **Which one of the following patients is most likely to have a good result after migraine surgery?**

   D. A patient with multiple trigger sites decompressed

   Five-year outcomes after migraine surgery were described by Guyuron's team.[4,5] They found that more than 80% of patients who had surgery reported improvement in terms of reduced frequency of attacks and improved symptoms. They found that patients who had multiple trigger sites treated were more likely to have a successful outcome. This applied to targeting both frontal and temporal trigger sites together and targeting all four sites where appropriate (including nasal and occipital).

   Factors associated with better outcomes also included an older age at first onset of migraine symptoms, fewer baseline migraines per month, and daily use of over-the-counter medications. Factors associated with worse outcomes included a history of head or neck injury, increased intraoperative bleeding, and single-site surgery that could result in inadequate treatment of all trigger sites.

REFERENCES

1. Janis JE, Barker JC, Javadi C, et al. A review of current evidence in the surgical treatment of migraine headaches. Plast Reconstr Surg 134(4 Suppl 2):131S-141S, 2014.
2. Cianchetti C, Cianchetti ME, Pisano T, et al. Treatment of migraine attacks by compression of temporal superficial arteries using a device. Med Sci Monit 15:CR185-188, 2009.
3. Chim H, Okada HC, Brown M, et al. The auriculotemporal nerve in etiology of migraine headaches: compression points and anatomical variations. Plast Reconstr Surg 130:336-341, 2012.
4. Guyuron B, Kriegler J, Davis J, et al. Five-year outcome of surgical treatment of migraine headaches. Plast Reconstr Surg 127:603, 2011.
5. Larson K, Lee M, Davis J, et al. Factors contributing to migraine headache surgery failure and success. Plast Reconstr Surg 128:1069, 2011.

Congenital Conditions

21. Craniosynostosis

See *Essentials of Plastic Surgery*, second edition, pp. 234-247.

CRANIAL GROWTH AND DEVELOPMENT

1. **Match each of the following descriptions to the age at which it most commonly occurs. (Each option may be used once, more than once, or not at all.)**
   A. The age at which the brain reaches 85% of adult size
   B. Closure of the anterior fontanelle
   C. Closure of the sagittal suture

   Options:
   a. 3 months
   b. 12 months
   c. 2 years
   d. 3 years
   e. 18 years
   f. 22 years
   g. 26 years

PATHOPHYSIOLOGY OF CRANIOSYNOSTOSIS

2. **Which one of the following statements is correct regarding craniosynostosis?**
   A. Most cases are syndromic and linked to the FGFR gene.
   B. Normal cranial growth occurs parallel to the suture lines.
   C. Virchow's law relates to changes in ICP with untreated synostoses.
   D. Appositional growth is part of normal cranial development.
   E. Cranial base theory fully explains all types of craniosynostoses.

DIAGNOSIS OF RAISED INTRACRANIAL PRESSURE

3. **Which one of the following is expected in a craniosynostosis patient with elevated intracranial pressure (ICP)?**
   A. Normal fundoscopic examination
   B. Soft fontanelles on physical examination
   C. Decreased optic nerve sheath diameter on transorbital ultrasound
   D. Decreased latency on measurement of visual evoked potentials
   E. Headaches, irritability, and an altered developmental progression

ELEVATED INTRACRANIAL PRESSURE IN CRANIOSYNOSTOSIS

4. **Which one of the following is correct regarding the pediatric population?**
   A. The normal ICP value in children is well documented.
   B. Fundoscopy is an unreliable tool for assessment of ICP in young children.
   C. A Chiari malformation is a vascular malformation resulting in elevated ICP.
   D. Cephalocranial disproportion is the sole cause of raised ICP in syndromic craniosynostosis.
   E. Elevated ICP is most likely in a single-suture craniosynostosis.

IMAGING IN CRANIOSYNOSTOSIS

5. **Which one of the following is correct regarding imaging of a patient who has nonsyndromic craniosynostosis?**
   A. Cortical thickening, fingerprinting, and loss of cisternae are early radiologic findings that suggest raised ICP.
   B. A CT scan is usually required in all cases of craniosynostosis, because plain radiographic films are unhelpful.
   C. The absence of suture lines on plain radiographic films is evidence of suture fusion.
   D. A copper-beaten appearance on CT is highly specific for elevated intracranial pressure.
   E. Serial MRI assessment is helpful for most cases of craniosynostosis.

DIAGNOSIS OF CRANIOSYNOSTOSIS

6. The parents of a 12-week-old baby have concerns about their child's head shape. On examination the child has a misshapen head with a triangular appearance when viewed from above. The child's eyes are close together. **What is the most likely suture involved in this craniosynostosis?**
   A. Unilateral coronal
   B. Metopic
   C. Lambdoid
   D. Sagittal
   E. Bilateral coronal

CLASSIFICATION OF SYNOSTOSIS

7. **Which one of the following is the most common craniosynostosis?**
   A. Unilateral coronal
   B. Metopic
   C. Lambdoid
   D. Sagittal
   E. Bilateral coronal

HARLEQUIN DEFORMITY

8. **Which one of the following sutures is associated with a harlequin deformity?**
   A. Unilateral coronal
   B. Metopic
   C. Lambdoid
   D. Sagittal
   E. Bilateral coronal

DEFORMATIONAL PLAGIOCEPHALY

9. A child is referred to clinic with a diagnosis of deformational plagiocephaly. **What head shape is typical of this condition?**
   A. Triangular
   B. Parallelogram
   C. Boat shaped
   D. Square
   E. Trapezoidal

10. A child is referred with an abnormal head shape but normal physical development. **When trying to differentiate between a deformational plagiocephaly and a true craniosynostosis, which anatomic structure will be positioned normally in only the deformational condition?**
    A. Cheek
    B. Chin
    C. Brow
    D. Nasal root
    E. Ear

MORPHOLOGICAL VARIANTS IN CRANIOSYNOSTOSIS

11. You see a syndromic child who has an untreated bicoronal synostosis. *Which one of the following would you expect to see on examination?*
    - A. Turribrachycephaly
    - B. Oxycephaly
    - C. Kleeblatschadel
    - D. Posterior plagiocephaly
    - E. Scaphocephaly

CROUZON SYNDROME

12. *Which one of the following is correct regarding Crouzon syndrome?*
    - A. The inheritance pattern is autosomal recessive.
    - B. Multiple different sutures may be involved.
    - C. ICP is rarely elevated.
    - D. Class I malocclusion is present.
    - E. Extremity abnormalities are common.

APERT SYNDROME

13. A child who has been diagnosed with Apert syndrome presents to clinic. *Which one of the following features will differentiate this condition from other similar synostototic syndromes?*
    - A. Normal intracranial pressure (ICP)
    - B. Cleft palate
    - C. Brachycephaly
    - D. Complex syndactyly
    - E. Midface hypoplasia

PFEIFFER SYNDROME

14. *Which one of the following is least expected during examination of a patient with Pfeiffer syndrome?*
    - A. Broad thumbs and halluces
    - B. Mild cutaneous syndactyly
    - C. Tracheostomy in situ
    - D. Mental impairment
    - E. Turribrachycephaly

SAETHRE-CHOTZEN SYNDROME

15. *Which one of the following is correct regarding Saethre-Chotzen syndrome?*
    - A. It has an incidence of 1:200,000.
    - B. It is associated with a TWIST gene mutation.
    - C. It involves symmetrical brachycephaly.
    - D. Patients have a relative absence of upper eyelid skin.
    - E. A high hairline is typically seen.

Answers

CRANIAL GROWTH AND DEVELOPMENT
1. *For the following descriptions, the best options are as follows:*
   A. *The age at which the brain reaches 85% of adult size*
      d. **3 years**
         The brain grows rapidly after birth and usually triples in size by the time a child is 1 year of age. It continues to rapidly increase in size, and by 3 years of age it is 85% of adult size.
   B. *Closure of the anterior fontanelle*
      b. **12 months**
         The posterior fontanelle is the first to close at 3 to 6 months, followed by the anterior fontanelle at 9 to 12 months.
   C. *Closure of the sagittal suture*
      f. **22 years**
         Most of the cranial sutures remain open until the third decade of life (sagittal: 22 years, coronal: 24 years, and lambdoidal: 26 years). The exception is the metopic suture, which typically closes in the first year of life (Fig. 21-1).

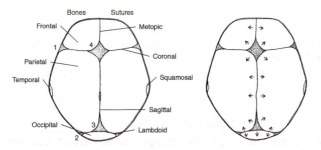

Fig. 21-1 Cranial sutures in the human fetus. Premature closure produces growth restriction perpendicular to the line of the suture and compensatory overgrowth parallel to it.

PATHOPHYSIOLOGY OF CRANIOSYNOSTOSIS
2. *Which one of the following statements is correct regarding craniosynostosis?*
   D. **Appositional growth is part of normal cranial development.**
      Cranial growth usually occurs through two processes, suture growth and appositional growth. Appositional growth involves bone resorption on the inner surface and deposition on the outer surface of the skull. Suture growth usually occurs perpendicular to the cranial sutures and premature suture fusion will result in predominantly parallel growth. This is known as Virchow's law and explains the deformities observed with fusion of a given suture.

      Only one third of craniosynostoses are syndromic. In cases that are syndromic, genetic mutations in the FGFR2, FGFR3, and TWIST1 genes may be identified. Various theories exist regarding abnormal suture fusion and include the cranial base theory and the intrinsic suture theory. The cranial base theory states that synostoses result from abnormal tension exerted by the cranial base through the dura, but this does not account for isolated synostoses. The intrinsic suture biology theory proposes that synostoses result from the osteoinductive properties of dura mater, which contains osteoblast-like cells.

DIAGNOSIS OF RAISED INTRACRANIAL PRESSURE

3. Which one of the following is expected in a craniosynostosis patient with elevated intracranial pressure (ICP)?

E. Headaches, irritability, and an altered developmental progression

Elevated intracranial pressure (ICP) is associated with craniosynostosis either due to cephalocranial disproportion or other factors such as intracranial venous congestion, hydrocephalus or upper airway obstruction. Early clinical findings that suggest a raised ICP include headache, irritability, nausea, vomiting, and sleeping difficulties. Later findings include mental impairment, delayed development, and visual disturbances. Fundoscopic examination may show papilledema and examination of the fontalles may show tense bulging, sometimes known as the *volcano sign*.

Raised ICP may be measured directly or indirectly. Transorbital ultrasound can be used to measure optic nerve sheath diameter, which will increase (not decrease) with raised ICP. Visual evoked potentials measure the latency time of an encephalographic response to visual stimuli and will also be increased with raised ICP and axonal injury. Other modalities used to assess raised ICP include plain radiographs which may show late signs of a copper-beaten appearance or thumb printing from pressure of the gyri on the inner table.

ELEVATED INTRACRANIAL PRESSURE IN CRANIOSYNOSTOSIS

4. Which one of the following is correct regarding the pediatric population?

B. Fundoscopy is an unreliable tool for assessment of ICP in young children.

No universal definition exists for raised ICP in children. Fundoscopy is a useful tool for assessing raised ICP in many cases, but it should be interpreted with caution in children. Across all age groups it has a specificity of 98% and a sensitivity of 100%. However, in children younger than 8 years of age, the sensitivity is around 22%. A Chiari malformation is not a vascular malformation, but it can result in a raised ICP. It is present when the cerebellar tonsils are displaced downward through the foramen magnum. This malformation may be a cause of hydrocephalus and neurodevelopmental injury. It is commonly seen in patients with Crouzon or Pfeiffer syndrome. Cephalocranial disproportion refers to a decreased intracranial volume and restriction of brain growth. It is one cause of raised ICP; others include intracranial venous congestion, hydrocephalus, and airway obstruction. The incidence of elevated ICP is affected by the number of sutures involved in craniosynostosis. The incidence of elevated ICP with single suture involvement is 13% and 42% when multiple sutures are involved.

IMAGING IN CRANIOSYNOSTOSIS

5. Which one of the following is correct regarding imaging of a patient who has nonsyndromic craniosynostosis?

C. The absence of suture lines on plain radiographic films is evidence of suture fusion.

Plain radiographs are useful to show an absence of suture lines and are usually the only imaging modality required for patients with craniosynostoses. In syndromic cases, however, CT can be helpful to diagnose associated abnormalities, to plan surgery, and to monitor hydrocephalus. MRI is typically unnecessary except in patients with selected syndromes such as Aperts or Pfeiffers, when associated brain abnormalities are suspected.

Radiographs may show other signs of synostosis. For example, a copper-beaten appearance on radiograph is also known as *Luckenschadel* and is a characteristic late sign (with a low specificity) of raised ICP in craniosynostosis. Other late findings are cortical thickening, fingerprinting, and loss of cisternae.

DIAGNOSIS OF CRANIOSYNOSTOSIS

6. The parents of a 12-week-old baby have concerns about their child's head shape. On examination the child has a misshapen head with a triangular appearance when viewed from above. The child's eyes are close together. **What is the most likely suture involved in this craniosynostosis?**
   B. Metopic
   The appearance described is known as *trigonocephaly*. This is caused by premature fusion of the metopic suture. A spectrum of deformities occurs, including bitemporal narrowing, hypotelorism, and bilateral supraorbital retrusion.

CLASSIFICATION OF SYNOSTOSES

7. **Which one of the following is the most common craniosynostosis?**
   D. Sagittal
   Sagittal synostosis represents half of all synostoses. They are four times as common in males and clinically present with an increased AP cranial diameter and decreased biparietal width. This appearance is described as *scaphocephaly*, meaning "boat shaped." Coronal synostoses represent approximately one third of all synostoses, and they are usually unilateral. Metopic synostoses are a little less common than coronal synostoses, and affected babies develop trigonocephaly. The least common form is lambdoid, which is extremely rare (Fig. 21-2).

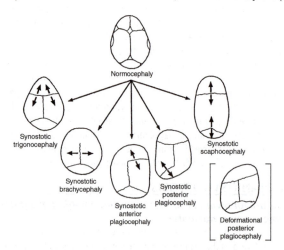

Fig. 21-2 Skull shapes and affected sutures in craniosynostosis.

HARLEQUIN DEFORMITY

8. Which one of the following sutures is associated with a harlequin deformity?
A. Unilateral coronal

A harlequin deformity results from a lack of descent of the greater wing of the sphenoid on the affected side. It is seen on radiographs of patients with a unilateral coronal synostosis. Physical findings in unilateral synostosis include an anterior plagiocephaly that involves ipsilateral frontal and occipitoparietal flattening, contralateral frontal and parietal bossing, and posterior displacement of the ipsilateral ear (Fig. 21-3).

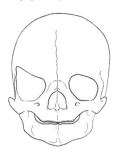

Fig. 21-3 Harlequin deformity.

DEFORMATIONAL PLAGIOCEPHALY

9. A child is referred to clinic with a diagnosis of deformational plagiocephaly. What head shape is typical of this condition?
B. Parallelogram

The characteristic head shape in deformational plagiocephaly is a parallelogram appearance (see Fig. 21-2).

Deformational plagiocephaly can be mistaken for either posterior (lambdoidal) or anterior (unilateral coronal) synostoses, but is not a true craniosynostosis. It is relatively common with an incidence of 1 in 300 and occurs secondary to external forces applied through the baby's head. It has recently become more common and this may be due to the fact that infants are increasingly nursed in a supine position in order to minimize risk of sudden infant death syndrome. A triangular head shape is characteristic of metopic synostosis (see question 6). A boat-shaped head is associated with a sagittal synostosis. A square, broad head shape is associated with a bicoronal synostosis. A trapezoidal head shape is associated with anterior or posterior plagiocephaly (lambdoidal or coronal synostoses, respectively).

10. A child is referred with an abnormal head shape but normal physical development. When trying to differentiate between a deformational plagiocephaly and a true craniosynostosis, which anatomic structure will be positioned normally in only the deformational condition?
D. Nasal root

As described in question 9, deformational plagiocephaly is distinguished from a true craniosynostoses by the presence of a parallelogram configuration with flattening of the occiput (Table 21-1). The nasal root will be unaffected in this condition and therefore remain in the midline. In contrast, the nasal root will be moved towards the ipsilateral side in a true craniosynostosis. The cheek, chin, ear, and brow position are all affected in both deformational and synostotic conditions. In general, the direction of their movement is opposite in each of two conditions.

Table 21-1 *Anatomic Features That Differentiate Synostotic and Deformational Plagiocephaly*

Anatomic Feature	Synostotic	Deformational
Ipsilateral superior orbital rim	Up	Down
Ipsilateral ear	Anterior and high	Posterior and low
Nasal root	Ipsilateral	Midline
Ipsilateral cheek	Forward	Backward
Chin deviation	Contralateral	Ipsilateral
Ipsilateral palpebral fissure	Wide	Narrow
Anterior fontanel deviation	Low contralateral	High none

MORPHOLOGICAL VARIANTS IN CRANIOSYNOSTOSIS

11. You see a syndromic child who has an untreated bicoronal synostosis. *Which one of the following would you expect to see on examination?*
   A. Turribrachycephaly
   Turribrachycephaly is where there is excessive skull height and vertical forehead secondary to an untreated brachycephaly. *Oxycephaly* refers to a pointed head with a retroverted forehead secondary to a pansynostosis. *Kleeblatschadel* refers to a cloverleaf deformity secondary to involvement of all sutures except squamosal. Posterior *plagiocephaly* occurs secondary to lambdoid synostosis. *Scaphocephaly* (or *dolichocephaly*) is secondary to premature fusion of the sagittal suture.

CROUZON SYNDROME

12. *Which one of the following is correct regarding Crouzon syndrome?*
   B. Multiple different sutures may be involved.
   Crouzon is the most common syndromic craniosynostosis that occurs 1 in 25,000 live births. It most commonly involves the coronal sutures but may involve other sutures including the sagittal and metopic. It is an autosomal dominant condition and ICP is elevated in approximately 65% of cases. Crouzon patients have normal extremities and this is a key finding that helps to differentiate this condition from some other synostotic conditions. Midface hypoplasia with exorbitism and turribrachycephaly is a typical finding. This results in a class III malocclusion in most cases.

APERT SYNDROME

13. A child who has been diagnosed with Apert syndrome presents to clinic. *Which one of the following features will differentiate this condition from other similar synostotic syndromes?*
   D. Complex syndactyly
   Apert syndrome is an autosomal dominant condition that affects 1:100,000 to 1:160,000 live births.[1] The presence of a complex symmetrical syndactyly distinguishes this syndrome from

other craniosynostoses which may have the other features described. Apert syndactyly has three distinct subtypes and was classified by Upton[1] in 1991. Type I is a spade hand with the thumb and little finger separate and a syndactyly of the second and third web spaces. Type II is a mitten hand with the thumb free and syndactyly between the second, third, and fourth web spaces. Type III is a rosebud hand with all digits involved in the syndactyly (Fig. 21-4).

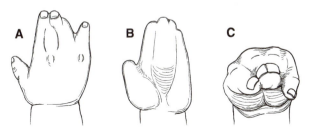

Fig. 21-4 **A,** Typical type I or spade-shaped hand. **B,** Type II or mitten hand. **C,** Type III or rosebud hand.

Raised ICP is seen in more than three quarters of patients with Apert syndrome and ventriculoperitoneal (VP) shunts are often required. Many patients have decreased intelligence. Apert syndrome is associated with bicoronal synostoses with significant turribrachycephaly and midface hypoplasia, therefore patients have some features in keeping with both Crouzon and Pfeiffer syndromes. Cleft palate is also a feature of many different craniosynostotic syndromes so it is not a good differentiating factor.

PFEIFFER SYNDROME

14. Which one of the following is least expected during examination of a patient with Pfeiffer syndrome?

D. Mental impairment

Patients with Pfeiffer syndrome usually have a normal mental status, although this may be decreased in the most severe cases.

Pfeiffer syndrome is a rare craniofacial condition involving synostoses in conjunction with extremity deformities and hydrocephalus. Incidence is 1:100,000 and is a result of mutations in the FGFR genes. Three different subtypes have been described according to clinical features and syndrome severity.[2]

Type I features include brachycephaly, midface hypoplasia, finger, toe abnormalities, and normal intelligence. Type 2 features a cloverleaf skull, proptosis, major finger/toe abnormalities. Developmental delay may be present. Type 3 patients are similar to type 2 but without the cloverleaf skull.

SAETHRE-CHOTZEN SYNDROME

15. Which one of the following is correct regarding Saethre-Chotzen syndrome?

B. It is associated with a TWIST gene mutation.

Saethre-Chotzen syndrome occurs in 1:25,000 to 1:50,000 live births. It is inherited in an autosomal dominant fashion and is associated with the TWIST gene mutation. Patients have asymmetrical brachycephaly, eyelid ptosis, and a low hairline.

REFERENCES

1. Upton J. Apert syndrome. Classification and pathologic anatomy of limb anomalies. Clin Plast Surg 18:321-355, 1991.
2. Cohen MM Jr. Pfeiffer syndrome update, clinical subtypes, and guidelines for different diagnosis. Am J Med Genet 45:300-307, 1993.

22. Craniofacial Clefts

See *Essentials of Plastic Surgery*, second edition, pp. 248-257.

CRANIOFACIAL EMBRYOLOGY

1. **Which one of the following statements is correct regarding facial embryology?**
   A. Development of the face occurs between weeks 2 and 10.
   B. The frontonasal prominence derives from the primitive forebrain.
   C. The lateral nasal prominence forms the nasal ala and premaxilla.
   D. The basic facial features are clearly recognizable by week 4.
   E. The external ear is formed entirely from the mandibular arch.

TESSIER CLEFTS

2. **Which one of the following statements is correct regarding Tessier clefts?**
   A. All clefts are numbered in increasing order according to their position relative to the midline.
   B. Cleft numbers 10-14 are described as *cranial clefts*.
   C. The lateral facial clefts are the most common subtypes.
   D. Fifteen different types of cleft are described in Tessier's classification.
   E. Oral-ocular clefts (numbers 4-6) usually disrupt nasal integrity.

3. **Match the following descriptions of Tessier clefts to the most appropriate option. (Each option may be used once, more than once, or not at all.)**
   A. This cleft is postulated to arise secondary to disruption of the stapedial artery in embryogenesis.
   B. This cleft can involve colobomas and encephaloceles.
   C. This is the most common of all craniofacial clefts.

   Options:
   a. Cleft number 3
   b. Cleft number 5
   c. Cleft number 7
   d. Cleft number 8
   e. Cleft number 10
   f. Cleft number 13
   g. Cleft number 30

4. Match the following descriptions of Tessier clefts to the most appropriate option. (Each option may be used once, more than once, or not at all.)
   A. This cleft passes through the nasolacrimal duct, leading to epiphora, and is associated with globe malposition.
   B. This midline cleft can continue as cleft number 14.
   C. This disruptive and complicated oral-ocular cleft passes between the upper lateral incisor and the canine. The medial canthal ligament and nasolacrimal duct are usually intact.

   Options:
   a. Cleft number 0
   b. Cleft number 3
   c. Cleft number 4
   d. Cleft number 7
   e. Cleft number 10
   f. Cleft number 14
   g. Cleft number 30

TREACHER COLLINS SYNDROME

5. A patient is referred to clinic with a diagnosis of Treacher Collins syndrome. **Which one of the following is associated with this condition?**
   A. Bilateral oronasal Tessier clefts
   B. A mitochondrial inheritance pattern
   C. A genetic abnormality on chromosome 12
   D. An incidence of 1 in 1000 live births
   E. A high risk of airway compromise

6. A patient with a diagnosis of Treacher Collins syndrome requests cosmetic surgery to improve their facial appearance. **Which one of the following procedures is least likely to be required based on the clinical features of this condition?**
   A. Lower eyelid surgery
   B. Cheek reconstruction
   C. Ear reconstruction
   D. Rhinoplasty
   E. Upper eyelid blepharoplasty

GOLDENHAR'S SYNDROME

7. A patient presents to clinic with a diagnosis of Goldenhar's syndrome. On examination they have two polypoid soft tissue protuberances on the cheek which the parents would like removed. **What is the most likely diagnosis?**
   A. Pedunculated papillomas
   B. Epibulbar dermoids
   C. Colobomas
   D. Lipomas
   E. Auricular appendages

CLEFT NUMBER 14

8. Which one of the following is expected in a patient with a cleft 14?
A. A normal life expectancy
B. A coexisting cleft through the alar rim
C. A short frontal midline hairline
D. Midline herniation of the intracranial contents
E. A decreased intraorbital distance

CLEFT NUMBER 30

9. A five-year-old child is noted to have a bifid tongue and notching of the lower lip. Which one of the following findings would you also expect to be present on examination of this child?
A. An absent thyroid
B. An absent hyoid
C. A hypoplastic thyroid
D. Absence of the central incisors
E. Notching of the upper lip

Answers

CRANIOFACIAL EMBRYOLOGY
1. **Which one of the following statements is correct regarding facial embryology?**
   B. The frontonasal prominence derives from the primitive forebrain.
   Facial development occurs between weeks 3 and 8 (see Fig. 22-1, *Essentials of Plastic Surgery*, second edition). Key facial features such as the mouth, ears, eyes, and nose are clearly recognizable by week 8. They become progressively defined beginning in week 6. The lateral nasal prominence forms the nasal alae, but the premaxilla is formed from the medial nasal prominences. Both medial and lateral nasal prominences are formed from the frontonasal prominence, a derivative of the forebrain. The mandibular arch bifurcates to form the mandibular and maxillary processes. The external ear is formed from the mandibular (first) and hyoid (second) branchial arches (see Chapters 27 and 28).

TESSIER CLEFTS
2. **Which one of the following statements is correct regarding Tessier clefts?**
   B. Cleft numbers 10-14 are described as *cranial clefts*.
   Tessier described cleft numbers 0-14 relative to the midline and subgrouped them according to their location as oral-nasal, oral-ocular, lateral facial, and cranial (see Fig. 22-2, *Essentials of Plastic Surgery*, second edition). An additional cleft number 30 does not fit into this subcategorization. It passes inferiorly from the lower lip toward the neck and is not numbered according to the midline per se, although it is a midline cleft. This totals 16 clefts of which the most common is a lateral cleft (number 7). The other lateral clefts (numbers 8 and 9), however, are rare. Oral-ocular clefts do not disrupt the integrity of the nose. They occur lateral to Cupid's bow and extend through the cheek and maxillary process. This is called *meloschisis*.[1]

3. **For the following descriptions, the best options are as follows:**
   A. This cleft is postulated to arise secondary to disruption of the stapedial artery in embryogenesis.
   c. Cleft number 7
   Cleft number 7 is a lateral cleft that passes from the oral commissure toward the ear. It stops at the anterior border of the masseter. It is the most common overall cleft and may occur because of disruption of the stapedial artery. This cleft is bilateral in 1 of 10 cases.
   B. This cleft can involve colobomas and encephaloceles.
   e. Cleft number 10
   Cleft 10 is a cranial cleft positioned in the center of the upper eyelid, brow, and orbit. It corresponds to facial cleft number 4 and is associated with hypertelorism, encephaloceles, and colobomas.
   C. This is the most common of all craniofacial clefts.
   c. Cleft number 7
   Cleft number 7 is a lateral cleft that passes from the oral commissure toward the ear. It stops at the anterior border of the masseter. It is the most common overall cleft and may occur because of disruption of the stapedial artery. This cleft is bilateral in 1 of 10 cases.

Chapter 22 ▪ Craniofacial Clefts

4. *For the following descriptions, the best options are as follows:*
   A. *This cleft passes through the nasolacrimal duct, causing epiphora, and is associated with globe malposition.*
      b. Cleft number 3
         The most common oral-nasal cleft is probably cleft number 3. This passes from the lateral margin of Cupid's bow and across the alar base through the frontal process of the maxillary process, extending through the nasolacrimal duct. The lacrimal system is often blocked, which leads to tearing onto the cheek.
   B. *This midline cleft can continue as cleft number 14.*
      a. Cleft number 0
         The lower facial clefts (numbers 0-4) may continue as cranial clefts (numbers 14-10), respectively, totaling 14. Cleft number 0 can be tissue deficient or have an excess of tissue within midline structures. Deficiencies involve soft tissues of the upper lip and nose and absence of the premaxilla with partial or total absence of the nasal bones. Cases of tissue excess can have a bifid nose and diastema of the upper incisors with broad nasal bones and septum. Cleft numbers 0 and 14 are both midline clefts, and 14 are associated with CNS abnormalities, hypotelorism or hypertelorism, and frontonasal encephaloceles.
   C. *This disruptive and complicated oral-ocular cleft passes between the upper lateral incisor and the canine. The medial canthal ligament and nasolacrimal duct are usually intact.*
      c. Cleft number 4
         The oral-ocular clefts are numbers 4, 5, and 6. Cleft number 4 begins lateral to Cupid's bow, between the oral commissure and the philtral crest. It passes onto the cheek lateral to the nasal ala, and curves into the lower eyelid to terminate medial to the punctum. Although most of the lower eyelid supporting structures are disrupted, the lacrimal apparatus is usually intact.

TREACHER COLLINS SYNDROME

5. A patient is referred to clinic with a diagnosis of Treacher Collins syndrome. ***Which one of the following is associated with this condition?***
   E. A high risk of airway compromise
      Treacher Collins described this syndrome in 1900. It has an incidence of 1 in 10,000 live births. A genetic alteration occurs on chromosome 5, and the condition is inherited in an autosomal dominant pattern. Bilateral oral ocular and lateral facial clefts are typically seen, and the airway is a major priority in these patients, many of whom will require long-term tracheostomy placement.[2]

6. A patient with a diagnosis of Treacher Collins syndrome requests cosmetic surgery to improve their facial appearance. ***Which one of the following procedures is least likely to be required based on the clinical features of this condition?***
   D. Rhinoplasty
      The clinical findings in Treacher Collins syndrome include upper and lower eyelid deformity, absence of the zygomatic arch with a malar deficiency, and varying degrees of microtia. Patients do, however, generally have normal nasal development and would be least likely to require a rhinoplasty given the other options listed.
      The lower eyelid has coloboma and retraction which may require reconstruction and the lateral canthi are displaced inferiorly and therefore may benefit from canthal elevation. The lack of cheek projection due to absence of the zygomatic arch and malar bone hypoplasia may require cheek

reconstruction using flaps or lipofilling techniques. Formal ear reconstruction may be required using costal cartilage and local flaps. Upper eyelid surgery may be required as patients have an excess of upper eyelid skin laterally giving a false impression of ptosis. (see Fig. 22-7, *Essentials of Plastic Surgery*, second edition).

GOLDENHAR'S SYNDROME

7. A patient presents to clinic with a diagnosis of Goldenhar's syndrome. On examination they have two polypoid soft tissue protuberances on the cheek which the parents would like removed. ***What is the most likely diagnosis?***
   E. Auricular appendages
   Goldenhar's syndrome is a type of hemifacial microsomia with sporadic occurrence in which patients have a constellation of abnormalities including bilateral accessory auricular appendages, varying degrees of microtia, epibulbar dermoids, vertebral anomalies, a low anterior hairline, and mandibular hypoplasia. The description in this patient is most in keeping with auricular appendages and these may well comprise of skin and underlying cartilage. They can safely be excised under general anesthetic on an elective basis. Pedunculated papillomas and subcutaneous lipomas can have a similar appearance but are not typical of Goldenhar's syndrome. Epibulbar dermoids and colobomas are characteristic of Goldenhar's syndrome but affect the eye, not the cheek (see Fig. 22-8, *Essentials of Plastic Surgery*, second edition).[3,4]

CLEFT NUMBER 14

8. ***Which one of the following is expected in a patient with a cleft 14?***
   D. Midline herniation of the intracranial contents
   Cleft 14 is one of the cranial clefts and has a very poor prognosis. It is a midline cleft with associated central nervous system abnormalities including a midline encephalocele, holoprosencephaly, and microcephaly. It is often paired with a facial midline cleft 0 (not a cleft 3 as discussed in question 4, which would pass through the alar rim). Hypertelorism is present because the cleft increases the distance between the bony orbits. A Harlequin deformity may be seen on radiographs due to upslanting of the anterior cranial fossa (see Fig. 21-3).

CLEFT NUMBER 30

9. A five-year-old child is noted to have a bifid tongue and notching of the lower lip. ***Which one of the following findings would you also expect to be present on examination of this child?***
   B. An absent hyoid
   Tessier described cleft 30 in his original 1976 publication.[1] It is a very rare anomaly, with fewer than 70 cases described in the literature. In its milder form it may be limited to a defect of soft tissue in the lower lip. In more severe forms it may involve a cleft of the mandibular symphysis, absence of the hyoid, and hypoplasia of the thyroid cartilage, or strap muscles. The tongue abnormality ranges from total absence to a bifid anterior portion or complete duplication. A cleft of the mandibular symphysis usually passes between the central incisors, which are present. The thyroid gland itself is not involved, although the thyroid cartilage can be hypoplastic.

REFERENCES

1. Tessier P. Anatomical classification facial, cranio-facial, and latero-facial clefts. J Maxillofac Surg 4:69-92, 1976.
2. Treacher Collins E. Case with symmetrical congenital notches in the outer part of each lower eyelid and defective development of the malar bones. Trans Opthalmol Soc Uk 20:191-192, 1900.
3. Gorlin RJ, Pindborg JJ. Syndromes of the Head and Neck. New York: McGraw-Hill, 1964.
4. Mellor DH, Richardson JE, Douglas DM. Goldenhar's syndrome. Oculoauriculo-vertebral dysplasia. Arch Dis Child 48:537-541, 1973.

23. Distraction Osteogenesis

See *Essentials of Plastic Surgery*, second edition, pp. 258-263.

GENERAL PRINCIPLES
1. **Which one of the following statements is correct regarding distraction osteogenesis?**
   A. It is a single-stage surgical technique used to generate new bone.
   B. It relies on the principle that growth is stimulated when compressive stress is placed across tissue.
   C. Successful outcome requires the application of a consistent, moderate increase in tension.
   D. It often causes atrophy to the surrounding soft tissues.
   E. It results in bone whose characteristics are different from those of normal, mature bone.

BONE PHYSIOLOGY
2. **Which one of the following represents a single zone within the bony generate in distraction osteogenesis?**
   A. Cellular proliferation zone
   B. Mineralization front
   C. Zone of vasculogenesis
   D. Osteoid paracentral zone
   E. Mature bone zone

THE DISTRACTION PROCESS
3. An 18-month-old infant has micrognathia secondary to Treacher Collins syndrome. **After performing an osteotomy and placement of a mandibular distractor, which one of the following strategies should be part of the distraction process?**
   A. The activation phase should begin immediately following placement of the distraction device and should last for six months.
   B. The latency period should be 3 weeks between osteotomy and commencement of distraction.
   C. The distractor should be adjusted every other day to optimize the quality and volume of new bone.
   D. The distraction rate should be maintained at around 1 mm per day throughout the distraction process.
   E. The consolidation period should be 16 weeks once the desired distraction has been achieved, with the distractor left in place.

DISTRACTION DEVICES

4. Which one of the following represents the main advantage of using an external distractor over an internal distractor on the mandible?
A. Multidirectional distraction can be achieved.
B. Only one general anesthetic will be required.
C. It is less likely to disrupt tooth buds.
D. Cutaneous scarring will be reduced.
E. Fewer postoperative complications are observed.

MANDIBULAR DISTRACTION

5. Which one of the following is not achieved with distraction of the mandible?
A. Lengthening of the ramus/body
B. Reconstruction of a mandibular defect
C. Normalization of a retroplaced tongue base
D. Correction of class III malocclusion
E. Improvement of airway patency

COMPLICATIONS OF CRANIOFACIAL DISTRACTION OSTEOGENESIS

6. You are consenting the parents of a one-year-old child for craniofacial distraction osteogenesis using a single-vector external device. *Which one of the following is the most common complication of craniofacial distraction?*
A. Bleeding
B. Pin tract infection
C. Nerve damage
D. Inappropriate vector
E. Premature consolidation

Answers

GENERAL PRINCIPLES

1. **Which one of the following statements is correct regarding distraction osteogenesis?**
   C. Successful outcome requires the application of a consistent, moderate increase in tension.
   Distraction osteogenesis is a staged procedure that takes many months to complete. It relies on the principle that tissue generation is stimulated when tissues are placed under consistent, moderate tensile forces. The application of these principles allows bone to be lengthened after an osteotomy, and then progressive distraction of the divided bone ends using a surgically placed device. Soft tissues respond well to the process and typically hypertrophy, not atrophy. The characteristics of bone formed during distraction osteogenesis are identical to those of normal mature bone. Not only are these principles applicable to patients with micrognathia such as hemifacial microsomia and Treacher Collins syndrome, they are useful for bone transport in long bones after segmental loss of the tibia or femur.

BONE PHYSIOLOGY

2. **Which one of the following represents a single zone within the bony generate in distraction osteogenesis?**
   A. Cellular proliferation zone
   The bone gap in distraction osteogenesis is similar to callus, but it has collagen fibers that run parallel to the vector of distraction. This area is called the *generate*. It has the following five key components, all of which are duplicated except the central cellular proliferation zone (see Fig. 23-1, *Essentials of Plastic Surgery*, second edition):
   1. A **central zone** in which proliferation of mesenchymal cells occurs
   2. Two **transitional zones** of vasculogenesis that sandwich the central zone
   3. Two **paracentral zones** in which osteoid production occurs
   4. Two **mineralization fronts** in which primary mineralization occurs
   5. Two **mature bone zones** in which bone is progressively calcified to form cortical and cancellous elements

THE DISTRACTION PROCESS

3. **An 18-month-old infant has micrognathia secondary to Treacher Collins syndrome. After performing an osteotomy and placement of a mandibular distractor, Which one of the following strategies should be part of the distraction process?**
   D. The distraction rate should be maintained at around 1 mm per day throughout the distraction process.
   The distraction process begins with an osteotomy and application of a distraction device. Distraction is delayed for about 1 week after placement of the distractor to allow a callus to form at the fracture site. This is called the *latency period*. The latency period may be reduced to around three days in patients younger than one year of age. The period of active distraction is termed the *activation phase* and does not commence until the latency period is complete. Active distraction is usually complete within six weeks when distraction rates of 1 mm per day are used. Once

distraction is complete, the distractor is left in situ for eight weeks or until bone healing is evident radiologically. This is termed the *consolidation phase*. Distraction is usually increased at a rate of 1 mm per day because this avoids premature ossification or local ischemia. In neonates and infants less than one year of age it may be increased to 2 to 4 mm per day. The rhythm describes the number of times per day the distractor is increased. Usually this is done two to four times each day as this provides the best volume and quality of new bone formation.

DISTRACTION DEVICES

4. Which one of the following represents the main advantage of using an external distractor over an internal distractor on the mandible?
A. Multidirectional distraction can be achieved.

The benefits of external craniofacial distractors are that they provide flexibility for alteration of distraction vectors; they can prevent formal reoperation to remove the device. However, a second general anesthetic is still often required to facilitate removal of the percutaneous pins. Furthermore, these pins will leave visible external scarring at the pin sites.

In contrast, internal devices involve an intraoral approach, thus avoiding cutaneous scarring. However, they provide distraction only in a single vector that cannot be altered after insertion, and a second procedure will always be required for their removal. Careful planning should prevent disruption of the tooth buds in all distraction approaches. Complication rates are similar with either device.

MANDIBULAR DISTRACTION

5. Which one of the following is not achieved with distraction of the mandible?
D. Correction of class III malocclusion

Mandibular distraction can help patients achieve proper occlusion, but it does not correct a class III deformity which is essentially where the mandibular dentition is prominent with respect to the maxillary dentition (i.e., the patient is prognathic).

Correction requires orthodontic intervention, resetting of the mandible posteriorly, or advancement of the maxilla, depending on the underlying pathology. Mandibular distraction is often performed to improve the airway in patients with disorders such as Pierre Robin sequence. It provides more space for the tongue and moves the base more anteriorly.

COMPLICATIONS OF CRANIOFACIAL DISTRACTION OSTEOGENESIS

6. You are consenting the parents of a one-year-old child for craniofacial distraction osteogenesis using a single-vector external device. Which one of the following is the most common complication of craniofacial distraction?
D. Inappropriate vector

A review of 3278 cases of craniofacial distraction published in 2001 showed that an inappropriate vector was the most common complication, occurring in almost 9% of cases in which a single vector device was used.[1] This complication occurred in 7.2% of cases in which multivector devices were used (see Table 23-1, *Essentials of Plastic Surgery,* second edition). Other complications included pin tract infection (5.2%), compliance problems (4.7%), and hardware failure (4.5%).

REFERENCE

1. Mofid MM, Manson PN, Robertson BC, et al. Craniofacial distraction osteogenesis. A review of 3278 cases. Plast Reconstr Surg 108:1103-1114, 2001.

24. Cleft Lip

See *Essentials of Plastic Surgery*, second edition, pp. 264-274.

DEMOGRAPHICS

1. Which one of the following statements is correct regarding cleft lip/palate?
A. It most commonly affects the right side.
B. The overall incidence is 1:350.
C. Males are affected twice as often as females.
D. Incidence is unaffected by race.
E. One in four patients have an associated syndrome.

ANATOMY OF THE NORMAL UPPER LIP

2. Match each of the following anatomic descriptions to the most appropriate option. (Each option may be used once, more than once, or not at all.)
A. This prominent ridge is just above the cutaneous-vermilion border.
B. This is the junction between the wet and dry vermilion.
C. This structure is formed by the dermal insertion of orbicularis oris.

Options:
a. Philtral column
b. Philtral dimple
c. White roll
d. Vermilion
e. Red line
f. Cupid's bow
g. Gray line

CLEFT LIP ANATOMY

3. Which one of the following statements regarding the anatomy of the cleft lip is correct?
A. Vertical lip height and projection are increased.
B. Deep and superficial parts of orbicularis oris insert on the cleft side alar base.
C. The prolabium usually contains muscle fibers.
D. Muscle continuity is maintained in a microform lip.
E. A Simonart's band is a skin bridge devoid of muscle.

ANATOMY OF THE CLEFT NASAL DEFORMITY

4. You are examining the nose of a 2-month-old infant with a unilateral incomplete cleft lip deformity. Which one of the following findings is expected to be present on the cleft lip side of this infant?
A. A more acute angle between the medial and lateral crura
B. Flattening of the alar-facial angle
C. Narrowing of the nostril floor
D. Deviation of the tip towards this side
E. A normal columellar length

RISK OF FAMILIAL RECURRENCE IN CLEFT LIP/PALATE

5. You are advising a young couple in clinic who are planning to start a family. The lady has an isolated cleft lip that was repaired as a child. **What is the approximate risk of this couple having a child with a cleft lip/palate assuming the father is unaffected?**
   A. 1%
   B. 4%
   C. 12%
   D. 20%
   E. 33%

FEEDING CLEFT PALATE INFANTS

6. **What is the best feeding modality for a patient with a cleft lip deformity?**
   A. A normal bottle with a Haberman nipple
   B. A squeezable bottle with a normal nipple
   C. A pigeon nipple with a normal bottle
   D. A pigeon nipple with a soft squeezable bottle
   E. A normal bottle/nipple or breast-feeding

PRESURGICAL ORTHOPEDICS

7. **Which one of the following statements is correct regarding presurgical orthopedics?**
   A. A Latham device is a passive type of presurgical orthopedic device.
   B. Lip adhesion is an alternative to presurgical orthopedics, but it has a high risk of dehiscence.
   C. Nasoalveolar molding can improve the nasal deformity but does not improve arch alignment.
   D. A Latham device promotes maxillary growth.
   E. A Latham device is mainly used for mild deformities.

TIMING OF CLEFT LIP REPAIR

8. **Which one of the following is performed at the time of primary lip repair?**
   A. Full rhinoplasty
   B. Tip rhinoplasty
   C. Palatoplasty
   D. Primary alveolar bone grafting
   E. Correction of a whistle tip deformity

TYPES OF CLEFT LIP REPAIR

9. Select the technique of cleft lip repair that is described in each of the following statements. (Each option may be used once, more than once, or not at all.)
   A. This straight-line repair is described for unilateral cleft lip repair.
   B. This rotation advancement repair for cleft lip incorporates a superiorly placed Z-plasty.
   C. This technique for repair of a bilateral cleft lip uses the prolabium for the white roll and vermilion reconstruction.

   Options:
   a. LeMesurier
   b. Tajima technique
   c. Rose-Thompson
   d. Randall-Tennison
   e. Millard
   f. Modified Manchester
   g. McComb

THE MILLARD REPAIR FOR UNILATERAL CLEFT LIPS (BYRD MODIFICATION)

10. *For each of the following components of the Millard repair, select the most likely flap option. (Each option may be used once, more than once, or not at all.)*
    A. This flap is used to lengthen the columella.
    B. This flap is used to augment the nasal lining.
    C. This flap is used to augment the gingivolabial sulcus.

    Options:
    a. L flap
    b. C flap
    c. R flap
    d. Triangular lateral vermilion flap
    e. Z flap
    f. M flap
    g. V-Y flap

WHISTLE TIP DEFORMITY

11. A patient who presents to clinic after a cleft lip repair has a whistle tip deformity. *Which one of the following structures is deficient?*
    A. Buccal sulcus
    B. Vermilion
    C. White roll
    D. Upper lip skin
    E. Cupid's bow

… Chapter 24 ▪ Cleft Lip   191

Answers

DEMOGRAPHICS
1. **Which one of the following statements is correct regarding cleft lip/palate?**
   C. Males are affected twice as often as females.
   Cleft lip/palate is more frequent in males with a 2:1 ratio, although isolated cleft lip is seen equally in both sexes. Left-sided cleft defects are more common than right-sided cleft defects, and the ratio is 6:3:1 in the order left/right/bilateral. The overall incidence is 1:750 and ranges from 1 in 500 to 1 in 2000, depending on race. Cleft lip/palate is significantly more common in patients of Asian descent (1 in 500) and is least common in Afro-Caribbeans (1 in 2000). The incidence among white individuals is 1:1000. An incidence of 1:350 is more in keeping with hypospadias rather than cleft lip/palate (see Chapter 54). Associated syndromes are seen in 10% of patients with cleft lip/palate (not 25%).

ANATOMY OF THE NORMAL UPPER LIP
2. **For the following descriptions, the best options are as follows:**
   A. This prominent ridge is just above the cutaneous-vermilion border.
   c. White roll
   The white roll represents the junction between the skin and vermilion. It is an important landmark to realign precisely during cleft lip and general lip repair after trauma or tumor resection.
   B. This is the junction between the wet and dry vermilion.
   e. Red line
   The lip comprises skin, muscle, fat, and mucosa. The vermilion is the red part of the lip and is divided into wet and dry components by the red line. The dry component is keratinized, whereas the wet part is not. The wet component is continuous with the oral cavity lining.
   C. This structure is formed by the dermal insertion of orbicularis oris.
   a. Philtral column
   The philtral columns are vertical bulges that laterally frame the philtral dimple, a midline area of the lip with a relative deficiency of the orbicularis oris muscle. The philtral columns are formed by the insertion of orbicularis oris fibers into the dermis. Cupid's bow is the curved midline section of the white roll between the philtral columns. The gray line refers to the eyelid margin, not the lip (see Chapter 92).

CLEFT LIP ANATOMY
3. **Which one of the following statements regarding the anatomy of the cleft lip is correct?**
   E. A Simonart's band is a skin bridge devoid of muscle.
   A cleft lip is the projection and outward rotation of the premaxilla, with retropositioning of the lateral maxillary segment. The vertical lip height is reduced, and the philtrum is short. Only the superficial part of orbicularis oris inserts into the alar base on the cleft side. The deep portion is interrupted but does not abnormally insert. Neither the prolabium in a bilateral cleft lip nor the Simonart's band contains muscle. The continuity of muscle is disrupted in a microform cleft.

ANATOMY OF THE CLEFT NASAL DEFORMITY

4. You are examining the nose of a 2-month-old infant with a unilateral incomplete cleft lip deformity. *Which one of the following findings is expected to be present on the cleft lip side of this infant?*

B. Flattening of the alar-facial angle

The cleft nasal deformity comprises a collection of specific abnormalities. They can be remembered by considering anatomical subgroups as shown in Box 24-1.

Flattening of the alar facial angle is a key finding on the cleft side. There is a more obtuse angle between the medial and lateral crura (not acute), there is widening of the cleft nostril with a deficiency of the sill. The nasal tip deviates away from (not towards) the cleft side. Columellar length is reduced on the cleft side.

Box 24-1 *ANATOMIC CHARACTERISTICS OF CLEFT NASAL DEFORMITY*

Cartilaginous Deformities

The caudal septum is deviated to the noncleft side.
The posterior septum is convex on the cleft side and can block the cleft-side airway.
Lower lateral cartilages are attenuated and displaced caudally on the cleft side.
The medial crura are separated from one another at the dome.
The angle between medial and lateral crura is more obtuse on the cleft side.

Soft Tissue and Bone

The nasal tip and columellar base deviate to the noncleft side.
The cleft-side alar base is displaced laterally, posteriorly, and caudally.
The maxilla is hypoplastic with a posteriorly displaced piriform margin on the cleft side.
The nostril sill is deficient, and the nostril is widened on the cleft side.
The cleft alar-facial angle is flattened.
The vestibular lining is deficient on the cleft side.
The columella is shorter on the cleft side.

RISK OF FAMILIAL RECURRENCE IN CLEFT LIP/PALATE

5. You are advising a young couple in clinic who are planning to start a family. The lady has an isolated cleft lip that was repaired as a child. *What is the approximate risk of this couple having a child with a cleft lip/palate assuming the father is unaffected?*

B. 4%

If one parent is affected, the risk of cleft lip/palate in the first child is 4%. If an affected parent already has an affected child the risk increases to 17% for the second child. If unaffected parents have one affected child, the risk of having subsequent affected children is 4%. When unaffected parents have two affected children, the risk of having other affected children is 9%. It is important to have an idea of relative risk for cleft lip and palate development as patients and families are likely to ask about this during the consultation.

FEEDING CLEFT PALATE INFANTS

6. *What is the best feeding modality for a patient with a cleft lip deformity?*
   E. A normal bottle/nipple or breast-feeding
   The best method of feeding a baby with an isolated cleft lip is either directly from the breast or with a regular bottle. The need for specialized bottles or nipples is only for infants with a cleft palate. There are three types of bottles used to feed cleft palate infants: the Mead-Johnson cleft palate nurser, the Haberman feeder, and the Pigeon nipple. The Mead-Johnson device is a soft squeezable bottle with a long cross-cut nipple. The Haberman feeder has a one-way valve and does not require a squeezable bottle. The Pigeon nipple works by compression and can be used with normal or squeezable bottles and has a faster flow than other feeding systems.

PRESURGICAL ORTHOPEDICS

7. *Which one of the following statements is correct regarding presurgical orthopedics?*
   B. Lip adhesion is an alternative to presurgical orthopedics, but it has a high risk of dehiscence.
   Lip adhesion is a surgical procedure in which preliminary closure of the lip is performed around 2 months of age to reduce the lip/nasal deformity and facilitate definitive closure in wide cleft lips. Not only is dehiscence a risk, the scars created can interfere with subsequent definitive lip repair.
   Presurgical orthopedics are used to narrow the cleft margin and improve arch alignment before surgery. They can be either active or passive. The Latham device is an active appliance that is placed and secured with pins while the patient is under a general anesthetic. Screw activation will expand the plate and retract the premaxilla, but this process can adversely affect maxillary growth and should be reserved for severe deformities.

TIMING OF CLEFT LIP REPAIR

8. *Which one of the following is performed at the time of primary lip repair?*
   B. Tip rhinoplasty
   Primary repair of a cleft lip is performed around the age of 3 months. During this surgery the primary cleft nasal repair and gingivoperiosteoplasty are usually performed. A nasal repair involves release and repositioning of the cleft nasal components and alar cartilages (tip rhinoplasty). Tajima or McComb sutures may be used to support the lower lateral cartilage in primary cleft rhinoplasty. A gingivoperiosteoplasty involves the primary closure of an alveolar cleft using mucoperiosteal flaps.
   Palatoplasty is typically performed at 9 to 12 months of age (see Chapter 25). Alveolar bone grafting involves harvesting cancellous bone from the iliac crest and is most successful between ages 8 and 12 years, because this coincides with eruption of the canine teeth. Orthognathic surgery and secondary or full rhinoplasty are usually performed once facial growth and secondary dentition is complete.

TYPES OF CLEFT LIP REPAIR

9. *For the following statements, the best options are as follows:*
A. *This straight-line repair is described for unilateral cleft lip repair.*
   c. Rose-Thompson
   Several different techniques are available for cleft lip repair. Techniques such s the Rose-Thompson technique involve a straight line and are no longer commonly used because they have been replaced with techniques involving Z-plasties to improve lip height.

B. *This rotation advancement repair for cleft lip incorporates a superiorly placed Z-plasty.*
   e. Millard
   The Millard repair is one of the most commonly used techniques and involves a superiorly placed Z-plasty. The Randall-Tennison repair uses a Z-plasty at the vermilion border and can result in excessive vertical lip height. LeMesurier modified a quadrangular flap repair first described by Hagedorn. The McComb and Tajima techniques are suture techniques that are performed to correct a cleft nasal deformity.

C. *This technique for repair of a bilateral cleft lip uses the prolabium for the white roll and vermilion reconstruction.*
   f. Modified Manchester
   Bilateral cleft lip can be repaired using Millard or Modified Manchester techniques. In the Millard technique the central skin of the prolabium is used to reconstruct the philtral dimple, but the white roll and vermilion are discarded. The modified Manchester technique preserves the white roll and vermilion from the prolabium to reconstruct Cupid's bow and tubercle.

THE MILLARD REPAIR FOR UNILATERAL CLEFT LIPS (BYRD MODIFICATION)

10. *For the following scenarios, the best options are as follows (see Fig. 24-3, Essentials of Plastic Surgery, second edition):*
A. *This flap is used to lengthen the columella.*
   b. C flap
   The markings and steps of the Millard rotation advancement repair are shown in Fig. 24-1, *A* through *F*. The key flaps used in this repair are as follows: The C flap is known as the columellar flap and is a triangle of skin that begins inferiorly at the high point of Cupid's bow. It is used to close the nasal sill or lengthen the columella.

B. *This flap is used to augment the nasal lining.*
   a. L flap
   The L flap is known as the lateral flap and is a superiorly based flap from the lateral lip that is used to line the nasal vestibule.

C. *This flap is used to augment the gingivolabial sulcus.*
   f. M flap
   The M flap is known as the medial or mucosal flap and is a rectangular flap of mucosa from the medial lip. It is used to line the gingivobuccal sulcus.

   The R flap is the rotation flap based on the noncleft side (medial) lip that rotates into place during cleft lip repair to join with the cleft side lip (lateral). The A flap is the advancement flap based on the cleft side lip. It advances to join the R flap from the noncleft side. There is no named Z flap, although the repair design does incorporate a Z-plasty. V-Y flaps are sometimes used to correct residual deformities after cleft lip repair, but are not part of the Millard repair.[2,3]

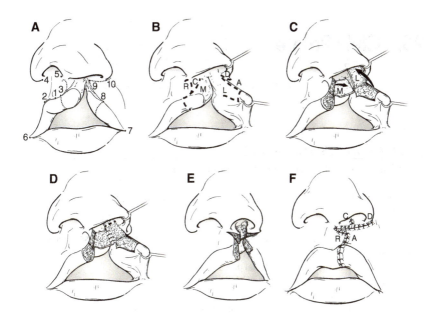

Fig. 24-1 A, Flaps are marked using the alar base, columella, lip margins, philtral columns, and Cupid's bow. **B** and **C,** The R, C, M, L, and A flaps are incised and elevated. **D,** The M and L flaps are sutured into place. **E** and **F,** Rotation-advancement is completed with interposition of C flap above A flap.

WHISTLE TIP DEFORMITY

11. A patient who presents to clinic after a cleft lip repair has a whistle tip deformity.
Which one of the following structures is deficient?
B. Vermilion

The whistle deformity is normally secondary to a deficiency in the central part of the vermilion often in conjunction with abnormal orbicularis alignment.

Various methods have been described for the surgical management of this condition and technique selection will depend on the precise nature and extent of the deformity. For example, if the deficiency is mild, the upper lip itself can be used for reconstruction, such as Z-plasty, V-Y advancement, double pendulum flaps, bilateral lateral vermilion border transposition flaps, and bilobed mucosal flaps. If the deformity is more severe then adjacent tissue such as the tongue and lower lip (Abbé flap) may be required. More novel approaches include fat grafting, palmaris longus tendon grafting and dermofat grafts.[1]

REFERENCES

1. Choi WY, Yang JY, Kim GB, et al. Surgical correction of whistle deformity using cross-muscle flap in secondary cleft lip. Arch Plast Surg 39:470-476, 2012.
2. Millard DR. A radical rotation in single harelip. Amer J Surg 95:318-322, 1958.
3. Byrd HS. Unilateral cleft lip. In Aston SJ, Beasley RW, Thorne CHM, eds. Grabb and Smith's Plastic Surgery, ed 5. Philadelphia: Lippincott-Raven, 1997.

25. Cleft Palate

See *Essentials of Plastic Surgery*, second edition, pp. 275-287.

EMBRYOLOGY OF THE PALATE

1. **Which one of the following is part of the secondary palate?**
   A. Lip
   B. Nostril sill
   C. Alveolus
   D. Anterior hard palate
   E. Posterior hard palate

2. **Which one of the following statements is correct regarding the secondary palate?**
   A. It is formed from the medial palatal processes of the maxilla.
   B. Before 8 weeks of gestation, the palatal shelves are horizontal.
   C. Embryologic development may explain a higher incidence of cleft palate in females.
   D. Rotation of the palatal shelves is unaffected by tongue development.
   E. Both palatal processes become horizontal at the same time.

MUSCLES OF THE SOFT PALATE

3. **Which one of the velum muscles is innervated by the fifth cranial nerve?**
   A. Levator veli palatini
   B. Superior pharyngeal constrictor
   C. Palatopharyngeus
   D. Tensor veli palatini
   E. Palatoglossus

BLOOD SUPPLY TO THE PALATE

4. **Which one of the following is the main blood supply to the hard palate?**
   A. Nasopalatine artery from the maxillary artery
   B. Lesser palatine artery from the maxillary artery
   C. Greater palatine artery from the facial artery
   D. Greater palatine artery from the maxillary artery
   E. Ascending pharyngeal artery from the external carotid artery

SUBMUCOUS CLEFT PALATE

5. **Which one of the following represents the triad seen in submucous cleft palate?**
   A. Absent uvula, zona pellucida, and soft palate notch
   B. Absent uvula, zona pellucida, and hard palate notch
   C. Bifid uvula, lower lip pits, and hard palate notch
   D. Bifid uvula, lower lip pits, and zona pellucida
   E. Bifid uvula, hard palate notch, and zona pellucida

CLEFT PALATE DEFECTS

6. Which one of the following is the most common palatal deformity?
- A. Midline isolated cleft
- B. Complete primary palate cleft
- C. Complete secondary palate cleft
- D. Bifid uvula
- E. Submucous cleft

DEMOGRAPHICS OF CLEFT

7. Match each of the following descriptions to the most appropriate option. (Each option may be used once, more than once, or not at all.)
- A. This is the combined overall incidence of cleft lip, cleft palate, or cleft lip and palate.
- B. This is the incidence of isolated cleft palate in white patients.
- C. This is the incidence of cleft lip or cleft lip and palate in Asians.

Options:
- a. 1:250 live births
- b. 1:500 live births
- c. 1:750 live births
- d. 1:1000 live births
- e. 1:1250
- f. 1:2000

RISK OF DEVELOPING CLEFT LIP/PALATE

8. You see a couple in clinic that have two children and are interested in having one more child. The father has a cleft lip/palate that was repaired as a child and the mother is unaffected. They have one unaffected child and one with a cleft lip/palate. **What is the risk of their next child having a cleft lip/palate deformity?**
- A. 2%
- B. 10%
- C. 17%
- D. 25%
- E. 42%

RISK OF DEVELOPING AN ISOLATED CLEFT PALATE

9. For each of the following scenarios, select the most appropriate likely risk from the options listed. (Each option may be used once, more than once or not at all)
- A. A couple with no personal history of cleft palate has one child with a cleft palate. What is the risk of their next child having a cleft palate?
- B. A woman has a cleft palate and her partner does not. What is the chance of their first child having a cleft palate deformity?
- C. If the woman described in scenario B has one child with a cleft palate, what is the risk of her next child having a cleft palate?

Options:
- a. 2%
- b. 6%
- c. 15%
- d. 30%
- e. 50%

CLEFT SUBTYPES

10. Which one of the following types of cleft is most commonly associated with another anomaly?
- A. Unilateral cleft lip
- B. Bilateral cleft lip
- C. Isolated cleft palate
- D. Unilateral cleft lip and palate
- E. Bilateral cleft lip and palate

PIERRE ROBIN SEQUENCE

11. While on call for the pediatric plastic surgical team, you are referred an infant with a diagnosis of Pierre Robin sequence. *Which one of the following is the most likely reason for the infant to require an acute admission?*
  A. Failure to thrive
  B. Feeding issues
  C. Renal failure
  D. Airway compromise
  E. Chest infection

SYNDROMIC CLEFTS

12. A patient is referred with a syndromic cleft palate, ocular malformations, hearing loss, and arthropathies. They have a proven genetic mutation for type II collagen. *What syndrome does this specifically represent?*
  A. Stickler syndrome
  B. Shprintzen's syndrome
  C. Velocardiofacial syndrome
  D. Van der Woude syndrome
  E. Pierre Robin sequence

ENVIRONMENTAL RISK FACTORS IN CLEFT PALATE

13. *Which one of the following is associated with an increased risk of developing an isolated oral cleft?*
  A. Maternal smoking
  B. Maternal alcohol
  C. Maternal caffeine ingestion
  D. Increased paternal age
  E. Folic acid supplements

SURGICAL REPAIR OF CLEFT PALATE

14. *For each of the following descriptions, select the most likely surgical procedure. (Each option may be used once, more than once, or not at all.)*
  A. This technique involves reorientation of the levator veli palatini and palatopharyngeus muscles across the midline to reconstruct the levator sling.
  B. This technique uses two local flaps that are comprised of different constituents. It can lengthen the soft palate but reduces its transverse dimension, causing difficult closure of wide clefts.
  C. This technique involves bilateral mucoperiosteal flaps based on the greater palatine arteries, which are closed in a V-Y fashion.

Options:
  a. von Langenbeck palatoplasty
  b. Intravelar veloplasty
  c. Pharyngeal flap
  d. Veau-Wardill-Kilner pushback palatoplasty
  e. Furlow's double-opposing technique
  f. Vomer flaps

POSTOPERATIVE CARE OF CLEFT PALATE PATIENTS

15. Which one of the following is often part of the postoperative regimen after cleft palate repair?
   A. Discharge home on day of surgery
   B. The use of intranasal oxymetazoline (Afrin)
   C. Nursing supine without pillows
   D. Institution of a normal diet at day 3
   E. Heavy sedation for the first 48 hours

COMPLICATIONS OF CLEFT PALATE REPAIR

16. Which one of the following statements is correct regarding cleft palate repairs?
   A. Maxillary growth is normalized by cleft palate repair.
   B. Palatal fistulas should be surgically repaired.
   C. Fistula rates are consistent between series.
   D. Operative mortality risk remains above 2%
   E. Fistulas most commonly form at the junction of the hard and soft palates.

Answers

EMBRYOLOGY OF THE PALATE

1. Which one of the following is part of the secondary palate?
E. Posterior hard palate
The primary palate includes the lip, nostril, alveolus, and hard palate anterior to the incisive foramen. It is formed from the frontonasal prominence. The palate posterior to the incisive foramen is part of the secondary palate and is formed from the maxillary prominence.

2. Which one of the following statements is correct regarding the secondary palate?
C. Embryologic development may explain a higher incidence of cleft palate in females.
The secondary palate develops from the lateral palatal processes of the maxilla (not the medial palatal processes) from weeks 5 to 12. In week 8, the lateral palatal processes are vertical and progress to a horizontal position as the tongue moves caudally. The palatal shelves rotate at different times, with the right moving before the left. This may explain the higher incidence of left-sided clefts. Fusion of the palatal processes takes longer in females (approximately 1 week), which may explain the increased incidence of cleft palate in females.

MUSCLES OF THE SOFT PALATE

3. Which one of the velum muscles is innervated by the fifth cranial nerve?
D. Tensor veli palatini
With the exception of the tensor veli palatini muscle, all of the muscles of the soft palate are innervated by the pharyngeal plexus, with contributions from cranial nerves IX, X, and XI. The tensor veli palatini muscle originates from the first pharyngeal arch and functions to open the Eustachian tube. This is logical embryologically, because the first arch forms the second and third parts of the trigeminal nerve.

BLOOD SUPPLY TO THE PALATE

4. Which one of the following is the main blood supply to the hard palate?
D. Greater palatine artery from the maxillary artery
The greater palatine artery passes through the greater palatine foramen to supply the hard palate. It originates from the maxillary artery via the descending palatine artery. The hard palate is also supplied by the nasopalatine artery and the anterior and posterior superior alveolar arteries, all of which arise from the maxillary artery. The soft palate is supplied by the lesser palatine artery (from the maxillary artery) and the ascending pharyngeal artery (from the external carotid artery) more laterally.

SUBMUCOUS CLEFT PALATE

5. Which one of the following is absent in a patient with a submucous cleft palate?
E. Bifid uvula, hard palatte notch, and zona pellucida
Submucous clefts have a triad of posterior hard palate notch (not anterior), a bifid uvula, and a zona pellucida. The zona pellucida is a thin central area created by a diastasis of the soft

palate musculature. It has a typical translucent appearance. The triad is sometimes referred to as Calnan's triad, as it was described by him in 1954.[1,2] Surgery is reserved for patients with velopharyngeal incompetence and may go unnoticed unless this is evident. Lower lip pits in conjunction with cleft palate is typical for Van der Woude syndrome, which is an autosomal dominant condition representing one fifth of all syndromic cleft palates. It is not a feature of submucous cleft palate.

CLEFT PALATE DEFECTS

6. Which one of the following is the most common palatal deformity?
   D. Bifid uvula

   A bifid uvula is effectively a partial cleft of the uvula and is traditionally regarded as a marker for submucous cleft palate. The connection between the two findings was discussed in question 5, where submucous clefts are associated with the triad of bifid uvula, notching of the hard palate, and muscular diastasis of the soft palate.[3] Bifid uvula can however occur spontaneously in many healthy and otherwise normal individuals. In fact it is estimated that a bifid uvula is present in around 2% of the population. The frequency of the other clefts is far less common and is discussed in question 7.

DEMOGRAPHICS OF CLEFT

7. For the following descriptions, the best options are as follows:
   A. This is the combined overall incidence of cleft lip, cleft palate, or cleft lip and palate.
      c. 1:750 live births
   B. This is the incidence of isolated cleft palate in white patients.
      f. 1:2000
   C. This is the incidence of cleft lip or cleft lip and palate in Asians.
      b. 1:500 live births

   The overall incidence of cleft lip or cleft palate deformities is 1:750 live births. The incidence in Asians is increased at 1:500 because of their increased risk of cleft lip/palate deformities. It is less common in whites (1:1000) and blacks (1:2000). In contrast, the incidence of cleft palate is unaffected by race (1:2000 live births for all races).

RISK OF DEVELOPING CLEFT LIP/PALATE

8. You see a couple in clinic that have two children and are interested in having one more child. The father has a cleft lip/palate that was repaired as a child and the mother is unaffected. They have one unaffected child and one with a cleft lip/palate. What is the risk of their next child having a cleft lip/palate deformity?
   C. 17%

   The baseline risk for developing a cleft lip/palate (CL/P) deformity is dependent on race and varies between 0.05% and 0.2% (0.5:1000 to 2:1000). The risk of having a child with a CL/P is significantly increased by either a parent or sibling having a cleft deformity. If one parent has CL/P with no affected children, the risk is 4%. However, if an affected parent has one child with CL/P the risk increases to 17%. The risk for normal parents with two CL/P children increases to 9%. Risks of 30% and 50% do not relate to CL/P development.

RISK OF DEVELOPING AN ISOLATED CLEFT PALATE

9. For the following scenarios, the best options are as follows:
   A. A couple with no personal history of cleft palate has one child with a cleft palate. What is the risk of their next child having a cleft palate?
      a. 2%
   B. A woman has a cleft palate and her partner does not. What is the chance of their first child having a cleft palate deformity?
      b. 6%
   C. If the woman described in scenario B has one child with a cleft palate, what is the risk of her next child having a cleft palate?
      c. 15%

   The standard risk for developing cleft palate is around 0.5% or 1 in 2000. The risk of having a child with an isolated cleft palate is significantly increased by either the parent or sibling having a cleft palate deformity. If unaffected parents have a child with a cleft palate, the risk of having another increases to 2%. If one parent has a cleft palate with no affected children, the risk for the first child is 6%. However, if an affected parent has one child with a cleft palate, the risk for the next child increases to 15%. These risks are relevant to clinical practice as parents will often wish to discuss risks during consultation.

CLEFT SUBTYPES

10. Which one of the following types of cleft is most commonly associated with another anomaly?
    C. Isolated cleft palate

    Cleft palate can be syndromic or nonsyndromic. Nonsyndromic clefts are characterized by one defect or multiple anomalies that are the result of a single initiating event or primary malformation. Syndromic clefts are characterized by more than one malformation involving more than one developmental field. Associated anomalies are most commonly seen with isolated cleft palates. This can be as high as 70% where Pierre Robin sequence is included. Anomalies are also higher in bilateral cleft patients. Syndromic clefts include syndromes such as Stickler, velocardiofacial, and Van der Woude.

PIERRE ROBIN SEQUENCE

11. While on call for the pediatric plastic surgical team, you are referred an infant with a diagnosis of Pierre Robin sequence. **Which one of the following is the most likely reason for an infant requiring an acute admission?**
    D. Airway compromise

    The clinical features of Pierre Robin sequence are micrognathia/retrognathia and glossoptosis often with cleft palate. These can lead to significant airway problems, especially in young babies that require acute admission. The risk of airway compromise usually improves with age but in the acute setting needs meticulous care. Treatment includes lateral or prone positioning, and careful observation. In some cases a nasopharyngeal airway or CPAP is required for a short duration. Occasionally tracheostomy is required. Infants with Pierre Robin sequence do not always have a cleft palate, but when one is present it tends to be wide and U-shaped as opposed to the normal V-shaped cleft.

SYNDROMIC CLEFTS

12. A patient is referred with a syndromic cleft palate, ocular malformations, hearing loss, and arthropathies. They have a proven genetic mutation for type II collagen. *What syndrome does this specifically represent?*
A. Stickler syndrome
 There are a number of syndromes associated with cleft palate. The most common is Stickler syndrome which represents 25% of all syndromic cases. This is an autosomal dominant condition with a mutation in the gene for type II collagen. The clinical presentation may include Pierre Robin sequence (but this is not specific to the other factors listed), ocular malformations, hearing loss, and arthropathies, each due to the collagen abnormality.
 Velocardiofacial and Shprintzen's syndrome are different terms used to describe the same condition and represent 15% of syndromic CP. This autosomal dominant condition is associated with a deletion on chromosome 22. It is also therefore known as 22q11 deletion. It involves cardiovascular abnormalities, abnormal facies, and developmental delay. Van der Woude syndrome represents around 20% of all syndromic cleft palate cases. This is also autosomal dominant and is associated with lower lip pits. Other syndromes associated with cleft palate include Apert syndrome and Crouzon syndrome (see Chapter 21).

ENVIRONMENTAL RISK FACTORS IN CLEFT PALATE

13. *Which one of the following is associated with an increased risk of developing an isolated oral cleft?*
D. Increased paternal age
 The risk of developing an isolated oral cleft increases with increased age of the parents, particularly if both are over the age of 30 years. Paternal age has the most profound effect. The data on maternal smoking are inconsistent regarding the increased risk of clefts. Neither maternal alcohol nor caffeine ingestion is associated with increased risk. The use of oral folic acid and multivitamin supplements is associated with a lower incidence of cleft lip or cleft lip and palate births for pregnant women with a family history of cleft lip/palate.

SURGICAL REPAIR OF CLEFT PALATE

14. *For the following descriptions, the best options are as follows:*
A. *This technique involves reorientation of the levator veli palatini and palatopharyngeus muscles across the midline to reconstruct the levator sling.*
 b. Intravelar veloplasty
B. *This technique uses two local flaps that are comprised of different constituents. It can lengthen the soft palate but reduces its transverse dimension, causing difficult closure of wide clefts.*
 e. Furlow's double-opposing technique
C. *This technique involves bilateral mucoperiosteal flaps based on the greater palatine arteries, which are closed in a V-Y fashion.*
 d. Veau-Wardill-Kilner pushback palatoplasty
  The soft palate can be repaired using an intravelar veloplasty or a double-opposing Z-plasty, as described by Furlow.[4] Both of these techniques should improve functional outcomes in terms of speech and feeding. The intravelar veloplasty involves reorientation of the levator veli

palatini muscle and palatopharyngeus muscle complex transversely following their dissection from the abnormal insertion. Furlow's technique uses double-opposing Z-plasties based on the cleft midline. The anteriorly based flaps contain only mucosa, while the posteriorly based flaps contain mucosa and levator muscle complex. Nasal mucosal flaps are transposed and closed, the levator sling is reoriented transversely, and the oral mucosal flaps are transposed and closed. Although the soft palate is lengthened, as per Z-plasty techniques in general, the transverse dimension is reduced, thereby making closure of wide clefts more difficult and increasing the risk of subsequent fistula formation (see Fig. 25-4, *Essentials of Plastic Surgery*, second edition). The hard palate can be repaired with the von Langenbeck technique, the Veau-Wardill-Kilner technique (V-Y pushback palatoplasty), or the Bardach technique (two-flap palatoplasty). Selection of technique is often based on personal preference. The V-Y pushback technique involves bilateral mucoperiosteal flaps based on the greater palatine arteries. It incorporates a V-Y closure anteriorly to lengthen the palate as well as fracture of the hamulus, levator muscle repair, and closure of the nasal and oral mucosa in separate layers. It has been associated with a high incidence of fistula formation and growth disturbances, and has fallen out of favor in many centers (see Fig. 25-6, *Essentials of Plastic Surgery*, second edition).[5]

The von Langenbeck palatoplasty uses bilateral bipedicled mucoperiosteal flaps with parallel incisions made along the cleft margin and lingual side of the alveolus. Nasal and oral mucosal flaps are mobilized and approximated in the midline. Poor speech outcomes have been attributed to the creation of a short immobile palate. These outcomes can be improved when combined with an intravelar veloplasty[2] (see Fig. 25-5, *Essentials of Plastic Surgery*, second edition).

Vomer flaps can be used to close hard palate defects. They can be either inferiorly or superiorly based and are useful in wide or bilateral clefts. Their use early in palatoplasty is controversial because of the risk of facial growth disturbance. Pharyngeal flaps are used to address poor speech in velopharygeal dysfunction and are described in Chapter 26.

POSTOPERATIVE CARE OF CLEFT PALATE PATIENTS

15. Which one of the following is often part of the postoperative regimen after cleft palate repair?

B. The use of intranasal oxymetazoline (Afrin)

The key concerns after cleft palate repair are: (1) airway monitoring, (2) control of postoperative bleeding, and (3) encouragement of early feeding.

Bleeding can be controlled by meticulous intraoperative hemostasis and injection of local anesthetic that contains epinephrine, with packing of raw areas. Postoperative application of oxymetazoline (Afrin) can also reduce bleeding and is a popular adjunct. Oxymetazoline is a direct-acting sympathomimetic amine that acts on alpha-adrenergic receptors in the arterioles of the oronasal mucosa, resulting in decreased blood flow. Patients should be placed with the head gently elevated using pillows after cleft palate repair and not supine. Airway management involves continuous pulse oximetry and sedation is stopped as early as possible to minimize risk of respiratory compromise. Early feeding should be arranged, with liquid for the first 24 hours followed by a soft diet until day 10. Often, feeding can be the determining factor in discharge timing and all patients will stay overnight after surgery.

COMPLICATIONS OF CLEFT PALATE REPAIR
16. *Which one of the following statements is correct regarding cleft palate repairs?*
  E. Fistulas most commonly form at the junction of the hard palate and the soft palate.
  Palatal fistulas by definition occur posterior to the incisive foramen. They most often occur at the junction of the soft and hard palates. The most common long-term complication after cleft palate repair is development of a palatal fistula, but rates are diverse (5% to 60%). They are likely to depend on many factors, including cleft severity, previous surgery, and surgical technique. The most common anatomic site is the junction of hard and soft palates. Fistulas can be treated surgically (with local or distant flaps) but alternatively may be managed nonsurgically with or without an obturator. The operative mortality in cleft palate repair is approximately 0.5%. Cleft palate repair can interfere with maxillary growth and does not normalize it. This can display as midface hypoplasia or problems with occlusion.

REFERENCES
1. Calnan J. Submucous cleft palate. Br J Plast Surg 6:264-282, 1954.
2. Trier WC, Dreyer TM. A comparison of palatoplasty techniques. Cleft Palate J 21:251-253, 1984.
3. Shprintzen RJ, Schwartz RH, Daniller A, et al. Morphologic significance of bifid uvula. Pediatrics 75:553-561, 1985.
4. Furlow L. Cleft palate repair by double opposing Z-plasty. Plast Reconstr Surg 78:724-738, 1986.
5. Afifi GY, Kaidi AA, Hardesty RA. Cleft palate repair. In Evans GR, ed. Operative Plastic Surgery. New York: McGraw-Hill, 2000.

26. Velopharyngeal Dysfunction

See *Essentials of Plastic Surgery*, second edition, pp. 288-294.

VELOPHARYNGEAL DYSFUNCTION

1. **Which one of the following is correct regarding velopharyngeal dysfunction?**
   A. It results from incomplete closure of the velum against the hypopharyngeal walls.
   B. It can be exacerbated by adenoidectomy.
   C. It rarely presents after satisfactory cleft palate repair.
   D. It is usually associated with a small nasopharynx.
   E. It is most often due to an abnormal bow-tie sphincter closure pattern.

TERMINOLOGY

2. **What is the most accurate term to describe impaired neuromotor control of the velum or pharyngeal wall resulting in abnormal velopharyngeal function?**
   A. Velopharyngeal disproportion
   B. Velopharyngeal insufficiency
   C. Velopharyngeal mislearning
   D. Velopharyngeal incompetence
   E. Velopharyngeal dysfunction

SPEECH ASSESSMENT

3. **Which one of the following is associated with abnormal production of vowels during speech in a patient with velopharyngeal dysfunction?**
   A. Nasal substitution
   B. Compensatory substitution
   C. Sibilant distortion
   D. Hypernasality
   E. Nasal emission

4. A speech and language therapist is testing specific speech sounds with a child in the cleft palate clinic. **Which one of the following is described as a "plosive"?**
   A. f
   B. v
   C. s
   D. sh
   E. t

5. You observe abnormal facial movements in an isolated cleft palate patient during speech. **What are they trying to achieve by doing this?**
   A. Prevent abnormal nasal airflow by constricting the nares
   B. Seal the lips and achieve oral competence
   C. Close the palatal defect by moving the tongue to the roof of the mouth
   D. Facilitate lift of the soft palate against the posterior pharyngeal wall
   E. Trying to convey their words by expression

6. When listening to a patient with velopharyngeal dysfunction you note that when trying to say "b" an "m" sound is heard instead. **What is the term used to describe this problem?**
   A. Nasal rustle
   B. Nasal turbulence
   C. Sibilant distortion
   D. Nasal substitution
   E. Compensatory articulation

EVALUATION

7. You have a 2-year-old child in clinic with velopharyngeal dysfunction. **Which one of the following modalities will provide a noninvasive, instrumented assessment of both the type and extent of velopharyngeal closure?**
   A. Nasometry
   B. Nasoendoscopy
   C. MRI
   D. Videofluoroscopy
   E. Perceptual speech evaluation

8. **In which one of the following cases of velopharyngeal dysfunction is MRA indicated before surgery?**
   A. Myasthenia gravis
   B. Post adenoidectomy
   C. Cleft palate fistula
   D. Velocardiofacial syndrome
   E. Submucosal cleft

TREATMENT

9. *According to recent evidence, what is the most effective surgical intervention in velopharyngeal dysfunction?*
   A. Furlows double-opposing Z-plasty
   B. Sphincter pharyngoplasty
   C. Intravelar veloplasty
   D. Pharyngeal flap
   E. Posterior pharyngeal wall augmentation

10. **Which one of the following has a limited success and a high complication rate in treating velopharyngeal dysfunction?**
    A. Furlow's double-opposing Z-plasty
    B. Sphincter pharyngoplasty
    C. Intravelar veloplasty
    D. Pharyngeal flap
    E. Posterior pharyngeal wall augmentation

11. *What do the Hynes and Orticochea pharyngoplasty techniques have in common?*
    A. The number of flaps utilized
    B. The muscle included within the flaps
    C. The point of insertion of the flaps
    D. The creation of a sphincter at the velopharyngeal port
    E. The use of Z-plasties

POSTOPERATIVE CARE

12. *In which patient group is postoperative airway management particularly important?*
    A. Secondary palate repair
    B. Post adenoidectomy
    C. Pierre Robin sequence
    D. Velocardiofacial syndrome
    E. Stickler syndrome

13. A six-year-old girl has velopharyngeal insufficiency with poor speech, in spite of continued speech therapy. Velopharyngeal surgery is subsequently planned. **When taking consent from the parents, which one of the following complications is it particularly important to discuss?**
 A. Dysphagia
 B. Sleep apnea
 C. Odynophagia
 D. Gastric reflux
 E. Chest infection

Answers

VELOPHARYNGEAL DYSFUNCTION

1. **Which one of the following is correct regarding velopharyngeal dysfunction?**
   B. It can be exacerbated by adenoidectomy.
   Velopharyngeal dysfunction occurs when closure of the velum against the nasopharyngeal walls (not hypopharyngeal walls) is incomplete. Normal velopharyngeal function involves composite movements of the velum posterosuperiorly, posterior pharyngeal wall ventrally, and the lateral pharyngeal wall medially. Dysfunction can be caused by a short or immobile velum or a large nasopharynx with poor function. It leads to poor speech quality and nasal regurgitation of food and is seen in patients following cleft palate repair, LeFort I/II advancement, or adenoidectomy. Other patients at risk of velopharyngeal dysfunction are those with a relatively large nasopharynx. Normal closure patterns of the velopharyngeal sphincter are classified as coronal, sagittal, circular, or bow tie. Any of these patterns can be involved in dysfunction of the sphincter, but a bow tie is not the most common.

TERMINOLOGY

2. **What is the most accurate term to describe impaired neuromotor control of the velum or pharyngeal wall resulting in abnormal velopharyngeal function?**
   D. Velopharyngeal incompetence
   Velopharyngeal dysfunction is a general descriptive term to describe any abnormal velopharyngeal function regardless of the cause. A more accurate description for a neuromotor control problem is velopharyngeal incompetence. In contrast, velopharyngeal insufficiency describes a structural abnormality resulting in dysfunction. Velopharyngeal dysfunction can result from a learned response that is neither structural nor neuromotor and this is termed velopharyngeal mislearning. Velopharyngeal disproportion describes a situation where the velum is small relative to the nasopharyngeal space as may be seen in patients with velocardiofacial syndrome.

SPEECH ASSESSMENT

3. **Which one of the following is associated with abnormal production of vowels during speech in a patient with velopharyngeal dysfunction?**
   D. Hypernasality
   Hypernasality occurs secondary to reverberation of nasally escaping air in a confined postnasal space. It occurs most commonly during the production of vowels. Other distinct signs of abnormal speech associated with abnormal production of consonants include nasal emission, nasal rustle, nasal substitution, compensatory articulation, and sibilant distortion (see question 6).

4. A speech and language therapist is testing specific speech sounds with a child in the cleft palate clinic. **Which one of the following is described as a "plosive"?**
   E. t
   Consonants may be categorized as plosives, fricatives, or affricates. Plosives include b, t, d, and k. Fricatives include f, v, s, z, sh, and th. Affricates include ch and j. During formation of these sounds, nasal emissions may be evident if closure of the nasopharynx is incomplete.

5. You observe abnormal facial movements in an isolated cleft palate patient during speech. **What are they trying to achieve by doing this?**
   A. Prevent abnormal nasal airflow by constricting the nares
   Clear phonation involves the generation of a column of air pressure passing from the subglottis into the upper airway. This airflow passes through the oral cavity for most sounds in the English language and nasal air emission is necessarily restricted. Exceptions are the sounds m, n, and ng, which require nasal airflow. When velopharyngeal closure is impaired, air can escape through the nose, when generating consonant sounds such as p, b, and t, clarity of speech is therefore impaired. Grimacing represents a subconscious attempt by the patient to inhibit abnormal nasal airflow and is evidenced by aberrant facial muscle movements during speech.

6. When listening to a patient with velopharyngeal dysfunction you note that when trying to say "b" an "m" sound is heard instead. **What is the term used to describe this problem?**
   D. Nasal substitution
   When a patient with velopharyngeal dysfunction tries to produce an oral consonant with appropriately positioned articulators the sound is converted into its nasal equivalent. In this case a "b" becomes an "m" and a "d" becomes an "n". This is termed nasal substitution. Nasal rustle and nasal turbulence are equivalent. They refer to a distinct fricative sound on the voiced pressure consonants b, d, and g. Sibilant distortion is the production of sounds "s" and "z" with incorrect tongue placement and often is secondary to malocclusion. Compensatory articulation is the production of plosives or fricatives in spite of velopharyngeal dysfunction by inappropriately positioned articulators and closure at the glottal or pharyngeal level.

EVALUATION

7. You have a 2-year-old child in clinic with velopharyngeal dysfunction. **Which one of the following modalities will provide a noninvasive, instrumented assessment of both the type and extent of velopharyngeal closure?**
   D. Videofluoroscopy
   Instrumental assessment of velopharyngeal dysfunction is directed at identification of the cause and severity of the speech problem. Multiview videofluoroscopy is a useful modality for semi-quantitatively assessing both the type and extent of velopharyngeal closure. It involves static and dynamic frontal and lateral views of the velopharynx. It can be performed at an early age (usually from age 2 onward) and avoids the need for an invasive approach. Nasometry is performed from age 3 onward and involves placement of air pressure transducers inside the nostril and mouth. This enables measurement of oral and nasal air pressure, nasal airflow, and also facilitates calculation of the velopharyngeal port size. Nasoendoscopy can be performed from age 4 onward and allows qualitative assessment of velopharyngeal closure patterns and port size. MRI is used as an adjunct to velopharyngeal dysfunction and provides only static rather than dynamic views. Perceptual speech evaluation is not an instrumented assessment. It is undertaken by the speech and language therapist. Both spontaneous speech and provocative speech samples are assessed.

8. **In which one of the following cases of velopharyngeal dysfunction is MRA indicated before surgery?**
   D. Velocardiofacial syndrome
   MRA is used to define neck vascular anatomy before surgical intervention and is indicated in patients with velocardiofacial and DiGeorge syndromes because these conditions are associated with medialization of the internal carotid arteries. Without prior localization, there is a significant risk of injury to these vessels during surgical procedures involving the posterior nasopharyngeal wall.

Chapter 26 ■ Velopharyngeal Dysfunction 211

TREATMENT

9. According to recent evidence, what is the most effective surgical intervention in velopharyngeal dysfunction?
   D. Pharyngeal flap
   Some authorities propose an algorithmic approach to the surgical management of velopharyngeal dysfunction. This is dependent on the location of the velopharyngeal port closure deficiency:
   Minimal circular gap—Furlow double-opposing Z-plasty or intravelar veloplasty
   Moderate circular gap or sagittal gap—pharyngeal flap
   Large circular, coronal, or bow-tie gap—sphincter pharyngoplasty
   However, a recent meta-analysis refutes the effectiveness of this theoretical approach and suggests that a pharyngeal flap is the superior choice in most cases.[1]

10. Which one of the following has a limited success and a high complication rate in treating velopharyngeal dysfunction?
   E. Posterior pharyngeal wall augmentation
   Posterior wall augmentation creates a static posterior obstruction and can be achieved using injectable substances such as fat, collagen, or Teflon. Although it is quick and relatively simple, it is less effective than other surgical techniques and there is a risk of migration, extrusion, or embolization of the injected material. This is of particular concern where the internal carotid arteries are medialized and lie just deep to the posterior pharyngeal wall as can occur in velocardiofacial syndrome.

11. What do the Hynes and Orticochea pharyngoplasty techniques have in common?
   D. The creation of a sphincter at the velopharyngeal port
   The Hynes and Orticochea procedures are both types of sphincter pharyngoplasty. Although they are based on the same principle of raising pharyngeal wall flaps to create a sphincter at the velopharyngeal port, they differ in a number of ways. The Hynes technique involves bilateral superiorly based salpingopharyngeus musculomucosal flaps where the Orticochea technique involves bilateral superiorly based palatopharyngeus musculomucosal flaps. In addition, the Orticochea technique utilizes a third, inferiorly based, posterior pharyngeal wall flap. The flaps from the Orticochea technique are attached in an overlapped fashion to the posterior pharyngeal wall and covered by the third flap. Neither technique involves Z-plasties.[2,3]

POSTOPERATIVE CARE

12. In which patient group is postoperative airway management particularly important?
   C. Pierre Robin sequence
   The most significant complication following velopharyngeal surgery is airway obstruction and this occurs in approximately 10% of patients. Approximately 1% will require reintubation. The risk will be affected by other factors such as mandibular size, age at surgery, and respiratory function. Therefore airway monitoring is vital in all postoperative patients undergoing velopharyngeal surgery. However, Pierre Robin patients are particularly at risk because the sequence includes the triad of micrognathia/retrognathia, glossoptosis, and airway obstruction that can be exacerbated by speech surgery. Adenoidectomy can exacerbate VPD, as it can increase the physical distance required to achieve VP closure during speech. Velocardiofacial syndrome may be associated with VPD in conjunction with abnormal facies and cardiovascular abnormalities. Stickler syndrome often involves cleft palate in conjunction with a collagen gene mutation, leading to ocular

malformations, hearing loss, and arthropathies. VPD may also be present. These conditions do not specifically predispose to airway issues.

13. A six-year-old girl has velopharyngeal insufficiency with poor speech, in spite of continued speech therapy. Velopharyngeal surgery is subsequently planned. **When taking consent from the parents, which one of the following complications is particularly important to discuss?**

B. Sleep apnea

The most common early complication following velopharyngeal surgery is obstructive sleep apnea and this can occur in as many as 90% of cases during the first 1 to 2 days. It usually resolves spontaneously as postoperative edema decreases and is managed conservatively. However, in some circumstances (less than 1%) intubation is required in the short term. Either way, it is vital to discuss this preoperatively as the effects can be life threatening and even if not it can be alarming for the family to observe. Other potential complications include intraoperative and postoperative bleeding, wound dehiscence, and failure to significantly improve speech. Life-threatening bleeds can occur when injury to the internal carotid artery occurs. This is a risk when the vessel is placed aberrantly toward the midline as occurs in certain conditions such as velocardiofacial syndrome. Swallowing problems are unlikely following velopharyngeal surgery. General complications such as chest infection are also unlikely in most cases.

REFERENCES

1. Collins J, Cheung K. Farrokhyar F, et al. Pharyngeal flap versus sphincter pharyngoplasty for the treatment of velopharyngeal insufficiency: a meta-analysis. J Plast Reconstr Aesthet Surg 65:864-868, 2012.
2. Hynes W. Pharyngoplasty by muscle transplantation. Br J Plast Surg 3:128-135, 1950.
3. Orticochea M. Construction of a dynamic muscle sphincter in cleft palates. Plast Reconstr Surg 41:323-327, 1968.

27. Microtia

See *Essentials of Plastic Surgery*, second edition, pp. 295-303.

DEMOGRAPHICS OF MICROTIA

1. **Which one of the following statements is correct regarding microtia?**
   A. Males and females are equally affected.
   B. There are no racial differences in incidence.
   C. It most commonly affects the left ear.
   D. Risk increases in a mother's fifth child.
   E. The incidence is approximately 1:2500 births worldwide.

EMBRYOLOGY AND PATHOPHYSIOLOGY OF MICROTIA

2. **Which one of the following statements is correct regarding the embryology of external ear development?**
   A. The ear develops from the second and third branchial arches.
   B. Nine identifiable hillocks are involved in normal ear development.
   C. Retinoic acid supplement during pregnancy can reduce microtia risk.
   D. Teratogens that are present in the third trimester have most profound effects on microtia.
   E. Three anterior hillocks form the tragus, helical root, and superior helix.

ASSOCIATED HEARING ABNORMALITIES WITH MICROTIA

3. **Which one of the following statements is correct regarding microtia?**
   A. Middle ear and external auditory canal defects are rarely involved.
   B. The severity of the external ear defect is strongly correlated with middle ear function.
   C. Sensorineural defects are more common than conductive defects.
   D. CT imaging is strongly indicated in microtia patients with aural atresia.
   E. Unilateral microtia commonly results in bilateral hearing loss.

CURRENT CLASSIFICATION OF MICROTIA

4. A child presents with a remnant ear lobule that has a concha, acoustic meatus, and tragus. **What type of microtia does this represent when using current terminology?**
   A. Anotia type
   B. Conchal type
   C. Lobular type
   D. Small conchal type
   E. Atypical type

CONSIDERATIONS FOR RECONSTRUCTION IN MICROTIA

5. *When considering approaches to ear reconstruction, which one of the following statements is correct?*
   A. Middle ear surgery should be performed before autologous ear reconstruction.
   B. Silastic frameworks are a popular, reliable alternative to autologous reconstruction.
   C. Porous polyethylene has acceptable short-term results, but longer term outcomes are unproven.
   D. Osseointegrated prosthetic reconstruction should only be considered after failed reconstruction.
   E. Bone-anchored hearing devices have a limited role for microtia patients with hearing loss.

COMMON TECHNIQUES FOR EAR RECONSTRUCTION

6. *Which one of the following is common to both the Nagata and Brent techniques for autologous ear reconstruction?*
   A. The timing of surgery
   B. The number of stages involved
   C. The ribs used for cartilage harvest
   D. The soft tissue cover used
   E. The method of stabilizing projection

THE BRENT TECHNIQUE FOR EAR RECONSTRUCTION

7. You are performing a first-stage ear reconstruction for microtia using the original Brent technique. *Which one of the following is correct regarding this stage of reconstruction?*
   A. The child will be at least four years of age.
   B. Two further stages will be required.
   C. The lobule will be transposed during the procedure.
   D. Ipsilateral rib cartilage will be harvested.
   E. A superficial temporal artery flap will be elevated.

THE NAGATA TECHNIQUE FOR EAR RECONSTRUCTION

8. You are performing a Nagata technique autologous ear reconstruction. *Which one of the following statements is correct?*
   A. The process will typically require three stages.
   B. Reconstruction can begin at an earlier age than with the Brent technique.
   C. No perichondrium is included when harvesting the costal graft.
   D. Split-skin graft is harvested from the hip or thigh during the second stage.
   E. Both the lobule and tragus are reconstructed in the first stage.

COMPLICATIONS OF EAR RECONSTRUCTION

9. You are consenting the parents of a child for autologous ear reconstruction. *Which one of the following statements is correct?*
   A. If skin loss develops over the construct, a further surgical procedure will be required.
   B. The procedure carries a relatively high risk of postoperative infection.
   C. The risk of chest wall deformity can be reduced by delaying the age at first surgery.
   D. Hematoma formation is rare and is usually self-limiting.
   E. The reconstructed ear will remain a static size as the child continues to grow.

Answers

DEMOGRAPHICS OF MICROTIA
1. *Which one of the following statements is correct regarding microtia?*
   D. Risk increases in a mother's fifth child.

   The risk of microtia increases with maternal parity beyond four pregnancies, especially with anotia (the most severe form). Microtia displays significant racial variance with increased incidence in people of Japanese and Hispanic descent, compared with whites. Males are twice as likely to have microtia, compared with females of the same race. The overall incidence varies from 7 to 23:100,000. Right-sided microtia is most common, with a ratio of 5:3:1 for right/left/bilateral cases.

EMBRYOLOGY AND PATHOPHYSIOLOGY OF MICROTIA
2. *Which one of the following statements is correct regarding the embryology of external ear development?*
   E. Three anterior hillocks form the tragus, helical root, and superior helix.

   The ear develops from the first and second branchial (pharyngeal) arches (not the second and third). It arises from six buds of mesenchyme, known as the hillocks of His. These are numbered from 1 to 6 with the first three formed by the first arch and the second three formed by the second arch. Each hillock relates to an adult component of the ear (see Fig. 27-2, *Essentials of Plastic Surgery*, second edition):

   Hillock 1: Tragus
   Hillock 2: Helical root
   Hillock 3: Ascending helical rim
   Hillock 4: Superior scapha and helical rim
   Hillock 5: Inferior scapha and conchal bowl
   Hillock 6: Lobule

   The external auditory canal is formed by the first branchial (pharyngeal) cleft. The pharyngeal arch derivatives are described in more detail in Chapter 19, *Essentials of Plastic Surgery*, second edition.

   The first 6 to 8 weeks of gestation (i.e., the first trimester) are the most significant with regard to development of microtia. Teratogens include Accutane, retinoic acid, and thalidomide and should be avoided during pregnancy. Insults that occur beyond the first trimester are less likely to have a major effect.

ASSOCIATED HEARING ABNORMALITIES WITH MICROTIA
3. *Which one of the following statements is correct regarding microtia?*
   D. CT imaging is strongly indicated in microtia patients with aural atresia.

   Many patients with microtia also have aural atresia which itself is associated with hearing loss and canal cholesteatoma. Patients with aural atresia should undergo CT imaging as part of their workup. CT findings form part of the Jahrsdoerfer criteria which can help predict the likely hearing outcomes following surgery in patients with aural atresia. The Jahrsdoerfer grading system[1] is based on the appearance of the external ear and the findings on temporal CT including the appearance of the stapes. The grade assigned preoperatively has been shown to correlate well

with the patient's chance of successful outcome in terms of postoperative speech reception. Knowledge of these specifics is highly relevant to plastic surgeons working with microtia patients and highlights the multidisciplinary approach required for such patients.

Although middle ear and external auditory canal defects are commonly associated with microtia, no specific isolated correlation exists between the severity of the external defect and middle ear function. The most common type of hearing loss is conductive (80% to 90% of cases), not sensorineural. Conductive loss can be caused by absence or fusion of the ossicles. Unilateral microtia typically results in unilateral hearing loss.

CURRENT CLASSIFICATION OF MICROTIA

4. A child presents with a remnant ear lobule that has a concha, acoustic meatus, and tragus. *What type of microtia does this represent using current terminology?*

B. Conchal type

The currently favored classification system for microtia is based on the surgical correction of the deformity. The classification system is as follows:

Anotia: Absence of auricular tissue
Lobular type: A remnant ear with a lobule and helix but without a concha, acoustic meatus, or tragus
Conchal type: A remnant ear and lobule with a concha, acoustic meatus, and tragus
Small conchal type: A remnant ear and lobule with a small indentation of the concha
Atypical microtia: Cases that do not fall into the previous categories

A further classification worth knowing for exam purposes is that described by Tanzer[2] who previously classified auricular deformities into five types, some of which are then further subclassified. Type IV is subdivided into a, b, and c. The constricted ear is IVa, cryptocia (buried ear) is type IVb, and a hypoplastic upper one third is IVc. The full classification is as follows:

Type I: Anotia
Type IIa: Microtia with atresia of the external auditory meatus
Type IIb: Microtia without atresia of the external auditory meatus
Type III: Hypoplasia of the middle third of the ear
Type IVa: Constricted ear
Type IVb: Cryptocia
Type IVc: Hypoplasia of the entire upper third of the ear
Type V: Prominent ear

In clinical practice, it is entirely reasonable to accurately describe the appearance of the microtia and support this pictorially with photographic images rather than try to use one of the classification schemes.

CONSIDERATIONS FOR RECONSTRUCTION IN MICROTIA

5. *When considering approaches to ear reconstruction, which one of the following statements is correct?*

C. Porous polyethylene has acceptable short-term results, but longer term outcomes are unproven.

Porous polyethylene implants for ear reconstruction have good short-term aesthetic results and low rates of extrusion, but no longer term data is available. In contrast, silastic frameworks as described by Cronin[3] have high extrusion rates, so are not currently used in spite of the early excellent aesthetic appearance. Osseointegrated prosthetic reconstruction has a role in many cases and should not be reserved solely for cases in which autologous reconstruction has failed. Although outcomes will be affected by the availability of skilled anaplastologists and manufacturing procedures, prostheses can provide very good aesthetic outcomes. They are particularly useful following trauma, cancer, irradiation, and in the elderly.

Middle ear surgery is usually performed after autologous auricular reconstruction but if not, it is important to liaise with the otologist to plan access so flap vascularity is not compromised and optimal aesthetic positioning can be achieved. Conductive hearing loss is more common than sensorineural loss in microtia patients and is often treated with bone-anchored hearing devices.

COMMON TECHNIQUES FOR EAR RECONSTRUCTION

6. *Which one of the following is common to both the Nagata and Brent techniques for autologous ear reconstruction?*
   E. **The method of stabilizing projection**
   The two main techniques used for autologous ear reconstruction are those described by Brent and Nagata. They differ in many ways including the timing of surgery, the number of stages involved, the side and number of ribs used for cartilage harvest and the method of soft tissue cover. The theme common to both is that projection is achieved as a staged procedure by elevating the cartilage framework and placing a cartilage block underneath to act as a wedge beneath the framework.[4,5]

THE BRENT TECHNIQUE FOR EAR RECONSTRUCTION

7. You are performing a first-stage ear reconstruction for microtia using the original Brent technique. *Which one of the following statements is correct regarding this stage of reconstruction?*
   A. **The child will be at least four years of age.**
   Children undergoing the Brent[4] technique for ear reconstruction should be at least age four in order to have sufficient rib cartilage to construct the ear framework. The technique described by Brent was originally four stages but has since been reduced to three by incorporating the tragal component into the initial framework. In the first stage a framework is fabricated from the sixth to eighth contralateral (not the ipsilateral) costochondral cartilages. This construct is buried within a subcutaneous pocket. The lobule is not transposed until the second stage several months after the first. As discussed in question 6, projection is achieved in the third stage by placing a wedge of cartilage behind the construct. In this stage, soft tissue cover is achieved with split-skin graft from the hip and not a superficial temporal artery fascial flap. The original fourth stage involved tragal reconstruction using the contralateral conchal vault.

THE NAGATA TECHNIQUE FOR EAR RECONSTRUCTION

8. You are performing a Nagata technique autologous ear reconstruction. *Which one of the following statements is correct?*
   E. **Both the lobule and tragus are reconstructed in the first stage.**
   The Nagata[5] technique for ear reconstruction is a two-stage procedure (not three) that uses ipsilateral costal cartilage from ribs five through nine. It cannot usually be performed until 10 years of age, because cartilage volume is insufficient before this time. The first stage involves creation of a cartilage construct from ribs six to nine. Most but not all of the perichondrium is left in the chest wall to minimize residual deformity. The construct is placed in a subcutaneous pocket, and simultaneous lobule transposition is performed. Tragal reconstruction is also performed during this stage. The second stage is usually performed 6 months later, and further cartilage is harvested from the fifth rib. A temporoparietal fascial flap is elevated and inset to cover the grafts. This is then covered with split-skin graft from the scalp rather than the thigh.

COMPLICATIONS OF EAR RECONSTRUCTION

9. You are consenting the parents of a child for autologous ear reconstruction. *Which one of the following statements is correct?*

C. The risk of chest wall deformity can be reduced by delaying the age at first surgery.

The most common late complication in ear reconstruction is chest wall deformity, which occurs in approximately two thirds of cases. It is affected by age at the time of surgery and is reduced when surgery is performed later. The most significant early complications are skin loss, infection, and hematoma, all of which are rare. However, each must be identified early and managed accordingly to prevent extrusion of the cartilage framework. Areas of skin loss should be debrided and only reconstructed if the area is greater than 1 cm. Smaller defects can be managed with dressings. Avoiding pressure dressings and replacing them with small suction drains has been shown to reduce skin-related complications from 33% to 1% in Brent's series.[4] Hematomas are not self-limiting and must be drained immediately to minimize risk of skin loss. Reconstructed ears commonly remained the same size over time (48%) but many increased in size as the child developed (42%) in Brent's series.

REFERENCES

1. Jahrsdoerfer RA, Yeakley JW, Aguilar EA, et al. Grading system for the selection of patients with congenital aural atresia. Am J Otol 13:6-12, 1992.
2. Tanzer RC, ed. Reconstructive Plastic Surgery, ed 2. Philadelphia: WB Saunders, 1977.
3. Cronin TD. Use of a Silastic frame for total and subtotal reconstruction of the external ear: preliminary report. Plast Reconstr Surg 37:399, 1966.
4. Brent B. Auricular repair with autogenous rib cartilage grafts: two decades of experience with 600 cases. Plast Reconstr Surg 90:355-374, 1992.
5. Nagata S. A new method for total reconstruction of the auricle for microtia. Plast Reconstr Surg 92:187, 1993.

28. Prominent Ear

See *Essentials of Plastic Surgery*, second edition, pp. 304-314.

NORMAL EAR ANATOMY
1. **Which one of the following is true regarding the anatomy of the external ear?**
   A. The medial skin is adherent and thin.
   B. The ear grows to 95% of adult size by 2 years of age.
   C. Mature width is achieved in both sexes at the same age.
   D. The lateral skin is loose and thick.
   E. Length and height mature at different ages.

VASCULARITY OF THE EAR
2. **In addition to the posterior auricular artery, which other branch of the external carotid artery represents a significant vascular supply to the ear?**
   A. Maxillary
   B. Facial
   C. Occipital
   D. Superficial temporal
   E. Deep temporal

INNERVATION TO THE EAR
3. **Select the nerve that is described in each of the following statements. (Each option may be used once, more than once, or not at all.)**
   A. Transection of this nerve results in numbness to the tragus and helical root.
   B. This nerve contributes to sensation of the external auditory meatus, along with the facial, great auricular, and glossopharyngeal nerves.
   C. This is a branch of the cervical plexus that supplies sensation to the lower lateral part of the ear.

   Options:
   a. Glossopharyngeal
   b. Greater occipital
   c. Auriculotemporal
   d. Great auricular
   e. Facial
   f. Lesser occipital
   g. Vagus

NORMAL EAR AESTHETIC PROPORTIONS

4. Select the best option that is described in each of the following statements about normal ears. (Each option may be used once, more than once, or not at all.)
   A. In the lateral view, the long axis of the ear typically inclines approximately this amount posteriorly.
   B. This represents a typical conchoscaphal angle.
   C. When viewed from directly behind, the long axis of the ear typically inclines this amount laterally from the scalp.

   Options:
   a. 5 degrees
   b. 25 degrees
   c. 40 degrees
   d. 60 degrees
   e. 90 degrees
   f. 110 degrees
   g. 130 degrees

ASSESSMENT OF PROMINENT EARS

5. Which one of the following is probably least relevant during the clinical assessment of a patient with prominent ears?
   A. Depth and size of the conchal bowl
   B. Strength and spring of the auricular cartilage
   C. The angle between helical rim and mastoid plane
   D. Posterior inclination of the ear from the vertical plane
   E. Lobular deformity

CLINICAL FINDINGS IN PROMINENT EARS

6. Which one of the following is a typical finding in prominent ears?
   A. Overdevelopment of the antihelical fold
   B. A small conchal bowl
   C. A conchoscaphal angle of less than 90 degrees
   D. A helical rim to mastoid distance of less than 2 cm
   E. Helical rim projection laterally beyond the antihelical fold

TECHNIQUES FOR CORRECTION OF PROMINENT EARS

7. Select the pinnaplasty technique that is described by each of the following statements. (Each option may be used once, more than once, or not at all.)
   A. This suture technique is used for patients with upper pole prominence caused by a poorly defined antihelical fold.
   B. This suture technique is used to correct deformities of the upper two thirds caused by conchal excess.
   C. This technique involves a fishtail excision and may be used to correct a prominent lobule.

   Options:
   a. Nagata
   b. Wood-Smith
   c. Furnas
   d. Converse–Wood-Smith
   e. Chongchet
   f. Brent
   g. Mustarde
   h. Stenstroem

GIBSON'S PRINCIPLE

8. *Which one of the following pinnaplasty techniques is based on Gibson's principle?*
   A. Wood-Smith
   B. Converse–Wood-Smith
   C. Furnas
   D. Chongchet
   E. Mustarde

EAR ABNORMALITY IN CLINICAL PRACTICE

9. A patient is reviewed in clinic with concerns about the appearance of their right ear. On examination, the following findings are noted: From behind, the helix to mastoid distance is 12 mm superiorly and 20 mm inferiorly. From the front, the helix extends just beyond the antihelix all the way down. From the side, the ear is angled posteriorly at 30 degrees and there is a pointed thickening at the anterior junction of the upper and middle third of the helix. *What is the diagnosis in this case?*
   A. A normal ear
   B. A prominent ear
   C. A Stahl's ear
   D. A mastoid prominence
   E. A Darwin's tubercle

Answers

NORMAL EAR ANATOMY
1. **Which one of the following is true regarding the anatomy of the external ear?**
   E. Length and height mature at different ages.
   The medial skin is loose and thick, whereas the lateral skin is adherent and thin. The ear grows to 85% of adult size by 3 years of age. Timing of ear development differs between the sexes. Ear development is complete 1 year earlier in girls. Maximum height and width occur at different developmental stages. In boys, maximum width typically occurs at age 7 years and maximum height at age 13 years. In girls, these occur at ages 6 and 12 years, respectively.

VASCULARITY OF THE EAR
2. **In addition to the posterior auricular artery, which other branch of the external carotid artery usually represents a significant vascular supply to the ear?**
   D. Superficial temporal
   The external ear receives its vascular supply from terminal branches of the external carotid artery. These are the posterior auricular (dominant supply) and the superficial temporal arteries. The occipital artery also contributes in a small number (7%) of patients (see Fig. 28-2 and Chapter 38 of *Essentials of Plastic Surgery*, second edition).

INNERVATION TO THE EAR
3. **For the following statements, the best options are as follows:**
   A. Transection of this nerve results in numbness to the tragus and helical root.
      c. Auriculotemporal
   B. This nerve contributes to sensation of the external auditory meatus, along with the facial, great auricular, and glossopharyngeal nerves.
      g. Vagus
   C. This is a branch of the cervical plexus that supplies sensation to the lower lateral part of the ear.
      d. Great auricular
      The auriculotemporal nerve is a branch of the trigeminal nerve (V_3) that supplies sensation to the tragus and crus helicis. The glossopharyngeal, vagus, and facial nerves contribute to Arnold's nerve, which supplies sensation to the external auditory canal. The greater and lesser occipital nerves originate from the cervical plexus, as does the great auricular nerve. The lesser occipital nerve supplies the superior surface of the ear, whereas the greater occipital supplies the scalp above the ear. The great auricular nerve runs up the superficial surface of sternocleidomastoid to supply the lower lateral portion and inferior cranial surface of the ear (see Fig. 28-3, *Essentials of Plastic Surgery*, second edition).

NORMAL EAR AESTHETIC PROPORTIONS
4. **For the following statements, the best options are as follows:**
   A. In the lateral view, the long axis of the ear typically inclines approximately this amount posteriorly.
      b. 25 degrees

B. *This represents a typical conchoscaphal angle.*
   e. 90 degrees
C. *When viewed from directly behind, the long axis of the ear typically inclines this amount laterally from the scalp.*
   b. 25 degrees
   In a normal ear, the long axis inclines posteriorly approximately 20 to 30 degrees from the vertical plane. In addition, the long axis of the ear when viewed from behind also inclines at a similar angle laterally (20 to 30 degrees). There is interpatient variability but if the angle is greater than 30 degrees then the ear will appear abnormally prominent. The conchoscaphal angle is usually 90 degrees and angles greater than this will also give the appearance of a prominent ear (see Fig. 28-4, *Essentials of Plastic Surgery*, second edition).

ASSESSMENT OF PROMINENT EARS

5. *Which one of the following is probably least relevant during the clinical assessment of a patient with prominent ears?*
   D. Posterior inclination of the ear from the vertical plane
   A full assessment of the characteristics of the external ear should be made in clinic when assessing a patient for pinnaplasty. All abnormalities need to be identified and documented preoperatively as they will have bearing on surgical approach and likely outcome. Of all of the factors described, the inclination in the vertical plane is probably least important with specific reference to ear prominence. But some techniques will allow the lateral prominence and the inclination in the vertical plane to be altered. For example, if a postauricular pocket (mastoid region) is created then the conchal bowl can be rotated posterosuperiorly into this, thereby decreasing prominence and posterior inclination. It can then be secured with a conchomastoid suture (see Fig. 28-4, *Essentials of Plastic Surgery*, second edition).

CLINICAL FINDINGS IN PROMINENT EARS

6. *Which one of the following is a typical finding in prominent ears?*
   E. Helical rim projection laterally beyond the antihelical fold
   In a normal ear the helical rim projects 2 to 5 mm higher than the antihelical fold. This is often exaggerated in prominent ears. The main causes of prominent ears are underdevelopment of the antihelical fold and conchal bowl excess. Often patients have a combination of both abnormalities. These result in conchoscaphal angles of more than 90 degrees and an increased helical-mastoid distance. Techniques used for prominent ear correction aim to address these issues (see question 7).

TECHNIQUES FOR CORRECTION OF PROMINENT EARS

7. *For the following statements, the best options are as follows:*
   A. *This suture technique is used for patients with upper pole prominence caused by a poorly defined antihelical fold.*
      g. Mustarde
   B. *This suture technique is used to correct deformities of the upper two thirds caused by conchal excess.*
      c. Furnas
   C. *This technique involves a fishtail excision and may be used to correct a prominent lobule.*
      b. Wood-Smith
         Techniques for the correction of prominent ears can be classified as those involving sutures, cartilage scoring, or cartilage breaking. Techniques can be combined in a single procedure, for

example, scoring and suturing. The Mustarde technique[1] is a suture technique that is used to correct an underdeveloped antihelical fold. Mattress sutures are placed on either side of the planned fold to re-create it (Fig. 28-1, A and B). The Furnas technique[2] is a suture technique that is used to reduce conchal bowl prominence. Sutures are placed between the mastoid and conchal bowl to reset the ear closer to the head (Fig. 28-1, C and D). The Converse–Wood-Smith[3] is a cartilage-breaking technique for correction of prominence of the entire ear. It also involves re-creation of the antihelical fold with mattress sutures. Correction of the lobule can be combined with any of the techniques described by using a fishtail excision of skin from the posterior aspect of the lobule using the Wood-Smith technique (Fig. 28-1, E). Chongchet's technique[4] involves anterior blade scoring without sutures. Stenstroem's technique[5] involves anterior rasping of the antihelical fold without sutures.[6] Brent has described a technique for ear reconstruction rather than prominent ear correction.

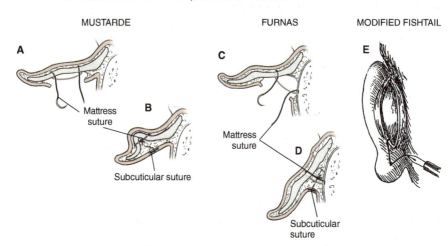

Fig. 28-1 The Mustarde technique: **A,** The skin excision is carried down to cartilage. After hemostasis is obtained, several sutures are placed through the full thickness of cartilage. Usually two or three well-placed sutures are all that are required. **B,** The sutures are tied simultaneously. A subcuticular 4-0 nylon suture is used for closure. The Furnas technique: **C** and **D,** Several mattress sutures are used to attach conchal cartilage to the mastoid fascia. The mattress sutures should be placed through the full thickness of conchal cartilage. The sutures are tied simultaneously. Modified fishtail excision: **E,** A V-extension of the posterior auricular incision is drawn on the posterior surface of the lobule.

GIBSON'S PRINCIPLE

8. Which one of the following pinnaplasty techniques is based on Gibson's principle?

D. Chongchet

Gibson's principle is based on the observation that cartilage will curl away from a cut surface, because interlocking stresses are released when perichondrium is incised. Gibson and Davis[7] published this work in 1958. Techniques that employ scoring are based on these principles. Cartilage is known to maintain its position because of the balancing forces of perichondrium on each side. When the perichondrium is incised on one side, the balance of forces is no longer equal and the cartilage moves away from the incision. For this reason anterior rather than posterior scoring has been more commonly performed. The Mustarde and Furnas techniques[1,2] rely solely on the ability of sutures to overpower the interlocking stresses rather than break or unbalance them. The Converse–Wood-Smith[3] is a cartilage-breaking technique, and the Wood-Smith is a technique that is used to set back the lobule.

EAR ABNORMALITY IN CLINICAL PRACTICE

9. A patient is reviewed in clinic with concerns about the appearance of their right ear. What is the diagnosis in this case?

E. A Darwin's tubercle

Darwin's tubercle is a pointed thickening at the junction of the upper and middle third of the helix present in one in ten individuals. This can be surgically treated with a full-thickness excision of the skin and the underlying prominent cartilage (Fig. 28-2). Aside from the description of Darwin's tubercle, the other measurements are all in keeping with a normal ear (see Fig. 28-4 and Box 28-1, *Essentials of Plastic Surgery*, second edition).

Stahl's ear refers to the presence of a third and/or horizontal superior crus with a pointed upper helix. This results in upper and mid third prominence and while a number of surgical options exist for addressing this problem, it remains difficult to satisfactorily treat. A mastoid prominence will alter the appearance of the postauricular valley and can be surgically managed with either soft tissue or bone resection of this area.

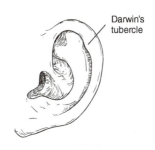

Fig. 28-2 Darwin's tubercle.

REFERENCES

1. Mustarde JC. The correction of prominent ears using mattress sutures. Br J Plast Surg 16:170, 1963.
2. Furnas DW. Correction of prominent ears by conchamastoid sutures. Plast Reconstr Surg 42:189, 1968.
3. Converse JM, Wood-Smith D. Technical details in the surgical correction of the lop ear deformity. Plast Reconstr Surg 31:118, 1963.
4. Chongchet V. A method of antihelix reconstruction. Br J Plast Surg 16:268, 1963.
5. Stenstroem SJ. A natural technique for correction of congenitally prominent ears. Plast Reconstr Surg 32:509, 1963.
6. Janis JE, Essentials of Plastic Surgery, ed 2. St Louis: Quality Medical Publishing, 2014.
7. Gibson T, Davis W. The distortion of autogenous cartilage grafts: its cause and prevention. Br J Plast Surg 10:257-274, 1958.

Traumatic Injuries

29. Facial Soft Tissue Trauma

See *Essentials of Plastic Surgery*, second edition, pp. 315-322.

GENERAL PRINCIPLES IN THE MANAGEMENT OF SOFT TISSUE FACIAL WOUNDS

1. **When managing patients with soft tissue facial wounds, which one of the following is correct?**
   A. Formal assessment begins with administration of local anesthetic.
   B. Tetanus boosters are required for all patients with contaminated wounds.
   C. Abrasions are partial-thickness skin defects, often managed with dressings.
   D. Permanent tattooing may be the result of inadequate debridement.
   E. Local flaps are often useful for closing wounds in the acute setting.

MANAGEMENT OF BITE WOUNDS

2. **In a patient with a human bite wound to the face, which one of the following is correct?**
   A. The wound should be debrided and left to heal by secondary intention.
   B. A course of amoxicillin should be prescribed for seven days.
   C. *Pasteurella multocida* is the most likely pathogen to cause infection.
   D. Antibiotic coverage should target *Eikenella* and *Streptococcus*.
   E. The risk of developing infection is greater than with animal bites.

MANAGING SCALP WOUNDS

3. **Which one of the following methods of wound closure is recommended for the skin of the hair-bearing scalp to minimize alopecia?**
   A. Absorbable monofilament sutures
   B. Absorbable braided sutures
   C. Nonabsorbable monofilament sutures
   D. Nonabsorbable braided sutures
   E. Skin staples

WOUNDS TO THE PERIORAL AREAS

4. You see a patient with a soft tissue injury involving the lip, cheek, and tongue. **Which one of the following is correct?**
   A. Wharton's duct may be injured and should be repaired with microsurgical techniques.
   B. Divisions of the facial nerve close to the oral commissure require neurosyntheses.
   C. The parotid papilla should be located intraorally at the level of the canine to assess duct injury.
   D. The white roll should be marked with methylene blue following local anesthetic infiltration.
   E. Smaller lacerations of the tongue heal satisfactorily without surgical intervention.

ANATOMY OF THE FACIAL DUCTAL SYSTEMS

5. Select the structure that is described in each of the following statements. *(Each option may be used once, more than once, or not at all.)*
   A. This structure continues as the lacrimal duct.
   B. This structure drains directly into the common canaliculus and is often damaged in lower eyelid injuries.
   C. The parotid papilla can help to identify the location of this structure.

   Options:
   a. Lacrimal gland
   b. Wharton's duct
   c. Stensen's duct
   d. Inferior canaliculus
   e. Superior canaliculus
   f. Lacrimal sac

CLINICAL SCENARIOS IN SOFT TISSUE FACIAL TRAUMA

6. A 30-year-old man sustains an avulsion flap injury to the scalp in a motor vehicle accident. **To what depth is the injury most likely to pass?**
   A. Frontal bone
   B. Periosteum
   C. Frontalis
   D. Subcutaneous tissue
   E. Skin

NERVE INJURY IN SOFT TISSUE TRAUMA

7. A young male presents after an altercation in a bar. He was struck with a broken glass bottle and has a soft tissue wound that passes vertically from the mandibular body to the zygomatic arch. The wound does not breach the oral mucosa. **Which one of the following is least likely to be present on examination?**
   A. Weakness of the frontalis muscle
   B. Paresthesia to the ipsilateral ear helical root and lobule
   C. Weakness of the corrugator and procerus
   D. Saliva in the wound
   E. Loss of oral competence

Answers

GENERAL PRINCIPLES IN THE MANAGEMENT OF SOFT TISSUE FACIAL WOUNDS

1. **When managing patients with soft tissue facial wounds, which one of the following is correct?**
   D. Permanent tattooing may be the result of inadequate debridement.

   The principles of soft tissue wound management are careful examination of the patient and assessment of the injury, followed by meticulous sharp debridement, irrigation, and defect closure with repair of any specialized structures such as nerves and ducts. Inadequate debridement can lead to permanent tattooing of the skin. An example is road rash in a partial-thickness abrasion, where gravel left in the wound will be permanently visible as black pigment. Although local anesthetic is useful to help fully assess and treat many wounds, it must not be used until nerve function has been assessed.

   Although all patients should have their tetanus status checked, not all will need further tetanus doses. Current guidelines differ, with some advocating a booster every ten years or at the time of an injury if no booster has been given within a five-year period[1] (see Table 29-1, *Essentials of Plastic Surgery,* second edition). The source text describes recommendations in Table 29-1 which suggest that even patients with tetanus-prone injuries do not require boosters, providing they have undergone complete immunization and received a booster within five years. Current National Health Service U.K. guidelines[2] state that once the five injections are given, further boosters are not required except for high-risk injuries.

   There is often confusion regarding descriptions for soft tissue wounds. An abrasion is a scraped area of skin but may be partial or full thickness. Partial-thickness abrasions are generally treated with dressings, while full-thickness abrasions may require grafts or flaps for closure. Local flaps are not recommended for use in the acute setting, especially in wounds with crush components and should therefore be preserved for secondary reconstruction.[3,4]

MANAGEMENT OF BITE WOUNDS

2. **In a patient with a human bite wound to the face, which one of the following is correct?**
   D. Antibiotic coverage should target *Eikenella* and *Streptococcus*.

   The most common pathogens implicated in infection in human bites are *Eikenella* and *Streptococcus viridans,* so antibiotics should be selected to target these organisms. Amoxicillin alone is not a suitable antibiotic for bite injuries and needs to be combined with clavulanate (Augmentin) to provide extended spectrum beta lactam coverage.

   Most bite injuries should be left open to heal after debridement, but bites to the face should be closed primarily after debridement. An exception to this rule is where there is evidence of infection. In this case, delayed primary closure is indicated after debridement and antibiotic treatment. *Pasteurella canis* and *Pasteurella multocida* are frequently associated with canine and feline bites, respectively. Although human bites can lead to severe infections, cat bites are those most commonly associated with infection because of the deep, puncture type wounds and the virulent bacteria involved.

Chapter 29 ▪ Facial Soft Tissue Trauma   229

MANAGING SCALP WOUNDS

3. *Which one of the following methods of wound closure is recommended for the skin of the hair-bearing scalp to minimize alopecia?*
   E. Skin staples
   When closing scalp defects a layered approach is advised so the galea is approximated with interrupted absorbable sutures before skin closure. Skin closure can then be achieved with any of the above sutures; however staples may cause the least tissue necrosis, provide adequate wound-edge eversion, and less subsequent scalp alopecia than other forms of closure. Another advantage to staples is the ease and speed with which they can be placed. This is particularly useful in reducing bleeding from scalp wound edges. Alopecia may be further minimized by careful use of cautery at the wound edges. When planned incisions are made in the scalp, beveling the blade may also help reduce alopecia as this allows hair regrowth through the scar.

WOUNDS TO THE PERIORAL AREAS

4. *You see a patient with a soft tissue injury involving the lip, cheek, and tongue. Which one of the following is correct?*
   E. Smaller lacerations of the tongue heal satisfactorily without surgical intervention.
   Larger lacerations of the tongue notoriously break down because of the strength of the tongue musculature. For this reason layered closure is advocated in larger lacerations. However, smaller lacerations can be left to heal by secondary intention.
   Although microsurgical repair of the parotid duct (Stensen's duct) is advocated, lacerations to Wharton's ducts, which are found on the floor of the mouth, are usually managed with marsupialization. The parotid duct opens into the oral cavity at the level of the upper second molar (not canine) and should be identified in cases involving cheek or intraoral injury. Once the opening is identified, the duct can be stented with a 24-gauge angiocatheter and extravasation of saline indicates an injury that warrants repair. When managing lip injuries, it is vital to ensure that close approximation of the white roll is achieved, as even small malalignments of 1 mm can be noticeable at short distances. For this reason marking the white roll with methylene blue or a skin marking pen before (not after) infiltration with local anesthesia is recommended. Once the local anesthetic has been infiltrated, distortion occurs that may limit the ability to accurately identify the white roll. Facial nerve lacerations medial to the lateral canthus do not usually require repair because of the significant arborization of the buccal and zygomatic branches.

ANATOMY OF THE FACIAL DUCTAL SYSTEMS

5. *For the following statements, the best options are as follows:*
   A. This structure continues as the lacrimal duct.
   f. Lacrimal sac
   B. This structure drains directly into the common canaliculus and is often damaged in lower eyelid injuries.
   d. Inferior canaliculus
   C. The parotid papilla can help to identify this structure.
   c. Stensen's duct
   The lacrimal apparatus is clinically relevant to soft tissue facial trauma as it can be damaged during periorbital injuries. Tears drain from the upper and lower eyelids through puncta and then pass along the superior or inferior canaliculus respectively towards the lacrimal sac. The lacrimal sac drains into the lacrimal duct and then enters the nasal cavity at the valve of Hasner (see Fig. 29-2, *Essentials of Plastic Surgery,* second edition). Injury to the ductal

system is most commonly seen with lower medial eyelid injuries and will result in epiphora. It can be managed with surgical repair over a stent by the ophthalmology team. The parotid duct is also known as Stensen's duct and drains into the oral cavity at the parotid papilla.

CLINICAL SCENARIOS IN SOFT TISSUE FACIAL TRAUMA

6. A 30-year-old man sustains an avulsion flap injury to the scalp in a motor vehicle accident. *To what depth is the injury most likely to pass?*
   B. Periosteum
   Avulsion injuries of the scalp are common and often referred to plastic surgery for evaluation. The soft tissues of the scalp have five layers: skin, subcutaneous tissue, galea, loose areolar tissue, and pericranium. Avulsion injuries most commonly occur at the level of the scalping plane between the galea and pericranium. Other common injury types are burst injuries in young children. With this mechanism of injury the patient falls onto the head and bangs it on a furniture corner or the floor. Wounds are deep and often pass down to bone, stripping a small amount of pericranium. In some instances these injuries cause an underlying fracture, and this should be excluded. Wounds should be examined under anesthesia, debrided, and closed in layers with absorbable sutures.

NERVE INJURY IN SOFT TISSUE TRAUMA

7. A young male presents after an altercation in a bar. He was struck with a broken glass bottle and has a soft tissue wound that passes vertically from the mandibular body to the zygomatic arch. The wound does not breach the oral mucosa. *Which one of the following is least likely to be present on examination?*
   B. Paresthesia to the ipsilateral ear helical root and lobule
   This patient is at risk of damage to any of the five main branches of the facial nerve and therefore can have symptoms ranging from mild to complete unilateral facial paralysis (see Fig. 29-1, *Essentials of Plastic Surgery*, second edition). The paralysis can account for a loss in oral competence, which may be amplified by damage to the buccinator muscle itself. Although the wound is not full thickness, saliva can be present because of injury to the parotid gland or division of Stensen's duct. The auriculotemporal branch of the trigeminal nerve is at risk of injury. This supplies the superior lateral aspect of the ear. Sensation to the lobule should be spared, because this is supplied by the great auricular nerve.

REFERENCES

1. Mayo Clinic. Tetanus: prevention. Available at *http://www.mayoclinic.com/health/tetanus/DS00227/DSECTION5prevention*.
2. NHS Choices. Tetanus. Available at *http://www.nhs.uk/Conditions/Tetanus/Pages/Prevention.aspx*.
3. Centers for Disease Control and Prevention (CDC). Deferral of routine booster doses of tetanus and diphtheria toxoids for adolescents and adults. MMWR Morb Mortal Wkly Rep 50:481, 427, 2001.
4. Update on adult immunization. Recommendations of the Immunization Practices Advisory Committee (ACIP). MMWR Recomm Rep 40(RR-12):1-94, 1991.

30. Facial Skeletal Trauma

See *Essentials of Plastic Surgery*, second edition, pp. 323-348.

FACIAL FRACTURES

1. Which one of the following facial bones requires the greatest force to fracture?
- A. Mandible
- B. Nasal bone
- C. Maxilla
- D. Frontal bone
- E. Zygoma

MANAGEMENT AFTER SEVERE HEAD TRAUMA

2. Which one of the following is correct regarding life-threatening hemorrhage after a major facial injury?
- A. The external maxillary artery is the most common source of severe hemorrhage in facial fractures.
- B. Angiography and embolization are recommended for uncontrolled bleeding in an unstable patient.
- C. Ligation of the common carotid artery may be required.
- D. Nasal packing and immediate fracture reduction are key steps to control hemorrhage.
- E. Ligation of the external carotid artery risks ischemia to ipsilateral facial structures.

FRONTAL SINUS ANATOMY

3. Which one of the following is correct regarding the frontal sinus?
- A. It is normally present at birth.
- B. Drainage typically occurs through the nasofrontal duct.
- C. Adult size is achieved by age 5.
- D. It may be easily identified radiologically in all age groups.
- E. It usually drains into the inferior meatus.

DUCTAL INJURY IN FRONTAL SINUS FRACTURES

4. A patient is seen in the emergency department with a suspected frontal sinus fracture after an assault with a baseball bat to the forehead. A CT head scan is performed to confirm the diagnosis. **Which one of the following cannot be directly assessed by the CT scan?**
- A. Involvement of the anterior and posterior tables
- B. The presence of a nasofrontal duct injury
- C. Evidence of pneumocephalus
- D. The degree of posterior table involvement
- E. The injury level relative to the superior orbital rim

MANAGEMENT OF FRONTAL SINUS FRACTURES

5. For each of the following clinical scenarios, select the most appropriate management plan. (Each option may be used once, more than once, or not at all.)
   A. A patient presents with an undisplaced anterior table fracture.
   B. A patient presents with a displaced anterior table fracture and no nasofrontal duct involvement.
   C. A patient presents with anterior and posterior table fractures and significant displacement of the posterior wall (more than one width of the table); a CSF leak is present.

Options:
   a. No operative intervention.
   b. No operative intervention for 1 week, then reassess.
   c. Reduce and stabilize anterior wall, but preserve the sinus.
   d. Reduce and stabilize anterior wall, but obliterate the sinus.
   e. Reduce and stabilize the anterior wall and perform cranialization.

OPERATIVE MANAGEMENT OF FRONTAL SINUS FRACTURES

6. When undertaking surgical reduction of a frontal sinus fracture, which one of the following is correct?
   A. Surgical access should be achieved through a bicoronal approach.
   B. Dissection should proceed in the subperiosteal plane.
   C. Sinus obliteration should be achieved with either bone/fat grafts or bone cement.
   D. Cranialization simply involves removing mucosa and obliterating the ducts.
   E. When cranialization is required, the nasal and cranial cavities are separated with a pericranial flap.

NASOORBITAL ETHMOID FRACTURES

7. For management of patients with nasoorbital ethmoidal fractures, which one of the following applies?
   A. These are technically simple fractures to repair but commonly affect facial appearance.
   B. Thermoplastic splints should be used postoperatively to reduce soft tissue thickening.
   C. The Markowitz classification is used and is based on movement of the superior bony fragment.
   D. Surgical fixation is usually achieved with plates and bone graft alone.
   E. Bone grafts are favored in pediatric patients to minimize future growth disturbances.

MANAGEMENT OF NASAL FRACTURES

8. A patient is seen in clinic following an assault where they were punched in the face. Their nose is now deviated and flattened at the nasal bridge. The left airway is no longer patent and the septum appears abnormally positioned. There is no evidence of septal hematoma or significant swelling. *What is the next step in management of this case in order to optimize long-term outcome?*
   A. Elevation and ice with reassessment in 5 days.
   B. Order a CT scan with 3 mm slices.
   C. Request a radiographic series of the skull base.
   D. Proceed with manipulation under anesthesia.
   E. Perform an open rhinoplasty

Chapter 30 ■ Facial Skeletal Trauma

ANATOMY OF THE BONY ORBIT

9. The lamina papyracea is the thinnest part of the orbital floor. **Which bone is it formed by?**
   A. Palatine
   B. Ethmoid
   C. Sphenoid
   D. Frontal
   E. Lacrimal

ORBITAL FRACTURES

10. You see a patient with a suspected orbital fracture. **Which one of the following statements is correct?**
    A. Increased intraorbital volume would be the sole cause of enophthalmos in this patient.
    B. Nausea and vomiting with limited eye excursion are highly suggestive of extraocular muscle entrapment.
    C. Dystopia most commonly refers to horizontal globe malposition.
    D. Entrapment of the extraocular muscles is most common in adults and leads to diplopia.
    E. Surgical access should be obtained through a subciliary approach.

ANATOMY OF THE ZYGOMA

11. **Which one of the following bones does not articulate with the zygoma?**
    A. Frontal
    B. Maxilla
    C. Sphenoid
    D. Temporal
    E. Ethmoid

ZYGOMATICOMAXILLARY COMPLEX FRACTURES (ZMC)

12. **For management of a patient with an unstable ZMC fracture, which one of the following statements is correct?**
    A. All four articulations must be reduced and stabilized with monocortical miniplates and screws.
    B. The patient is likely to have permanent deformity even if accurate reduction and stabilization is achieved.
    C. Fixation of the zygomaticofrontal articulation should ideally be performed first following reduction.
    D. The best surgical approach is through a combination of intraoral and lower blepharoplasty incisions.
    E. Accurate reduction of the zygomaticotemporal articulation is most important.

MAXILLARY FRACTURES

13. **Which one of the following statements is correct regarding maxillary fractures?**
    A. The maxilla contains three vertical and four horizontal buttresses.
    B. Dentoalveolar and LeFort I fractures are essentially the same.
    C. Their management in children follows different principles.
    D. Closed reduction and maxillomandibular fixation are recommended for LeFort fractures.
    E. Rowe forceps are useful for management of impacted fractures.

SURGICAL MANAGEMENT OF PANFACIAL FRACTURES

14. **When operating on a patient with panfacial fractures, which one of the following fracture sites should normally be stabilized first?**
    A. Maxilla
    B. Zygoma
    C. Mandible
    D. Orbital floor
    E. Nasal bone

TEMPORAL BONE FRACTURES

15. A patient presents with a transverse temporal bone fracture. **What is the most likely finding on clinical examination?**
    A. Trigeminal neuralgia
    B. Facial nerve paresis
    C. CSF otorrhea
    D. Hearing loss
    E. Vestibular dysfunction

OPHTHALMIC CONSEQUENCES OF FACIAL FRACTURES

16. **For each of the following clinical scenarios, select the most appropriate option from those listed. (Each option may be used once, more than once, or not at all.)**
    A. A patient presents with ipsilateral ptosis of the upper lid, proptosis, ophthalmoplegia, numbness to the forehead and nose, and a dilated ipsilateral pupil.
    B. A patient presents with the findings as in (A) but also experiences loss of vision.
    C. A patient presents with proptosis, chemosis, ophthalmoplegia, and an ocular bruit.

    Options:
    a. Traumatic optic neuropathy
    b. Orbital apex syndrome
    c. Anterior segment injury
    d. Sympathetic ophthalmia
    e. Superior orbital fissure syndrome
    f. Posterior segment trauma
    g. Traumatic carotid-cavernous sinus fistula

17. **Which one of the following conditions requires treatment within minutes?**
    A. Corneal abrasion
    B. Iridodialysis
    C. Traumatic mydriasis
    D. Hyphema
    E. Central retinal artery occlusion

CLINICAL ASSESSMENT IN FACIAL TRAUMA

18. You see a patient with suspected frontal bone fracture and CSF leak from the ears. **Which test is most helpful to confirm the diagnosis?**
    A. Alpha transferrin
    B. Beta transferrin
    C. Glucose
    D. Albumin
    E. Prealbumin

19. A patient sustains a high impact trauma to the face and trunk. A CT confirms a maxillary fracture involving the frontonasal junction with movement of the upper jaw and nasal bones as a single unit. *What type of fracture does this represent?*
  A. LeFort I
  B. LeFort II
  C. LeFort III
  D. Dentoalveolar
  E. Alveolar

20. You are asked to assist your head and neck colleague with reduction and stabilization of a facial fracture using a Gillies approach. *What type of fracture is involved?*
  A. Frontal
  B. Zygomatic
  C. Nasal
  D. Maxilla
  E. Mandible

21. A patient presents with bruising over the mastoid process with persistent headache 2 days following facial trauma. A CT scan of the head demonstrates a fracture. *Injury to which bone is associated with this bruising pattern?*
  A. Maxilla
  B. Mandible
  C. Zygoma
  D. Temporal
  E. Parietal

LONG-TERM COMPLICATIONS FOLLOWING FACIAL INJURY

22. A patient presents to clinic with bilateral inflammation of the uvea 3 months following a severe soft tissue injury to the right eye. *Which one of the following is the most likely diagnosis?*
  A. Sympathetic opthalmia
  B. Vitreous hemorrhage
  C. Traumatic optic neuropathy
  D. Iridodialysis
  E. Orbital apex syndrome

Answers

FACIAL FRACTURES
1. **Which one of the following facial bones requires the greatest force to fracture?**
   D. Frontal bone
   In 1975 Nahum[1] presented the forces necessary to fracture various bones in the facial skeleton. The forces required to fracture the frontal bone were three times greater than those required to fracture the zygoma, maxilla, or mandible. The force required was 800 to 1600 pounds for the frontal sinus versus 300 to 750 pounds for the mandibular angle, 550 to 900 pounds for the mandibular symphysis, 200 to 400 pounds for the zygomatic arch, and 150 to 300 pounds for the maxilla. Frontal bone fractures therefore illustrate the high-energy trauma that has occurred and are likely to be associated with other coexisting injuries.

MANAGEMENT AFTER SEVERE HEAD TRAUMA
2. **Which one of the following is correct regarding life-threatening hemorrhage after a major facial injury?**
   D. Nasal packing and immediate fracture reduction are key steps to control hemorrhage.
   The internal maxillary artery is the most common source of bleeding in facial fractures. This should be managed with posterior nasal packing and immediate fracture reduction. Angiography and selective embolization are only recommended once a patient has been stabilized. If a patient is hemodynamically unstable, ligation of the external carotid artery may be indicated. This does not risk ischemia to the ipsilateral facial structures because of the considerable arterial networks in the head and neck.

FRONTAL SINUS ANATOMY
3. **Which one of the following is correct regarding the frontal sinus?**
   B. Drainage typically occurs through the nasofrontal duct.
   The focal point of frontal sinus drainage is commonly the osteomeatal complex, which comprises the maxillary, frontal, and anterior ethmoid ostia and is located in the middle meatus.[2] Drainage is usually through the nasofrontal ducts into the middle meatus, but this can occur directly. There is some evidence that the frontal sinus may have an independent drainage pattern in some patients. The frontal sinus does not develop until after birth. Development begins at about age 2, and it typically reaches adult size after age 12. It may be visible radiographically from age 8 onward.

DUCTAL INJURY IN FRONTAL SINUS FRACTURES
4. A patient is seen in the emergency department with a suspected frontal sinus fracture after an assault with a baseball bat to the forehead. A CT head scan is performed to confirm the diagnosis. **Which one of the following cannot be directly assessed by the CT scan?**
   B. The presence of a nasofrontal duct injury
   A CT scan is an important imaging tool for suspected frontal sinus fractures. It allows assessment of the bony injury in terms of the table involved, the level of injury, and the degree of fracture displacement. All of these are important factors in the management algorithm. It also helps to identify associated neurologic injuries and pneumocephalus. A CT scan will only provide indirect

evidence of a ductal injury, and injury should be assumed unless the CT shows transverse anterior and posterior table fractures above the sinus floor or an isolated anterior table fracture.

MANAGEMENT OF FRONTAL SINUS FRACTURES

5. *For the following scenarios, the best options are as follows:*
   A. *A patient presents with an undisplaced anterior table fracture.*
      a. **No operative intervention.**
   B. *A patient presents with a displaced anterior table fracture and no nasofrontal duct involvement.*
      c. **Reduce and stabilize anterior wall, but preserve the sinus.**
   C. *A patient presents with anterior and posterior table fractures and significant displacement of the posterior wall (more than one width of the table); a CSF leak is present.*
      e. **Reduce and stabilize the anterior wall and perform cranialization.**

   Frontal sinus fractures are high-energy injuries that present with upper-face edema and bruising. There is often a palpable deformity of the frontal bone with parasthesias of the supraorbital and supratrochlear nerves. CSF leak rhinorrhea may occur where dural laceration is present. The globe may be displaced forward and inferiorly.

   Management of frontal sinuses depends on a number of key factors built into the algorithm shown in Figs. 30-2 and 30-3, *Essentials of Plastic Surgery,* second edition. These will depend on the skull wall involved, the degree of fracture displacement, the presence or absence of CSF leak, and whether the nasofrontal duct is involved.

OPERATIVE MANAGEMENT OF FRONTAL SINUS FRACTURES

6. *When undertaking surgical reduction of a frontal sinus fracture, which one of the following is correct?*
   E. **When cranialization is required, the nasal and cranial cavities are separated with a pericranial flap.**

   Although access is commonly through a bicoronal approach, access through existing lacerations may be used. Subgaleal dissection is performed to preserve a pericranial flap in case the sinus requires obliteration or cranialization. Obliteration of the sinus may be achieved with bone or fat grafts as alternatives to a pericranial flap, but bone cement should not be used because of potential complications from infection. Cranialization not only involves removal of mucosa and obliteration of the ducts, but also includes removal of the posterior table. The nasal cavity is isolated from the cranial cavity by interposing a pericranial flap, and the anterior table is then reconstructed.

NASOORBITAL ETHMOID FRACTURES

7. *For management of patients with nasoorbital ethmoidal fractures, which one of the following applies?*
   B. **Thermoplastic splints should be used postoperatively to reduce soft tissue thickening.**

   Nasoethmoidal fractures are complex to manage and are associated with changes in postinjury facial appearance due to their involvement with the nasal dorsum, nasoorbital valley, and medial canthus. Use of either bolsters or thermoplastic nasal splints postoperatively is advised to help optimize soft tissue outcomes.

   Nasoethmoidal fractures have been classified by Markowitz into three groups according to the involvement of a central bony fragment (see Fig. 30-4, *Essentials of Plastic Surgery,* second edition). The relevance of this is that the central fragment is the site of attachment of the medial

canthal tendon. Disruption of this tendon results in telecanthus. Type I fractures do not involve telecanthus as they represent simple fractures of the central fragment without disruption of the canthal tendon. In type II fractures there is comminution of the central fragment but the tendon is not disrupted and may or may not involve telecanthus. Type III fractures involve severe comminution and disruption of the medial canthal tendon. These will display telecanthus. Treatment involves either a direct or bicoronal approach and stabilization requires a combination of plates, wires, and bone graft. In children, bone grafts are avoided where possible and these patients are at high risk of growth disturbances, given that the septum is a major growth center.

MANAGEMENT OF NASAL FRACTURES

8. A patient is seen in clinic following an assault where they were punched in the face. Their nose is now deviated and flattened at the nasal bridge. The left airway is no longer patent and the septum appears abnormally positioned. There is no evidence of septal hematoma or significant swelling. *What is the next step in management of this case in order to optimize a long-term outcome?*
   ### D. Proceed with manipulation under anesthesia.
   Isolated nasal fractures are the most common fracture of the facial skeleton and early accurate management is essential to minimize long-term deformity and morbidity. The key to achieving good long-term outcomes is to ensure accurate reduction of both the nasal bones and septum in the acute period.

   Manipulation should therefore be performed in a controlled environment to ensure accuracy of reduction, particularly as in this case where the septum is disrupted. Therefore a general anesthetic is advised. Where there is minimal swelling as in this case, the reduction is best performed as soon as possible. If there is significant swelling, then elevation and ice should be used and the patient reassessed in 3 to 5 days. Imaging is not required for isolated nasal bone fractures. A CT scan however, is warranted in cases of suspected NOE fractures or other head injury. Open rhinoplasty is reserved for cases with residual problems after manipulation under anesthesia.

   Rohrich and Adams[3] describe an algorithm for the management of nasal fractures which may be a useful guide in clinical practice. Fractures are classified from I through V, where I through III represents isolated nasal bone fractures, type IV has additional septal disruption (as in this case) and type V corresponds to NOE fractures. This algorithm is shown in Fig. 30-5, *Essentials of Plastic Surgery,* second edition.

   Septal fractures (type IV injuries) may require specific attention with reduction, with or without reconstruction/resection. Septal hematomas are associated with type IVa injuries and require early intervention to avoid necrosis to the septum.

ANATOMY OF THE BONY ORBIT

9. The lamina papyracea is the thinnest part of the orbital floor. *Which bone is it formed by?*
   ### B. Ethmoid
   The orbit consists of seven bones that also include the maxilla and zygoma. The thinnest area is the lamina papyracea, and this is part of the ethmoid. It is so named as it is paper thin.

Chapter 30 ▪ Facial Skeletal Trauma 239

ORBITAL FRACTURES

10. You see a patient with a suspected orbital fracture. *Which one of the following statements is correct?*
    B. Nausea and vomiting with limited eye excursion are highly suggestive of extraocular muscle entrapment.
    Enophthalmos and dystopia may occur following an orbital fracture. Enophthalmos is posterior displacement of the globe and occurs either from an increase in the bony orbital volume or a decrease in volume of the globe and surrounding structures. Dystopia refers to a vertical globe malposition. Entrapment of the periocular muscles is rare in adults but is more common in children because of the elastic characteristics of pediatric bone. Entrapment will cause limited eye excursion and diplopia and is a surgical emergency because of potential ischemic muscle damage. Nausea and vomiting in association with pain and limited eye excursion are highly suggestive of entrapment. Surgical access for orbital fractures is best achieved through subtarsal or transconjunctival approaches. A subciliary approach should be avoided because of a risk of lower lid deformity.

ANATOMY OF THE ZYGOMA

11. *Which one of the following bones does not articulate with the zygoma?*
    E. Ethmoid
    The zygoma has four articulations; these are with the frontal, maxilla, sphenoid, and temporal bones. There are left and right zygomas that each comprise the cheek and malar regions. The zygoma is a commonly fractured bone that is reduced for a cosmetic rather than functional benefit in most cases. The exception is when the fracture impedes mandibular excursion by interfering with the coronoid process. It is usual to stabilize three of the articulations.

ZYGOMATICOMAXILLARY COMPLEX FRACTURES (ZMC)

12. *For management of a patient with an unstable ZMC fracture, which one of the following statements is correct?*
    C. Fixation of the zygomaticofrontal articulation should ideally be performed first following reduction.
    Although the zygomaticomaxillary complex has four articulations, it is common practice to stabilize just three of these. When treated properly, these fractures do not leave deformities. The AO foundation guidelines recommend that the zygomaticofrontal articulation is plated first, as this allows more control to accurately reduce the remaining articulations.[4] It should also ensure the zygomaticosphenoid suture is well aligned and this is the most important to assess.
    Surgical access will depend on the complexity of the fracture but a common approach involves intraoral and upper blepharoplasty (not lower) incisions. Wide exposure using a bicoronal approach may be indicated. The Carroll-Girard screw is a percutaneous T-bar–shaped device that can be used as a joystick to reduce and control the fracture.

MAXILLARY FRACTURES

13. *Which one of the following statements is correct regarding maxillary fractures?*
    E. Rowe forceps are useful for management of impacted fractures.
    The maxilla contains three vertical and three horizontal (AP) buttresses. A fourth horizontal (AP) buttress is provided by the mandible. Dentoalveolar and LeFort fractures are different. Dentoalveolar fractures pass through the dentition where LeFort fractures separate the entire

alveolus and dentition from the midface. The fracture line is above the dentition. Malocclusion of the maxilla is commonly seen as an anterior open bite and this is secondary to posterior-inferior displacement of the maxilla. LeFort fractures should be reduced and fixed with miniplates and screws through an open approach. Closed reduction and fixation to the mandible is not recommended, because this leads to facial lengthening from the downward pull of the mandible. Rowe forceps are used to facilitate disimpaction of maxillary fractures (see Fig. 30-13, *Essentials of Plastic Surgery,* second edition).

SURGICAL MANAGEMENT OF PANFACIAL FRACTURES

14. When operating on a patient with panfacial fractures, which one of the following fracture sites should normally be stabilized first?
   C. Mandible
   Panfacial fractures involve the upper and midfacial skeleton in association with fractures of the mandible. Management of these injuries is challenging, because there is no stable reference from which to begin reduction and stabilization. It may be useful to begin with the mandible to provide a stable base from which to reconstruct the midface. Reconstruction of the zygomas should then be undertaken to provide normal facial projection. Reconstruction then proceeds inferiorly from the stable frontal process to the level of the maxilla. Fixation of the maxilla as a LeFort fracture is the last to be stabilized.

TEMPORAL BONE FRACTURES

15. A patient is seen with a transverse temporal bone fracture. *What is the most likely finding on clinical examination?*
   D. Hearing loss
   Temporal bone fractures can result in hearing loss, facial nerve paresis, vestibular dysfunction and CSF leak. Of these, hearing loss is the most common complication, occurring in the vast majority of patients with temporal bone fractures. The risk is related to the fracture configuration with all transverse fractures resulting in hearing loss compared with two thirds of longitudinal fractures. Hearing loss is either sensorineural or conductive. Sensorineural hearing loss does not improve, whereas conductive hearing loss may, unless there is disruption of the ossicular chain. Fracture pattern is also relevant to the risk of developing facial nerve paresis. Loss of facial nerve function is more likely when the fracture pattern is transverse[5] (Table 30-1).

Table 30-1 *Fracture Patterns and Complications in Temporal Bone Fractures*

Fracture Pattern	Representative Proportion of All Cases	Facial Nerve Involvement As a Proportion of Fracture Subtype	Hearing Loss As a Proportion of Fracture Subtype
Longitudinal	80% to 90%	20%	67%
Transverse	10% to 20%	40%	100%

Vestibular dysfunction can result in vertigo and nystagmus. This has a varied incidence and usually resolves spontaneously once the patient is mobilizing normally. CSF leaks occur in approximately 25% of cases following temporal bone fracture and settle spontaneously within 24 hours. Involvement of the trigeminal nerve is unusual.

Chapter 30 ▪ Facial Skeletal Trauma

OPHTHALMIC CONSEQUENCES OF FACIAL FRACTURES

16. *For the following scenarios, the best options are as follows:*
  A. *A patient presents with ipsilateral ptosis of the upper lid, proptosis, ophthalmoplegia, numbness to the forehead and nose, and a dilated ipsilateral pupil.*
  e. Superior orbital fissure syndrome
  B. *A patient presents with the findings as in (A) but also experiences loss of vision.*
  b. Orbital apex syndrome
  C. *A patient presents with proptosis, chemosis, ophthalmoplegia, and an ocular bruit.*
  g. Traumatic carotid-cavernous sinus fistula

  Superior orbital fissure syndrome occurs in association with LeFort II/III or zygomatic orbital fractures. It involves the oculomotor, trochlear, abducens, and trigeminal nerves and the ophthalmic vein. With reduction of fractures recovery typically occurs over weeks. Orbital apex syndrome is similar, but also includes a loss of vision, because the optic nerve is involved at the apex.

  Traumatic cavernous sinus fistula occurs with arterial bleeding so blood shunts from the internal carotid artery to the cavernous sinus. Angiography will provide the diagnosis. Fistulas typically close spontaneously. Treatment may include surgical ligation of the carotid artery, or placement of coils by an interventional radiologist.

  Traumatic optic neuropathy (TON) is a traumatic loss of vision without external or initial opthalmoscopic evidence of injury to the eye or the optic nerve. It may occur secondary to globe injury, retinal vascular occlusion, or orbital compartment syndrome. The only objective finding is the presence of a relative afferent pupillary defect. Anterior segment trauma includes corneal abrasions, traumatic mydriasis, and hyphema. Posterior segment trauma includes vitreous hemorrhage and scleral rupture. Sympathetic opthalmia is a bilateral granulomatous inflammation of the uvea occurring as a complication of penetrating trauma.

17. *Which one of the following conditions requires treatment within minutes?*
  E. Central retinal artery occlusion

  There are two ocular emergencies that require treatment within minutes. They are chemical burns and central retinal artery occlusion. The other injuries can be treated quickly but less urgently. Corneal abrasions are treated conservatively. They usually reepithelialize in 24 hours. Traumatic mydriasis is pupillary sphincter rupture resulting in a permanently dilated pupil. This is also treated nonoperatively. Hyphema is blood in the anterior eye chamber. This is treated by prevention of a rebleed, bed rest, and atropine to decrease iris movement.

CLINICAL ASSESSMENT IN FACIAL TRAUMA

18. *You see a patient with suspected frontal bone fracture and CSF leak from the ears. Which test is most helpful to confirm the diagnosis?*
  B. Beta transferrin

  Diagnosis of CSF leak in patients following head injury is based on clinical examination of the nose and external ear, backed up by CT scanning or laboratory tests. Beta transferrin is a carbohydrate-free form of transferrin, which is almost exclusively found in the CSF. Beta transferrin is not present in blood, nasal mucus, tears or mucosal discharge, so is specific to CSF even where the fluid is bloodstained and difficult to assess clinically. It has been shown to have a sensitivity of near 100% and a specificity of about 95% for CSF leak in a large retrospective study.[6]

Detection of glucose in the sample fluid using Glucostix test strips is another traditional test for CSF in nasal and ear discharge, but is not recommended as a confirmatory test because of its lack of specificity and sensitivity.[7] Interpretation of the results is confounded by various factors such as contamination from glucose-containing fluid (tears, nasal mucus, blood in nasal mucus) or relatively low CSF glucose levels.

The other tests listed do not relate to CSF leak tests. Albumin and prealbumin are used as markers of nutritional state.

19. A patient sustains a high impact trauma to the face and trunk. A CT confirms a maxillary fracture involving the frontonasal junction with movement of the upper jaw and nasal bones as a single unit. **What type of fracture does this represent?**
B. LeFort II

Maxillary fractures may be classified using the LeFort system. There are three types of LeFort fracture as shown in Fig. 30-1, *A* through *C*.

They differ in their extent. A LeFort I (Fig. 30-1, *A*), separates the tooth-bearing maxilla from the midface. It extends from the piriform aperture posteriorly through the nasal septum, lateral nasal walls and maxillary wall through the maxillary tuberosity or pterygoid plates. The LeFort II (Fig. 30-1, *B*) is a pyramidal fracture that extends through the frontonasal junction along the medial orbital wall, usually passing through the inferior orbital rim at the ZM suture. It continues posteriorly through the pterygoid plates. It leaves the upper jaw and nasal bones as a mobile solitary unit. The LeFort III (Fig. 30-1, *C*), fracture represents craniofacial disjunction extending through the frontonasal junction along the medial orbital wall and inferior orbital fissure and out the lateral orbital wall. Dentoalveolar fractures involve the teeth and supporting osseous structures alone.

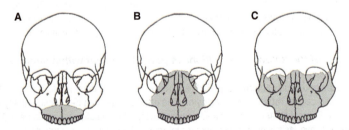

Fig. 30-1 LeFort midfacial fractures. **A,** LeFort I fracture separating the inferior portion of the maxilla in horizontal fashion, extending from the piriform aperture of the nose to the pterygoid maxillary suture area. **B,** LeFort II fracture involving separation of the maxilla and nasal complex from the cranial base, zygomatic orbital rim area, and pterygoid maxillary suture area. **C,** LeFort III fracture (i.e., craniofacial separation) is complete separation of the midface at the level of the NOE complex and ZF suture area. It extends through the orbits bilaterally.

20. You are asked to assist your head and neck colleague with reduction and stabilization of a facial fracture using a Gillies approach. **What type of fracture is involved?**
    B. Zygomatic
    A Gillies lift is an approach to elevate a zygomatic arch fracture through a temporal hairline incision. The elevator is passed beneath the deep temporal fascia under the arch and the arch is elevated, taking care not to lever against the underlying temporal bone (see Fig. 30-11, *Essentials of Plastic Surgery*, second edition). An alternative approach as described by Keen involves a 1 to 2 cm incision made lateral to the buccal sulcus. Subperiosteal elevation allows the elevator to be placed behind the arch.

21. A patient presents with bruising over the mastoid process with persistent headache 2 days following facial trauma. A CT scan of the head demonstrates a fracture. **Injury to which bone is associated with this bruising pattern?**
    D. Temporal
    This patient has *Battle's sign,* which is ecchymosis over the mastoid process and seen in conjunction with a skull base fracture. It is associated with temporal bone fractures but is not exclusive to them. For example, it is also seen in fractures of the occipital, sphenoid, and ethmoid bones. *Battle's sign* typically appears 2 to 3 days following injury and may be associated with other signs of skull base fracture such as otorrhea, rhinorrhea, facial nerve palsy, nystagmus, hemotympanum, and deafness. Raccoon eyes may also be present, which are black patches in the periorbital region secondary to ecchymosis.

LONG-TERM COMPLICATIONS FOLLOWING FACIAL INJURY

22. A patient presents to clinic with bilateral inflammation of the uvea 3 months following a severe soft tissue injury to the right eye. **Which one of the following is the most likely diagnosis?**
    A. Sympathetic opthalmia
    Sympathetic opthalmia is a bilateral granulomatous inflammation of the uvea. It occurs as a consequence of penetrating trauma. The nontraumatized eye becomes inflamed within 1 year of injury, and a severely traumatized eye should be enucleated early to prevent this.

REFERENCES

1. Nahum AM. The biomechanics of maxillofacial trauma. Clin Plast Surg 2:59-64, 1975.
2. Wallace R, Salazar JE, Cowles S. The relationship between frontal sinus drainage and osteomeatal complex disease: a CT study in 217 patients. AJNR Am J Neuroradiol 11:183-186, 1990.
3. Rohrich RJ, Adams WP. Nasal fracture management: minimizing secondary nasal deformities. Plast Reconstr Surg 106:266, 2000.
4. AO Foundation. Available at *https://www2.aofoundation.org/wps/portal/surgery.*
5. Tos M. [Practura ossi temporalis. The course and sequelae of 248 fractures of the temporal bones] Ugeskr Laeger 133:1449-1456, 1971.
6. Skedros DG, Cass SP, Hirsch BE, et al. Sources of error in use of beta-2 transferrin analysis for diagnosing perilymphatic and cerebral spinal fluid leaks. Otolaryngol Head Neck Surg 109:861, 1993.
7. Chan DT, Poon WS, IP CP, et al. How useful is glucose detection in diagnosing cerebrospinal fluid leak? The rational use of CT and Beta-2 transferrin assay in detection of cerebrospinal fluid fistula. Asian J Surg 27:39-42, 2004.

31. Mandibular Fractures

See *Essentials of Plastic Surgery*, second edition, pp. 349-357.

ANATOMY OF THE MANDIBLE

1. *Match each of the following descriptions of the mandible to the correct anatomic subunit. (Each option may be used once, more than once, or not at all.)*
   A. *The midline region of the mandible between the central incisors*
   B. *The region of the mandible between the mental foramen and the second molar*
   C. *The region of the mandible between the angle and the condyle*

   Options:
   a. Condyle
   b. Body
   c. Coronoid
   d. Ramus
   e. Angle
   f. Sigmoid
   g. Symphysis
   h. Alveolus
   i. Parasymphysis

FRACTURE SITES OF THE MANDIBLE

2. A patient is involved in an assault and sustains a mandibular fracture. **What is the most commonly fractured site in this situation?**
   A. Condyle
   B. Coronoid
   C. Ramus
   D. Angle
   E. Body

CLINICAL FINDINGS IN MANDIBULAR FRACTURES

3. A patient comes to the emergency department following an assault. On examination the following findings are present. **Which one of them is pathognomonic of a mandibular fracture?**
   A. Malocclusion
   B. Mental nerve paresthesia
   C. Ecchymosis to the floor of mouth
   D. Trismus
   E. Loose teeth

IMAGING IN MANDIBULAR FRACTURES

4. **When requesting imaging of a patient after an isolated mandibular fracture, which one of the following is true?**
   A. A panoramic radiograph alone provides adequate views of the fractured mandible.
   B. CT imaging is commonly required to confirm the fracture sites involved prior to stabilization.
   C. CT is preferable for imaging in most cases.
   D. The single best radiograph for mandibular screening is the panoramic view.
   E. Imaging will confirm diagnosis of sensory nerve damage.

INDICATIONS FOR DENTAL EXTRACTION IN MANDIBULAR FRACTURES

5. **Which one of the following is not usually an indication for the removal of teeth in conjunction with a mandibular fracture?**
   A. Gross mobility with periodontal disease
   B. Periapical radiolucency
   C. Root fracture
   D. Exposure of the apices
   E. Complete bony impaction

THE CHAMPY SYSTEM

6. An 18-year-old male is admitted after a fall onto his chin during a vasovagal attack. Examination and imaging confirm the presence of an isolated symphyseal fracture. **Which one of the following statements is correct regarding the Champy system?**
   A. ORIF will require the use of biocortical miniplates.
   B. ORIF will require a submental approach.
   C. Two miniplates will be required to stabilize the fracture.
   D. Temporary arch bars are likely to be required.
   E. The principles of fixation are based on neutralization of compression forces.

MANAGEMENT OF MANDIBULAR FRACTURES

7. **For the management of patients with mandibular fractures, which one of the following is correct?**
   A. Preoperative and postoperative broad-spectrum antibiotics should be prescribed.
   B. Oral chlorhexidine mouthwash should be used to reduce postoperative infections.
   C. Open reduction and internal fixation will be required.
   D. Principles of reduction, fixation, and early mobilization should be followed.
   E. Fracture reduction and stabilization should be achieved within 72 hours.

8. A 25-year-old male is admitted following an alleged assault. Examination confirms tenderness and swelling over the left TMJ. The mouth opening is reduced but occlusion is preserved. Radiographs show a unilateral extraarticular fracture of the left condyle. **How should this injury best be managed?**
   A. Application of arch bars
   B. MMF screws and elastics
   C. ORIF via a preauricular approach
   D. ORIF via an intraoral approach
   E. Soft diet and close observation

COMPLICATION RATES IN MANDIBULAR FRACTURES

9. **Which site is associated with the highest complication rate in mandibular fractures?**
   A. Angle
   B. Body
   C. Symphysis
   D. Condyle
   E. Sigmoid notch

Answers

ANATOMY OF THE MANDIBLE

1. **For the following descriptions, the best options are as follows:**
   A. The middle region of the mandible between the central incisors
   g. Symphysis
   B. The region of the mandible between the mental foramen and the second molar
   b. Body
   C. The region of the mandible between the angle and the condyle
   d. Ramus

   The mandible has a number of discrete anatomic subunits and fracture sites are classified according to these locations. The condyle forms part of the TMJ. The coronoid is the site of attachment of the temporalis. The sigmoid notch is found between these two points. The symphysis is the midline region between the incisors. The parasymphysis is the region on either side of the symphysis between the midline and mental foramen. The body forms the horizontal part of the mandible between the first or second premolar and the third molar. The ramus is the vertical component and the angle is the site between the body and ramus. The alveolus is the site where dentition is located (Fig. 31-1).

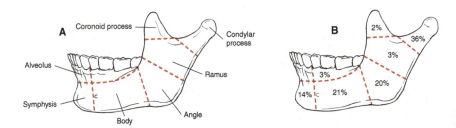

Fig. 31-1 **A,** Anatomic regions of the mandible. **B,** Frequency of fractures in those regions.

FRACTURE SITES OF THE MANDIBLE

2. A patient is involved in an assault and sustains a mandibular fracture. **What is the most commonly fractured site in this situation?**
   D. Angle

   Mandible fractures are classified by location. The most common sites are the condyle, body, angle, and symphysis. The fracture site is dependent upon the mechanism of injury and is related to both the direction and magnitude of force. For example, assaults commonly result in angle fractures, while motor vehicle crashes commonly result in body fractures. The mandible frequently fractures at two sites simultaneously. The coronoid is the least commonly fractured site representing around 2% of cases.

Chapter 31 ■ Mandibular Fractures   247

CLINICAL FINDINGS IN MANDIBULAR FRACTURES

3. A patient comes to the emergency department following an assault. On examination the following findings are present. *Which one of them is pathognomonic of a mandibular fracture?*
   C. Ecchymosis to the floor of mouth
   All of the above may be seen in conjunction with a mandibular fracture but ecchymosis to the floor of the mouth is said to be pathognomonic of this condition. When assessing patients with suspected mandibular fractures, external and internal examinations are required. A visible step-off is often visible between the teeth in addition to the bruising. Asking patients whether their bite feels normal is very useful and a highly sensitive test. The mental nerve is a continuation of the inferior alveolar nerve that supplies sensation to the skin overlying the anterior mandible. Paresthesia in this region indicates that the fracture has resulted in damage to this nerve. This must be documented preoperatively. Trismus refers to a reduced ability to open the mouth and is often seen following a mandibular fracture as a result of pain and swelling. It may also be due to a mechanical problem where a displaced fracture is present. Loose teeth are common following facial trauma and must be documented during initial assessment. Dental assessment is advised in such cases.

IMAGING IN MANDIBULAR FRACTURES

4. *When requesting imaging of a patient after an isolated mandibular fracture, which one of the following is true?*
   D. The single best radiograph for mandibular screening is the panoramic view.
   Although the panoramic view of the mandible is excellent and will enable the vast majority of fractures to be diagnosed, it should be supplemented with a mandibular series. This will typically include a PA and lateral skull view, right and left lateral oblique views, Towne projection, and submental vertex views. CT scans are not usually required for isolated mandibular fractures, but they may be useful in situations where plain radiographs are inadequate, such as when cervical collars are still in place. Radiographs may be useful to identify the inferior alveolar nerve relationships, but nerve injury is diagnosed during clinical examination.

INDICATIONS FOR DENTAL EXTRACTION IN MANDIBULAR FRACTURES

5. *Which one of the following is not usually an indication for the removal of teeth in conjunction with a mandibular fracture?*
   E. Complete bony impaction
   There are five typical indications for tooth removal:
   1. Grossly mobile teeth in which *periapical* pathology or advanced periodontal disease is present
   2. Partially erupted third molars with an associated dental pathologic condition
   3. Teeth that prevent adequate reduction of the fracture
   4. Teeth with fractured roots
   5. Teeth with exposed root apices

   Nonrestorable teeth and bony impactions should be retained if this assists in reduction. For example, extraction of bony impactions can result in removal of excessive amounts of bone that may compromise both the fracture site and the potential placement points for plate or screw fixation.

THE CHAMPY SYSTEM

6. An 18-year-old male is admitted after a fall onto his chin during a vasovagal attack. Examination and imaging confirm the presence of an isolated symphyseal fracture. *Which one of the following statements is correct regarding the Champy system?*
   C. Two miniplates will be required to stabilize the fracture.
   The Champy system was first described by Michelet et al[1] in 1973 and later validated by Champy et al[2] in 1978. It advocates the use of monocortical (not bicortical) miniplates and is based on the concept that only tensile stresses are harmful to fracture healing, as these tend to open up the fracture line. Compressive forces, however, tend to pull the fracture lines together and can be used to help fracture reduction and stabilization. The system involves placement of miniplates to counteract the tensile or opening forces and utilize the compressive forces. Anterior to the first premolar, two miniplates are required, one above the other, as there are multidirectional forces acting across this site. Fractures posterior to the first premolar normally only require single plate fixation. The standard approach to ORIF of a symphyseal fracture is intraoral (not submental) within the lower lip sulcus. Care should be taken to ensure that the incision is placed away from the attached gingiva to ensure there is sufficient nonadherent mucosa to facilitate tension-free soft tissue closure. Temporary arch bars are usually only required where there are two concomitant fractures such as a symphyseal, condyle, or angle.

MANAGEMENT OF MANDIBULAR FRACTURES

7. *For the management of patients with mandibular fractures, which one of the following is correct?*
   D. Principles of reduction, fixation, and early mobilization should be followed.
   Prophylactic antibiotic use in mandibular fractures has been proved to significantly reduce the incidence of postoperative infection. However, antibiotics only need to be prescribed until definitive fixation. Further antibiotic use does not affect infection rates, nor does the use of oral chlorhexidine, even though it can reduce bacterial counts. Not all fractures will require surgical fixation; for example, some condylar fractures may be managed conservatively with a soft diet and physical rehabilitation exercises. There is usually no urgency to stabilize mandibular fractures if antibiotics and analgesics are being given. The AO has comprehensive guidance on its website that includes approaches and fixation placement that can be a useful reference.[3]

8. A 25-year-old male is admitted following an alleged assault. Examination confirms tenderness and swelling over the left TMJ. The mouth opening is reduced but occlusion is preserved. Radiographs show a unilateral extraarticular fracture of the left condyle. *How should this injury be managed?*
   E. Soft diet and close observation
   Fractures of the condyle require early active ROM to rehabilitate TMJ articulation. In fractures such as this, where occlusion is maintained, soft diet and close observation represent the best treatment. If malocclusion subsequently develops, then arch bars or MMF should be placed and occlusion controlled with elastics. ORIF is indicated for some condylar fractures, such as bilateral cases or cases where there is significant displacement of the fracture and where occlusion cannot be established. Access to the TMJ and condyle are commonly through a preauricular approach and this can be difficult and risks damage to the facial nerve.

COMPLICATION RATES IN MANDIBULAR FRACTURES

9. Which site is associated with the highest complication rate in mandibular fractures?

A. Angle

The angle has the highest complication rate of any single region of the mandible. These fractures can also be difficult to reduce and stabilize accurately. Approaches include transbuccal, intraoral, and MMF.

REFERENCES

1. Michelet FX, Deymes J, Dessus B. Osteosynthesis with miniaturized screwed plates in maxillo-facial surgery. J Maxillofac Surg 1:79-84, 1973.
2. Champy M, Lodde JP, Schmitt R, et al. Mandibular osteosynthesis by miniature screwed plates via a buccal approach. J Maxillofac Surg 6:14-21, 1978.
3. Available at *www.aofoundation.org*.

32. Basic Oral Surgery

See *Essentials of Plastic Surgery*, second edition, pp. 358-370.

CRANIAL NERVE FORAMINA

1. For each part of the trigeminal nerve, identify the correct exit foramen from the skull. (Each answer may be used once, more than once, or not at all.)
   A. Ophthalmic division (V_1)
   B. Maxillary division (V_2)
   C. Mandibular division (V_3)

   Options:
   a. Hypoglossal foramen
   b. Jugular foramen
   c. Foramen rotundum
   d. Foramen spinosum
   e. Internal acoustic meatus
   f. Superior orbital fissure
   g. Optic foramen
   h. Foramen ovale

2. For each of the cranial nerves listed, identify the correct exit foramen from the skull. (Each answer may be used once, more than once, or not at all.)
   A. Optic nerve (CN II)
   B. Oculomotor nerve (CN III)
   C. Glossopharyngeal nerve (CN IX)

   Options:
   a. Jugular foramen
   b. Styloid foramen
   c. Hypoglossal foramen
   d. Foramen spinosum
   e. Internal acoustic meatus
   f. Superior orbital fissure
   g. Optic foramen
   h. Infraorbital foramen

CRANIAL NERVE RELATIONS

3. Which one of the following statements is correct regarding cranial nerve anatomy?
   A. The ophthalmic branch of the trigeminal nerve and the oculomotor nerve are the only nerves to pass through the superior orbital fissure.
   B. The glossopharyngeal nerve exits the skull through the jugular foramen with the hypoglossal nerve.
   C. The vestibulocochlear nerve is the only nerve to pass through the internal acoustic meatus.
   D. The accessory and vagus nerves both exit the skull through the jugular foramen.
   E. The olfactory and optic nerves share the same foramen as they exit the skull.

PRIMARY AND SECONDARY DENTITION

4. Match each of the following descriptions to the most appropriate choice. (Each option may be used once, more than once, or not at all.)
   A. The total number of teeth in primary dentition
   B. The total number of teeth in secondary dentition
   C. The reference number for the adult upper left incisor

   Options:
   a. 1
   b. 7
   c. 9
   d. 11
   e. 20
   f. 22
   g. 24
   h. 28
   i. 32

ERUPTION SEQUENCE FOR SECONDARY DENTITION

5. A 6-year-old child is seen in clinic following eruption of their first adult teeth, which are first molars. **Which tooth type would be most likely to erupt next?**
   A. Canine
   B. Incisor
   C. First molar
   D. Second premolar
   E. Second molar

DENTAL TERMINOLOGY

6. When using oral surgery terminology to describe a patient's dentition, what does the term **distal** *refer to?*
   A. Away from the cheek
   B. Towards the feet
   C. Towards the midline
   D. Away from the tongue
   E. Away from the midline

MALOCCLUSION

7. A patient is referred to the aesthetic clinic concerned about her lack of chin projection. On examination you note that the patient has excessive overjet with normal angulation of the incisors. **What type of occlusion does this likely represent?**
   A. Class I
   B. Class II
   C. Class III
   D. Class IV
   E. Normal occlusion

SENSORY NERVE BLOCKS

8. For each of the following descriptions, select the correct nerve block administered using the options listed. (Each option may be used once, more than once, or not at all.)
   A. This block may be given intraorally or extraorally and produces anesthesia of the upper lip, medial cheek, lower eyelid, nose, and buccal gingiva.
   B. This block is given intraorally to the anterior surface of the mandibular ramus, 1 cm above the occlusal plane, and produces anesthesia of the entire mandibular hemidentition and buccal mucosa anterior to the second premolar.
   C. This block is given intraorally in the midline approximately 5 mm behind the upper incisors and produces anesthesia of the palatal mucosa from canine to canine.

   Options:
   a. Infraorbital
   b. Greater palatine
   c. Inferior alveolar
   d. Lingual
   e. Buccal
   f. Mental
   g. Nasopalatine

ODONTOGENIC INFECTIONS

9. A patient presents to the emergency department with a 24-hour history of facial swelling, trismus, and severe pain to the dentition. You suspect the symptoms are caused by an odontogenic infection. **Which one of the following is correct in this case?**
   A. The infection is most likely caused by a single organism.
   B. The infection is most likely to be periodontal in origin.
   C. The likely organism will be anaerobic bacteria.
   D. The symptoms are consistent with a parapharyngeal space infection.
   E. Antibiotics are the mainstay of treatment in this case.

SOFT TISSUE CEPHALOMETRIC LANDMARKS

10. **Which one of the following soft tissue cephalometric points refers to the most anterior soft tissue point on the chin?**
    A. Pogonion
    B. Stomion superioris
    C. Menton
    D. Gnathion
    E. Labrale

BONY CEPHALOMETRIC LANDMARKS

11. When reviewing a bony cephalogram, **which one of the following is used as a guide to the external auditory meatus?**
    A. Sella turcica
    B. Porion
    C. Articulare
    D. Gonion
    E. Nasion

ARCH BARS

12. A patient has a dentoalveolar fracture which is unstable and displaced. ***Which one of the following is correct when using arch bars in this scenario?***
A. They should normally be placed from the first molar to the first molar.
B. The wires should normally be twisted anticlockwise to tighten.
C. The first wires are usually placed posteriorly then progressively placed towards the midline.
D. 5-gauge wires are normally used to secure the bar to the dentition.
E. Each wire should be fully tightened as it is placed.

CORRECTION OF BONY DEFORMITY

13. A young adult patient who had previous Pierre Robin sequence as an infant presents with class II malocclusion and is concerned with regard to their lack of chin prominence. ***Which one of the following procedures may be most helpful in this scenario?***
A. LeFort I osteotomy
B. LeFort II osteotomy
C. LeFort III osteotomy
D. Bilateral sagittal split osteotomies
E Intraoral vertical ramus osteotomies

Answers

CRANIAL NERVE FORAMINA

1. For each part of the trigeminal nerve, the correct exit foramina are as follows:
   A. **Ophthalmic division (V_1)**
      f. **Superior orbital fissure**
   B. **Maxillary division (V_2)**
      c. **Foramen rotundum**
   C. **Mandibular division (V_3)**
      h. **Foramen ovale**

   The trigeminal nerve has three divisions: ophthalmic, maxillary, and mandibular. The ophthalmic and maxillary divisions are purely sensory, while the mandibular division is both motor and sensory. The ophthalmic division exits the cranial vault through the superior orbital fissure. It supplies sensation to the upper third of the face including the forehead, scalp, upper eyelid, nose conjunctiva, and cornea. The maxillary division exits the cranial vault through the foramen rotundum and supplies sensation to the lower eyelids, cheek, and upper dentition. The mandibular division exits the cranium through the foramen ovale and supplies sensation to the lower lip, chin, jaw, and lower dentition. It also supplies the muscles of mastication including the temporalis, masseter, and pterygoids (see Table 32-1, *Essentials of Plastic Surgery,* second edition).

2. For each of the cranial nerves listed, the correct exit foramina are as follows:
   A. **Optic nerve (CN II)**
      g. **Optic foramen**
   B. **Oculomotor nerve (CN III)**
      f. **Superior orbital fissure**
   C. **Glossopharyngeal nerve (CN IX)**
      a. **Jugular foramen**

   The optic nerve supplies specialized sensation to the retina with information regarding brightness, contrast, and color. It exits the cranium through the optic foramen. The oculomotor nerve supplies motor function to the extraocular muscles: superior rectus, inferior rectus, medial rectus, inferior oblique, and the ciliary and sphincter muscles. It exits the cranium through the superior orbital fissure and can be compromised in conditions such as superior orbital fissure syndrome, leading to ptosis, proptosis, opthalmoplegia, paresthesia, and a dilated pupil (see Chapter 30). The glossopharyngeal nerve supplies sensation to the oropharynx and motor supply to the pharynx. It exits the cranium through the jugular foramen (see Table 32-1, *Essentials of Plastic Surgery,* second edition).

CRANIAL NERVE RELATIONS

3. Which one of the following statements is correct regarding cranial nerve anatomy?
   D. **The accessory and vagus nerves both exit the skull through the jugular foramen.**

   The accessory, vagus, and glossopharyngeal nerves all pass through the jugular foramen along with the sigmoid sinus, which becomes the internal jugular vein, but the hypoglossal nerve passes through the hypoglossal canal. The trochlear and abducens nerves also pass through the superior orbital fissure, in addition to V_1 and the oculomotor nerve. The vestibulocochlear nerve leaves the posterior cranial fossa with the facial nerve through the internal auditory canal. The olfactory nerve passes through the cribriform plate, and the optic nerve passes through the optic foramen.

PRIMARY AND SECONDARY DENTITION

4. For the following descriptions, the best choices are as follows:
   A. The total number of teeth in primary dentition
      e. 20
   B. The total number of teeth in secondary dentition
      i. 32
   C. The reference number for the adult upper left incisor
      c. 9

   The number of teeth present differs between primary and secondary dentition. The normal primary dentition includes the central and lateral incisors, the canines, and the first and second molars. This gives a total of 20 teeth (10 per arch). The secondary dentition includes the first and second premolars and third molars. This gives a total of 32 teeth (16 per arch).
   There are different ways to number the teeth. The method described in *Essentials of Plastic Surgery,* second edition, numbers the adult teeth from the right upper third molar to the left upper third molar then continues from the left lower third molar through to the third right lower molar. So the left first upper incisor is the ninth tooth from the upper right. An alternative method uses four quadrants: right upper, left upper, right lower, left lower, numbered one to eight beginning at the midline.[1,2] In this case the left upper incisor would be LU1 (Figs. 32-1 and 32-2).

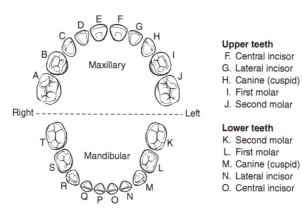

Upper teeth
F. Central incisor
G. Lateral incisor
H. Canine (cuspid)
I. First molar
J. Second molar

Lower teeth
K. Second molar
L. First molar
M. Canine (cuspid)
N. Lateral incisor
O. Central incisor

Fig. 32-1 Primary (pediatric) dentition.

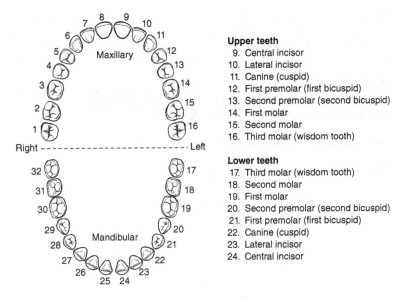

Fig. 32-2 Secondary (adult) dentition.

ERUPTION SEQUENCE FOR SECONDARY DENTITION

5. A 6-year-old child is seen in clinic following eruption of their first adult teeth, which are first molars. **Which tooth type would be most likely to erupt next?**
   B. Incisor
   The adult eruption sequence is commonly first molars, central incisors, lateral incisors, first premolars, canines, second then third molars. This can be remembered as an eight digit code: 612 453 78. Where each quadrant is labeled from one to eight, commencing with the central incisor.

DENTAL TERMINOLOGY

6. When using oral surgery terminology to describe a patient's dentition, what does the term **distal** refer to?
   E. Away from the midline
   In dental terminology *distal* means *away from the midline* and *mesial* means *towards the midline*. The term *buccal* means *towards the cheek* and *lingual* means *towards the tongue*. These terms can sometimes be confusing. For example, when describing teeth, the terms *distal* and *mesial* are applied to the dental arches, and as the arches are followed from the molars to the incisors, the teeth are becoming progressively more *mesial*. In more traditional anatomy we might describe this relationship as the incisors being more anterior and also more medial to the molars (Fig. 32-3).

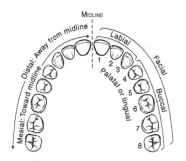

Fig. 32-3 Dental relationships.

MALOCCLUSION

7. A patient is referred to the aesthetic clinic concerned about her lack of chin projection. On examination you note that the patient has excessive overjet with normal angulation of the incisors. ***What type of occlusion does this likely represent?***
B. Class II

Occlusion refers to the relationship of the teeth to one another. Normal occlusion is based on the relationship of the upper and lower first permanent molars. It was described by Edward Angle who identified that in normal occlusion the mesiobuccal cusp of the maxillary first molar interfaces with the buccal groove of the mandibular first molar. Malocclusion is where this relationship is altered in some way and is split into three subtypes: class I, II, and III. The descriptions of the three classes of malocclusion are:

Class I: The mesiobuccal cusp of the first maxillary molar occludes in the buccal groove of the mandibular molar but the teeth are malpositioned or malrotated.
Class II: The mandibular molar is distally positioned relative to the maxillary molar.
Class III: The mandibular molar is mesially positioned relative to the maxillary molar.

In general terms, patients with small or retruded mandibles have a class II occlusion and patients with prognathism have class III occlusion. The patient described in this scenario has class II malocclusion which can either be subdivided as division I or division II depending on the angulation of the incisors and the degree of overjet and overbite. Overjet refers to the amount of horizontal overlap of the incisal edges, while overbite refers to the amount of vertical overlap.

SENSORY NERVE BLOCKS

8. For the following descriptions, the best options are as follows:
   A. This block may be given intraorally or extraorally and produces anesthesia of the upper lip, medial cheek, lower eyelid, nose, and buccal gingiva.
      a. Infraorbital
   B. This block is given intraorally to the anterior surface of the mandibular ramus, 1 cm above the occlusal plane, and produces anesthesia of the entire mandibular hemidentition and buccal mucosa anterior to the second premolar.
      c. Inferior alveolar
   C. This block is given intraorally in the midline approximately 5 mm behind the upper incisors and produces anesthesia of the palatal mucosa from canine to canine.
      g. Nasopalatine

   Local anesthetic blocks are very useful when performing intraoral surgery. Typically a dental syringe is used, which gives good control for the injection and provides adequate reach for areas deeper in the oral cavity such as the posterior dentition. Lidocaine 2% is commonly used within small vials (2.2 ml each) that are combined with epinephrine 1:80,000. This concentration differs from the 1:200,000 dilution typically used and has the theoretical advantage of reducing bleeding while working in this highly vascular area.

   Local anesthetic blocks are not only useful for procedures where patients are fully conscious, but are also useful combined with general anesthesia as they can reduce the requirements for anesthetic agents and systemic pain relief requirements such as opiates. They can also help reduce bleeding as discussed above, and help with dissection of soft tissues. Knowledge of the main local anesthetic blocks, such as those described, is therefore useful in clinical practice.

   The Infraorbital block is particularly useful when performing surgery on the nose under local anesthesia because injection at this site can reduce pain on subsequent external nasal injections. The inferior alveolar block is mainly used for dental procedures of the lower dentition, while the nasopalatine block is usually used for dental procedures of the upper dentition or in orthognathic surgery. The greater palatine block is injected into the hard palate at the level of upper second molar to block the upper dentition and palate. The lingual block is performed during an inferior alveolar nerve block by withdrawing the needle 5 mm and depositing local anesthetic in this region. It provides a block to the entire lingual musculature and half of the tongue. A mental nerve block is also part of the inferior alveolar nerve block, but can be given as an isolated block in the lower buccal sulcus at the level of the second premolar. It provides anesthesia of the buccal mucosa and gingiva anterior to the first premolar. A buccal block is performed at the mandibular ramus after withdrawing and confirming no aspiration of blood. It provides anesthesia of the buccal mucosa and gingiva anterior to the first premolar.

Chapter 32 ■ Basic Oral Surgery   259

ODONTOGENIC INFECTIONS

9. A patient presents to the emergency department with a 24-hour history of facial swelling, trismus, and severe pain to the dentition. You suspect the symptoms are caused by an odontogenic infection. **Which one of the following is correct in this case?**
   D. The symptoms are consistent with a parapharyngeal space infection.
   When examining a patient with a suspected odontogenic infection, trismus may be the only indication of a parapharyngeal space abscess. Examination must include a thorough review of the oropharynx. Odontogenic infections can range from localized conditions to severe life-threatening infections. Almost all are polymicrobial and are not limited to anaerobic organisms alone. In more than half of cases, infections will be a mixed aerobic/anaerobic combination. Odontogenic infections arise from two major sources: periapical and periodontal, of which the former is most common. Although antibiotics are a component of treatment, the main management is drainage of the abscess and this is undertaken by a dentally trained professional.

SOFT TISSUE CEPHALOMETRIC LANDMARKS

10. **Which one of the following soft tissue cephalometric points refers to the most anterior soft tissue point on the chin?**
    A. Pogonion
    The most anterior soft tissue point on the chin is the soft tissue pogonion. The *menton* refers to the lowest point on the contour of the soft tissue chin, while the *gnathion* refers to the midpoint between the pogonion and menton. The *stomion superioris* refers to the lowest point of the lower lip vermilion and the *labrale* refers to the mucocutaneous border of the lip in the midsaggital plane. (See Fig. 32-9 and Box 32-1, *Essentials of Plastic Surgery,* second edition.)

BONY CEPHALOMETRIC LANDMARKS

11. **When reviewing a bony cephalogram, which one of the following is used as a guide to the external auditory meatus?**
    B. Porion
    Bony cephalometric landmarks may be useful for analysis of the facial and cranial skeleton with reference to orthodontics and mandibular/maxillary deformity. The *porion* is the most superior point of the external auditory meatus. The *sella turcica* represents the center of the pituitary fossa. The *articulare* represents the junction of the basisphenoid and the posterior part of the mandibular condyle. The *gonion* is the point at the angle of the mandible that is directed most inferiorly and posteriorly. The *nasion* is the most anterior point at the junction of the nasal and frontal bones in the midsaggital plan. (See Fig. 32-9 and Box 32-2, *Essentials of Plastic Surgery,* second edition.)

ARCH BARS

12. A patient has a dentoalveolar fracture which is unstable and displaced. **Which one of the following is correct when using arch bars in this scenario?**
    A. They should normally be placed from first molar to first molar.
    Arch bars may be used to stabilize dentoalveolar fractures. They provide a stable base from which to institute maxillomandibular fixation and control occlusion in the posttraumatic period. When using arch bars they are usually placed from first molar to first molar and applied starting in the

midline to prevent redundancy within the arch bar. Twenty-five-gauge wires (not 5-gauge) are used and are conventionally twisted clockwise to tighten. Proper occlusion and fracture reduction must be established before complete tightening of all wires within the quadrant of the fracture to prevent malreduction. This is facilitated by tightening the wires in the fracture segment after reducing the fracture. For this reason, complete tightening of each individual wire as it is placed is not performed.

CORRECTION OF BONY DEFORMITY

13. A young adult patient who had previous Pierre Robin sequence as an infant presents with class II malocclusion and is concerned with regard to their lack of chin prominence. *Which one of the following procedures may be most helpful in this scenario?*

D. Bilateral sagittal split osteotomies

Orthognathic surgery involves correction of the components of the facial skeleton to restore proper functional and aesthetic relationships such as occlusion and normal facial appearance. The *bilateral sagittal split osteotomy* (BSSO) is a useful and commonly used orthognathic technique for the correction of dentofacial abnormalities such as in patients with mandibular deficiency who had Pierre Robin sequence as an infant. It can also be used to treat mandibular excess. BSSO is achieved through an intraoral approach with an incision made through the mucosa overlying the anterior border of the mandibular ramus. Extensive soft tissue dissection is performed at a subperiosteal level to adequately expose the angle, ramus, and body for the osteotomy and release the soft tissues adequately to allow mandibular advancement (or set-back). Osteotomies are performed such that key neurovascular structures and dental roots are preserved. Once freed, the mandible can be advanced or set back as required and stabilized in place using plates and screws.[3]

A LeFort I osteotomy is typically performed to correct maxillary excess or maxillary deficiency. This also involves an intraoral approach with a mucosal incision made in the upper buccal sulcus from first molar to first molar. An osteotomy is made to separate the tooth-bearing maxilla from the midface. This will extend from the piriform aperture through the anterior maxilla and posteriorly to the pterygoid plates. Again, preservation of key neurovascular structures and dental roots as well as the nasal mucosa must be ensured. Once adequate soft tissue and bone release have been achieved the desired position of the maxilla can be achieved and fixation is performed with mini plates and screws.[4] LeFort II and III osteotomies are not routinely used to correct mandibular or maxillary deficiencies. Intraoral vertical ramus osteotomies may be used to correct mandibular excess in some cases.

REFERENCES

1. Tooth numbering system. Available at *www.drbunn.com/faq/tooth-numbering*.
2. Tooth eruption: the permanent teeth. Available at *www.ada.org/sections/scienceAndResearch/pdfs/patient_58. pdf*.
3. Monson L. Bilateral sagittal split osteotomy. Semin Plast Surg 27:145–148, 2013.
4. Buchanan EP, Hyman CH. LeFort I osteotomy. Semin Plast Surg 27:149–154, 2013.

Acquired Deformities

33. Principles of Head and Neck Cancer: Staging and Management

See *Essentials of Plastic Surgery*, second edition, pp. 371-381.

INCIDENCE/ETIOLOGIC FACTORS

1. **What is the most common tumor type in head and neck cancers?**
   A. Adenoid cystic
   B. Squamous cell
   C. Adenocarcinoma
   D. Lymphoma
   E. Melanoma

EXAMINATION/WORKUP

2. A 50-year-old male smoker presents with a 4-week history of a 3 cm diameter left-sided neck mass without any other obvious signs or symptoms. **After the initial history and examination, what would the next most appropriate investigation be?**
   A. Excision biopsy of the mass
   B. Incision biopsy to the tongue base
   C. CT scan of the head, neck, and chest
   D. Panendoscopy to view the pharynx, larynx, esophagus, and bronchial tree
   E. Fine-needle aspiration cytology of the mass in the clinic

LEVELS OF THE NECK

3. **When undertaking a selective neck dissection (I through III), which one of the following represents the inferior limit of the dissection?**
   A. Carotid bifurcation
   B. Clavicle
   C. Omohyoid
   D. Posterior belly of digastric
   E. Hyoid bone

4. You are undertaking a neck dissection for a patient with a floor-of-mouth SCC. Your professor has asked you to include level IIa within the dissection but says that IIb can be preserved. **Which structure will subdivide these two areas?**
   A. Hypoglossal nerve
   B. Marginal mandibular nerve
   C. Phrenic nerve
   D. Spinal accessory nerve
   E. Vagus nerve

TUMOR STAGING WITH THE AJCC CLASSIFICATION

5. *For each of the following tumor descriptions, select the correct staging using the current AJCC system. (Each option may be used once, more than once, or not at all.)*
   A. A tumor of the lip measuring 2.3 cm in diameter, with multiple positive ipsilateral nodes 3 cm in diameter, but no evidence of metastatic spread to distant organs.
   B. A tumor of the nasopharynx that involves the skull base, a single ipsilateral node 2 cm in diameter, and no obvious metastases.
   C. An oropharyngeal tumor invading the larynx and tongue base, with a single 6 cm node in level II and lung metastases.

   Options:
   a. T1N1M0
   b. T1N0M1
   c. T2N2aM0
   d. T2N2bM0
   e. T3N2M0
   f. T3N1M0
   g. T4aN2aM1
   h. T3N2bM0

6. *For each of the following tumor descriptions, select the correct staging using the current AJCC system. (Each option may be used once, more than once, or not at all.)*
   A. A supraglottic tumor of the larynx limited to one subsite of the supraglottis with normal vocal cord mobility, no palpable neck disease, and no metastases.
   B. A subglottic laryngeal tumor with vocal cord fixation, multiple positive ipsilateral positive nodes less than 6 cm in diameter, and no evidence of metastasis.
   C. A squamous cell carcinoma of the lateral tongue 2 cm in diameter with radiologic changes evident in the mandibular alveolus. No palpable lymphadenopathy or metastatic disease is evident.

   Options:
   a. T1N0M1
   b. T1M0N0
   c. T2N2aM0
   d. T2N2bM0
   e. T3N2bM0
   f. T3N1M0
   g. T4aN3M1
   h. T4aN0M0
   i. T3N2cM0

7. For each of the following clinical scenarios involving the parotid gland, select the most likely T stage. (Each option may be used once, more than once, or not at all.)
   A. A patient presents with a parotid gland swelling that is invading the skin and mandible but not the facial nerve.
   B. A patient presents with a 2 cm tumor of the parotid that does not have any extraparenchymal spread.
   C. A patient presents with a parotid tumor invading the skull base and pterygoid plate. It also encases the carotid sheath.

Options:
a. T1
b. T2
c. T2a
d. T3
e. T4
f. T4a
g. T4b

TREATMENT OF THE NECK

8. Correctly match each of the following descriptions of neck dissection techniques. (Each option may be used once, more than once, or not at all.)
   A. Sometimes called a Bocca neck dissection, this procedure preserves all nonlymphatic structures but removes levels I through V.
   B. This dissection removes levels I through V and the sternocleidomastoid muscle, internal jugular vein, and spinal accessory nerve.
   C. In this procedure not all levels are taken, and some nonlymphatic structures may be preserved.

Options:
a. Radical neck dissection
b. Modified radical neck dissection type I
c. Functional neck dissection
d. Extended neck dissection
e. Comprehensive neck dissection
f. Modified radical neck dissection type II
g. Selective neck dissection

9. Which one of the following statements is true when considering salivary gland tumors?
   A. Most salivary gland tumors can be managed nonsurgically.
   B. Half of all salivary gland tumors involve the parotid gland.
   C. Parotid gland pathology must be excluded in all preauricular masses.
   D. Minor salivary gland tumors are more likely to be benign than malignant.
   E. More than 90% of solid salivary gland tumors in children are benign.

10. A child is seen in clinic with confirmed salivary gland tumor. **Which one of the following statements is correct regarding salivary gland masses in children?**
    A. Most salivary gland masses are of vascular origin.
    B. Fewer than 10% of solid tumors are malignant.
    C. Lymphangiomas normally involute without treatment.
    D. Pleomorphic adenomas are rare in children. Tumors are most commonly pleomorphic adenomas.
    E. Most malignant tumor subtypes are adenoid cystic.

11. **Which one of the following statements is correct regarding pleomorphic adenomas?**
    A. They represent half of all benign parotid tumors in adults.
    B. They commonly present with facial paralysis and a palpable swelling.
    C. They have low rates of recurrence, even when incompletely excised.
    D. When adenomas recur, they tend to reappear as nodular tumor implants within extraglandular tissue.
    E. The responses to radiotherapy are consistently good.

12. A patient is referred with a diagnosis of a low-grade malignant tumor. **Which one of the following tumor subtypes is most likely to be a low-grade malignancy?**
    A. Adenoid cystic carcinoma
    B. Squamous cell carcinoma
    C. Adenocarcinoma
    D. Undifferentiated
    E. Acinic cell carcinoma

SALIVARY TUMORS

13. For each of the following clinical scenarios, select the most likely diagnosis. (Each option may be used once, more than once, or not at all.)
    A. An 80-year-old man presents with small bilateral nontender swellings at the angle of the mandible.
    B. A 35-year-old woman presents with a slowly enlarging painless swelling of the right preauricular region. She has normal facial nerve function.
    C. A 48-year-old woman presents with a 1 cm firm tumor involving the hard palate; there is no cervical lymphadenopathy. The tumor is surgically excised and sent for histologic analysis. The pathology report describes a cribriform tumor with a swiss-cheese appearance.

    Options:
    a. Adenoid cystic carcinoma
    b. Papillary cystadenoma lymphomatosum (Warthin's tumor)
    c. Sebaceous adenoma
    d. Oncocytoma
    e. Mucoepidermoid carcinoma
    f. Carcinoma ex-pleomorphic adenoma
    g. Acinic cell tumor
    h. Pleomorphic adenoma

14. A patient is undergoing laryngectomy for a T4 tumor. **What is the benefit of performing intraoperative cricophryngeal myotomy?**
    A. Improve surgical margins
    B. Improve swallowing
    C. To reduce surgical time
    D. To avoid a tracheostomy
    E. To improve airway patency

Answers

INCIDENCE/ETIOLOGIC FACTORS

1. *What is the most common tumor type in head and neck cancers?*
   B. Squamous cell
   The most common tumor subtype in head and neck cancer is the squamous cell carcinoma. This represents more than 90% of all head and neck cancers. Head and neck malignancies are increasingly common and represent around 7% of all cancers in the US. They represent around 4% of all US cancer deaths. Squamous cell carcinomas may originate from the skin or mucosal surfaces of the upper aerodigestive tract. Other common tumor types include adenocarcinoma, adenoid cystic, and mucoepidermoid.

EXAMINATION/WORKUP

2. A 50-year-old male smoker presents with a 4-week history of a 3 cm diameter left-sided neck mass without any other obvious signs or symptoms. *After the initial history and examination, what would the next most appropriate investigation be?*
   E. Fine-needle aspiration cytology of the mass in the clinic
   In this case the initial step would be to undertake fine-needle aspiration cytology to provide information on the nature of the mass. The subsequent steps would include baseline blood tests, panendoscopy, and a CT scan of the head, neck, chest, and abdomen. If malignancy is proven on the cytology sample, it would be appropriate to consider an ipsilateral tonsillectomy, biopsies to the base of tongue and nasopharynx, or excision biopsy if the malignancy is lymphoma. This case would then require multidisciplinary team discussion. PET is also a useful tool for evaluation of an unknown primary tumor as it highlights tissues displaying an increased metabolic rate.

LEVELS OF THE NECK

3. *When undertaking a selective neck dissection (I through III), which one of the following represents the inferior limit of the dissection?*
   C. Omohyoid
   There are seven levels used to describe the neck with reference to head and neck oncology. Primary tumors tend to metastasize in a predictable manner to specific areas of the neck. For example, floor of mouth and tongue tumors tend to spread to levels I through III, while laryngeal tumors tend to spread to levels II through IV. This means that treatment of neck disease can be targeted to specific levels. The levels of the neck are separated by key anatomical structures. The omohyoid is highly relevant to neck dissection as it crosses the lower part of the neck. It marks the junction between levels III and IV and is often included within the dissection specimen when undertaking a I through III dissection. As it passes into level V, it also subdivides this region into Va and Vb.

   The carotid bifurcation is the surgical landmark for the junction of levels II and III. The clavicle is the inferior border for both levels IV and V. The hyoid is an important landmark for many levels. It represents a boundary for levels I, II, III, and VI.

4. You are undertaking a neck dissection for a patient with a floor-of-mouth SCC. Your professor has asked you to include level IIa within the dissection but says that IIb can be preserved. **Which structure will subdivide these two areas?**
   D. **Spinal accessory nerve**

   The boundaries of level II are the sternohyoid, the sternocleidomastoid, the skull base, and the carotid bifurcation. The accessory nerve is a key structure to locate when undertaking a level II neck dissection. It can be identified in levels II, III, and V. In level II it is identified by elevating the anterior border of the sternocleidomastoid, until it is seen passing obliquely into the muscle belly. Once identified, it is traced cranially to the posterior belly of digastric which marks the superior extent of a standard dissection. The area below the nerve represents level IIa and the level above the nerve represents level IIb. It is also seen during level V dissection after passing through SCM. Again it should be preserved here, otherwise it will result in weakness of the trapezius leading to shoulder discomfort and instability.

TUMOR STAGING WITH THE AJCC CLASSIFICATION

5. *For each of the following descriptions, the best options are as follows (see Fig. 33-2, Essentials of Plastic Surgery, second edition):*
   A. *A tumor of the lip measuring 2.3 cm in diameter, with multiple positive ipsilateral nodes 3 cm in diameter, but no evidence of metastatic spread to distant organs*
      d. **T2N2bM0**
   B. *A tumor of the nasopharynx that involves the skull base, a single ipsilateral node 2 cm in diameter, and no obvious metastases*
      f. **T3N1M0**
   C. *An oropharyngeal tumor invading the larynx and tongue base with a single 6 cm node in level II, and lung metastases*
      g. **T4aN2aM1**

   The TNM classification is well known for many different tumor sites and types. The T stands for tumor size, the N stands for nodal disease, and the M stands for metastatic disease. The T grading will differ according to the site in question, although the general principles remain consistent. For example, a lip tumor T1 is less than 2 cm diameter. Whereas a nasopharyngeal T1 tumor is confined to the nasopharynx but no specific dimension is recorded. Tumors of the larynx are T1 if they are limited to one subsite. The full description for each tumor type is shown in Box 33-1.

Box 33-1 *Tumor Staging: AJCC 7th Edition, 2010*[1]

- **T: Extent of primary tumor**
  - **Lip and oral cavity**
    - Tx: No available information on primary tumor
    - T0: No evidence of primary tumor
    - Tis: Carcinoma in situ
    - T1: Greatest diameter of primary tumor ≤2 cm
    - T2: Greatest diameter of primary tumor >2 cm but ≤4 cm
    - T3: Greatest diameter of primary tumor >4 cm
    - T4a: Moderately advanced local disease:
      - Lip: Invades through cortical bone, inferior alveolar nerve, floor of mouth, skin of face
      - Oral cavity: Invades adjacent structures only (cortical bone of mandible/maxilla, deep extrinsic muscles of tongue—genioglossus, hyoglossus, palatoglossus, styloglossus—maxillary sinus, skin of face)
    - T4b: Very advanced local disease that invades masticator space, pterygoid plates, skull base; encases internal carotid artery

- **Nasopharynx**
  - T1: Tumor confined to nasopharynx
  - T2: Parapharyngeal extension
  - T3: Involves skull base or paranasal sinuses
  - T4: Intracranial extension, involves cranial nerves, hypopharynx, orbit, infratemporal fossa/masticator space.
- **Oropharynx**
  - T1: Greatest diameter of tumor <2 cm
  - T2: Tumor 2-4 cm in greatest dimension
  - T3: Tumor >4 cm in greatest diameter or extension to lingual epiglottis
  - T4a: Moderately advanced local disease:
    - Tumor invades larynx, tongue, medial pterygoid, hard palate, mandible
  - T4b: Very advanced local disease:
    - Invades lateral pterygoid, pterygoid plates, lateral nasopharynx, skull base; encases internal carotid artery
- **Larynx**
  - Supraglottis:
    - T1: Tumor limited to one subsite of supraglottis with normal vocal cord mobility
    - T2: Invades more than one adjacent subsite without fixation of larynx
    - T3: Limited to larynx with vocal cord fixation and/or invades postcricoid space, preepiglottic space, paraglottic space, inner cortex of thyroid cartilage
    - T4a: Invades through thyroid cartilage and/or tissues beyond larynx
    - T4b: Invades prevertebral space; encases internal carotid artery, mediastinal structures
  - Glottis:
    - T1a: Tumor limited to one vocal cord with normal mobility
    - T1b: Tumor involves both true vocal cords with normal mobility
    - T2: Extends to supraglottis or subglottis and/or impairs vocal cord mobility
    - T3: Limited to larynx with vocal cord fixation, invasion of paraglottic space, inner cortex of thyroid cartilage
    - T4a: Invades through outer cortex of thyroid cartilage and/or tissues beyond larynx
    - T4b: Invades prevertebral space; encases carotid artery, mediastinal structures
  - Subglottis:
    - T1: Limited to subglottis
    - T2: Extends to vocal cords
    - T3: Limited to larynx with vocal cord fixation
    - T4a: Invades cricoid or thyroid cartilage or tissues beyond larynx
    - T4b: Invades prevertebral space, mediastinal structures; encases carotid artery
  - Major salivary glands:
    - T1: Tumor ≤2 cm in greatest dimension without extraparenchymal extension
    - T2: Tumor 2-4 cm without extraparenchymal extension
    - T3: Tumor >4 cm and/or extraparenchymal extension
    - T4a: Moderately advanced disease that invades skin, mandible, ear canal, or facial nerve
    - T4b: Very advanced disease that invades skull base, pterygoid plates, or encases internal carotid artery

Continued

Box 33-1 *TUMOR STAGING: AJCC 7TH EDITION, 2010[1] — CONT'D*

- N: Regional lymph nodes[1,2]
  - Single greatest influence on survival is presence of nodal metastasis.
  - Nodal staging system is generally the same for upper aerodigestive tumors (except nasopharynx) (Fig. 33-1).
    - Nx: Nodes cannot be assessed
    - N0: No nodes containing metastasis
    - N1: A single ipsilateral node metastasis, ≤3 cm in diameter
    - N2a: A single ipsilateral positive node 3-6 cm in diameter
    - N2b: Multiple positive ipsilateral nodes <6 cm in diameter
    - N2c: Bilateral or contralateral positive nodes <6 cm in diameter
    - N3: Nodes >6 cm in diameter

NOTE: Older designations such as fixed nodes and matted nodes are no longer used.

- M: Distant metastasis
  - M0: No distant metastasis
  - M1: Distant metastasis

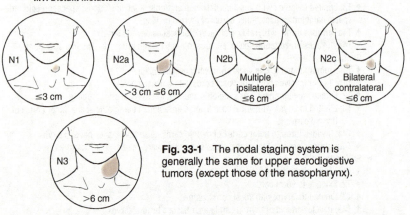

Fig. 33-1 The nodal staging system is generally the same for upper aerodigestive tumors (except those of the nasopharynx).

6. *For each of the following descriptions, the best options are as follows:*
   A. *A supraglottic tumor of the larynx limited to one subsite of the supraglottis with normal vocal cord mobility, no palpable neck disease, and no metastases.*
      b. T1N0M0
   B. *A subglottic laryngeal tumor with vocal cord fixation, multiple positive ipsilateral positive nodes less than 6 cm in diameter, and no evidence of metastasis.*
      e. T3N2bM0
   C. *A squamous cell carcinoma of the lateral tongue, 2 cm in diameter, with radiologic changes evident in the mandibular alveolus. No palpable lymphadenopathy or metastatic disease is evident.*
      h. T4aN0M0

The classification for laryngeal tumors is based initially on their relation to the glottis. They can therefore be supraglottic, glottis, or subglottic tumors. For example, a supraglottic T1 tumor would be confined to one subsite of the supraglottis with normal vocal cords. A T1 glottic tumor involves the vocal cords with normal cord mobility. Subglottic T1 tumors are limited to the subglottic region (see Fig. 33-1, *Essentials of Plastic Surgery,* second edition).

7. *For the following scenarios, the most likely T stages are as follows:*
   A. *A patient presents with a parotid gland swelling that is invading the skin and mandible but not the facial nerve.*
      f. **T4a**
   B. *A patient presents with a 2 cm tumor of the parotid that does not have any extraparenchymal spread.*
      b. **T2**
   C. *A patient presents with a parotid tumor invading the skull base and pterygoid plate. It also encases the carotid sheath.*
      g. **T4b**

      As with other head and neck TNM classifications, those for the salivary gland are different. The AJCC staging of parotid tumors is as follows[3]:
      T1: Less than 2 cm without extraparenchymal extension
      T2: 2-4 cm and without extraparenchymal extension
      T3: Greater than 4 cm and/or having extraparenchymal extension
      T4: Greater than 6 cm or extension into extraglandular tissues
      T4a: Invades the skin, mandible, ear canal, or facial nerve
      T4b: Invades the skull base and/or pterygoid plates and/or encases the carotid artery

TREATMENT OF THE NECK

8. *For the following descriptions, the best options are as follows:*
   A. *Sometimes called a Bocca neck dissection, this procedure preserves all nonlymphatic structures but removes levels I through V.*
      c. **Functional neck dissection**
   B. *This dissection removes levels I through V and the sternocleidomastoid muscle, internal jugular vein, and spinal accessory nerve.*
      a. **Radical neck dissection**
   C. *In this procedure not all levels are taken and some nonlymphatic structures may be preserved.*
      g. **Selective neck dissection**

      Neck dissections are commonly classified as selective or comprehensive. Comprehensive dissections involve resection of lymph node basins I through V. They include radical, modified radical, functional, and extended neck dissections. Modified radical nodal dissections (MRND) include three subtypes:
      MRND I (preserves the spinal accessory nerve)
      MRND II (preserves spinal accessory nerve and internal jugular vein)
      MRND III (preserves spinal accessory nerve, internal jugular vein, and sternocleidomastoid)
      A functional (Bocca) dissection is also called a *modified radical neck dissection type III*. Selective neck dissections involve clearing some but not all of the lymphatic neck levels, and selection is according to the nature and site of the primary tumor.

9. **Which one of the following statements is true when considering salivary gland tumors?**
   C. Parotid gland pathology must be excluded in all preauricular masses.
   All preauricular masses are considered to be of parotid origin unless proven otherwise and should be thoroughly investigated. Most salivary gland tumors require surgical intervention. The most commonly involved gland is the parotid where 80% of all salivary gland tumors (benign and malignant) are located. The submandibular glands represent 10% to 15% of all salivary gland tumors. The sublingual or minor salivary glands constitute the remaining 5% to 10%. The ratio of benign to malignant salivary tumor type is related to gland size with a higher incidence of malignancy in smaller glands. Around half of all solid salivary gland tumors in children are malignant.

10. **Which one of the following statements is correct regarding salivary gland neoplasms in children?**
    A. Most salivary gland masses are of vascular origin.
    Most salivary gland masses in children are vascular and hemangiomas represent the most common overall tumor type in children. Pleomorphic adenomas are the most common solid subtype in children, but are not the most common overall. Half of all solid salivary gland tumors are malignant and the most common subtype is mucoepidermoid, not adenoid cystic. Lymphangiomas present within the first year of life rarely involute. They are treated with surgery or sclerosing agents such as OK 432.

11. **Which one of the following statements is correct regarding pleomorphic adenomas?**
    D. When adenomas recur, they tend to reappear as nodular tumor implants within extraglandular tissue.
    Pleomorphic adenomas are the most common benign tumor of the parotid, representing 70% (not 55%) of all tumors. It is rare to have facial nerve involvement except in recurrent tumors, and most present as asymptomatic painless masses. Treatment involves surgical excision with parotidectomy. These tumors are radioresistant and tend to recur if surgical excision is incomplete. For this reason enucleation is not recommended.

12. A patient is referred with a diagnosis of a low-grade malignant tumor. **Which one of the following tumor subtypes is most likely to be a low-grade malignancy?**
    E. Acinic cell carcinoma
    Acinic cell carcinomas are low-grade tumors. In fact, they were previously considered to be benign tumors because of their behavioral characteristics of slow growth and a high degree of differentiation. The prognosis for acinic cell carcinomas is probably the best of all malignant salivary tumors. High-grade tumors include:
    High-grade mucoepidermoid
    Adenoid cystic carcinoma
    Squamous cell carcinoma
    Adenocarcinoma
    Carcinoma ex-pleomorphic adenoma

SALIVARY TUMORS

13. For the following clinical scenarios, the best diagnoses are as follows:
    A. An 80-year-old man presents with small bilateral nontender swellings at the angle of the mandible.
       b. Papillary cystadenoma lymphomatosum (Warthin's tumor)
    B. A 35-year-old woman presents with a slowly enlarging painless swelling of the right preauricular region. She has normal facial nerve function.
       h. Pleomorphic adenoma
    C. A 48-year-old woman presents with a 1 cm firm tumor involving the hard palate; there is no cervical lymphadenopathy. The tumor is surgically excised and sent for histological analysis. The pathology report describes a cribriform tumor with a swiss-cheese appearance.
       a. Adenoid cystic carcinoma

14. A patient is undergoing laryngectomy for a T4 tumor. *What is the benefit of performing intraoperative cricophryngeal myotomy?*
    B. Improve swallowing
    The main purpose of performing a cricopharyngeal myotomy at the time of laryngectomy is to improve postoperative swallow. A secondary benefit may be observed with respect to speech when an implantable speech valve. It has no benefit on airway patency or surgical margins. The technique involves surgical sectioning of the cricopharyngeus muscle which normally acts as a sphincter to the upper esophagus from the distal pharynx. If left intact it can inhibit free flow of saliva and secretions into the upper esophagus postlaryngectomy or total pharyngolaryngectomy and reconstruction.

REFERENCES

1. Edge SB, Byrd DR, Compton CC, et al, eds. American Joint Committee on Cancer Staging Handbook, ed 7. New York: Springer, 2010.
2. Candela FC, Shah J, Jacques DP, et al. Patterns of cervical node metastases from squamous carcinoma of the larynx. Arch Otolargyngol Head Neck Surg 116:432-435, 1990.
3. Salivary gland cancer. Available at *http://www.cancer.gov/cancertopics/pdq/treatment/salivarygland/HealthProfessional/page1.*

34. Scalp and Calvarial Reconstruction

See *Essentials of Plastic Surgery*, second edition, pp. 382-391.

APPLIED ANATOMY

1. **Which component of the scalp provides most strength during layered repair?**
   A. Epidermis
   B. Dermis
   C. Aponeurotic layer
   D. Subgaleal fascia
   E. Pericranium

2. **Which one of the following statements is correct regarding the blood supply to the scalp?**
   A. The anterior scalp is supplied by the supraorbital and supratrochlear vessels from the external carotid artery.
   B. The supratrochlear vessels are lateral to the supraorbital vessels.
   C. The posterior territory is the largest area and is supplied by the occipital vessels.
   D. The lesser occipital artery supplies the posterolateral scalp.
   E. The lateral territory is supplied by the superficial temporal artery, which arises from the external carotid artery.

3. **Which one of the following statements is correct regarding scalp innervation?**
   A. The supraorbital nerve has both superficial and deep divisions.
   B. The zygomaticofacial nerve is a branch of the ophthalmic division of trigeminal nerve.
   C. The auriculotemporal nerve supplies the posterior and lateral scalp.
   D. The lesser occipital nerve emerges from the semispinalis muscle, 3 cm below the occipital protuberance.
   E. The muscles of the scalp are supplied by the facial and trigeminal nerves.

SKIN BIOMECHANICS

4. **Which one of the following specifically requires the application of a constant force intraoperatively in order to assist in closure of a tight scalp wound?**
   A. Tissue creep
   B. Stress relaxation
   C. Galeal scoring
   D. Undermining
   E. Tissue expansion

GUIDELINES FOR RECONSTRUCTION

5. **Which one of the following statements is correct regarding the use of Orticochea flaps to reconstruct a scalp defect?**
   A. They are based entirely on the superficial temporal vessels.
   B. They are useful for reconstructing large parietal defects.
   C. Their classical description was for reconstruction of the frontal scalp.
   D. Commonly, they involve elevation of three local pericranial flaps.
   E. Modification of this technique to include more flaps can improve flap vascularity and reduce alopecia.

6. **Which one of the following statements is correct regarding parietal defects?**
   A. They are commonly reconstructed using flaps based on the terminal branch of the external carotid artery.
   B. They are less likely to involve bone exposure, compared with vertex defects.
   C. They are at low risk of displacement of the sideburn and distortion of the hair pattern.
   D. They are challenging to reconstruct given the limited scalp mobility.
   E. They frequently require importation of distant tissue for closure.

7. **In which scenario might the pinwheel flap be particularly useful to reconstruct a small scalp defect in a patient with a full head of hair?**
   A. A circular defect on the vertex
   B. A longitudinal defect on the occiput
   C. A triangular defect on the parietal area
   D. A rectangular defect on the forehead
   E. An elliptical defect on the temple

CALVARIAL RECONSTRUCTION

8. **When harvesting split calvarial bone for calvarial reconstruction, which anatomic area is normally preferred?**
   A. Occipital
   B. Frontal
   C. Parietal
   D. Temporal
   E. No specific region is preferred

CLINICAL SCENARIOS IN SCALP RECONSTRUCTION

9. An 85-year-old woman has a 1.5 by 2 cm defect on her anterior scalp with exposed bone after excision of a basal cell carcinoma. The defect is within the hair-bearing skin. **Which one of the following is the best reconstructive option for this patient?**
   A. Leave to heal by secondary intention
   B. Direct layered closure with undermining
   C. Burring of the outer table and full-thickness skin graft
   D. Integra and a split-thickness skin graft
   E. A posteriorly based scalp rotation flap

10. A 4-year-old patient with a full head of hair requires reconstruction of a congenital nevus to the vertex of the scalp. The lesion covers 30% of the scalp. **Which one of the following is the best reconstructive option?**
    A. Serial excision and direct closure
    B. Tissue expansion and local flap reconstruction
    C. Transposition flap and skin graft to the donor site
    D. Orticochea flaps with galeal scoring
    E. Free tissue muscle transfer and split-skin graft

11. *For each of the following cases, select the most appropriate reconstruction modality. (Each option may be used once, more than once, or not at all.)*
    A. *A 75-year-old man requires reconstruction of a full-thickness calvarial defect after necrosis of a craniotomy measuring 7 by 7 cm.*
    B. *A 20-year-old patient has a near-total scalp defect after excision of an angiosarcoma. Some of the outer table has been removed (4 by 4 cm surface area), but the inner table is intact. The patient is otherwise fit and well.*
    C. *A frail, elderly bald man had a 3 cm squamous cell carcinoma excised from the vertex of his scalp. The pericranium is involved.*

    Options:
    a. Full-thickness skin graft
    b. Transposition flap and skin graft to the donor site
    c. Orticochea flap
    d. Tissue expansion and local flap reconstruction
    e. Free tissue transfer with latissimus dorsi and a split-thickness skin graft ± titanium plate
    f. Titanium mesh, methylmethacrylate, and scalp transposition flap with a skin graft to the donor site
    g. Split calvarial graft and a scalp rotation flap
    h. Direct, layered closure with undermining

Chapter 34 ▪ Scalp and Calvarial Reconstruction   275

Answers

APPLIED ANATOMY

1. **Which component of the scalp provides most strength during layered repair?**
   C. Aponeurotic layer

   The scalp comprises five layers, each of which can be remembered using the mnemonic *SCALP*: **S**kin, sub**C**utaneous tissue, **A**poneurotic layer, **L**oose areolar tissue, **P**ericranium.

   The aponeurotic layer is also known as the galea and connects the frontalis and occipitalis muscles. It is also contiguous with the SMAS of the face and neck. It should be approximated during closure of scalp wounds as it provides deep support to the repair.

   The terms *subgaleal fascia* and *innominate fascia* are used interchangeably with the term *loose areolar layer* which provides scalp mobility rather than strength. It is at this layer that most injuries are sustained and it is described as the *scalping plane*. Skin thickness varies from 3 to 8 mm according to anatomic location on the scalp and provides additional strength to the repair. The pericranium is the deepest layer and is tightly adherent to the calvarium. It tends to be thin and can easily tear. Therefore approximation does not add to the strength of a scalp repair.

   Skin comprises the dermis and the epidermis. Overall thickness varies from 3 to 8 mm according to anatomic location on the scalp, and placement of sutures or clips through the skin provides additional strength to the repair and reapproximates the wound edges, but does not represent the most strength.

2. **Which one of the following statements is correct regarding the blood supply to the scalp?**
   E. The lateral territory is supplied by the superficial temporal artery, which arises from the external carotid artery.

   The scalp derives its blood supply from both the internal and external carotid systems. It is divided into four zones: anterior, posterior, lateral, and posterolateral. Each zone has its own blood supply, with collateralization between zones. This is clinically relevant with respect to scalp reconstruction using local flaps.

   The anterior scalp is supplied by the supraorbital and supratrochlear vessels. These derive from the internal carotid vessels (not the external carotid vessels). The supratrochlear vessels lie medial (not lateral) to the supraorbital vessels. The posterior territory is supplied by the occipital vessels and perforators from the splenius capitis and trapezius, but it is not the largest territory. The largest is the lateral territory, which is supplied by the superficial temporal arteries. A lesser occipital artery does not exist. The greater and lesser occipital nerves supply sensation to the occipital territory. The posterolateral scalp is the smallest territory and is supplied by the posterior auricular artery.

3. **Which one of the following statements is correct regarding scalp innervation?**
   A. The supraorbital nerve has both superficial and deep divisions.

   The supraorbital nerve has superficial and deep divisions. The superficial component supplies sensation to the forehead anterior to the hairline. The deep component supplies sensation posterior to the hairline. This has clinical relevance in brow-lift procedures, bicoronal cranial flaps, and trauma in which the nerves may be damaged, leaving an area of paresthesia. The zygomaticofacial nerve derives from the maxillary division (not the ophthalmic division) of the trigeminal nerve. It supplies a region of skin lateral to the brow. The auriculotemporal nerve derives from the mandibular division of the trigeminal nerve and supplies the lateral scalp. The greater and lesser occipital nerves supply the occipital territory, but it is the greater occipital nerve that emerges from the semispinalis 3 cm below the occipital protuberance. The facial nerve supplies the scalp muscles. The trigeminal nerve supplies the muscles of mastication and the tensor tympani.

SKIN BIOMECHANICS

4. **Which one of the following specifically requires the application of a constant force intraoperatively in order to assist in closure of a tight scalp wound?**
   A. **Tissue creep**

   The biomechanics of the skin and different viscoelastic properties of the scalp layers can be used to assist in closure of scalp defects. Tissue creep and stress relaxation are terms used to describe the viscoelastic properties of skin that enable on-table closure of tight wounds and also apply to tissue expansion techniques. The two terms are often confused but have different meanings. Stress relaxation occurs when a force is applied to the skin that causes it to stretch to a given length. After a short amount of time, the load required to achieve the desired length or stretch reduces. In contrast, creep occurs when the force applied remains constant and this causes a continued stretch over time. Skin can be placed under tension intraoperatively by either placing temporary sutures or using skin hooks to partially close the wound.

   The skin has more stretch or elasticity than the underlying galea. Therefore multiple perpendicular incisions or scores to the undersurface of the galea can significantly increase the amount of stretch within this layer. Simple undermining can also be helpful to close some defects because this allows redistribution of the available skin.[1]

GUIDELINES FOR RECONSTRUCTION

5. **Which one of the following statements is correct regarding the use of Orticochea flaps to reconstruct a scalp defect?**
   D. **Commonly, they involve elevation of three local pericranial flaps.**

   The Orticochea technique uses either three or four subgaleal flaps to reconstruct large scalp defects. The three-flap technique comprises two lateral flaps based on the superficial temporal vessels, combined with a posterior flap based on the occipital vessels. This technique can improve flap vascularity and reduce alopecia, compared with the four-flap technique. Orticochea flaps were classically described for occipital defects and are not suitable for vertex or lateral defects.

6. **Which one of the following statements is correct regarding parietal defects?**
   B. **They are less likely to involve bone exposure, compared with vertex defects.**

   The parietal scalp has a high degree of mobility, which facilitates closure with direct suturing or local flap reconstruction. Bone exposure is less common, because the temporalis muscle and fascia provide an additional layer of soft tissue cover anteriorly. Local flaps are at risk of changing the orientation of hair and affecting the hairline or sideburn. The parietal scalp is supplied by the superficial temporal artery, the terminal branch of the external carotid artery. The superficial temporal artery is unlikely to be the vascular supply to flaps used in reconstruction of this area, because it is likely to have been sacrificed already. Because of the excellent mobility of local tissues, distant tissue use is limited.

Chapter 34 ▪ Scalp and Calvarial Reconstruction

7. In which scenario might the pinwheel flap be particularly useful to reconstruct a small scalp defect in a patient with a full head of hair?
   A. A circular defect on the vertex
   The pinwheel flap is a type of local flap that uses three or four advancing triangular flaps which are arranged around a circular defect (see Fig. 34-8, *Essentials of Plastic Surgery*, second edition). It may be particularly useful in small defects less than 2 cm^2 on the vertex to recreate a whorl pattern at the patient's crown while disguising the remaining scars within the hair. It can be used in other sites on the scalp including nonhair-bearing areas, but is probably less useful as the long flap limbs result in more noticeable scars.

CALVARIAL RECONSTRUCTION

8. When harvesting split calvarial bone for calvarial reconstruction, which anatomic area is normally preferred?
   C. Parietal
   Split calvarial bone graft is useful for reconstructing bony defects of the scalp as it has the same contour and can be harvested from the same operative site. Grafts are either taken full-thickness then split, or harvested at the level of the diploic space. The parietal region is the preferred donor site for calvarial bone harvest because it is thickest and minimizes risk of damage to dura or dural venous sinuses. Most split calvarial grafts are nonvascularized, and have a good take; however, it is possible to harvest a vascularized graft. This is based on the superficial temporal vessels by maintaining attachment to the superficial temporal fascia and pericranium.[2]

CLINICAL SCENARIOS IN SCALP RECONSTRUCTION

9. An 85-year-old woman has a 1.5 by 2 cm defect on her anterior scalp with exposed bone after excision of a basal cell carcinoma. The defect is within the hair-bearing skin. *Which one of the following is the best reconstructive option for this patient?*
   B. Direct layered closure with undermining
   Small defects of the anterior scalp can often be closed directly with undermining of surrounding tissues. This avoids the need for a skin graft which will leave a bald patch and a contour defect at the surgical site. A scalp rotation flap is usually preserved for larger defects following triangulation of the defect (see Fig. 4-11, *Essentials of Plastic Surgery*, second edition). Small defects can be left to heal by secondary intention, but are best for nonhair-bearing regions of the scalp such as the forehead when there is a deep layer of vascularized tissue covering bone. Integra can be a useful adjunct when reconstructing scalp defects, as it adds tissue depth, but in this situation it would not provide any benefit.

10. A 4-year-old patient with a full head of hair requires reconstruction of a congenital nevus to the vertex of the scalp. The lesion covers 30% of the scalp. *Which one of the following is the best reconstructive option?*
   B. Tissue expansion and local flap reconstruction
   The primary aim in this case is to fully remove the nevus and provide soft tissue cover while retaining a full head of hair. Two approaches to the management of congenital nevi on the scalp are serial excision or excision and tissue expansion. Serial excision is best suited to smaller defects that can be excised within three or four sessions. A defect of 30% is best treated with tissue expansion and local flap closure. Defects up to 50% of the hair-bearing scalp can be closed

with tissue expansion and avoid bald patches. A transposition flap and skin graft would create a large bald area and would not be aesthetically pleasing. Free tissue transfer would be reserved for near-total scalp defects, particularly where bone is exposed. The Orticochea flap is not well suited to vertex defects because the location does not allow a large third flap to cover the donor defect.

11. *For the following scenarios, the best options are as follows:*
    A. *A 75-year-old man requires reconstruction of a full-thickness calvarial defect after necrosis of a craniotomy measuring 7 by 7 cm.*
       f. **Titanium mesh, methylmethacrylate, and scalp transposition flap with skin graft to the donor site**
          This patient could have a free-tissue transfer as suggested in answer option E, but given the size of the soft tissue defect it is not necessary and a more simple local flap approach is probably a better option for him.
    B. *A 20-year-old patient has a near-total scalp defect after excision of an angiosarcoma. Some of the outer table has been removed (4 by 4 cm surface area), but the inner table is intact. The patient is otherwise fit and well.*
       e. **Free tissue transfer with latissimus dorsi and a split-thickness skin graft skin graft ± titanium plate**
    C. *A frail, elderly bald male has a 3 cm squamous cell carcinoma excised from the vertex of his scalp. The pericranium is involved.*
       b. **Transposition flap and skin graft to the donor site**
          Several algorithms have been developed for scalp reconstruction. However, as with most reconstructions, the selection requires common sense and is based on each patient's needs. The goals are to reconstruct like with like tissue and to minimize deformity and alopecia. It is not always necessary to reconstruct the calvarium, provided that soft tissue cover is adequate.

REFERENCES

1. Jackson IT. Local Flaps in Head and Neck Reconstruction, ed 2. St Louis: Quality Medical Publishing, 2007.
2. Freund RM. Scalp, calvarium and forehead reconstruction. In Aston SJ, Beasley RW, Thorne CH, eds. Grabb and Smith's Plastic Surgery. Philadelphia: Lippincott Williams & Wilkins, 1997.

35. Eyelid Reconstruction

See *Essentials of Plastic Surgery*, second edition, pp. 392-402.

EYELID ANATOMY

1. *Which one of the following statements is correct?*
   A. The outer lamella consists of skin only.
   B. The middle lamella consists of orbital septum and capsulopalpebral fascia.
   C. The inner lamella includes the medial and lateral canthal tendons.
   D. Eyelid skin is usually thicker than postauricular skin.
   E. Hypertrophic scarring is often seen after surgery to the eyelid.

2. *Which one of the following statements is correct regarding eyelid anatomy?*
   A. The tarsal plate of the upper lid is slightly shorter in height than that of the lower lid.
   B. The tarsus is located at the orbital rim.
   C. The inferior margin of the upper lid tarsus is the attachment for Müller's muscle and the levator aponeurosis.
   D. The tarsus is connected to the orbital rim by the orbital septum.
   E. The palpebral portion of the conjunctiva lines the sclera.

ORBICULARIS OCULI MUSCLE

3. *Which one of the following statements is correct?*
   A. This muscle has two components: orbital and pretarsal.
   B. This muscle is innervated by CN III.
   C. Pretarsal fibers are solely responsible for involuntary blinking.
   D. Orbital fibers overlie the bony rim and provide forceful voluntary contraction.
   E. Innervation is via the superficial surface of the muscle.

EYELID RETRACTORS

4. *Which one of the following statements is correct regarding elevation of the upper eyelid?*
   A. Müller's muscle is innervated by CN III.
   B. Loss of Müller's muscle function typically results in 5 to 6 mm of upper lid ptosis.
   C. The levator palpebrae superioris originates from the greater wing of the sphenoid.
   D. Müller's muscle arises from the superior surface of the levator palpebrae superioris and inserts onto the superior edge of the tarsal plate.
   E. Whitnall's ligament redirects the vector of the levator palpebrae superioris to provide superior lid retraction.

BLOOD SUPPLY TO THE EYELIDS

5. **Which one of the following statements is correct regarding the vascular anatomy of the eyelid?**
   A. The upper lids are primarily supplied by branches of the facial artery.
   B. Contributions are made from the internal and external carotid arteries.
   C. The lower lids are primarily supplied by branches of the ophthalmic artery.
   D. The angular artery is a continuation of the zygomaticofacial artery.
   E. Only the marginal arcades provide blood supply to the eyelids.

GENERAL PRINCIPLES OF EYELID RECONSTRUCTION

6. **Which one of the following statements is correct regarding reconstruction of eyelid defects?**
   A. Only defects of less than 20% can be closed directly.
   B. Defects greater than 75% can often be closed with canthotomy and cantholysis alone.
   C. Defects of 50% to 75% can usually be closed using myocutaneous advancement flaps.
   D. Selection of reconstructive technique is based on whether the defect is partial-thickness or full-thickness only.
   E. The lower lid is best reconstructed using the upper lid as a donor site.

EYELID RECONSTRUCTION

7. **Which one of the following statements is correct regarding reconstruction of the eyelid?**
   A. The contralateral upper lid should not be used as a full-thickness skin graft donor site for upper lid reconstruction.
   B. Conjunctival losses are best replaced with advancement of adjacent conjunctiva.
   C. Buccal mucosal grafts are preferred over nasal mucosal grafts for conjunctival reconstruction because of their reduced rate of contraction.
   D. Skin grafts to the conjunctiva are a reasonable alternative to a mucosal graft.
   E. The only option for tarsal reconstruction is to use palatal mucosal grafts.

FULL-THICKNESS TISSUE LOSS OF THE EYELIDS

8. **Which one of the following statements is correct?**
   A. Primary closure of small (less than 25%) defects can be satisfactorily achieved with a triangular-shaped excision.
   B. A Tenzel semicircular flap combines lateral canthotomy and cantholysis with a medially based skin flap.
   C. A single-stage Cutler-Beard flap is useful for replacing tarsal plate and conjunctiva.
   D. A Fricke flap is a type of advancement flap that is useful for lower eyelid reconstruction.
   E. A paramedian forehead flap can be used for upper lid reconstruction if it is combined with a mucosal graft.

RECONSTRUCTIVE OPTIONS

9. *For each of the following clinical scenarios, select the best option for reconstruction. (Each option may be used once, more than once, or not at all.)*
   A. A patient has a partial-thickness defect of the lower eyelid (50% width) with an intact conjunctiva and tarsal plate.
   B. A patient has a full-thickness defect of the upper eyelid (25% width).
   C. A patient has a full-thickness defect of the lower lid (60% width).

   Options:
   a. Split-thickness skin graft from the scalp
   b. Full-thickness skin graft from the groin
   c. Full-thickness skin graft from the upper eyelid
   d. Direct closure
   e. Direct closure with canthopexy
   f. Direct closure with cantholysis
   g. Tenzel semicircular flap with a lateral cantholysis and canthopexy
   h. Cutler-Beard flap

Answers

EYELID ANATOMY
1. *Which one of the following statements is correct?*
   C. The inner lamella includes the medial and lateral canthal tendons.
   The eyelid can be considered to have an outer and an inner lamella. Sometimes a further middle layer is considered. The inner layer consists of the tarsal plate, medial and lateral canthal tendons, capsulopalpebral fascia, and conjunctiva. The outer lamella consists of skin and orbicularis oculi. The middle layer is a term sometimes used to describe the orbital septum only. The eyelid skin is the thinnest on the body (300 to 800 μ). Postauricular skin is around 800 μ thick. Hypertrophic scarring is seen typically in burns, sites of delayed healing, or undue tension on wounds. In contrast, surgery to the eyelids usually results in very high-quality scars.

2. *Which one of the following statements is correct regarding eyelid anatomy?*
   D. The tarsus is connected to the orbital rim by the orbital septum.
   The tarsal plate of the upper lid has a greater vertical height (12 to 15 mm) than that of the lower lid (4 to 10 mm). The tarsus is separated from the orbital rim by the orbital septum. The superior margin of the upper lid tarsus is the attachment for Müller's muscle and the levator aponeurosis. The bulbar portion of the conjunctiva lines the sclera, and the palpebral portion lines the inner surface of the eyelids.

ORBICULARIS OCULI MUSCLE
3. *Which one of the following statements is correct?*
   D. Orbital fibers overlie the bony rim and provide forceful voluntary contraction.
   The orbicularis oculi acts as a sphincter and has three components: orbital, pretarsal, and preseptal. Orbital fibers are responsible for voluntary closure of the eye, and pretarsal fibers are responsible for involuntary blinking, assisted by preseptal fibers. The orbicularis oculi receives innervation from the facial nerve (CN VII) via its deep surface, as do most of the facial mimetic muscles. Only three of them are innervated via their superficial surfaces: the buccinator, levator anguli oris, and mentalis.

EYELID RETRACTORS
4. *Which one of the following statements is correct regarding elevation of the upper eyelid?*
   E. Whitnall's ligament redirects the vector of the levator palpebrae superioris to provide superior lid retraction.
   Müller's muscle is innervated by the sympathetic nervous system, which is carried along with the ophthalmic nerve through the cavernous sinus. The fibers originate from the superior cervical ganglion. The muscle arises from the inferior (not superior) surface of the levator palpebrae superioris and inserts into the superior edge of the tarsal plate. Loss of Müller's muscle function results in 2 to 3 mm of ptosis. The levator palpebrae superioris arises from the lesser wing of the sphenoid (not the greater wing) and inserts into the superior edge of the tarsal plate. It receives its innervation from CN III.

BLOOD SUPPLY TO THE EYELIDS

5. Which one of the following statements is correct regarding the vascular anatomy of the eyelid?

B. Contributions are made from the internal and external carotid arteries.

Blood supply contributions to the eyelid include the following:

Facial artery: This vessel forms the angular, lateral nasal, and inferior medial palpebral arteries.

Transverse facial artery: This vessel forms the zygomaticofacial and inferior palpebral arteries.

Superficial temporal artery: This vessel forms the superior medial palpebral artery (peripheral arcade).

Ophthalmic artery: This vessel forms the lacrimal, supraorbital, medial palpebral, and dorsal nasal vessels.

The upper lids are primarily supplied by branches of the ophthalmic artery (the first branch of the internal carotid). The lower lids are mainly supplied by branches of the facial artery (a branch of the external carotid). The angular artery is a continuation of the facial artery as it passes lateral to the nose. (This later becomes the lateral nasal artery, which anastomoses with the dorsal nasal artery from the ophthalmic artery.) Both marginal and peripheral arcades supply the eyelids (see Fig. 35-4, *Essentials of Plastic Surgery,* second edition).

GENERAL PRINCIPLES OF EYELID RECONSTRUCTION

6. Which one of the following statements is correct regarding reconstruction of eyelid defects?

C. Defects of 50% to 75% can usually be closed using myocutaneous advancement flaps.

Defects of up to 30% can be usually be closed directly, but this depends on individual patient factors such as lid laxity, tissue quality, and age. Defects larger than 75% typically require importation of tissue from the opposite lid or adjacent regions such as the cheek, forehead, or temple. Selection of a reconstruction technique requires knowledge of the defect size and the tissue layers involved. Techniques that borrow tissue from the upper lid should be performed with caution, because this structure contributes significantly to eyelid function.

EYELID RECONSTRUCTION

7. Which one of the following statements is correct regarding reconstruction of the eyelid?

B. Conjunctival losses are best replaced with advancement of adjacent conjunctiva.

Full-thickness skin grafts from the contralateral upper eyelid ensure good thickness and color match. Buccal and nasal mucosal grafts are options for reconstruction of the conjunctiva, but nasal grafts tend to contract less than buccal mucosal grafts (20% versus 50%, respectively). Skin grafts are contraindicated, because they irritate the cornea. Several options exist for reconstruction of the tarsal plate. These include palatal mucosa grafts, autologous cartilage, and allografts such as AlloDerm.

FULL-THICKNESS TISSUE LOSS OF THE EYELIDS

8. Which one of the following statements is correct?

E. A paramedian forehead flap can be used for upper lid reconstruction if it is combined with a mucosal graft.

Defects of less than a third should be closed directly with a shield-shaped excision. A Tenzel semicircular flap is laterally based. A Cutler-Beard is a two-stage flap used for total upper lid reconstruction. It involves advancement of a full-thickness lower lid flap that is passed under the lower lid margin and sutured into the defect. Division is usually performed at 3 to 6 weeks. A Fricke flap is a type of transposition (not advancement) flap that is also known as a *temporal forehead flap.*

RECONSTRUCTIVE OPTIONS

9. *For the following clinical scenarios, the best options are as follows:*
   A. *A patient has a partial-thickness defect of the lower eyelid (50% width) with an intact conjunctiva and tarsal plate.*
      c. **Full-thickness skin graft from the upper eyelid**
         The general principles for eyelid reconstruction follow the principles common to most reconstructions: analyze the defect site and tissue structures involved, then reconstruct, replacing like with like where possible. The selection of a technique for eyelid reconstruction will therefore depend on the site; e.g., upper versus lower eyelid, and the width, height and depth of the defect. Partial-thickness defects (anterior lamella) can be reconstructed with a full-thickness skin graft, providing there is a well-vascularized bed such as orbicularis oculi. This is the case in scenario 1. A full-thickness graft is preferable to a split-thickness graft because there will be less secondary contraction which can risk development of ectropion. Many patients, particularly the elderly, will have an excess of upper eyelid skin and this can make a good graft donor site, as the skin is thin and a good color match for the contralateral eyelid.
   B. *A patient has a full-thickness defect of the upper eyelid (25% width).*
      d. **Direct closure**
         Full-thickness defects of up to 30% of the eyelid width can often be closed directly; defects from 30% to 50% can usually be closed directly with a lateral canthotomy and cantholysis. Defects of 50% to 70% eyelid width can often be closed with myocutaneous flaps, while defects larger than this require importation of tissue from the cheek or forehead. The patient in this scenario has a relatively small defect and even though it is full-thickness, according to these principles, this can be reconstructed with direct closure. Where such a defect is planned surgically, a shield excision is recommended. A canthopexy or cantholysis would not be required.
   C. *A patient has a full-thickness defect of the lower lid (60% width).*
      g. **Tenzel semicircular flap with a lateral cantholysis and canthopexy**
         The patient in this scenario has a defect that is too large to be reconstructed with direct closure, even where a canthotomy and cantholysis are performed. This defect can be reconstructed using a myocutaneous flap such as the Tenzel flap which was described in question 8. This is a semicircular rotation flap that can be used for either upper or lower lid reconstruction. It involves rotation and advancement of skin and soft tissue lateral to the eye in order to reconstruct the defect. When combined with canthotomy and canthoplasty, defects of up to 60% can be reconstructed. (See Fig. 35-12, *Essentials of Plastic Surgery,* second edition.) A Cutler-Beard flap is used for upper lid reconstruction and was also described in question 8. It involves advancement of a full-thickness lower lid flap that is passed under the lower lid margin and sutured into the defect. Division is usually performed at 3 to 6 weeks.

36. Nasal Reconstruction

See *Essentials of Plastic Surgery*, second edition, pp. 403-419.

BLOOD SUPPLY
1. **Which blood vessel is the main supply to the nasal sill and septum?**
   A. Angular artery
   B. Lateral nasal artery
   C. Maxillary artery
   D. Superior labial artery
   E. Ophthalmic artery

SENSORY INNERVATION
2. **Which one of the following is supplied by the maxillary division of the trigeminal nerve?**
   A. Radix
   B. Rhinion
   C. Cephalic portion of the nasal sidewalls
   D. Dorsal skin to the tip
   E. Columella

LINING RECONSTRUCTION
3. **Which one of the following statements is correct regarding reconstruction of a nasal lining defect?**
   A. Folding of an extranasal flap is only possible with staged forehead flap techniques.
   B. The septal door flap described by de Quervain involves removal of septal mucosa from the contralateral side to the defect.
   C. Skin grafts applied to the posterior surface of flaps are associated with high failure rates and stricture formation.
   D. Septal mucoperichondrial flaps involve harvesting a rectangle of mucosa with the underlying perichondrium from the ipsilateral septum.
   E. The mucosal advancement flap described by Burget and Menick involves an unipedicled advancement flap with a medial blood supply.

TECHNIQUES FOR PROVISION OF NASAL SKELETAL SUPPORT

4. *For each of the following descriptions, select the most appropriate technique. (Each option may be used once, more than once, or not at all.)*
   A. A longitudinal piece of bone or cartilage is seated on the nasal radix and extends along the dorsum to the tip, where it is bent sharply to rest on the anterior nasal spine.
   B. A longitudinal piece of bone is secured at a single point to either the frontal or nasal bone or both and extends along the dorsum of the nose.
   C. This composite flap provides nasal lining and dorsal skeleton support and is based on a branch of the superior labial artery.

   Options:
   a. Hinged septal flap
   b. Rieger dorsal nasal flap
   c. Gillies strut technique
   d. Cantilever graft
   e. Gull-winged flap
   f. Axial frontonasal flap
   g. Septal pivot flap

TECHNIQUES FOR PROVISION OF ALAR SUPPORT

5. *For each of the following descriptions, select the most appropriate technique. (Each option may be used once, more than once, or not at all.)*
   A. In this technique cartilage is placed via an infracartilaginous approach into an alar vestibular pocket inferior and lateral to the rim of the crus.
   B. In this technique a bar or triangular-shaped cartilage graft is placed to push the lateral crura apart.
   C. In this technique a cartilage graft is placed between the deep surface of the lateral crus and the vestibular skin and is sutured to the crus.

   Options:
   a. Alar batten graft
   b. Alar spreader graft
   c. Lateral crural turnover graft
   d. Alar contour graft
   e. Composite alar rim graft
   f. Lateral crural strut graft

SKELETAL AND CARTILAGINOUS SUPPORT

6. A 37-year-old woman presents with a pinched-tip deformity of her nose and difficulty breathing at night. On examination she has a bilateral positive Cottle's test. **Which one of the following techniques is most likely to address both of her symptoms?**
   A. Alar batten graft
   B. Lateral crural strut graft
   C. Alar spreader graft
   D. Alar contour graft
   E. Cantilever graft

RECONSTRUCTION OF SKIN AND SOFT TISSUE

7. Which one of the following flaps used in nasal reconstruction can be based on the supratrochlear vessels?
   A. Washio/Temporomastoid flap
   B. Frontotemporal flap
   C. Rieger dorsal nasal flap
   D. Forehead flap
   E. Converse scalping flap

8. **For each of the following scenarios, select the most appropriate reconstruction. (Each option may be used once, more than once, or not at all.)**
   A. A 56-year-old woman is referred by the local Mohs surgeon after excision of an infiltrative basal cell carcinoma from her nose 1 week earlier. On examination she has a full-thickness defect of her left ala measuring 2 by 1.5 cm. The nasal tip, dorsum, and caudal lateral sidewall are spared.
   B. A 24-year-old woman develops a 3 mm nodular basal cell carcinoma on her medial canthus. The edges are well defined. You plan to excise this with a 3 mm margin.
   C. A 70-year-old man develops an 8 mm microcystic basal cell carcinoma on the dorsum of his nose, just below the nasal bridge. Following a staged excision with 4 mm margins, histology confirms complete excision.

Options:
a. Staged paramedian forehead flap and mucoperichondrial flap
b. Healing by secondary intent
c. Glabellar flap
d. Nasolabial flap and conchal cartilage graft
e. Staged paramedian forehead flap with conchal cartilage and mucoperichondrial flap
f. Single-stage paramedian forehead flap with full-thickness graft underneath
g. Banner flap

SOFT TRIANGLE RECONSTRUCTION

9. A patient is referred with a soft triangle defect 3 months after a dog bite injury to the nose. The original injury was cleaned and sutured in the emergency department. On examination an isolated, unilateral, soft triangle defect is present, with both mucosal and soft tissue deficiencies. There is no skin loss evident. **Which one of the following reconstructions is this patient most likely to require?**
   A. Composite conchal bowl graft
   B. Paramedian forehead flap
   C. Paramedian forehead flap, folded in for lining and cartilage graft
   D. Nasolabial flap
   E. Nasolabial flap and cartilage graft

DORSUM AND SIDEWALL RECONSTRCTION

10. **Which one of the following statements is correct when planning a bilobed flap for reconstruction of a circular alar tip defect that measures 1.3 cm in diameter?**
    A. The defect should be triangulated.
    B. The ideal rotation for each lobe is 90 degrees.
    C. The pivot point should be 1.3 cm from the defect.
    D. The vascular supply is the ipsilateral angular artery.
    E. All lobes should be of equal width.

RHINOPHYMA

11. A patient is examined in clinic with a diagnosis of rhinophyma. *Which one of the following statements is correct?*
- A. Rhinophyma is approximately twice as common in men as women.
- B. Patients carry a generalized increased risk of BCC development.
- C. Dermabrasion is the gold standard for surgical management.
- D. Surgical treatment is the mainstay treatment for stage IV disease.
- E. Patients are likely to be heavy drinkers and smokers.

SKIN DISORDERS OF THE NOSE

12. A 63-year-old man presents with skin discoloration involving the tip of his nose and cheeks. He says that it has progressively worsened over the past 5 years and wishes to have it treated. On examination multiple erythematous pustules and papules are present on his nasal tip and cheeks. *Which one of the following is part of the first-line treatment for this patient?*
- A. Topical metronidazole gel
- B. Retinoic acid
- C. Tetracycline
- D. Surgery
- E. Zinc oxide and sunscreen

Answers

BLOOD SUPPLY

1. Which blood vessel is the main supply to the nasal sill and septum?

D. Superior labial artery

The external nose is supplied by branches of the facial, ophthalmic, and maxillary arteries. The superior labial artery is a branch of the facial artery that supplies the nasal sill, the nasal septum, and the columellar base. The angular artery arises from the facial artery and supplies the lateral surface of the nose. The maxillary artery supplies the dorsum and lateral sidewalls. The ophthalmic artery also supplies the nasal dorsum through the dorsal artery from the supratrochlear vessels (see Fig. 36-2, *Essentials of Plastic Surgery*, second edition).

SENSORY INNERVATION

2. Which one of the following is supplied by the maxillary division of the trigeminal nerve?

E. Columella

The radix, rhinion, cephalic portion of the nasal sidewalls, dorsum, and tip are supplied by the ophthalmic division of the trigeminal nerve (V_1). The columella and caudal portion of the lateral nasal sidewalls are supplied by the maxillary division of the trigeminal nerve (V_2). When performing surgery on the nose under local anesthesia, it is often a painful area to inject. For this reason it is often helpful to begin with an intraoral injection of the infraorbital nerve. This is achieved by lifting the upper lip and passing a needle cranially in line with the pupil, just lateral to the lateral incisor. Slow injection here followed by a short pause, can help to ensure patients remain comfortable during subsequent injections around the nose.

LINING RECONSTRUCTION

3. Which one of the following statements is correct regarding reconstruction of a nasal lining defect?

D. Septal mucoperichondrial flaps involve harvesting a rectangle of mucosa with the underlying perichondrium from the ipsilateral septum.

The mucosal surface of the nasal vestibule can be reconstructed in several ways. When external tissue is used, such as a forehead or nasolabial flap, a full-thickness skin graft can be sutured to the underside of the flap before inset. These grafts are associated with good outcomes and are not prone to stricture formation. Alternatively, if the lining is deficient close to or at the alar rim, then the tip of the flap can be turned over and sutured to itself. This can be successful, but it requires thinning of the flap to attain closure. In most cases a second procedure is needed to further thin the alar rim.

Other reconstructive options include mucosal flaps harvested as composites with either cartilage or perichondrium. The septal door flap as described by de Quervain[1] involves removal and discarding of mucosa from the ipsilateral septum and then hinging of the septum and remaining contralateral mucosa to cover the mucosal defect.

The mucosal advancement flap as described by Burget and Menick[2,3] involves a bipedicled (not unipedicled) mucosal flap based medially on the remaining septum and laterally at the piriform aperture. It is used to resurface small lining defects of the nasal ala. (See Figs. 36-4 through 36-7, *Essentials of Plastic Surgery*, second edition.)

TECHNIQUES FOR PROVISION OF NASAL SKELETAL SUPPORT

4. For the following descriptions, the best options are as follows:
    A. *A longitudinal piece of bone or cartilage is seated on the nasal radix and extends along the dorsum to the tip, where it is bent sharply to rest on the anterior nasal spine.*
        c. **Gillies strut technique**
        The Gillies strut technique[4] is used to provide midline cartilaginous or skeletal support for the reconstructed nose. It involves placement of a longitudinal piece of bone or cartilage (often rib) onto the radix with extension along the nasal dorsum to the tip, where it is bent sharply to rest on the anterior nasal spine.
    B. *A longitudinal piece of bone is secured at a single point to either the frontal or nasal bone or both and extends along the dorsum of the nose.*
        d. **Cantilever graft**
        The cantilever graft as described by Converse[5] and Millard[6] is another technique used to provide midline nasal support. This involves placement of a longitudinal piece of bone (typically rib) fixed to the frontal or nasal bones. Unlike the strut technique it does not fix to the anterior nasal spine, hence the cantilever effect.
    C. *This composite flap provides nasal lining and dorsal skeleton support and is based on a branch of the superior labial artery.*
        g. **Septal pivot flap**
        The septal pivot flap described by Burget and Menick[7,8] is used to reconstruct the nasal lining and can be used to provide dorsal cartilage support (see Fig. 36-7, *Essentials of Plastic Surgery*, second edition). Millard's hinged septal flap is an L-shaped flap of septum that is hinged superiorly to augment the nasal angle.[9] Millard's gull-wing flap is a modification of the forehead flap that combines a generous amount of skin for reconstruction of the skin and soft tissues of the nose.[10] The axial frontonasal flap described by Marchac and Toth[11] is used for reconstruction of the skin of the nose. It is based on vessels at the inner canthus. Rieger's dorsal nasal flap is a laterally based flap[12] for reconstruction of nasal lobule defects smaller than 2 cm in diameter. It is based on the angular arteries.

TECHNIQUES FOR PROVISION OF ALAR SUPPORT

5. For the following descriptions, the best options are as follows:
    A. *In this technique cartilage is placed via an infracartilaginous approach into an alar vestibular pocket inferior and lateral to the rim of the crus.*
        d. **Alar contour graft**
    B. *In this technique a bar or triangular-shaped cartilage graft is placed to push the lateral crura apart.*
        b. **Alar spreader graft**

C. In this technique a cartilage graft is placed between the deep surface of the lateral crus and the vestibular skin and is sutured to the crus.
   f. Lateral crural strut graft
      Alar support can be provided with anatomic or nonanatomic cartilage grafts. Contour grafts are placed caudally in the alar rim to improve external nasal valve function and to provide support to the alar rim contour. Spreader grafts are placed between the lateral crura to push them apart and thereby reduce nasal valving. Lateral crural strut grafts prevent alar rim retraction and lateral crural malposition. Alar batten grafts are used to treat alar collapse and external valve obstruction. They are placed cephalad to the alar rim and fashioned to span the collapse. Lateral crural turnover grafts are used to improve the strength and position/shape of the lateral crura. They involve a procedure where the cephalic portion of the lateral crura is turned over onto the remaining caudal lateral crura. Composite alar rim grafts are used to correct severe alar notching and are placed intranasally at the alar rim (see Chapter 96, *Question and Answer* and Figs. 36-9 through 36-12, *Essentials of Plastic Surgery*, second edition).

SKELETAL AND CARTILAGINOUS SUPPORT

6. A 37-year-old woman presents with a pinched-tip deformity of her nose and difficulty breathing at night. On examination she has a bilateral positive Cottle's test. **Which one of the following techniques is most likely to improve her symptoms?**
   C. Alar spreader graft
      Nonanatomic cartilage grafts can help to stiffen the nasal ala and improve patency. Alar spreader grafts involve placement of cartilage between the vestibular surface and the undersurface of the lateral crura to force them apart (see Figs. 36-9, 36-10, 36-12, *Essentials of Plastic Surgery*, second edition). They correct pinched-tip deformities and internal valve collapse. Alar batten grafts involve placement of cartilage cephalad to the alar rim and can improve alar collapse and external nasal valve obstruction. With lateral crural strut grafts, cartilage is placed between the deep surface of the lateral crus and then sutured to the crus. They prevent rim retraction and lateral crural malposition. Alar contour grafts involve placement of cartilage into an alar vestibular pocket inferior and lateral to the rim of the crus. They provide a natural alar contour and improve external nasal valving.

RECONSTRUCTION OF SKIN AND SOFT TISSUE

7. **Which one of the following flaps used in nasal reconstruction can be based on the supratrochlear vessels?**
   D. Midline forehead
      The forehead flap is a workhorse flap for nasal reconstruction. It may be midline or paramedian. The blood supply to this flap can be from the supratrochlear or supraorbital vessels which run within it axially. These facilitate a long flap to width ratio such that nasal tip defects can be reliably reconstructed. When raising this flap it can initially be raised at the level of pericranium to include the frontalis muscle. When dissection gets close to the base at the superior orbital rim it is necessary to change plane and dissect deep to pericranium in order to preserve the blood supply. This flap defect can usually be closed directly with the exception of the most distal part. This is left to heal by secondary intention. In the first stage of this reconstruction, the flap is inset but not usually thinned. In a subsequent stage the flap is reelevated, thinned, and replaced. Cartilage grafts may be placed at this stage. The third stage typically involves division of the flap and reinset of the base to close the distal forehead region (Fig. 36-1).

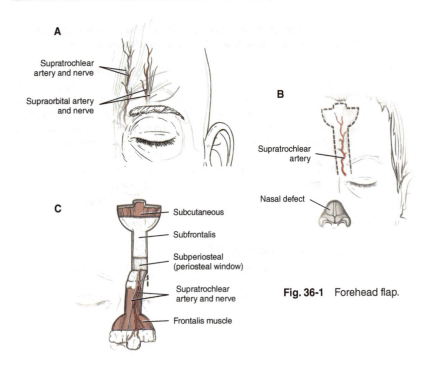

Fig. 36-1 Forehead flap.

The temporomastoid flap is also known as the Washio flap.[13,14] It is based on the superficial temporal vessels to transfer mastoid and auricular skin. It is not a commonly used flap and more often dissected on cadaver dissection courses. The frontotemporal flap[15] is a tubular flap with an internal supracilliary pedicle carrying lateral forehead skin with embedded ear cartilage. The dorsal nasal flap as described by Rieger[12] is a useful flap for reconstructing some distal nasal skin defects. It is based on the angular artery and involves elevation of the nasal dorsum skin which is rotated and advanced caudally. The scalping flap described by Converse[16] may be used to reconstruct large nasal defects in elderly patients. It is based on the superficial temporal vessels and is elevated through a coronal incision just behind the superficial temporal artery, extending to a skin paddle in the contralateral forehead (see Fig. 36-18, *Essentials of Plastic Surgery*, second edition).

8. **For the following scenarios, the best options are as follows:**
    A. A 56-year-old woman is referred by the local Mohs surgeon after excision of an infiltrative basal cell carcinoma from her nose 1 week earlier. On examination she has a full-thickness defect of her left ala measuring 2 by 1.5 cm. The nasal tip, dorsum, and caudal lateral sidewall are spared.
    e. **Staged paramedian forehead flap with conchal cartilage and mucoperichondrial flap**
    This patient requires reconstruction of all three layers: skin, mucosa, and cartilage (support). Skin can be obtained with a paramedian forehead flap. Mucosa can be provided by either a mucoperichondrial flap or a skin graft to the undersurface of the forehead flap. This will require a multistaged approach to optimize the cosmetic and functional result. Cartilage support is required to support the ala and limit nasal valving and airway problems. This can

be harvested from the conchal bowl with minimal morbidity and sandwiched between the reconstructed mucosa and skin layers. If lining is provided by a mucoperichondrial flap, the cartilage can safely be placed in the first stage. A nasolabial flap is an alternative option for this reconstruction, but it will blunt the nasojugal fold and may be undersized for this defect. A nasolabial flap and conchal cartilage graft does not include a lining option, so was unsuitable.

B. A 24-year-old woman develops a 3 mm nodular basal cell carcinoma on her medial canthus. The edges are well defined. You plan to excise this with a 3 mm margin.
   b. **Healing by secondary intent**
   This patient is likely to achieve the best cosmetic result if the area is left to heal. Some areas of the nose and surrounding area are best managed without formal reconstruction and instead allowing the area to heal by secondary intention. These include the glabellar, medial canthal regions, and upper lip (see Fig. 36-13, *Essentials of Plastic Surgery*, second edition). Alternative options are a full-thickness skin graft or a local transposition flap, but in this case each of these will result in additional, unnecessary scarring.

C. A 70-year-old man develops an 8 mm microcystic basal cell carcinoma on the dorsum of his nose, just below the nasal bridge. Following a staged excision with 4 mm margins, histology confirms complete excision.
   c. **Glabellar flap**
   This patient will have a defect that measures at least 1.5 cm given the excision includes 4 mm margins. This defect can be reconstructed with a full-thickness skin graft, but a glabellar flap is likely to provide a better cosmetic outcome with superior contour and skin color match. The Banner flap is typically used for reconstruction of small skin defects of the nasal dorsum using a triangular transposition flap from the adjacent nasal dorsum or cheek.[17]

SOFT TRIANGLE RECONSTRUCTION

9. A patient is referred with a soft triangle defect 3 months after a dog bite injury to the nose. The original injury was cleaned and sutured in the emergency department. On examination an isolated, unilateral, soft triangle defect is present, with both mucosal and soft tissue deficiencies. There is no skin loss evident. **Which one of the following reconstructions is this patient most likely to require?**
   A. **Composite conchal bowl graft**
   The soft triangle is a particularly difficult area to reconstruct because of its distal location on the nose and its complex shape. Defects are classified as type I, II, or III. Type I defects have intact skin but are deficient in soft tissue and mucosa. Type II defects have intact mucosa but are deficient in skin and soft tissue. Type III defects are deficient in all three layers. The patient described has a type I deformity. Constantine et al[18] have proposed an algorithm for reconstruction of soft triangle defects. According to this algorithm, the reconstruction of choice for this patient is a composite conchal bowl graft (see Fig. 36-20, *Essentials of Plastic Surgery*, second edition).

DORSUM AND SIDEWALL RECONSTRUCTION

10. **Which one of the following statements is correct when planning a bilobed flap for reconstruction of a circular alar tip defect that measures 1.3 cm in diameter?**
    D. **The vascular supply is the ipsilateral angular artery.**
    A bilobed flap is a useful technique for reconstructing defects that involve the nasal lobule or tip (Fig. 36-2). Using the Zitelli modification,[19] some key principles should be followed. The defect does not need to be triangulated (as is the case for a large rotation flap), but it requires

removal of a small triangle of tissue between the defect and the base of the first flap. This amounts to removal of a small dog-ear. The angle of rotation is a total of 90 to 100 degrees, split equally between the two transposing flaps. In this case the pivot point should be approximately 7 mm from the defect edge as this represents the defect radius. The blood supply for this flap will be from the ipsilateral angular artery, because the flap should be laterally based for tip reconstruction and medially based for alar reconstruction. It is usual to make the first flap equal in width to the defect and the second flap slightly narrower to facilitate direct closure.

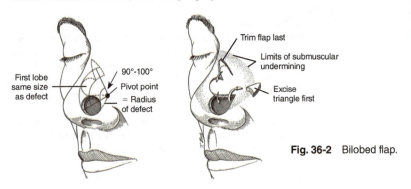

Fig. 36-2   Bilobed flap.

RHINOPHYMA

11. A patient is examined in clinic with a diagnosis of rhinophyma. *Which one of the following statements is correct?*

D. Surgical treatment is the mainstay treatment for stage IV disease.

Rhinophyma is a condition involving sebaceous hyperplasia of nasal skin with bulbous enlargement. It is typically seen in white men in their seventh decade. The male to female ratio is 12:1. Previously thought to be influenced by alcohol intake, this is no longer believed to be true.[20] Patients are at increased risk of developing basal cell carcinomas in the affected area only. Severe cases (such as stage IV disease) are treated surgically with blade excision, dermabrasion, dermaplaning, or CO_2 laser ablation. Outcomes appear to be similar for these various methods. Useful nonsurgical treatments for milder disease include tetracycline, isotretinoin, and metronidazole.

SKIN DISORDERS OF THE NOSE

12. A 63-year-old man presents with skin discoloration involving the tip of his nose and cheeks. He says that it has progressively worsened over the past 5 years and wishes to have it treated. On examination multiple erythematous pustules and papules are present on his nasal tip and cheeks. *Which one of the following is part of the first-line treatment for this patient?*

E. Zinc oxide and sunscreen

This patient has clinical signs of acne rosacea. Rohrich et al[20] have produced a treatment algorithm for management of this condition (see Fig. 36-21, *Essentials of Plastic Surgery,* second edition). First-line treatment involves sun avoidance, sunscreen, and topical zinc oxide cream. Second-line treatment involves prescription of topical metronidazole gel and retinoic acid. After this, oral medication can be considered with tetracycline, metronidazole, or Accutane. If malignant change is a concern, a biopsy specimen should be analyzed, as these patients are at risk of BCCs. If it is positive, surgical excision is warranted.

REFERENCES

1. de Quervain F. Ueber partielle seitliche Rhinoplastik. Zentralbl Chir 29:297, 1902.
2. Burget GC, Menick FJ. Nasal support and lining: the marriage of beauty and blood supply. Plast Reconstr Surg 84:189-202, 1989.
3. Burget GC, Menick FJ. Nasal reconstruction: seeking a fourth dimension. Plast Reconstr Surg 78:145-157, 1986.
4. Gillies HD, ed. Plastic Surgery of the Face. London: Oxford University Press, 1920.
5. Converse JM, ed. Reconstructive Plastic Surgery, vol 2, ed 2. Philadelphia: WB Saunders, 1977.
6. Millard DR Jr. Total reconstructive rhinoplasty and a missing link. Plast Reconstr Surg 37:167-183, 1966.
7. Menick F, ed. Nasal Reconstruction: Art and Practice. Philadelphia: Saunders Elsevier, 2009.
8. Burget GC, Menick FJ. The subunit principle in nasal reconstruction. Plast Reconstr Surg 76:239, 1985.
9. Millard DR Jr. Hemirhinoplasty. Plast Reconstr Surg 40:440-445, 1967.
10. Millard DR Jr. Reconstructive rhinoplasty for the lower half of a nose. Plast Reconstr Surg 53:133-139, 1974.
11. Marchac D, Toth D. The axial frontonasal flap revisited. Plast Reconstr Surg 76:686-694, 1985.
12. Rieger RA. A local flap for repair of the nasal tip. Plast Reconstr Surg 40:147-149, 1967.
13. Loeb R. Temporomastoid flap for reconstruction of the cheek. Rev Lat Am Chir Plast 6:185, 1962.
14. Washio H. Retroauricular temporal flap. Plast Reconstr Surg 124:826, 2009.
15. Meyer R. Aesthetic refinements in nose reconstruction. Aesthetic Plast Surg 24:241, 2000
16. Converse JM. New forehead flap for nasal reconstruction. Proc R Soc Med 35:811, 1942.
17. Elliot RA Jr. Rotation flaps of the nose. Plast Reconstr Surg 44:147, 1969.
18. Constantine FC, Lee MR, Sinno S, et al. Soft tissue triangle reconstruction. Plast Reconstr Surg 131:1045-1050, 2013.
19. Zitelli JA. The bilobed flap for nasal reconstruction. Arch Dermatol 125:957-959, 1989.
20. Rohrich RJ, Griffin JR, Adams WP Jr. Rhinophyma: review and update. Plast Reconstr Surg 110:860-869, 2002.

37. Cheek Reconstruction

See *Essentials of Plastic Surgery*, second edition, pp. 420-428.

AESTHETIC SUBUNITS OF THE CHEEK
1. **Which one of the following statements is correct regarding the aesthetic subunits of the cheek?**
   A. There are four overlapping zones.
   B. The buccomandibular zone is usually the largest.
   C. Zone 1 comprises three smaller subunits.
   D. Two borders in common are found between zones 2 and 3.
   E. Zone 3 is best reconstructed with a cervicofacial flap.

BOUNDARIES OF THE SUBORBITAL ZONE
2. **Which one of the following is not a boundary of the suborbital zone of the cheek?**
   A. Nasolabial line
   B. Posterior sideburn
   C. Gingival sulcus
   D. Lower eyelid skin
   E. Nose/cheek junction

RECONSTRUCTION OF THE CHEEK
3. **Which one of the following is most likely to produce the best cosmetic result reconstructing a 2 by 2 cm, 6 mm deep defect of the central cheek?**
   A. Preauricular full-thickness skin graft
   B. Supraclavicular full-thickness skin graft
   C. Superiorly based rhomboid flap
   D. Cervicofacial flap
   E. Inferiorly based transposition flap

CERVICOFACIAL FLAP RECONSTRUCTION
4. **When reconstructing a suborbital cheek defect with a cervicofacial flap, which one of the following statements is correct?**
   A. The vertical incision should be placed in the preauricular sulcus in all patients.
   B. Flap elevation should remain in the subcutaneous plane throughout.
   C. The superior limit of the flap should be level with the zygomatic arch.
   D. The flap should be anchored to the zygomatic arch and inferolateral orbital rim.
   E. Flap elevation should not continue beyond the lower border of the mandible.

TISSUE EXPANSION FOR CHEEK RECONSTRUCTION
5. You see a patient with a large nevus on the cheek which you are planning to excise and reconstruct using tissue expansion techniques. **Which one of the following is correct in this case?**
   A. More than one expander may be required for this procedure.
   B. Intraoperative filling of the expander(s) is unlikely to reduce seroma formation.

C. Formal expansion should commence four weeks following initial surgery.
D. Overexpansion is not usually required in this region of the face.
E. Capsulectomy should be undertaken during the second stage.

LOCAL FLAPS FOR INTRAORAL RECONSTRUCTION

6. You are planning to reconstruct an intraoral defect of the cheek using a local flap, following resection of a tumor. *Which one of the following is supplied by a branch of the external carotid other than the facial artery?*
A. Buccal fat pad flap
B. FAMM flap
C. Hemi-tongue flap
D. Inferiorly based nasolabial flap
E. Submental flap

RECONSTRUCTION OF LARGE INTRAORAL CHEEK DEFECTS

7. A 37-year-old woman presents with poor mouth opening (less than 2 cm intermaxillary distance) and a 3 by 4 cm ulcerated lesion involving the buccal mucosa. She regularly chews betel nut, is a nonsmoker, and is otherwise fit and well with a BMI of 23. Further investigations reveal a T4 squamous cell carcinoma involving the buccal mucosa and mandibular alveolus. Skin is not involved. Surgical excision of the tumor is planned, with a mandibular rim resection and selective neck dissection. *Which one of the following is the most acceptable reconstructive approach for this patient, with the lowest donor site morbidity?*
A. Pectoralis major pedicled flap
B. Combined tongue and buccal pad flaps
C. Free radial forearm flap
D. Free fibular osteocutaneous flap
E. Free ALT flap

RECONSTRUCTION OF CHEEK DEFECTS WITH LOCAL FLAPS

8. *For each of the following scenarios, select the most appropriate reconstruction method. (Each option may be used once, more than once, or not at all.)*
A. A 60-year-old woman has a 4 by 3.5 cm defect in the suborbital cheek, which also involves the lower two-thirds of the eyelid skin and orbicularis oculi following a wide excision of a melanoma.
B. A 34-year-old woman was bitten on the right side of her face by a dog. She has a full-thickness defect on her cheek (zone 3), overlying the mandible and involving the lower buccal sulcus. After early debridement the defect measures 3 cm in diameter.
C. A 79-year-old man has a 2 cm poorly differentiated squamous cell carcinoma on his central cheek. Excision with 1 cm margins is planned. The buccal mucosa is preserved.

Options:
a. Paramedian forehead flap
b. Cervicofacial flap
c. Superiorly based bilobed flap
d. Mustarde cheek advancement flap
e. Inferiorly based rhomboid flap
f. Nasolabial flap
g. Transposition flap from the submandibular region

SALVAGE FLAPS USED IN CHEEK RECONSTRUCTION

9. An elderly man has undergone a total parotidectomy and neck dissection for an aggressive, recurrent squamous cell carcinoma after radiotherapy. The overlying skin is involved. An 8 by 8 cm defect to the lower cheek and neck requires reconstruction. *Which one of the following potentially available flaps for reconstruction of this defect receives its major blood supply from the thoracoacromial vessels?*
   A. Deltopectoral
   B. Pectoralis major
   C. Sternocleidomastoid
   D. Trapezius
   E. Latissimus dorsi

Answers

AESTHETIC SUBUNITS OF THE CHEEK

1. *Which one of the following statements is correct regarding the aesthetic subunits of the cheek?*
   C. Zone 1 comprises three smaller subunits.
   The cheek can be divided into three (not four) overlapping aesthetic zones (Fig. 37-1). These zones are the suborbital (zone 1), preauricular (zone 2), and buccomandibular (zone 3). The largest one is probably the preauricular zone, because it overlaps zones 1 and 3. Zone 1 can be further subdivided into three zones: A, B, and C. **A** represents the cheek skin medial to the lateral edge of the brow, **B** represents the cheek skin lateral to the brow, and **C** represents the skin of the lower eyelid to the eyelid cheek interface. Zones 2 and 3 share only their inferior border, which corresponds to the lower border of the mandible. Zone 3 includes the lower cheek and oral lining in full-thickness defects. This zone cannot usually be reconstructed with a cervicofacial flap. However zones 1 and 2 often can be.

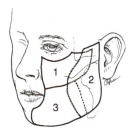

Fig. 37-1 Three overlapping zones of the cheek aesthetic unit.

BOUNDARIES OF THE SUBORBITAL ZONE

2. *Which one of the following is not a boundary of the suborbital zone of the cheek?*
   B. Posterior sideburn
   The posterior sideburn is not a boundary of the suborbital zone. The medial boundary is the nasolabial line and nasal cheek junction, the lateral boundary is the anterior sideburn, the superior boundary is the lower eyelid skin, and the inferior boundary is the gingival sulcus.

RECONSTRUCTION OF THE CHEEK

3. *Which one of the following is most likely to produce the best cosmetic result reconstructing a 2 by 2 cm, 6 mm deep defect of the central cheek?*
   E. Inferiorly based transposition flap
   Smaller cheek defects are generally best closed directly or with local flaps, particularly when they are deep, as in this case. This is because they provide superior color and texture match with avoidance of a contour defect. Inferiorly based flaps can reduce a trap-door effect and postoperative edema, because they facilitate flap drainage with gravity. When skin grafts are

used, full thickness is preferable to split thickness as there is less secondary contraction and the color match is superior. The optimal full-thickness graft location is probably the contralateral preauricular site as the color and texture match are good and the donor site may be well hidden at the junction of the ear and the cheek. Other sites are postauricular and supraclavicular. The location of this defect is not ideally suited to the cervicofacial flap and use of this flap is excessive for defects of this size, given the more conservative options available.

CERVICOFACIAL FLAP RECONSTRUCTION

4. When reconstructing a suborbital cheek defect with a cervicofacial flap, which one of the following statements is correct?

D. The flap should be anchored to the zygomatic arch and inferolateral orbital rim.

Placement of anchor sutures to the periosteum of the inferior orbital rim and zygomatic arch is very important to minimize subsequent development of ectropion. This approach may also be combined with a lateral canthopexy if inadequate lower lid support remains a concern.

A preauricular incision, as used in a face lift, can be ideal in some patients. However, in males the sideburn will be moved medially if this incision is performed. Therefore it is preferable to place an incision along the medial aspect of the sideburn only passing to the preauricular sulcus beneath the tip of the sideburn. The flap must be designed to extend above the zygomatic arch to ensure sufficient reach, as it has to both rotate and advance. The flap must be extensively undermined (often as far as the clavicle, when reconstructing large defects) to maximize reach and minimize tension during closure. The level of dissection should initially be in the subcutaneous plane, but should be subplatysmal in the neck to ensure adequate vascular supply to the flap. The marginal mandibular nerve must be carefully preserved during the dissection.

TISSUE EXPANSION FOR CHEEK RECONSTRUCTION

5. You see a patient with a large nevus on the cheek which you are planning to excise and reconstruct using tissue expansion techniques. *Which one of the following is correct in this case?*

A. More than one expander may be required for this procedure.

Tissue expansion offers the best color and texture match for reconstructing large defects of the cheek and multiple custom made expanders are often needed. Intraoperative filling may help to prevent hematoma and seroma formation. However, a balance is needed to prevent excessive tension during primary closure that will increase the risk of wound breakdown and subsequent extrusion.

Formal expansion should begin two weeks after the primary surgery and then continue on a weekly basis. Overexpansion by 30% to 50% is advised in the cheek area to overcome flap contraction. The capsule is a very vascular structure and should remain within the local tissue flaps that are used for closure. If the capsule is tight, it can be scored (capsulectomy) to allow more flap advancement but capsulectomy should not be performed.

LOCAL FLAPS FOR INTRAORAL RECONSTRUCTION

6. You are planning to reconstruct an intraoral defect of the cheek using a local flap, following resection of a tumor. *Which one of the following is supplied by a branch of the external carotid other than the facial artery?*

C. Hemi-tongue flap

Intraoral defects involving the cheek can be reconstructed using a number of different local flaps. Many of these receive blood supply from the facial artery. The hemi-tongue flap however, is based on the lingual artery. Flaps based on the facial artery include the facial artery myomucosal flap (FAMM), the submental artery flap (from branches passing through the submandibular gland),

Chapter 37 ▪ Cheek Reconstruction   301

and the random pattern nasolabial flap (predominantly from the angular branch of the facial artery). The buccal fat pad is based on a subcapsular plexus formed by both the facial artery and the internal maxillary artery and has good reported outcomes in reconstructing smaller intraoral defects.[1] The nasolabial region also receives blood supply from the infraorbital artery which is derived from the maxillary artery; however, this only supplies the superiorly based flap.

RECONSTRUCTION OF LARGE INTRAORAL CHEEK DEFECTS

7. A 37-year-old woman presents with poor mouth opening (less than 2 cm intermaxillary distance) and a 3 by 4 cm ulcerated lesion involving the buccal mucosa. She regularly chews betel nut, is a nonsmoker, and is otherwise fit and well with a BMI of 23. Further investigations reveal a T4 squamous cell carcinoma involving the buccal mucosa and mandibular alveolus. Skin is not involved. Surgical excision of the tumor is planned, with a mandibular rim resection and selective neck dissection. *Which one of the following is the most acceptable reconstructive approach for this patient, with the lowest donor site morbidity?*
   E. Free ALT flap

   The defect created in this reconstruction is likely to be 5 by 6 cm in diameter and will require importation of distant soft tissue. Bone will not be required unless a segmental mandibular resection is planned. The pectoralis major can be tunneled under the neck dissection flaps and used for intraoral reconstruction, but reach will be difficult and the donor site is poor for young female patients. It tends to be used as a salvage flap in elderly patients, where free tissue transfer is contraindicated. Local flaps such as the tongue, FAMM, and buccal fat pads can be useful for smaller intraoral defects, and in this case may be sacrificed during tumor resection. Either free radial forearm or free anterolateral thigh (ALT) flaps can be used in this case. An ALT flap is favorable because of its hidden scarring. One problem with ALT flaps for intraoral reconstruction is that they can be bulky, causing functional difficulties with speech and eating. In a patient with a low BMI, this should not be a major problem. Other reconstructive options for this patient include the scapula or parascapular flap or a groin flap.

RECONSTRUCTION OF CHEEK DEFECTS WITH LOCAL FLAPS

8. *For the following scenarios, the best options are as follows:*
   A. *A 60-year-old woman has a 4 by 3.5 cm defect in the suborbital cheek, which also involves the lower two-thirds of the eyelid skin and orbicularis oculi, following wide excision of a melanoma.*
      b. Cervicofacial flap

      This patient has a defect site (zone 1) that is well suited to cheek advancement flaps. If the defect were smaller, then either a McGregor or Mustarde-type flap could be used. Given the large size of the defect, a cervicofacial flap is most likely to be required. Smaller medial defects in zone 1 can be treated with a paramedian forehead flap.
   B. *A 34-year-old woman was bitten on the right side of her face by a dog. She has a full-thickness defect on her cheek (zone 3), overlying the mandible and involving the lower buccal sulcus. After early debridement the defect measures 3 cm in diameter.*
      g. Transposition flap from the submandibular region

      This patient's defect is too large to close directly without tissue distortion. In females, transposition of skin from the neck beneath the lower mandibular border can provide a good skin match with a relatively well-hidden donor scar. In this case it is necessary to suture a skin graft to the undersurface of the flap to reconstruct the intraoral buccal sulcus defect. However, in males this flap will alter the direction of beard growth and should be avoided.

C. *A 79-year-old man has a 2 cm poorly differentiated squamous cell carcinoma on his central cheek. Excision with 1 cm margins is planned. The buccal mucosa is preserved.*
   e. **Inferiorly based rhomboid flap**
      Several local flaps are options for this patient. These include bilobed, rhomboid, or V-Y advancement flaps. An inferior rhomboid flap is most preferable in this case and will minimize subsequent soft tissue edema, compared with a superiorly based bilobed flap. In many cases it is possible to achieve direct closure in the central cheek at the expense of a long scar.

SALVAGE FLAPS USED IN CHEEK RECONSTRUCTION

9. An elderly man has undergone a total parotidectomy and neck dissection for an aggressive, recurrent squamous cell carcinoma after radiotherapy. The overlying skin is involved. An 8 by 8 cm defect to the lower cheek and neck requires reconstruction. **Which one of the following potentially available flaps for reconstruction of this defect receives its major blood supply from the thoracoacromial vessels?**
   B. **Pectoralis major**
      The blood supply to the flaps listed is as follows:
      Pectoralis major: Internal mammary perforators, thoracoacromial vessels, and lateral thoracic vessels
      Deltopectoral: Internal mammary perforators
      Trapezius: Transverse cervical, dorsal scapular, and posterior intercostal vessels
      Sternocleidomastoid:
         Upper: Occipital artery
         Middle: Superior thyroid or external carotid artery
         Lower: Suprascapular artery from the transverse cervical artery
      Latissimus dorsi: Thoracodorsal and posterior intercostal perforators
   This defect can be reconstructed with a deltopectoral, pectoralis major, trapezius, or latissimus dorsi flap.[2] The sternocleidomastoid is unsuitable for this reconstruction because of its segmental blood supply and small size.[3,4] The pectoralis major muscle provides a reliable flap for reconstruction of the head and neck region. It can be muscle only or muscle and skin. The donor site can usually be closed directly by undermining adjacent tissue and rotating/advancing this into the donor defect. It will however distort the breast, particularly in women. The pedicle can be identified as it passes between the sternal and clavicular heads of the muscle, just below the clavicle. It is possible to dissect close to the vessel in this area in order to minimize bulk at the pivot point. The flap is then passed under a subcutaneous tunnel into the neck. The deltopectoral flap is usually reserved as a lifeboat flap and can be elevated and replaced during a pectoralis major flap harvest. The trapezius flap is particularly useful for posterior defects over the upper cervical spine as it has a reliable blood supply and easily reaches to provide muscle cover over the spinous processes. The donor site can usually be closed directly. A fasciocutaneous flap based on the transverse cervical vessels can be useful for head and neck reconstruction in both intraoral and skin defects. This is termed a supraclavicular artery perforator (a-SAP) flap.[5] The latissimus dorsi is not commonly used for head and neck reconstruction, although it may be incorporated into a free scapula flap when bone and soft tissue reconstruction is required (Fig. 37-2).

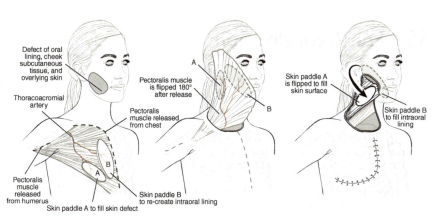

Fig. 37-2 Pectoralis major flap with two skin paddles: one for the intraoral defect and one for the cutaneous defect. (Although this was a common flap in years past, it is now mostly used as a salvage option.)

REFERENCES

1. Chakrabarti J, Tekriwal R, Ganguli A, et al. Pedicled buccal fat pad flap for intraoral malignant defects: a series of 29 cases. Indian J Plast Surg 42:26-42, 2009.
2. Yang D, Morris SF. Trapezius muscle: anatomic basis for flap design. Ann Plast Surg 41:52-57, 1998.
3. Kierner AC, Aigner M, Zelenka I, et al. The blood supply of the sternocleidomastoid muscle and its clinical implications. Arch Surg 134:144-147, 1999.
4. Freeman JL, Walker EP, Wilson JS, et al. The vascular anatomy of the pectoralis major myocutaneous flap. Br J Plast Surg 34:3-10, 1981.
5. Pallua N, Wolter TP. Moving forwards: the anterior supraclavicular artery perforator (a-SAP) flap: a new pedicled or free perforator flap based on the anterior supraclavicular vessels. J Plast Reconstr Aesthet Surg 66:489-496, 2013.

38. Ear Reconstruction

See *Essentials of Plastic Surgery*, second edition, pp. 429-439.

ANATOMY

1. **What is the dominant arterial blood supply to the ear?**
   A. Superficial temporal artery
   B. Deep temporal artery
   C. Posterior auricular artery
   D. Occipital artery
   E. Great auricular artery

2. **Which one of the following statements is correct regarding sensation to the ear?**
   A. The entire ear can be anesthetized with a circumferential ring block.
   B. Sensation to the lobule is provided by the lesser occipital nerve.
   C. The auriculotemporal nerve is the main nerve implicated in referred otalgia.
   D. Arnold's nerve is formed by cranial nerves IX through XII.
   E. The cervical plexus and trigeminal nerve supply the vast majority of the ear.

3. **Which one of the following tumor sites is most likely to have lymphatic drainage to the parotid nodes?**
   A. The antihelix
   B. The antitragus
   C. The lobule
   D. The superior helix
   E. The scapha

AESTHETIC RELATIONSHIPS OF THE EAR

4. **Which one of the following statements is correct regarding the normal position and size of the external ear?**
   A. The ear is normally located one ear width posterior to the lateral orbital rim.
   B. Ear height varies between 5.5 and 6.5 cm in adults.
   C. Ear width is usually less than one-third the height.
   D. Maximum projection from the mastoid to the helix occurs superiorly.
   E. The long axis tilt is consistently within 1 to 2 degrees in all individuals.

ACUTE INJURIES TO THE EAR

5. **Which one of the following statements is correct regarding soft tissue injuries involving the ear?**
   A. Dog bites in children frequently become infected secondary to viridans-group streptococci.
   B. Hematomas are the most common complication after blunt trauma and should be evacuated early to prevent cauliflower ear.
   C. Direct repair of the cartilage must be performed after debridement of a full-thickness ear laceration.
   D. Frostbite involving the ear should be managed with gentle rewarming using warm water.
   E. Thermal burns to the pinna usually warrant aggressive debridement in the early phases to prevent burn progression and cartilage desiccation.

TUMORS OF THE EAR

6. What is the most common site of a keloid tumor?
  A. The helix
  B. The concha
  C. The scapha
  D. The lobule
  E. The tragus

KELOID SCARRING TO THE EAR

7. Which one of the following statements regarding keloid scarring is correct?
  A. Keloids involving the ear are five times more common in dark-skinned patients.
  B. Recurrence after simple excision occurs in a third of cases.
  C. Outcomes are unpredictable after combined steroid injection and excision.
  D. The benefit of silicone therapy after excision is minimal.
  E. Radiation is a reliable first-line treatment for keloids.

8. Which one of the following is true of chondrodermatitis nodularis helicis (CDNH)?
  A. It is a malignant condition of the ear.
  B. Patients are unlikely to notice the condition themselves.
  C. Recurrence after excision is unlikely.
  D. Males and females are equally affected.
  E. It is usually caused by a pressure effect.

RECONSTRUCTION OPTIONS FOR EXTERNAL EAR DEFORMITIES

9. For each of the following clinical scenarios, select the most suitable reconstructive option. (Each option may be used once, more than once, or not at all.)
  A. A patient has a partial-thickness, 2 by 2 cm defect to the anterior surface of the conchal bowl after excision of a basal cell carcinoma and the underlying cartilage.
  B. An elderly man has a full-thickness, 1.8 cm high defect involving the midportion of the helical rim that was created during excision of a squamous cell carcinoma.
  C. A young woman has a 1.5 cm long, vertically split earlobe caused by wearing heavy earrings.

Options:
  a. Full-thickness skin graft
  b. Inferiorly based chondrocutaneous rotation flap
  c. Dieffenbach flap
  d. Antia-Buch flap
  e. Converse tunnel technique
  f. Direct repair with Z-plasty

10. For each of the following clinical scenarios, select the most suitable reconstructive option. (Each option may be used once, more than once, or not at all.)
   A. A patient has a 2 by 1.7 cm full-thickness defect to the middle third of the ear. It involves the helix, scapha, and antihelix but not the conchal bowl.
   B. A patient has a 4 cm high, healed helical rim defect 3 months after a human bite wound.
   C. A young nonsmoker has a guillotine amputation of the superior two thirds of the external ear.

Options:
   a. Prosthetic device
   b. Staged ear reconstruction
   c. Inferiorly based chondrocutaneous rotation flap
   d. Dieffenbach flap
   e. Staged tubed pedicle flap
   f. Antia-Buch flap
   g. Replantation using the superficial temporal artery

REPLANTATION OF THE EXTERNAL EAR

11. A thirty-year-old woman is involved in a motor vehicle accident during which her ear is amputated. She is taken immediately to the operating room for debridement and replantation. **Which one of the following is most likely to be part of the postoperative regimen specific to this procedure?**
    A. Cartilage banking
    B. Dextran
    C. Sulfamylon
    D. Hirudo medicinalis
    E. Aspirin

Answers

ANATOMY

1. What is the dominant arterial blood supply to the ear?
C. Posterior auricular artery
   The external ear is supplied by three main vessels: the posterior auricular (dominant), superficial temporal, and occipital. Good interconnections exist between the main source vessels. The ear can be replanted on either the superficial temporal or posterior auricular vessel (Fig. 38-1). The greater auricular artery does not exist (although there is a great auricular nerve).

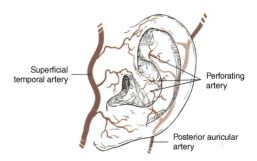

Fig. 38-1 Vascular supply to the external ear.

2. Which one of the following statements is correct regarding sensation to the ear?
E. The cervical plexus and trigeminal nerve supply the vast majority of the ear.
   The external ear receives sensory innervations from a number of nerves, but the main supply is from the cervical plexus (C2-3) and the trigeminal nerve (V3). Although most of the ear can be successfully anesthetized with a ring block, the concha and external auditory meatus would remain spared by this approach. The auriculotemporal nerve (V3) supplies the superior lateral surface of the ear and also contributes to the external auditory meatus. The lobule and lower part of the ear is supplied by the great auricular nerve (C2-3). The lesser occipital nerve (C2-3) supplies the superior cranial surface of the ear. Arnold's nerve receives contributions from the facial (CN VII), glossopharyngeal (CN IX), and vagus (CN X) nerves but not the eleventh or twelfth nerves. It supplies the external auditory canal and meatus as well as part of the conchal bowl. It is implicated in referred otalgia from other structures in the head and neck, and the initiation of coughing during manipulation of the ear canal.

3. Which one of the following tumor sites is most likely to have lymphatic drainage to the parotid nodes?
D. The superior helix
   The lymphatic drainage of the ear corresponds to the embryologic origins. The tragus, helical root, and superior helix all originate from the first branchial arch and drain to the parotid nodes. The antihelix, antitragus, and lobule all arise from the second branchial arch and drain to the cervical nodes (see Fig. 38-1). When examining patients with squamous cell carcinoma or

melanoma of the pinna, it is vital that the parotid and neck nodes are thoroughly assessed, given the pathway of spread in metastatic disease.

AESTHETIC RELATIONSHIPS OF THE EAR

4. Which one of the following statements is correct regarding the normal position and size of the external ear?

B. Ear height varies between 5.5 and 6.5 cm in adults.

The ear is located one ear height (not one width) posterior to the lateral orbital rim. The superior surface is usually level with the eyebrow. Height varies between 5.5 and 6.5 cm in adults, and width is usually a little over half the height. Projection varies among individuals but is usually greatest inferiorly (approximately 2 cm) from the mastoid to the helix. The long-axis tilts on average 20 degrees posteriorly, but this varies greatly.[1]

ACUTE INJURIES TO THE EAR

5. Which one of the following statements is correct regarding soft tissue injuries involving the ear?

B. Hematomas are the most common complication after blunt trauma and should be evacuated early to prevent cauliflower ear.

Cauliflower ear refers to a deformity that develops after a subperichondral hematoma in the pinna. It results in devascularization of the cartilage with permanent fibrosis and scarring. Preventative management involves early evacuation of the hematoma and application of a pressure dressing. Dog bites are commonly seen in children, but the pathogens involved in infection are most likely *Pasteurella multocida* or *P. canis*. Viridans-group streptococci are associated with human bites. Ear lacerations should be carefully debrided and repaired with skin-only closure. Frostbite should be managed with rapid rewarming using saline-soaked dressings. To preserve maximal tissue, thermal burns are usually treated conservatively with dressings and later debrided once demarcation has occurred.

TUMORS OF THE EAR

6. What is the most common site of a keloid tumor?

D. The lobule

Keloids represent fibroproliferative disorders of the skin that grow beyond the boundaries of the original wound. They can occur spontaneously but commonly occur secondary to localized trauma. The most common anatomic site for development of a keloid is the lobule and this is frequently secondary to ear piercing. Other trauma or surgery to the ear such as pinnaplasty risks development of keloid scarring and this must be communicated to patients before proceeding with such techniques. Other nonhead and neck sites that are affected include the anterior chest, lateral arm, and some flexor surfaces.

KELOID SCARRING TO THE EAR

7. Which one of the following statements regarding keloid scarring is correct?

C. Outcomes are unpredictable after combined steroid injection and excision.

As discussed in question 6, ear piercing is the most common cause of keloids on the ear. Keloids are 15 times (not 5 times) more frequent in dark-skinned individuals than in white individuals.[2] Keloids recur after simple excision in up to 100% of cases. Outcomes after combined excision and steroid therapy are unpredictable and vary from 0% to 100% recurrence.[3] Continuous silicone therapy for 3 months after surgery can significantly decrease potential keloid formation. Radiation should be reserved for resistant lesions because of the side effects. Alternatively, it may be combined with surgical excision.

8. **Which one of the following is true of chondrodermatitis nodularis helicis (CDNH)?**
   E. It is usually caused by a pressure effect.
      CDNH is a benign condition affecting the external ear resulting in a painful, chronic nodular, or ulcerative lesion. Patients notice these lesions because of the pain. This is in contrast to some asymptomatic ear lesions such as nodular BCC, where a patient's relatives often first notice the lesion. Males are four times more likely to develop CDNH, which is thought to be as a result of repeated external pressure being placed on the ear. When taking a history, a patient's sleeping position preference should be noted, as often they sleep lying on the affected side and this needs to be modified as part of the treatment plan. Lesions are treated surgically with a narrow margin excision. The key point is to remove the lesion while ensuring a smooth contour to the ear cartilage, such that no residual prominence remains. Recurrence rates vary between 10% and 30% according to series[4] and this can be affected by both surgical technique and subsequent pressure relief.

RECONSTRUCTION OPTIONS FOR EXTERNAL EAR DEFORMITIES

9. *For the following scenarios, the best options are as follows:*
   A. A patient has a partial-thickness, 2 by 2 cm defect to the anterior surface of the conchal bowl after excision of a basal cell carcinoma and the underlying cartilage.
   a. Full-thickness skin graft
      Use of a full-thickness graft works well on the ear, particularly when the anterior or posterior skin remains intact and can be grafted onto the ear. Often the defect is difficult to see once the graft has healed well and matured some months postoperatively.
   B. An elderly man has a full-thickness, 1.8 cm high defect involving the midportion of the helical rim that was created during excision of a squamous cell carcinoma.
   d. Antia-Buch flap
      The Antia-Buch flap[5] is a very useful technique for reconstruction of helical rim defects up to approximately 2 cm in height (Fig. 38-2). An incision is made in the helical sulcus through skin and cartilage and a posterior skin flap dissection is performed. This undermining allows advancement of the helix towards the defect. The helical root is also released and advanced as a V-Y flap.

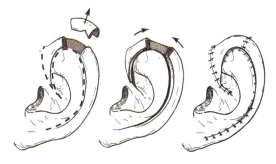

Fig. 38-2 The Antia-Buch procedure of helical rim advancement.

The swing flap is a variation on the superior part of the Anti-Buch flap that can be used for larger defects of the helical rim. It involves raising a helical root and superior rim flap on a mesentery without the posterior skin (which is elevated thinly). If the defect was greater than 2 cm then Converse's tunnel technique may be useful. This involves burying a piece of contralateral auricular cartilage under the postauricular skin and dividing and insetting the flap after 3 weeks.[6]

The Dieffenbach flap is used for middle third defects of the scapha and helical rim. It involves raising a postauricular skin flap placed over a contralateral auricular cartilage graft. This flap is also divided at 3 weeks.[6]

C. **A young woman has a 1.5 cm long, vertically split earlobe caused by wearing heavy earrings.**
   f. **Direct repair with Z-plasty**
      Although it is possible to repair split earlobes directly with a linear scar, many authorities believe that placement of a Z-plasty will reduce the risk of scar contraction and lobule deformity.

10. *For the following scenarios, the best options are as follows:*
    A. **A patient has a 2 by 1.7 cm full-thickness defect to the middle third of the ear. It involves the helix, scapha, and antihelix but not the conchal bowl.**
       d. **Dieffenbach flap**
          Dieffenbach's flap involves a contralateral auricular cartilage graft that is sutured to the defect and covered with a postauricular skin flap. The postauricular skin flap is divided 3 weeks later (see Fig. 38-9, *Essentials of Plastic Surgery,* second edition).
    B. **A patient has a 4 cm high, healed helical rim defect 3 months after a human bite wound.**
       e. **Staged tubed pedicle flap**
          Staged tubed pedicle flaps using the postauricular skin work well for reconstruction of the helical rim. They require three stages: in the first stage the skin is tubed; in the second stage one end is divided and inset into the helical rim; and in the third stage the flap is detached posteriorly and inset into the helical rim. If the rim is subsequently droopy, it may be necessary to insert a small cartilage graft within the reconstructed soft tissue in order to provide additional support.
    C. **A young nonsmoker has a guillotine amputation of the superior two thirds of the external ear.**
       g. **Replantation using the superficial temporal artery**
          Successful replantation can provide a superior aesthetic result compared with secondary reconstruction. It requires anastamosis of either the superficial temporal or posterior auricular artery. An additional venous anastomosis is preferable but not always technically possible, so venous drainage may be reliant on an external route into dressings.

REPLANTATION OF THE EXTERNAL EAR

11. A thirty-year-old woman is involved in a motor vehicle accident during which her ear is amputated. She is taken immediately to the operating room for debridement and replantation. **Which one of the following is most likely to be part of the postoperative regimen specific to this procedure?**
    D. **Hirudo medicinalis**
       As discussed in question 10, during replantation it may not be possible to achieve a satisfactory venous anastomosis. For this reason, leeches (Hirudo medicinalis) are commonly used as standard practice. They are typically used both in the presence or absence of a venous anastomosis. Sulfamylon (mafenide acetate) is used on ear burns as part of a conservative measure to minimize tissue loss and infection. Cartilage banking is performed in cases where replantation cannot be performed. It may be buried under a postauricular skin pocket or the

forearm. The success of this approach is variable. Dextran and heparin are part of the treatment of frostbite to the ear. They are intended to limit thrombosis and tissue loss. Either may be used in ear replantation but are not a core part of treatment. Aspirin may help the arterial anastomosis but is not evidence based (see Chapter 8).

References

1. Farkas L. Anthropometry of normal and anomalous ears. Clin Plast Surg 5:401-412, 1978.
2. Ogawa R. The most current algorithms for the treatment and prevention of hypertrophic scars and keloids. Plast Reconstr Surg 125:557-568, 2010.
3. Elsahy N. Acquired ear defects. Clin Plast Surg 29:175-186, 2002.
4. Wagner G, Liefeith J, Sachse MM. Clinical appearance, differential diagnoses, and therapeutical options of chondrodermatitis nodularis chronic helicis Winkler. J Dtsch Dermatol Ges 9:287-291, 2011.
5. Antia NH, Buch VI. Chondrocutaneous advancement flap for the marginal defect of the ear. Plast Reconstr Surg 39:472-477, 1967.
6. Aguilar EA. Traumatic total or partial ear loss. In Evans GR, ed. Operative Plastic Surgery. New York: McGraw-Hill, 2000.

39. Lip Reconstruction

See *Essentials of Plastic Surgery*, second edition, pp. 440-453.

LIP ANATOMY

1. *Match each of the following anatomic descriptions to the most appropriate option. (Each option may be used once, more than once, or not at all.)*
   A. This is the junction between the skin and the lip.
   B. This is the red mucosal portion of the lip and is divided into two parts.
   C. This muscle functions as the oral sphincter.

   Options:
   a. Philtral column
   b. White roll
   c. Vermilion
   d. Red line
   e. Commissure
   f. Deep portion of the orbicularis oris
   g. Superficial portion of the orbicularis oris

2. *Which one of the following is the same for both upper and lower lips?*
   A. The sensory innervation
   B. The blood supply
   C. The lymphatic drainage
   D. The number of subunit components
   E. The motor innervations to orbicularis

3. *At conversational distances, what minimum amount of white roll mismatch is typically evident?*
   A. 1 mm
   B. 2 mm
   C. 3 mm
   D. 4 mm
   E. 5 mm

REPAIR OF VERMILION DEFECTS

4. *Which one of the following statements is correct regarding defects of the vermilion?*
   A. Tongue flaps are useful single-stage procedures for defects that measure less than 50%.
   B. Total deficiency may be treated by advancing the buccal mucosa.
   C. Axial myomucosal advancement flaps are elevated superficial to the orbicularis.
   D. Vermilion lip switch is a single-stage procedure for subtotal defects.
   E. Tongue flaps provide the best aesthetic outcomes.

ALGORITHMIC APPROACH TO LIP RECONSTRUCTION

5. Which one of the following statements is correct regarding lip reconstruction?
A. Upper and lower lip defects that are smaller than a third should be closed directly.
B. Lower lip defects greater than 50% of total width require a two-stage reconstruction.
C. A V-Y flap is the first choice for reconstruction of a lower lip defect involving the commissure.
D. Perialar crescenteric advancement is a useful adjunct for the upper lip reconstruction.
E. Full-thickness defects larger than two thirds of the lip width require free flap reconstruction.

ABBÉ FLAP

6. Which one of the following statements is correct when using an Abbé flap for lip reconstruction?
A. The flap should be designed to be the same width as the defect.
B. The contralateral labial artery should be skeletonized during the dissection.
C. Reconstruction of the commissure is the main indication of this flap.
D. An advantage of this flap is that reconstruction is completed in a single stage.
E. The flap is particularly well suited for reconstruction of the philtral dimple.

ESTLANDER FLAP

7. Which one of the following statements is correct regarding an Estlander flap?
A. It is ideally suited to reconstruct central lip defects.
B. It is only suitable for defects less than half the lip width.
C. It is a two-stage process requiring division at two weeks.
D. Blood supply is from the contralateral labial artery of the opposite lip.
E. Postoperative commissure distortion is rarely observed.

KARAPANDZIC FLAP

8. Which one of the following statements is correct regarding the Karapandzic flap?
A. It should only be used for lower lip reconstruction.
B. Full-thickness dissection is required throughout.
C. Some branches of the facial nerve will have to be divided.
D. The flap is only full thickness medially.
E. Oral competence is preserved without microstomia.

TOTAL LIP RECONSTRUCTION

9. Which one of the following statements is incorrect regarding free flap total lower lip reconstruction with a radial forearm flap?
A. Preoperative assessment with an Allen's test should always be undertaken.
B. The tissue color match and aesthetics are often poor with this reconstruction.
C. Sensory innervation can be achieved by using the lateral cutaneous nerve of the forearm.
D. Motor function is well preserved ensuring oral competence.
E. Palmaris longus can be used as a sling to maintain lip height.

RECONSTRUCTIVE OPTIONS FOR LIP DEFECTS

10. For each of the following clinical scenarios, select the most suitable reconstructive option. (Each option may be used once, more than once, or not at all.)

   A. A 70-year-old man presents with a 3.5 cm wide defect in his lower lip following an excision of a moderately differentiated squamous cell carcinoma.

   B. A 19-year-old woman presents after a dog bite. She has a full-thickness, laterally placed upper lip defect that measures 40% of the width. The commissure is preserved.

   C. An 80-year-old man is referred after having Mohs surgery for a basal cell carcinoma that involved the central upper lip. He has a 1.5 cm defect with complete loss of his philtral dimple and columns.

   Options:
   a. Abbé flap
   b. Karapandzic flap
   c. Bernard-Burow flap
   d. Direct closure
   e. Tongue flap
   f. Estlander flap
   g. Radial forearm flap

Answers

LIP ANATOMY

1. **For the following descriptions, the best options are as follows:**
   A. This is the junction between the skin and the lip.
   b. White roll
   B. This is the red mucosal portion of the lip and is divided into two parts.
   c. Vermilion
   C. This muscle functions as the oral sphincter.
   f. Deep portion of the orbicularis oris

   The lip comprises skin, muscle, fat, and mucosa. The white roll marks the interface between the skin and vermilion (see Fig. 39-1, *Essentials of Plastic Surgery,* second edition). The vermilion is the red part of the lip and has wet and dry components based on the presence or absence of surface keratinization. The orbicularis oris has deep and superficial components. The superficial component is involved with speech and facial expression, whereas the deep portion is involved with oral competence. The oral commissure is the point where the upper and lower lips join. Lateral to this is the modeolus, where muscle fibers from other mimetic muscles attach, such as the depressor anguli oris, levator anguli oris, risorius, and zygomaticus major.

2. **Which one of the following is the same for both upper and lower lips?**
   E. The motor innervations to orbicularis

   The upper and lower lips differ in their vascular supply, sensory nerve supply, and their lymphatic drainage. However, orbicularis oris is innervated by the buccal branches of the facial nerve irrespective of whether the upper or lower lip is considered. The sensory innervation to the upper lip is from the second part of the trigeminal nerve (CN V_2) and the lower lip from the third part (CN V_3). The upper lip receives its main blood supply from the superior labial artery and the lower lip from the inferior labial artery. Each of these is a branch of the facial artery. The lower lip lymphatics drain to either the ipsilateral submandibular region (lateral part of the lip) or the submental and submandibular nodes (medial part of the lip). Drainage can be to either side so tumor spread can involve bilateral neck disease. In contrast, the upper lip primarily drains to the ipsilateral submandibular nodes and tends not to cross the midline. Drainage occasionally passes to the preauricular or parotid nodes.

   Although the upper lip has three subunits (right, left, and philtral dimple), the lower lip is a single unit. This is relevant to lip surgery, because it can increase the technical difficulty of upper lip reconstruction.

3. **At conversational distances, what minimum amount of white roll mismatch is typically evident?**
   A. 1 mm

   Malalignments of the white roll as small as 1 mm can be visualized at conversational distances. This highlights the importance of accurate lip repair after trauma or tumor resection. A good tip is to mark the white roll with ink before local anesthetic infiltration to ensure accurate alignment during reconstruction or repair.

REPAIR OF VERMILION DEFECTS

4. Which one of the following statements is correct regarding defects of the vermilion?

B. Total deficiency may be treated by advancing the buccal mucosa.

Smaller vermilion defects may be reconstructed using axial myovermilion advancement flaps, V-Y advancement flaps, or a two-stage (not single-stage) lip switch procedure. Defects that are larger than 50% require either a tongue flap or advancement of the buccal mucosa. Aesthetic outcomes after a tongue flap are suboptimal compared with those of vermilion or oral mucosa flaps. The blood supply to an axial myovermilion flap is the labial artery; therefore these flaps are elevated with the muscle deep to the arterial supply.

ALGORITHMIC APPROACH TO LIP RECONSTRUCTION

5. Which one of the following statements is correct regarding lip reconstruction?

D. Perialar crescenteric advancement is a useful adjunct for upper lip reconstruction.

Perialar crescenteric flaps are useful for reconstructing a range of defect sizes, particularly when combined with other procedures such as Abbé or Bernard-Burow flaps (Fig. 39-1).

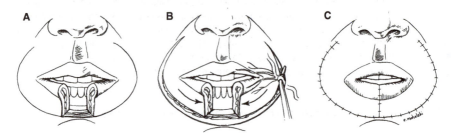

Fig. 39-1 Lower lip reconstruction with a Karapandzic flap. **A,** The width of the circumoral incision must be equal to the height of the defect at all points of the flap. **B,** The labial arteries and buccal nerve branches are identified and preserved bilaterally. **C,** Three-layer closure following medial advancement of the flaps.

Although lower lip defects of less than a third are closed directly, the same is not true for upper lip defects, because their reconstruction depends on the anatomic site. For example, lateral defects of the upper lip are commonly closed directly, but central defects may require perialar crescenteric excision, an Abbé flap, or both. Similarly, reconstruction of upper or lower lip defects that are larger than a half depends on the location of the defect. Some will require a two-stage procedure using an Abbé flap, but others can be reconstructed with single-stage techniques such as Estlander or Karapandzic flaps.

The first choice for reconstruction of a commissure defect that involves the lower lip is usually an Estlander flap (not a V-Y flap). Local flaps can be used in combination to reconstruct defects that are larger than two thirds of either lip. Free flaps are usually required in total lip reconstruction after radiation therapy or failed local flap reconstruction. However, free tissue transfer for lip reconstruction tends to give suboptimal functional and aesthetic results.

ABBÉ FLAP

6. Which one of the following statements is correct when using an Abbé flap for lip reconstruction?

E. The flap is particularly well suited for reconstruction of the philtral dimple.

Abbé[1] first described this flap for lip reconstruction in patients with double-hairlip deformities in 1898. It is particularly well suited for use in central defects of the upper lip. An Abbé flap is full thickness but not sensate and is not used for commissure defects. This flap is usually designed to be half the width of the original defect. It requires a two-stage process that requires division of the pedicle at 2 or 3 weeks. The flap receives its blood supply from the ipsilateral labial artery, which is within the orbicularis oris just deep to the white roll. To ensure safe preservation of the blood supply, a cuff of muscle should be maintained around the artery (see Fig. 39-1).

ESTLANDER FLAP

7. Which one of the following statements is correct regarding an Estlander flap?

D. Blood supply is from the contralateral labial artery of the opposite lip.

Estlander[2] originally described this flap in 1872 (Fig. 39-2). It is a good choice for reconstruction of defects of the oral commissure. The flap receives blood supply from the contralateral labial artery of the opposite lip and reconstruction is accomplished in a single stage, unlike the Abbé flap. The flap can be used for defects up to two thirds the lip width but does distort the lip and blunts the oral commissure.

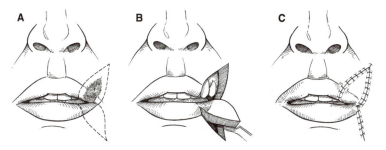

Fig. 39-2 Estlander flap for upper lip reconstruction. **A,** The lower lip flap is designed to be no more than half the size of the upper lip defect. **B,** The flap is rotated about the commissure. Blood supply is from the contralateral labial artery. **C,** Three-layer closure of the inset flap and donor site.

KARAPANDZIC FLAP

8. Which one of the following statements is correct regarding a Karapandzic flap?

D. The flap is only full thickness medially

The Karapandzic[3] flap may be used to reconstruct large central defects of either the upper or lower lips. A Karapandzic flap usually involves full-thickness dissection a short distance lateral to the defect. The remaining dissection is partial thickness with preservation of the neurovascular pedicle and oral mucosa. Hence all branches of the facial nerve should be preserved. This is achieved with gentle scissor dissection of the orbicularis oris fibers in the direction in which the nerves and vessels course. Oral competence is usually well maintained but microstomia is likely with larger defects following reconstruction with a Karapandzic flap (see Fig. 39-1). This may be particularly troublesome for patients who normally wear dentures as they may be unable to use them.

TOTAL LIP RECONSTRUCTION

9. Which one of the following statements is incorrect regarding free flap total lower lip reconstruction with a radial forearm flap?

D. Motor function is well preserved ensuring oral competence.

Total lower lip reconstruction can be achieved with a free radial forearm flap and a palmaris longus graft to support lip height. Sensory innervation can be provided with branches of the lateral cutaneous nerve. However, because this is not a functional muscle transfer, no motor innervation is achieved. For this reason, poor oral competence is observed. A preoperative Allen's test is required to assess the integrity of the radial and ulnar arterial supply to the hand. Smaller donor sites may be closed with a large hatchet flap, but larger flap defects require skin grafting. Although there are some benefits to using free tissue for lip reconstruction, the color match tends to be poor and it can be difficult to achieve aesthetically good reconstruction of specific lip landmarks.

RECONSTRUCTIVE OPTIONS FOR LIP DEFECTS

10. For the following scenarios, the best options are as follows:

A. A 70-year-old man presents with a 3.5 cm wide defect in his lower lip following an excision of a moderately differentiated squamous cell carcinoma.

b. Karapandzic flap

This defect is approximately 70% of the lower lip. The defect should be reconstructed with a Karapandzic flap.

B. A 19-year-old woman presents after a dog bite. She has a full-thickness, laterally placed upper lip defect that measures 40% of the width. The commissure is preserved.

a. Abbé flap

This defect is too large to be closed directly. It is best managed with a lower lip Abbé flap.

C. An 80-year-old man is referred after having Mohs surgery for a basal cell carcinoma that involved the central upper lip. He has a 1.5 cm defect with complete loss of his philtral dimple and columns.

a. Abbé flap

This defect can be closed directly, because it is less than a third of the lip. However, the patient's philtral dimple and columns are completely lost. A central lower lip Abbé flap will allow reconstruction of this central area and provide a better cosmetic outcome.

The Bernard-Burow flap is a complex flap reserved for reconstruction of much larger defects than described in scenarios A through C. It is shown in Fig. 39-16, *Essentials of Plastic Surgery,* second edition. The tongue flap is a two-stage procedure indicated in reconstruction of larger vermilion defects. It is associated with suboptimal appearance compared with vermilion or oral mucosal reconstructions. The radial forearm free flap as discussed in question 9 is used for total lip reconstruction so is not indicated in the scenarios described here.

REFERENCES

1. Abbé RA. A new plastic operation for the relief of deformity due to double harelip. Med Rec 53:477, 1898.
2. Estlander JA. Eine methode aus der einen lippe substanzverluste der anderen zu ersetzen. Arch Kim Chir 14:622, 1872.
3. Karapandzic M. Reconstruction of lip defects by local arterial flaps. Br J Plast Surg 27:93-97, 1974.

40. Mandibular Reconstruction

See *Essentials of Plastic Surgery*, second edition, pp. 454-461.

GENERAL PRINCIPLES

1. **What is the key reason why vascularized bone flaps are preferred for reconstruction of mandibular defects following resection of malignant tumors?**
   A. They are more resistant to the effects of radiotherapy.
   B. They encourage more radical excision margins.
   C. They facilitate reexcision where close margins are obtained.
   D. They are more cost effective than nonvascularized options.
   E. They have very low donor site morbidity.

COLLAPSING A MANDIBULAR DEFECT

2. A patient requires partial resection of the ascending ramus of the mandible, including the condylar head. **What is the main disadvantage of collapsing this defect rather than performing a bony reconstruction?**
   A. Technical difficulty
   B. Poor speech outcomes
   C. Long-term TMJ pain
   D. Difficulty swallowing
   E. Failure to reestablish a normal bite

MANDIBULAR RECONSTRUCTION PLATES

3. **Which one of the following is true of mandibular reconstruction plates as a single modality for mandibular reconstruction?**
   A. They are a reliable choice for most patients.
   B. They are ideal for reconstruction of central mandibular defects.
   C. They must be secured with nonlocking screws.
   D. They have relatively low rates of extrusion.
   E. They usually fail within 18 months following implantation.

SOFT TISSUE FLAPS FOR MANDIBULAR RECONSTRUCTION

4. **Which one of the following represents a disadvantage to using a pectoralis major flap to reconstruct a defect in the mandibular region?**
   A. The blood supply is unreliable.
   B. The vascular pedicle is too short.
   C. The flap is technically difficult to raise.
   D. The flap creates a bulge at the pivot point.
   E. A portion of the clavicle must be removed.

5. **Which one of the following is least relevant when determining the suitability for use of a nonvascularized bone graft in mandibular reconstruction?**
   A. Defect size
   B. Underlying pathology
   C. Subsequent treatment required
   D. Defect location
   E. Method of fixation

VASCULARIZED BONE FREE FLAPS

6. **Which one of the following represents a long-term advantage of using a vascularized bone graft in mandible reconstruction?**
   A. Increased strength
   B. Increased stiffness
   C. Better rates of union
   D. Superior functional outcomes
   E. All of the above

7. You are planning to use a free fibular osseocutaneous flap to reconstruct a composite mandibular body and floor of mouth defect. A 7 cm length of bone is required in conjunction with a 3 by 8 cm soft tissue skin paddle. **Which one of the following is correct?**
   A. A separate soft tissue flap is likely to be required as the skin paddle is unreliable.
   B. The bone will need to be double barreled to safely accept dental implants.
   C. Pedicle length will be limited to 5 cm when skin is being harvested.
   D. Osteotomies are safe but bone lengths greater than 2 to 3 cm should be preserved.
   E. Weight-bearing exercise should not be started before two weeks.

8. **Which one of the following is correct regarding the iliac crest free flap?**
   A. Blood supply is from the deep circumflex iliac artery, which arises from the internal iliac artery.
   B. A short pedicle length is a major disadvantage because it rarely exceeds 3 to 4 cm.
   C. Patients must be counseled regarding the risk of postoperative abdominal pain and hernia formation.
   D. Intraoral soft tissue cover is achieved by harvesting external oblique muscle with the flap.
   E. This flap provides excellent bone stock for implants and has thin pliable skin, useful for external cover.

9. **Which one of the following is considered an advantage of using a deep circumflex iliac artery (DCIA) flap over a fibula flap for reconstruction of a hemimandible?**
   A. Bone height
   B. Intraoral soft tissue cover
   C. Flap harvesting time
   D. Bone length
   E. Vessel diameter

10. **Which one of the following is correct regarding the scapular osseocutaneous flap?**
    A. The dominant blood supply is the suprascapular artery.
    B. Pedicle length is usually around 20 cm.
    C. Up to 8 cm of bone can be harvested in adult male patients.
    D. Soft tissue availability is less than that of a DCIA flap.
    E. Patient positioning can present a logistical disadvantage.

11. When raising an osseocutaneous scapula free flap, the triangular space must be located to identify the vascular pedicle. **What muscle forms the lateral border of this space?**
    A. Teres major
    B. Teres minor
    C. Rhomboid
    D. Long head of triceps
    E. Latissimus dorsi

12. **What is the major benefit of using computer-aided design for mandibular reconstruction?**
    A. Improved functional outcomes
    B. Decreased procedural costs
    C. Reduced duration of preoperative planning
    D. Improved accuracy of reconstruction
    E. Avoidance of multiple osteotomies

Answers

GENERAL PRINCIPLES
1. **What is the key reason why vascularized bone flaps are preferred for reconstruction of mandibular defects following resection of malignant tumors?**
   A. They are more resistant to the effects of radiotherapy.
   In general, patients likely to undergo postoperative radiotherapy should have autologous reconstruction, preferably using vascularized bone flaps. The principles of malignant tumor resection are that adequate margins are used to achieve complete resection irrespective of the chosen reconstruction method. Margins should not be compromised or tailored to a specific reconstruction type. The cost effectiveness of a reconstructive method is complex to assess and vascularized tissue transfer is expensive and time consuming and is unlikely to be more cost effective than other techniques. Donor site morbidity is a major consideration in any vascularized transfer and is never low.

COLLAPSING A MANDIBULAR DEFECT
2. A patient requires partial resection of the ascending ramus of the mandible, including the condylar head. **What is the main disadvantage of collapsing this defect rather than performing a bony reconstruction?**
   E. Failure to reestablish a normal bite
   Allowing the mandible to collapse without reconstruction may be acceptable for some ascending ramus or lateral defects, but will lead to deviation of the chin with malocclusion. The outcomes for speech and swallowing are generally good when using this technique. TMJ pain is not usually a problem following resection of the joint. Collapse of the mandible is a relatively straightforward procedure.

MANDIBULAR RECONSTRUCTION PLATES
3. **Which one of the following is true of mandibular reconstruction plates as a single modality for mandibular reconstruction?**
   E. They usually fail within 18 months following implantation.
   The advantages of using mandibular reconstruction plates alone are shorter operating times and avoidance of donor site morbidity. However, extrusion rates are high, especially when used in the anterior mandible. General consensus is that these techniques should be reserved for lateral defects in patients unable to tolerate longer procedures or those with short expected lifespans.

SOFT TISSUE FLAPS FOR MANDIBULAR RECONSTRUCTION
4. **Which one of the following represents a disadvantage to using a pectoralis major flap to reconstruct a defect in the mandibular region?**
   D. The flap creates a bulge at the pivot point.
   The pectoralis major is a workhorse flap for head and neck reconstruction, even with the increased popularity of free tissue transfer. It has many advantages such as the relative ease and speed with which it can be raised, the vascular supply is very reliable, reach is adequate for upper neck, and the mandibular region and the donor site is normally closed directly. It allows either muscle only or muscle and skin to be harvested and can be used to reconstruct mandibular, intraoral, or skin defects. The bulge created over the clavicle may be minimized by dissection of

the pedicle and reducing muscle bulk at the pivot point. Alternatively, the clavicle can be sectioned but this is not necessary and is rarely performed.

5. **Which one of the following is least relevant when determining the suitability for use of a nonvascularized bone graft in mandibular reconstruction?**
   E. Method of fixation
   The method of fixation is not a key consideration for determining the suitability of use in nonvascularized bone grafts as a standard approach is taken in all cases. Nonvascular bone grafts are indicated for reconstruction of mandibular defects up to 6 cm after trauma or benign tumor resection. Beyond that the failure rates of approximately 75% are just too high to justify their use. The site of defect is also important and use in lateral defects is acceptable but use in anterior mandibular defects should be avoided. Nonvascularized bone grafts are also contraindicated in cancer patients and those undergoing subsequent radiotherapy.

VASCULARIZED BONE FREE FLAPS

6. **Which one of the following represents a long-term advantage of using a vascularized bone graft in mandible reconstruction?**
   E. All of the above
   There are many advantages to using vascularized bone in reconstruction and this is why it remains the benchmark for reconstruction. Compared to nonvascularized alloplastic bone grafts, vascularized free flaps provide 40% more strength, 56% more stiffness, and superior functional outcomes.[1]

7. You are planning to use a free fibular osseocutaneous flap to reconstruct a composite mandibular body and floor of mouth defect. A 7 cm length of bone is required in conjunction with a 3 by 8 cm soft tissue skin paddle. **Which one of the following is correct?**
   D. Osteotomies are safe but bone lengths greater than 2 to 3 cm should be preserved.
   The fibula flap is a workhorse flap for mandibular reconstruction and can provide good volumes of soft tissue and bone. Because of the segmental vascular supply, it is safe to perform osteotomies when contouring to match the resected mandible, but it is advisable to maintain lengths of 3 cm and ensure the periosteum is intact in order to avoid vascular compromise. A separate soft tissue flap, such as a radial forearm, is not required in this case as the skin paddle for a fibula can provide the required skin paddle size. Although the skin island was originally thought to be unreliable, this is no longer considered to be the case, with survival rates close to 100%.
   The fibula is suitable for using osseointegrated dental implants, even though it does lack vertical height compared with the native mandible. It does not need to be double barreled in most instances, but some surgeons prefer to do so when reconstructing anterior midline defects. Pedicle length is an advantage of this flap and varies from 6 to 10 cm. The skin paddle is usually based on perforators at the junction of the mid to distal thirds of the leg and provides adequate pedicle length. Weight bearing can be commenced early in the postoperative period (between 2 and 5 days, according to surgeon and patient preference).

8. **Which one of the following is correct regarding the iliac crest free flap?**
   C. Patients must be counseled regarding the risk of postoperative abdominal pain and hernia formation.
   DCIA flaps have a role in mandibular reconstruction and some surgeons prefer to use them instead of the fibula flap. However, this flap has increased donor site complications compared with the fibula flap, including risk of postoperative hernia and lower abdominal/hip pain. Blood

supply is from the deep circumflex iliac artery which arises from the external iliac (not the internal) close to the deep inferior epigastric artery, used in a DIEP flap. A disadvantage of this flap is its short pedicle (up to 7 cm is typically quoted). This can be improved by moving the site of bone harvest more posteriorly. The skin paddle tends to be bulky and perforating vessels are not always present, but muscle can be harvested with the flap to provide intraoral cover. This muscle is the internal oblique (not the external oblique) and mucosalizes rapidly when placed intraorally. The DCIA bone flap provides an excellent foundation for the use of dental implants.

9. **Which one of the following is considered an advantage of using a deep circumflex iliac artery (DCIA) flap over a fibula flap for reconstruction of a hemimandible?**
   A. **Bone height**

   DCIA flaps provide superior bone height when compared with fibula flaps. This may be helpful for placing dental implants, although some surgeons feel that positioning a fibula flap more superiorly at the expense of the inferior mandibular contour or double barreling it anteriorly will address this problem. While a fibula flap can give more bone length (up to 25 cm in adult males), a DCIA gives adequate length for a hemimandible. Both flaps can provide intraoral soft tissue cover. The fibula flap achieves this with a pliable skin paddle, while the DCIA does so with muscle cover from the internal oblique. Harvest time is probably similar and depends on surgeon experience and patient body habitus. Both flaps have similar vessel diameter, typically 2 to 3 mm, so there would not normally be a significant difference in anastomotic difficulty between the two flaps.

10. **Which one of the following is correct regarding the scapular osseocutaneous flaps?**
    E. **Patient positioning can present a logistical disadvantage.**

    The dominant blood supply to the osseocutaneous scapula flap is the circumflex scapular artery arising from the subscapular vessels. The skin islands are termed scapular and parascapular and receive blood supply through the transverse or descending branches of the circumflex scapular artery, respectively. Bone is usually harvested from the lateral border of the scapula commencing 2 cm below the glenohumeral joint towards the scapular tip. In addition to the circumflex scapular artery, the scapula also receives blood supply through the thoracodorsal artery which normally provides the angular branch to the scapula tip. When raised on the thoracodorsal axis, the flap may include the latissimus dorsi muscle and the overlying skin. It is possible to raise a chimeric flap using both thoracodorsal and circumflex scapular vessels. For this reason, the scapular osseocutaneous flap offers a large amount of soft tissue cover in addition to length of bone, up to 14 cm in adult males. Two main disadvantages of this flap are that patients typically require intraoperatively turning, which may limit a two-team simultaneous approach, and that the bone harvested is thin compared with DCIA or fibula.

11. **When raising an osseocutaneous scapula free flap, the triangular space must be located to identify the vascular pedicle. What muscle forms the lateral border of this space?**
    D. **Long head of triceps**

    The circumflex scapular pedicle supplies the scapula flaps and passes through the triangular space. This space is formed from the following structures: superiorly, teres minor; inferiorly, teres major; laterally, long head of triceps (Fig. 40-1).

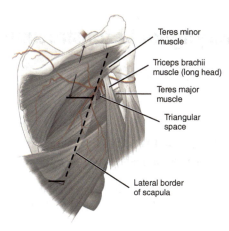

Fig. 40-1 The triangular space contains the vascular pedicle for the scapula flap. It can be identified by palpation approximately two fifths the distance from the midportion of the scapula spine to its inferior border.

12. **What is the major benefit of using computer-aided design for mandibular reconstruction?**
    D. Improved accuracy of reconstruction
    Computer-aided design is becoming popular as a tool to help plan and execute reconstruction of complex bony defects such as the mandible and maxilla. Three-dimensional computer images of the mandible and fibula are generated and a virtual mandibular defect is created. Cutting jigs are manufactured preoperatively to assist in bony resection and fibula harvest. The main advantages are that time in the OR is reduced and accuracy or reconstruction is improved. However, it is costly and requires additional time for preplanning. Whether this translates into improved functional outcomes is unknown.

REFERENCE

1. Goldberg VM, Shaffer JW, Field G, et al. Biology of vascularized bone grafts. Orthop Clin North Am 18:197-205, 1987

41. Pharyngeal Reconstruction

See *Essentials of Plastic Surgery*, second edition, pp. 462-477.

NASOPHARYNGEAL ANATOMY

1. **Which one of the following represents the posterior boundary of the nasopharynx?**
   A. Lower skull base (clivus) and C1 vertebra
   B. Sphenoid sinus and upper skull base
   C. Soft palate
   D. Choanae
   E. Retropharyngeal space

OROPHARYNGEAL ANATOMY

2. **Which one of the following represents the inferior boundary of the oropharynx?**
   A. Base of tongue
   B. Circumvallate papillae
   C. Hyoid and valleculae
   D. Pharyngeal wall
   E. Tonsillar fossa

HYPOPHARYNGEAL ANATOMY

3. **Which one of the following is a subsite of the hypopharynx?**
   A. Soft palate
   B. Tonsillar fossa
   C. Tongue base
   D. Palatoglossal folds
   E. Piriform sinus

REFERRED OTALGIA IN HEAD AND NECK CANCER

4. **Which one of the following cranial nerves accounts for a patient presenting with otalgia as the only symptom of a head and neck cancer?**
   A. Trigeminal nerve
   B. Vagus nerve
   C. Vestibulocochlear nerve
   D. Cervical plexus
   E. Accessory nerve

NASOPHARYNGEAL CARCINOMA

5. **Which one of the following is not a risk factor for the development of nasopharyngeal carcinoma?**
   A. A diet high in preservatives and nitrosamines
   B. Wood dust
   C. Epstein-Barr virus
   D. Genetic predisposition
   E. Tobacco smoking

CLINICAL ASSESSMENT OF NASOPHARYNGEAL CARCINOMA

6. A 50-year-old patient presents with nasal obstruction, epistaxis, and conductive hearing loss secondary to otitis media. You obtain a full history and perform a basic examination with fiberoptic nasoendoscopy, which reveals a suspicious area in the nasopharynx. *What is the next most appropriate step in management?*
   A. PET-CT scan
   B. Examination under anesthesia and biopsy
   C. Ultrasound-guided fine-needle aspiration cytology
   D. Multislice CT of the head, neck, and thorax
   E. MRI of the skull base

HUMAN PAPILLOMAVIRUS IN HEAD AND NECK CANCER

7. *Which one of the following tumor sites is strongly associated with human papillomavirus (HPV) 16 and 18 in younger patient groups?*
   A. Cervical esophagus
   B. Larynx
   C. Fossa of Rosenmüller
   D. Tonsils
   E. Nasopharynx

TYPES OF HEAD AND NECK TUMORS

8. For each of the following descriptions, select the most likely diagnosis. *(Each option may be used once, more than once, or not at all.)*
   A. This cancer has a much greater incidence in patients with Plummer-Vinson syndrome.
   B. Unilateral otitis media or bilateral level V nodes in an adult is particularly suspicious of this cancer subtype.
   C. This cancer is associated with Epstein-Barr virus and the Guangdong province of China.

   Options:
   a. Oropharyngeal
   b. Papillary thyroid
   c. Medullary thyroid
   d. Unknown primary
   e. Nasopharyngeal
   f. Hypopharyngeal
   g. Salivary gland

PHASES OF SWALLOWING

9. The process of swallowing has multiple phases. *Which one of the following represents the most important phase?*
   A. Oral preparatory
   B. Oral
   C. Pharyngeal
   D. Esophageal

EVALUATION OF SWALLOWING

10. Assessment of swallowing is vital in patients with pharyngeal carcinoma. *Which one of the following modalities provides the most comprehensive noninvasive assessment of all stages of swallowing?*
    A. Bedside assessment with colored fluids
    B. Videofluoroscopy
    C. MRI
    D. Endoscopy
    E. Contrast CT

MANAGEMENT OF HEAD AND NECK TUMORS

11. **Which one of the following is most likely to be avoided by performing robotic surgery in patients with pharyngeal carcinoma?**
    A. Radiotherapy
    B. Neck dissection
    C. Soft tissue reconstruction
    D. Mandibulotomy
    E. Dental extraction

12. **Which one of the following tumor sites is most likely to receive chemo/radiation therapy as its primary treatment modality?**
    A. Nasopharynx
    B. Oropharynx
    C. Hypopharynx
    D. Oral cavity
    E. Thyroid

OUTCOMES IN HEAD AND NECK CANCER

13. **In general, which site has the worst oncologic outcome of all the head and neck cancers?**
    A. Oral cavity
    B. Thyroid
    C. Oropharynx
    D. Hypopharynx
    E. Nasopharynx

RECONSTRUCTION OF THE HYPOPHARYNX

14. A patient has a circumferential defect after resection of a hypopharyngeal tumor. **According to the classification of Disa et al, what type of defect is this?**
    A. Type I
    B. Type II
    C. Type III
    D. Type IV
    E. Type V

RECONSTRUCTION FOLLOWING TOTAL LARYNGOPHARYNGECTOMY

15. You see a patient in clinic following a total laryngopharyngectomy with reconstruction and insertion of a speech valve for treatment of a T4 tumor. Their speech is now reasonably clear but they have a wet, coarse quality to their voice. **Which one of the following is the most likely reconstruction method used?**
    A. Pedicled pectoralis major flap
    B. Free radial forearm flap
    C. Free anterolateral thigh flap
    D. Laryngeal transplantation
    E. Free jejunum flap

16. **When reconstructing a circumferential defect of the hypopharynx with a free ALT flap, which one of the following should be undertaken to reduce the risk of early salivary fistula formation?**
    A. Early use of total parenteral nutrition (TPN)
    B. Use of nonabsorbable sutures at the esophageal anastomosis
    C. Delaying postoperative radiotherapy
    D. Use of a salivary pharyngeal bypass tube
    E. Use of a proton pump inhibitor

17. Which one of the following is correct when managing patients with posttumor resection defects of the oropharynx?
A. Most soft palate defects are well managed with prosthetic devices.
B. Larger tongue base defects are more safely treated with laryngectomy.
C. Pharyngeal wall defects usually require free tissue reconstruction.
D. Local flaps for tongue base reconstruction are associated with low complication rates.
E. Large tongue defects benefit from free muscle transfer with motor reinnervation.

Answers

NASOPHARYNGEAL ANATOMY

1. **Which one of the following represents the posterior boundary of the nasopharynx?**
   A. Lower skull base (clivus) and C1 vertebra
   The nasopharynx is a narrow space posterior to the nasal cavity and above the soft palate (Fig. 41-1). It is located immediately below the central skull base and has the following boundaries:
   Superior: Sphenoid sinus and upper skull base (clivus)
   Inferior: Soft palate
   Anterior: Choanae
   Posterior: Lower skull base (clivus) and first cervical vertebra
   The retropharyngeal space is located at the level of the hypopharynx, which forms its posterior boundary.

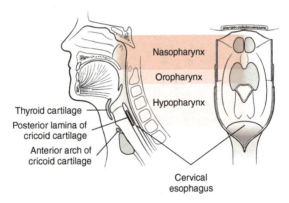

Fig. 41-1 Subdivisions of the pharynx.

OROPHARYNGEAL ANATOMY

2. **Which one of the following represents the inferior boundary of the oropharynx?**
   C. Hyoid and valleculae
   The oropharynx extends from the junction of the hard and soft palates to the aryepiglottic folds. With the hyoid and valleculae representing the inferior boundary. The base of tongue and the circumvallate papillae represent the ventral boundary, whereas the dorsal pharyngeal wall is the dorsal boundary. The lateral boundary is formed by the tonsillar fossa (see Fig. 41-1).

Chapter 41 ■ Pharyngeal Reconstruction   331

HYPOPHARYNGEAL ANATOMY

3. Which one of the following is a subsite of the hypopharynx?
E. Piriform sinus

The bilateral piriform sinuses represent subsites of the hypopharynx. The other subsites of the hypopharynx are the postcricoid area and the posterior hypopharyngeal wall. The soft palate, tonsils, tongue base, and oropharyngeal walls are subsites of the oropharynx.

REFERRED OTALGIA IN HEAD AND NECK CANCER

4. Which one of the following cranial nerves accounts for a patient presenting with otalgia as the only symptom of a head and neck cancer?
B. Vagus nerve

A patient may present with referred otalgia in the presence of a pharyngeal tumor. This occurs because sensory fibers from the pharyngeal plexus synapse in the jugular ganglion with Arnold's nerve, which supplies the external auditory meatus. Arnold's nerve is primarily formed from the vagus, with contributions from the facial and glossopharyngeal nerves.

NASOPHARYNGEAL CARCINOMA

5. Which one of the following is not a risk factor for the development of nasopharyngeal carcinoma?
E. Tobacco smoking

Although smoking is a risk factor for most head and neck cancers, this is not the case for nasopharyngeal tumors. The key risk factors are ethnicity (Eskimos, Polynesians, and indigenous Mediterraneans), genetic alterations with chromosomal deletions, dietary nitrosamines, and Epstein-Barr virus.

CLINICAL ASSESSMENT OF NASOPHARYNGEAL CARCINOMA

6. A 50-year-old patient presents with nasal obstruction, epistaxis, and conductive hearing loss secondary to otitis media. You obtain a full history and perform a basic examination with fiberoptic nasoendoscopy, which reveals a suspicious area in the nasopharynx. What is the next most appropriate step in management?
B. Examination under anesthesia and biopsy

Patients who have visible evidence of tumor during nasoendoscopy in the clinic should undergo examination under anesthesia for biopsy and formal assessment of the upper aerodigestive tract. Blind biopsies of the fossa of Rosenmüller should be performed at the same time. Once pathology is diagnosed, it should be staged using a multislice CT of the head, neck, and thorax. An MRI of the skull base is useful if the tumor is advanced. If an occult primary tumor of the nasopharynx is suspected, then a PET-CT scan before biopsy is indicated. If nodal neck disease is evident (which is not the case in this patient), the enlarged node or nodes can be investigated with ultrasound-guided fine-needle aspiration cytology.[1]

HUMAN PAPILLOMAVIRUS IN HEAD AND NECK CANCER

7. Which one of the following tumor sites is strongly associated with human papillomavirus (HPV) 16 and 18 in younger patient groups?
D. Tonsils

Oropharyngeal cancer has become increasingly common in recent years. Its incidence has doubled in the United States and the United Kingdom over the past decade. More than half of all new oropharyngeal cases are HPV-positive, and the tonsils and tongue base are particularly common subsites. HPV is also recognized in some oral cavity tumors such as the tongue, lip, and floor of the mouth. It also carries a better prognosis and treatment may be deescalated. HPV-associated squamous cell carcinoma disease typically presents in younger people in whom the usual risk factors for head and neck cancer (that is, high alcohol intake and smoking) are absent.

TYPES OF HEAD AND NECK TUMORS

8. For the following descriptions, the diagnoses are as follows:
   A. **This cancer has a much greater incidence in patients with Plummer-Vinson syndrome.**
      f. Hypopharyngeal
   B. **Unilateral otitis media or bilateral level V nodes in an adult is particularly suspicious of this cancer subtype.**
      e. Nasopharyngeal
   C. **This cancer that is associated with Epstein-Barr virus and the Guangdong province of China.**
      e. Nasopharyngeal

   Plummer-Vinson syndrome is a condition of unknown cause that is typically seen in postmenopausal women presenting with dysphagia, esophageal webs, and iron deficiency anemia. It is also associated with postcricoid cancer, glossitis, and splenomegaly.

   Nasopharyngeal cancer has an incidence of 1:100,000 in the United States and in white Europeans, but the incidence is much higher in inhabitants of the Guangdong province of China 30:100,000. The risk is reduced to approximately 1:100,000 in second-generation immigrants to Western societies. Suspicious findings suggestive of nasopharyngeal cancer include unilateral otitis media in an adult, bilateral level V nodes, an unknown primary lesion, and skull base symptoms. These findings should be investigated as discussed in question 6.

PHASES OF SWALLOWING

9. The process of swallowing has multiple phases. **Which one of the following represents the most important phase?**
   D. Pharyngeal

   Swallowing is the coordinated act that propels a bolus of food from the oral cavity to the esophagus while protecting the airway. It has four key phases which are the oral preparatory, oral, pharyngeal, and esophageal. Of these, the most important is the pharyngeal phase, as it involves the transit of food into the esophagus while providing airway protection. This key phase may be impaired in patients with pharyngeal tumors, either by the tumor mass itself or secondary to surgical or radiotherapy treatment. The pharyngeal phase is programmed and involves coordination between the medullary inputs of swallow and respiration. Respiration ceases for a fraction of a second during swallow. This requires some cortical input from tongue motion. Triggering of this phase programs five activities: closure of the velopharynx to prevent food reflux, retraction of the tongue base to propel food, contraction of the pharynx to clear residue, elevation and closure of the larynx, and opening of the cricoesophageal and upper esophageal sphincters to allow the food bolus to pass through.

EVALUATION OF SWALLOWING

10. Assessment of swallowing is vital in patients with pharyngeal carcinoma. **Which one of the following modalities provides the most comprehensive noninvasive assessment of all stages of swallowing?**
    B. Videofluoroscopy

    Swallowing may be assessed in a number of different ways. Clinically it may be assessed at the bedside using small volumes of fluid. During the assessment, the facial, lip, tongue, laryngeal, and respiratory control can be observed. When checking for postoperative fistula formation, the use of colored fluids can be helpful. The best modality for noninvasive assessment of all phases of the swallow is with videofluoroscopy using a contrast agent such as barium. Endoscopic assessment of swallow can be performed such as with the FEEST test. This is a "functional endoscopic evaluation of swallowing with sensory testing" where a trained observer uses an endoscope to watch the swallow process in real time. Sensation can be assessed with puffs of air.

MANAGEMENT OF HEAD AND NECK TUMORS

11. Which one of the following is most likely to be avoided by performing robotic surgery in patients with pharyngeal carcinoma?
D. Mandibulotomy

Mandibulotomy is a technique where the mandible is split in order to obtain access to the pharynx or oral cavity in major tumor resection. It generally involves an extended neck incision (as a continuation of a neck dissection wound) passing over the chin in the midline and through the full thickness of the lower lip. The mandible is then opened like a book (mandibular swing) for access. Minimally invasive surgery with robotic assistance can avoid the need for traditional transcervical access with a mandibulotomy and mandibular swing, thereby reducing postoperative morbidity and scarring.

Robotic surgery is one of a number of recent advances in the management of head and neck cancer patients. For example, free tissue transfer has allowed more complex defects to be functionally reconstructed, selective neck dissection has allowed preservation of unaffected lymph node basins and other key structures such as the IJV, spinal accessory, and sternocleidomastoid. Laser surgery has added another dimension to surgical tumor resection as an alternative to traditional blade dissection. Advances in radiotherapy with intensity modulated radiotherapy (IMRT) have meant that radiotherapy doses are more directed to the malignant tissues, resulting in less dosing to adjacent healthy tissues.

In spite of the benefits of minimally invasive robotic surgery, patients are likely to still require soft tissue reconstruction with local or free tissue transfer, neck dissection, and postoperative radiotherapy depending on tumor type. Dental extractions are not generally performed to help access but are indicated in patients expected to undergo postoperative radiotherapy or those with poor dentition.[2,3]

12. Which one of the following tumor sites is most likely to receive chemo/radiation therapy as its primary treatment modality?
A. Nasopharynx

Radiation therapy is the main treatment modality for nasopharyngeal carcinoma. Surgery is usually used only in the following selected circumstances:
- In salvage or recurrent cases
- To obtain tissue for diagnostic purposes
- To obtain tissue from clinically involved neck nodes
- To treat otitis media secondary to effusion

In contrast, surgery is more commonly the first-line treatment for the other head and neck tumor subsites, although this will depend on the tumor type and site, as radiotherapy is also used for many patients.

OUTCOMES IN HEAD AND NECK CANCER

13. *In general, which site has the worst oncologic outcome of all the head and neck cancers?*
   D. Hypopharynx
   In general, hypopharyngeal tumors have the worst outcomes. At least three quarters of patients with hypopharyngeal tumors present late with stage III or IV disease. Patients with early disease (that is, stage I or II) are asymptomatic at presentation. Patients with advanced disease most commonly present with a neck mass. Other symptoms include dysphagia, referred otalgia, and respiratory difficulties. The 5-year survival for patients with locally invasive cancer is less than 35%.

RECONSTRUCTION OF THE HYPOPHARYNX

14. A patient has a circumferential defect after resection of a hypopharyngeal tumor. *According to the classification of Disa et al, what type of defect is this?*
   B. Type II
   Disa et al[4] described a classification system for defects of the hypopharynx that require reconstruction. Type I defects involve less than 50% of the circumference, type II involve more than 50% of the circumference, and type III are extensive noncircumferential defects that involve multiple anatomic levels. This is clinically relevant as reconstruction options are based on the extent of the defect created by resection. Local flaps such as pectoralis major, are more often used for partial defects, while free tissue transfer flaps are used for larger and circumferential defects.

RECONSTRUCTION FOLLOWING TOTAL LARYNGOPHARYNGECTOMY

15. You see a patient in clinic following a total laryngopharyngectomy with reconstruction and insertion of a speech valve, for treatment of a T4 tumor. Their speech is now reasonably clear but they have a wet, coarse quality to their voice. *Which one of the following is the most likely reconstruction method used?*
   E. Free jejunum flap
   There are a number of reconstructive procedures used following total laryngopharyngectomy and they include free and pedicled tissue transfers. The primary purpose is to provide a conduit for food and saliva, a safe airway, and provide the potential for voice rehabilitation. A typical combination is to use a free flap, such as a tubed anterolateral thigh flap (ALT) or free jejunum, and then insert a prosthetic device containing a one-way valve between the posterior trachea and the anterior esophagus. This allows the creation of sound as air is diverted into the esophagus during speech. There remains debate as to the best flap for circumferential reconstruction of the pharynx, with ALT and jejunum remaining the most popular, each having different advantages. The ALT is useful in thinner patients and is particularly versatile where complex defects are present. Speech outcomes tend to be good and surgery avoids an intraabdominal approach. The free jejunum is a good size match and the moist mucosal tube with retained peristalsis may improve swallowing function. However, the mucus production can impair speech intelligibility and may result in a wet, coarse voice.

16. *When reconstructing a circumferential defect of the hypopharynx with a free ALT flap, which one of the following should be undertaken to reduce the risk of early salivary fistula formation?*
   D. Use of a salivary pharyngeal bypass tube
   When reconstructing the pharynx with a free ALT flap, the risk of salivary fistula formation can be reduced by inserting a salivary pharyngeal bypass tube within the neopharynx, bridging both

proximal and distal anastomoses. Salivary bypass tubes are clear silicone tubes, also called Montgomery[5] tubes that come in different sizes. The benefits of a bypass tube are to protect the anastomoses from saliva and stent open the neopharynx, thereby potentially also reducing the risk of stricture formation. The anastomoses are usually sutured with absorbable sutures such as Vicryl, as their presence is only required until healing has occurred, which should be one to two weeks during which time the patient is given nothing by mouth. Early feeding and hydration can begin with either a nasogastric or gastrostomy tube. There is no role for TPN where enteral feeding is possible. Use of a proton pump inhibitor has no direct effect on fistula formation. Many patients will require postoperative radiotherapy and this typically begins four to six weeks after surgery. Therefore, delaying postoperative radiotherapy is not required and of no routine benefit with regard to early fistula formation. Keeping to safe oncologic principles, radiotherapy should be started early once healing is complete. Long-term complications of radiotherapy include both stricture and fistula formation.

17. Which one of the following is correct when managing patients with posttumor resection defects of the oropharynx?
B. Larger tongue base defects are more safely treated with laryngectomy.
The tongue base is critical for airway protection and swallowing. As such, when much of the tongue base will be sacrificed during tumor resection, a laryngectomy should be considered to decrease the risk of aspiration after treatment. Although prosthetic devices are useful for isolated hard palate defects, soft palate defects are usually best reconstructed with local or imported soft tissue. Soft palate defects larger than 50% lead to velopharyngeal insufficiency. Small pharyngeal defects can be left to heal by secondary intention or closed directly. Large defects are often best reconstructed with free tissue flaps such as the radial forearm or ALT. Local flaps may be used for oropharyngeal reconstruction but are not usually recommended for the tongue, as they can cause deformation and tethering. Furthermore, they often lack the bulk required for adequate reconstruction, and flaps such as the platysma myocutaneous flap have high complication rates. Following total or subtotal glossectomy, outcomes for speech and swallowing are typically poor and there is no proven benefit in using muscle flaps with motor reinnervation.

REFERENCES

1. Roland NJ, Palleri V, eds. Head and Neck Cancer: Multidisciplinary Management Guidelines, ed 4. London: ENTUK, 2011.
2. Selber JC. Transoral robotic reconstruction of oropharyngeal defects: a case series. Plast Reconstr Surg 126:1978, 2010.
3. Selber JC, Serletti JM, Weinstein G, et al. Transoral robotic free flap reconstruction of oropharyngeal defects: a preclinical investigation. Plast Reconstr Surg 125:896, 2010.
4. Disa JJ, Pusic AL, Hidalgo DA, et al. Microvascular reconstruction of the hypopharynx: defect classification, treatment algorithm, and functional outcome based on 165 consecutive cases. Plast Reconstr Surg 111:652-660, 2003.
5. Montgomery WW. Plastic esophageal tube. Ann Otol Rhinol Laryngol 64:418-421, 1955.

42. Facial Reanimation

See *Essentials of Plastic Surgery*, second edition, pp. 478-497.

FACIAL NERVE ANATOMY

1. A patient presents with a progressive left-sided facial nerve palsy. Clinical examination reveals a complete unilateral paralysis of facial mimetic muscles and loss of taste to the anterior two thirds of the tongue. Hearing is bilaterally normal and sensation to the palate is preserved. ***At which anatomic location is the causal lesion likely to be present?***
   A. Intracranially at the facial nerve nucleus
   B. Within the labyrinthine segment
   C. Within the tympanic segment
   D. Within the mastoid segment
   E. Within the parotid gland

2. You receive a referral letter for a patient with a diagnosis of acoustic neuroma. The letter states the patient has evidence of Hitselberger's sign. ***What specifically would you expect to find when examining this patient?***
   A. Decreased taste sensation to the tongue
   B. Pain during facial movement
   C. Reduced sensation to the external auditory canal
   D. The inability to tolerate loud sounds
   E. A dry, gritty, inflamed eye

3. ***Which one of the following is correct regarding the anatomy of the facial nerve?***
   A. The facial nerve nucleus originates in the medulla with the geniculate ganglion.
   B. The first part of the extratemporal nerve lies deeper in children.
   C. There are nine different branching patterns of the extratemporal nerve.
   D. The frontal nerve usually passes 0.5 cm lateral to the lateral end of the brow.
   E. Risk of traumatic shearing is greatest at the junction of labyrinthine and tympanic segments.

FACIAL MUSCULATURE

4. ***The three deepest facial muscles receive innervation from their superficial surface and are the following:***
   A. Depressor anguli oris, zygomaticus major, and orbicularis oculi
   B. Depressor labii inferioris, risorius, and platysma
   C. Orbicularis oris, levator labii superioris, and levator labii superioris alaeque nasi
   D. Mentalis, levator anguli oris, and buccinator
   E. Mentalis, levator labii superioris, and buccinator

5. Match each of the following descriptions to the most appropriate choice from the options. (Each option may be used once, more than once, or not at all.)
   A. This muscle is the major contributor to production of a perceived smile.
   B. Patients may request botulinum toxin injection of this muscle to alleviate a frown.
   C. Patients who will have neck dissection need to be counseled about dysfunction of this muscle, which leads to weakness of the lower lip.

   Options:
   a. Levator labii superioris alaeque nasi
   b. Frontalis
   c. Corrugator supercilii
   d. Risorius
   e. Levator anguli oris
   f. Zygomaticus minor
   g. Zygomaticus major
   h. Depressor labii inferioris
   i. Mentalis

6. For each of the following clinical scenarios, select the most likely diagnosis from the options. (Each option may be used once, more than once, or not at all.)
   A. An 80-year-old farmer presents with a progressive global unilateral facial paralysis. On examination he has a firm palpable preauricular swelling and scarring from a partial pinnectomy.
   B. A 19-year-old pregnant woman presents to her general practitioner with new-onset complete unilateral facial paralysis. She first noticed the problem on awakening in the morning. On examination she has no other physical findings of note.
   C. A 51-year-old woman presents with her third episode of facial paralysis. On examination she has evidence of facial swelling and tongue fissures.

   Options:
   a. Primary parotid malignancy
   b. Pleomorphic salivary adenoma
   c. Metastatic squamous cell carcinoma
   d. Bell's palsy
   e. Ramsay Hunt syndrome
   f. Melkersson-Rosenthal syndrome
   g. Lyme disease
   h. Acoustic neuroma

PEDIATRIC FACIAL PALSY

7. Which one of the following statements is correct regarding facial palsy?
   A. Facial paralysis is common with hemifacial microsomia.
   B. All extratemporal facial nerve branches are affected in congenital unilateral lower lip palsy (CULLP).
   C. Hemifacial spasm is much more commonly observed in adults.
   D. Bell's palsy does not generally occur in children.
   E. Cholesteotoma is an infectious cause of facial palsy.

8. Which one of the following would not be expected in a patient with Möbius syndrome?
   A. Hyperacusis
   B. Limb abnormalities
   C. Inability to abduct the eye
   D. Strabismus
   E. Small jaw

GRADING FACIAL NERVE FUNCTION

9. A patient presents in the facial palsy clinic after being diagnosed with Bell's palsy. Examination shows complete eye closure with some effort, moderate weakness of the forehead, and the ability to achieve oral competence with maximum effort. **What is the most likely facial palsy grading according to the House-Brackmann scale?**
   A. II
   B. III
   C. IV
   D. V
   E. VI

SURGICAL MANAGEMENT OF FACIAL PALSY

10. For each of the following clinical scenarios, select the most appropriate treatment plan from the options. (Each option may be used once, more than once, or not at all.)
    A. A 40-year-old man presents with incompletely resolved Bell's palsy of 5 years duration that affects his left brow, resulting in ptosis on this side only. This is now starting to affect vision and cosmesis.
    B. A 53-year-old woman is unable to fully close her right eye 16 months after facial nerve injury. The eye is mildly inflamed, with evidence of epiphora.
    C. A patient has lower lid ectropion after a left-sided facial nerve palsy. Examination shows laxity of the lower lid soft tissues, corneal irritation, and epiphora.

    Options:
    a. Insertion of an upper lid gold weight
    b. Upper lid blepharoplasty
    c. Division of Müller's muscle
    d. Superciliary brow lift
    e. Cross-face nerve graft
    f. Corneal neurotization
    g. Canthoplasty or a lid-shortening procedure
    h. Endoscopic brow lift

11. For each of the following clinical scenarios, select the most appropriate treatment plan from the options. (Each option may be used once, more than once, or not at all.)
    A. A young patient presents 3 years after injury to the facial nerve and wishes to have facial reanimation surgery to improve resting symmetry and re-create a dynamic smile.
    B. A patient presents with partial facial nerve paralysis after a recent wound to the preauricular region.
    C. A frail, elderly patient presents 15 months after injury to the facial nerve during a parotidectomy. The buccal and zygomatic branches are completely paralyzed. The patient has significant cardiovascular problems and diabetes mellitus.

    Options:
    a. Babysitter procedure
    b. Static reanimation with fascia lata grafts
    c. Immediate surgical exploration and direct nerve repair or grafting
    d. Cross-face nerve graft
    e. Sliding temporalis myoplasty
    f. Cross-face nerve graft and delayed free functional muscle transfer
    g. No surgical intervention

SURGICAL MANAGEMENT OF FACIAL PALSY

12. In a 45-year-old patient with segmental extratemporal facial nerve loss following radical parotidectomy, which one of the following is the most suitable immediate reconstruction method?
    A. Direct nerve repair
    B. Cross-face nerve graft
    C. Ipsilateral facial nerve graft
    D. Temporalis transfer
    E. Free gracilis transfer

13. Which one of the following techniques may be useful in patients who have sustained marginal mandibular nerve injury?
    A. Temporalis transfer
    B. Masseter transfer
    C. Free gracilis transfer
    D. Digastric transfer
    E. Partial pectoralis minor transfer

Answers

FACIAL NERVE ANATOMY

1. A patient presents with a progressive left-sided facial nerve palsy. Clinical examination reveals a complete unilateral paralysis of facial mimetic muscles and loss of taste to the anterior two thirds of the tongue. Hearing is bilaterally normal and sensation to the palate is preserved. *At which anatomic location is the causal lesion likely to be present?*
   D. Within the mastoid segment
   The path of the facial nerve can be divided into three main segments: intracranial, intratemporal, and extratemporal. This is clinically relevant as knowledge of the anatomy can help identify the site of damage or compression of the nerve. There are no branches within the intracranial segment, so a lesion at this site would cause complete loss of facial nerve function with no sparing of individual branches. The intratemporal segment has three subdivisions: labyrinthine, tympanic, and mastoid (Fig. 42-1). Four nerve branches are given off within this region in the following order: the greater petrosal nerve (within the labyrinthine section), the nerve to stapedius, the sensory branch to the external auditory canal, and the branch to chorda tympani (within the mastoid section). The patient described has a lesion affecting the chorda tympani and the extratemporal nerve, with sparing of the greater petrosal nerve; the nerve to stapedius and the nerve to external auditory meatus. Therefore the lesion is located within the distal mastoid segment. A lesion within the parotid would spare all four of the intratemporal branches.

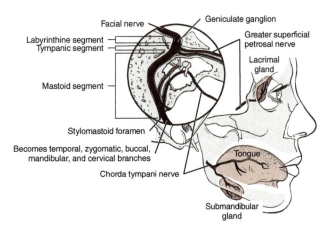

Fig. 42-1 Anatomy and relations of the facial nerve.

2. You receive a referral letter for a patient with a diagnosis of acoustic neuroma. The letter states the patient has evidence of Hitselberger's sign. **What specifically would you expect to find when examining this patient?**
   C. **Reduced sensation to the external auditory canal**
      Hitselberger's sign refers to hypesthesia of the external auditory canal, secondary to compression or damage to the sensory branch of the facial nerve within the mastoid segment of the intratemporal nerve pathway.[1] Hitselberger and House[1] described this in 1966 as an early diagnostic indicator of acoustic neuroma formation. Decreased taste sensation to the tongue would occur secondary to compression of the chorda tympani, which joins the lingual nerve to supply parasympathetic innervations to the submandibular and sublingual glands, as well as taste to the anterior two thirds of the tongue. Pain during facial movement is more likely to be associated with trigeminal or dental pain rather than facial nerve compression. Sound dampening is controlled by the nerve to stapedius which originates in the mastoid segment. A dry, gritty eye may well be present in association with a facial nerve palsy as a result of the incomplete eye closure and loss of the corneal reflex but is not specific to Hitselberger's sign.

3. *Which one of the following is correct regarding the anatomy of the facial nerve?*
   E. **Risk of traumatic shearing is greatest at the junction of labyrinthine and tympanic segments.**
      The junction between the labyrinthine and tympanic segments is formed by an acute angle, and shearing commonly occurs at this site. In addition, the labyrinthine segment is also the narrowest part so the nerve is at greatest risk of compression, secondary to edema at this site. The facial nerve nucleus is located in the dorsolateral pons, not the medulla; and the geniculate ganglion is present within the intratemporal segment. The first part of the extratemporal facial nerve lies more superficially in children under the age of 2 and is therefore more prone to injury at this site.
      Davis et al[2] described six (not nine) different extratemporal facial nerve branching patterns. Of these, a type III is the most common, representing 28% (see Fig. 42-2, *Essentials of Plastic Surgery*, second edition). The common theme is that after exiting the stylomastoid foramen, branches are given off to supply the posterior belly of digastrics and occipitalis muscle. Then the main nerve trunk divides into superior and inferior sections which collectively form the facial nerve branches most commonly recognized: temporal, zygomatic, buccal, marginal mandibular, and cervical. The surface marking for the temporal nerve passes from 0.5 cm below the tragus to 1.5 cm above the lateral brow. This is referred to as *Pitanguy's line*.[3] (See Fig. 42-4, *Essentials of Plastic Surgery*, second edition).

FACIAL MUSCULATURE

4. *The three deepest facial muscles receive innervation from their superficial surface and are the following:*
   D. **Mentalis, levator anguli oris, and buccinator**
      The mentalis, levator anguli oris, and buccinator muscles represent the deepest layer of facial musculature and receive their innervation on their superficial surfaces (see Fig. 42-5, *Essentials of Plastic Surgery*, second edition). All other muscles receive innervation on their deep surface. The facial musculature comprises 23 paired muscles and the orbicularis oris, grouped into four layers. Those described in A (depressor anguli oris, zygomaticus major, and orbicularis oculi) represent layer one and are the most superficial. Option B (depressor labii inferioris, risorius, and platysma) includes some of the muscles in layer two. Layer three contains only two muscles: orbicularis oris and levator labii superioris.

5. *For the following descriptions, the best options are as follows:*
   A. This muscle is the major contributor to production of a perceived smile.
   g. **Zygomaticus major**
   The major muscle involved in the production of a smile is the zygomaticus major. A recent study has shown that observers perceive a smile when the zygomaticus major functions to achieve 40% of its maximal movement.[4] Many other facial muscles are involved in smiling such as the orbicularis oculi, zygomaticus minor, and levator anguli oris.
   B. Patients may request botulinum toxin injection of this muscle to alleviate a frown.
   c. **Corrugator supercilii**
   Some patients are concerned about appearing tired or grumpy because of a frown and vertical forehead lines. This can be treated with botulinum toxin injections to the corrugator and procerus. A starting dose is upward of 20 units.
   C. Patients who will have neck dissection need to be counseled about dysfunction of this muscle, which leads to weakness in the lower lip.
   h. **Depressor labii inferioris**
   During a neck dissection (particularly level I clearance), the marginal mandibular nerve is at risk of damage, because it frequently lies below the lower mandibular border deep to platysma. Damage to this nerve results in elevation of the lower lip on the affected side from paralysis of the depressor labii inferioris and depressor anguli oris. Treatment can involve injection of botulinum toxin to the depressor labii inferioris on the unaffected side or surgical transfer of the anterior belly of digastric to the lower lip.[5]

6. *For the following scenarios, the best options are as follows:*
   A. An 80-year-old farmer presents with a progressive global unilateral facial paralysis. On examination he has a firm palpable preauricular swelling and scarring from a partial pinnectomy.
   c. **Metastatic squamous cell carcinoma**
   This man is likely to have a parotid malignancy. Benign parotid tumors such as pleomorphic salivary adenomas typically present in younger patients without facial nerve involvement. His presentation can indicate a primary malignancy. However, given his previous pinnectomy (presumably for a squamous cell carcinoma), he is likely to have recurrent disease that has spread to the parotid. This is a common pathway for such disease.
   B. A 19-year-old pregnant woman presents to her general practitioner with new-onset complete unilateral facial paralysis. She first noticed the problem on awakening in the morning. On examination she has no other physical findings of note.
   d. **Bell's palsy**
   The most common cause of facial palsy is Bell's palsy, and this is a diagnosis of exclusion. It is usually self-limiting and is treated with steroids with or without antiviral medications. The risk of Bell's palsy is significantly increased during pregnancy. Ramsay Hunt syndrome is an alternative diagnosis when otalgia or a facial rash is present.
   C. A 51-year-old woman presents with her third episode of facial paralysis. On examination she has evidence of facial swelling and tongue fissures.
   f. **Melkersson-Rosenthal syndrome**
   Melkersson-Rosenthal syndrome involves recurrent facial paralysis that may alternate sides. The cause is unknown, and treatment is usually conservative. Decompression should be considered in some cases. The most common cause of bilateral facial paralysis is Lyme disease.

Chapter 42 ▪ Facial Reanimation   343

PEDIATRIC FACIAL PALSY

7. Which one of the following is correct regarding pediatric facial palsy?
C. Hemifacial spasm is much more commonly observed in adults.

Hemifacial spasm is usually seen in middle-aged and elderly adults and reports in children are rare. It is a disorder of the seventh cranial nerve, characterized by irregular, involuntary, and recurrent tonic and clonic contractions of the ipsilateral muscles of facial expression. The cause is usually vascular compression at the brainstem, but can be seen secondary to other tumors.[6]

Facial paralysis is only present in a small proportion of patients with hemifacial microsomia. CULLP affects the marginal mandibular branch on one side only with the remainder of the facial nerve branches intact. It results in an asymmetrical appearance of the lower lip, particularly noticeable when the child cries. Bell's palsy is a diagnosis of exclusion and is observed in children as well as adults. Cholesteotoma is a localized expanding tumor of the middle ear that can cause facial nerve palsy in both children and adults.

8. Which one of the following would not be expected in a patient with Möbius syndrome?
A. Hyperacusis

Möbius syndrome is a congenital condition involving absence of the facial and abducens nerves. This results in facial paralysis, the inability to abduct the eye, and subsequent strabismus. Other cranial nerves may also be affected. Limb abnormalities such as club foot and micrognathia are quite often present. However, hyperacusis is not seen because the cell bodies of the nerve to stapedius are not located in the facial nerve nucleus, therefore its function is preserved.

GRADING FACIAL NERVE FUNCTION

9. A patient presents in the facial palsy clinic after being diagnosed with Bell's palsy. Examination shows complete eye closure with some effort, moderate weakness of the forehead, and the ability to achieve oral competence with maximum effort. *What is the most likely facial palsy grading according to the House-Brackmann scale?*
B. III

The House-Brackmann scale categorizes facial nerve function into six grades (I to VI) (see Table 42-3, *Essentials of Plastic Surgery*, second edition).[7] Grade I is normal facial nerve function, and grade VI is a total paralysis. The remaining grades pass from mild to severe. Each grade is based on gross appearance and motion. Gross appearance assesses muscle power, asymmetry, and tone. Motion assesses forehead, eye, and mouth movement. This patient is classified as having moderate dysfunction according to this scale. Other grading systems include the Burres-Fisch and Sunnybrook systems. The latter has become a popular alternative as an objective measuring tool in facial paralysis patients. It has three components: resting symmetry, symmetry of voluntary movement, and synkinesis (Fig. 42-2).[8,9] Comparison is based on the normal side. Assessment of the symmetry of voluntary movement involves five areas: the forehead wrinkle (raising eyebrows), gentle eye closure, open-mouth smile, snarl, and lip pucker. Patients with normal resting symmetry and those with no synkinesis will have a score of zero on this subsection. The composite or final score is calculated by assessing the symmetry of voluntary movement and then subtracting resting symmetry and synkinesis scores. A patient with no evidence of facial palsy should have a score of 100.

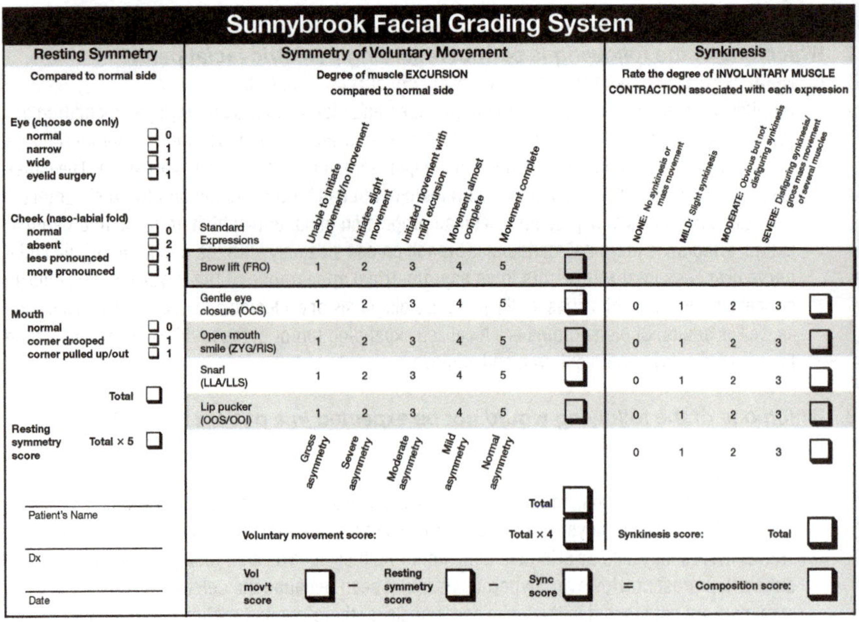

Fig. 42-2

SURGICAL MANAGEMENT OF FACIAL PALSY
10. For the following scenarios, the best options are as follows:
    A. A 40-year-old man presents with incompletely resolved Bell's palsy of 5 years duration that affects his left brow, resulting in ptosis on this side only. This is now starting to affect vision and cosmesis.
       d. **Superciliary brow lift**
          Patients with frontal branch weakness are at risk of brow ptosis, which can be treated with a brow-lift procedure. This candidate is young and probably prefers to minimize visible scarring on the brow. His options include a coronal, midforehead, or superciliary approach for a direct brow lift. An endoscopic lift probably will not offer a major benefit for this patient, given the unilateral ptosis.
    B. A 53-year-old woman is unable to fully close her right eye 16 months after facial nerve injury. The eye is mildly inflamed, with evidence of epiphora.
       a. **Insertion of an upper lid gold weight**
          Patients with long-standing facial nerve paralysis are at risk of damage to their eyes from incomplete eye closure. Insertion of a gold weight into the upper lid is a technique commonly used to assist closure. The disadvantages are that closure can remain incomplete when a patient is supine, because gravity is not acting to close the eye; the weight may be palpable and visible, and the weight can displace over time.

C. A patient has lower lid ectropion after a left-sided facial nerve palsy. Examination shows laxity of the lower lid soft tissues, corneal irritation, and epiphora.
  g. **Canthoplasty or a lid-shortening procedure**
   Lower lid laxity is a common problem in facial palsy patients because of atrophic changes in the orbicularis oculi. Various techniques can be used to tighten or shorten the lower lid to reduce ectropion and corneal exposure.

11. For the following scenarios, the best options are as follows:
A. A young patient presents 3 years after injury to the facial nerve and wishes to have facial reanimation surgery to improve resting symmetry and re-create a dynamic smile.
  f. **Cross-face nerve graft and delayed free functional muscle transfer**
B. A patient presents with partial facial nerve paralysis after a recent wound to the preauricular region.
  c. **Immediate surgical exploration and nerve repair**
   For treatment of the patients in scenarios A and B, the basic principles of facial reanimation surgery are followed to provide innervation to the mimetic muscles or to supplement them when absent. Therefore a motor unit (that is, a muscle) to perform the movement and a nerve to power this unit are both required. If the facial muscles are viable, then a nerve source should be provided by direct repair, nerve grafting to the ipsilateral side, or cross-face nerve grafting to the contralateral side. Alternatively, a different nerve such as the hypoglossal can be recruited to power the muscle. This can be done as a temporary measure to maintain functional motor endplates (babysitter procedure) or as a definitive treatment. In cases in which both nerve and muscle are lost, as in the first patient, regional or distant transfer of muscle is required.
C. A frail, elderly patient presents 15 months after injury to the facial nerve during a parotidectomy. The buccal and zygomatic branches are completely paralyzed. The patient has significant cardiovascular problems and diabetes mellitus.
  g. **No surgical intervention**
   This patient has many risk factors for surgery, and such cases should be approached with caution. Although options are available for this patient, for example, a static lift or a sliding temporalis myoplasty, the overall risks likely outweigh the benefits of surgery. No surgical intervention is advised.

SURGICAL MANAGEMENT OF FACIAL PALSY

12. In a 45-year-old patient with segmental extratemporal facial nerve loss following radical parotidectomy, which one of the following is the most suitable immediate reconstruction method?
  C. **Ipsilateral facial nerve graft**
   This patient should have both proximal and distal nerve stumps available for grafting and the motor end plates and facial mimetic muscles will be suitable for reinnervation given the immediate reconstruction planned. A cross-face nerve graft would only be required if the facial nerve was resected more proximally, thereby leaving no suitable stump for coaptation. Direct repair is clearly not an option given the nerve substance loss. A temporalis transfer, such as the Labbé procedure[10] may still be considered, particularly in older age groups where nerve regeneration is poorer and where postoperative radiotherapy is planned. Free gracilis transfer is not required because there is viable native muscle available for reanimation.

13. **Which one of the following techniques may be useful in patients who have sustained marginal mandibular nerve injury?**
   D. Digastric transfer
   Loss of marginal mandibular branch results in functional loss of the depressor anguli oris (DAO) muscle with the inability to pull the corner of the mouth downward. The anterior belly of the digastric muscle can be transferred and inserted into the lower lip, close to the insertion of DAO, just medial to the oral commissure. This provides restoration of lower lip depression.[5] Alternatively, botulinum toxin can be used on the unaffected side to provide better lower lip symmetry, as an alternative to surgery. The other procedures listed target the midface and upper lip in order to reproduce a smile, but do not provide a suitable vector to restore marginal nerve function.

REFERENCES

1. Hitselberger WE, House WF. Acoustic neuroma diagnosis. External auditory canal hypesthesia is an early sign. Arch Otolaryngol 83:218-221, 1966.
2. Davis RA, Anson BJ, Budinger JM, et al. Surgical anatomy of the facial nerve and parotid gland based upon a study of 350 cervicofacial halves. Surg Gynecol Obstet 102:385-412, 1956.
3. Pitanguy I, Ramos AS. The frontal branch of the facial nerve: the importance of its variations in face lifting. Plast Reconstr Surg 38:352-356, 1966
4. Penn JW, James A, Khatib M, et al. Development and validation of a computerized model of smiling: modeling the percentage movement required for perception of smiling in unilateral facial nerve palsy. J Plast Reconstr Aesthet Surg 6:345-351, 2013.
5. Tan ST. Anterior belly of digastric muscle transfer: a useful technique in head and neck surgery. Head Neck 24:947-954, 2002.
6. Masruha MR, Fialho LM, da Nóbrega MV. Hemifacial spasm as a manifestation of pilocytic astrocytoma in a pediatric patient. J Pediatr Neurosci 6:72-73, 2011.
7. House JW, Brackmann DE. Facial nerve grading system. Otolaryngol Head Neck Surg 93:146-147, 1985.
8. Ross BG, Fradet G, Nedzelski JM. Development of a sensitive clinical facial grading system. Otolaryngol Head Neck Surg 114:380-386, 1996.
9. Ross BG, Fradet G, Nedzelski JM. Sunnybrook facial grading system, 1992. Available at *http://sunnybrook.ca/uploads/FacialGradingSystem.pdf.*
10. Labbé D, Bussu F, Iodice A. A comprehensive approach to long-standing facial paralysis based on lengthening temporalis myoplasty. Acta Otorhinolaryngol Ital 32:145-153, 2012.

43. Face Transplantation

See *Essentials of Plastic Surgery*, second edition, pp. 498-506.

FACE TRANSPLANTATION
1. Which one of the following statements is correct regarding face transplant surgery?
A. There are no reported patient deaths after face transplant surgery.
B. Face transplants have yet to be combined with other VCA.
C. The recipient does not necessarily assume the appearance of the donor.
D. Face transplants remain rare, with fewer than 5 performed worldwide since 2000.
E. Most face transplants have been performed on female patients.

INDICATIONS FOR FACE TRANSPLANTATION
2. Which one of the following statements is correct regarding face transplant surgery?
A. At least 25% of the facial area should be involved to justify a face transplant.
B. The most common reason for face transplantation is major tumor resection.
C. Severe ballistic trauma is a poor indication for transplant surgery.
D. Patients must have a loss of the central face to warrant face transplantation.
E. Transplants are unsuitable for patients with failed free flap reconstruction.

SURGICAL PRINCIPLES IN FACE TRANSPLANTION
3. When undertaking face transplantation surgery, which one of the following statements is correct?
A. Vascular anastomoses must be undertaken bilaterally to the external carotid and internal jugular vessels.
B. Motor innervation is usually regained earlier than sensory innervation.
C. Procurement of the face takes priority over solid organ retrieval.
D. Immune suppression therapy is started soon after surgery to minimize rejection risk.
E. Synkinesis may be minimized by coaptation of nerves close to their target muscle.

CONTRAINDICATIONS TO FACE TRANSPLANT SURGERY
4. In which one of the following is it reasonable to proceed with face transplantation?
A. A patient with systemic lupus
B. A patient with a large intraoral SCC treated with radiotherapy
C. A patient who is legally blind
D. A patient with a known hypercoagulable disorder
E. A patient with severe depression

PREOPERATIVE EVALUATION IN FACE TRANSPLANT SURGERY

5. You have been asked to use the Cleveland Clinic FACES scoring system when assessing a patient for face transplant surgery. **Which one of the following statements is correct?**
   A. This is a validated scoring system to assess patient suitability before transplant surgery.
   B. Patients receive a score based on a prior surgical history and those having undergone less than five procedures score highest.
   C. Lateral and central defects make up the aesthetic scoring component and are equally weighted.
   D. The patient's functional status assessment is based solely on the Karnofsky score.
   E. Patients receive a composite score of 0 to 100, which is used postoperatively to monitor successful outcomes.

6. You are assessing a patient preoperatively for surgery using the Karnovsky performance score as part of the FACES scoring system, for which the patient receives a point score of 2. **What does this mean with regards to the patient's current health?**
   A. The patient is fit and well and leads an active life.
   B. The patient is capable of normal activity but this requires additional effort.
   C. The patient is mildly disabled and needs special care and assistance.
   D. The patient is very ill and needs hospital admission.
   E. The patient is a good candidate for face transplant.

MAJOR COMPLICATIONS AFTER FACE TRANSPLANT SURGERY

7. **Which one of the following complications is most common after face transplant surgery?**
   A. Microvascular failure with graft loss
   B. Systemic infection
   C. Poor social reintegration
   D. Acute graft rejection
   E. Death

THE PANEL REACTIVE ANTIBODY TEST

8. A patient awaiting face transplant surgery undergoes a panel reactive antibody test as part of their medical clearance. **What specific information does this test provide?**
   A. A prediction of hyperacute rejection risk
   B. A prediction of chronic rejection risk
   C. A prediction of whether antithymocyte globulin is required
   D. The blood group type of the patient
   E. The number of maintenance immunosuppressive drugs required

BANFF CLASSIFICATION OF REJECTION

9. A patient who has had face transplant surgery shows some abnormal skin changes in the transplanted area. A biopsy sample shows a dense perivascular infiltrate with mild epidermal and adnexal involvement. **According to the BANFF classification, what grade of rejection is present?**
   A. Grade 0 (minimal or no rejection)
   B. Grade I (mild rejection)
   C. Grade II (moderate rejection)
   D. Grade III (severe rejection)
   E. Grade IV (very severe rejection)

Answers

FACE TRANSPLANTATION

1. **Which one of the following statements is correct regarding face transplant surgery?**
   C. The recipient does not necessarily assume the appearance of the donor.
   An important point to consider when discussing face transplant surgery is that the recipient does not necessarily take on the facial appearance of the donor. The appearance will be dictated by the nature of the transplant and both donor and recipient features. For example, when the transplant is soft tissue only, the recipient will retain more of their own original appearance. However, where bony reconstruction is also involved, the donor appearance is more likely to be preserved. The site of the facial defect being transplanted is also likely to make a difference, for example, central face versus more peripheral regions.

   Over 25 face transplants have been performed since the first procedure was carried out in France in 2005. Of the first 17 patients, whose follow-up data were published in 2012, 15 are men and 2 are women. Face transplant has been combined with other VCA surgery and two deaths after face transplant have been reported. One patient had a bilateral hand transplant but later died from overwhelming postoperative infection. The other patient died within 2 years of surgery, and this was attributed to compliance issues with immune suppression therapy. Consequently, combining face transplant with other VCA remains controversial.[1]

INDICATIONS FOR FACE TRANSPLANTATION

2. **Which one of the following statements is correct regarding face transplant surgery?**
   A. At least 25% of the facial area should be involved to justify a face transplant.
   Face transplantation is used to reconstruct large facial defects that cannot be reconstructed with traditional techniques. The deficit should involve more than 25% of the facial area with or without loss of a central facial feature. Between 2005 and 2011, 17 patients underwent facial transplantation surgery worldwide. The most common etiology was ballistic trauma which had been the presenting injury in 8 patients. Other causes included animal bites in 2, burns in 3, congenital abnormality in 3, and benign tumor resection in 1. In general, malignant tumor resection is not a recognized indication for face transplantation. Having a failed free flap reconstruction is not a contraindication to transplant surgery. Many of the face transplant patients had undergone previous free tissue reconstruction.[1]

SURGICAL PRINCIPLES IN FACE TRANSPLANTATION

3. **When undertaking face transplantation surgery, which one of the following statements is correct?**
   E. Synkinesis may be minimized by coaptation of nerves close to their target muscle.
   Synkinesis refers to unwanted involuntary contractions that occur during voluntary muscle activation in another area of the face. It can occur secondary to aberrant regeneration after injury with resultant innervation of nonnative muscle groups. When undertaking face transplant surgery, coaptation of the motor nerve closer to the target muscle may help reduce subsequent synkinesis. Sensory reinnervation of nerve coaptation occurs earlier than motor reinnervation.

Because of the vascular networks within the head and neck, bilateral vascualar anastomoses are not usually required. Unilateral anastomoses to the internal jugular and external carotid are typically used. Immune suppression is started preoperatively to reduce the risk of acute rejection. This may be achieved with a depleting agent such as antithymocyte globulin (a monoclonal antibody) or alemtuzumad (a polyclonal antibody). These are known as depleting agents, as they reduce the number of lymphocytes. During harvest from the donor, VCA procurement may be halted if the donor becomes unstable to allow solid organ procurement. Once VCA procurement is complete the donor is fitted with a silicone prosthesis to cover the facial defect created.

CONTRAINDICATIONS TO FACE TRANSPLANT SURGERY

4. In which one of the following is it reasonable to proceed with face transplantation?
   C. A patient who is legally blind

There is debate as to whether blindness should be a contraindication to face transplant surgery. This stems from hand transplant surgery experience that has shown vision to be important in rehabilitation and not from the concern that a patient would be unable to view the result. A completely blind patient has already received a face transplant and there is no strong reason why a person who is legally blind should not receive a transplant.

There is a number of universally accepted contraindications to face transplant surgery. These can be subclassified as psychiatric, medical, or psychosocial. Psychiatric contraindications include an active psychiatric disorder, substance abuse, and cognitive and perceptual inability to understand the procedure. Medical contraindications include an active cancer diagnosis or risk of recurrence, immune deficiency (for example, human immunodeficiency virus–positive status), active infection (for example, hepatitis), scleroderma, systemic lupus erythematosus, pregnancy, and hypercoagulable disorders. Psychosocial contraindications include a history of poor compliance with medical therapy and a poor social support network.

PREOPERATIVE EVALUATION IN FACE TRANSPLANT SURGERY

5. You have been asked to use the Cleveland Clinic FACES scoring system when assessing a patient for face transplant surgery. *Which one of the following statements is correct?*
   B. Patients receive a score based on prior surgical history and those having undergone less than five procedures score highest.

The Cleveland Clinic FACES scoring system was developed as a tool to assist in the preoperative evaluation of a patient's suitability for face transplantation. It includes five key areas: functional status, aesthetic deficit, medical comorbidities, depth of tissue involvement, and previous surgical procedures. The system has not been formally validated. The functional status component is based on both the Karnofsky and Strauss-Bacon stability scores. The latter assesses aspects of a patient's social status, including long-term relationships and/or employment. Patients receive a score of 10 to 60 (not 0 to 100). A higher score is more favorable for surgery. The analysis tool alone does not represent a complete assessment for the decision-making process. Central defects are weighted more highly than lateral defects.

Chapter 43 ▪ Face Transplantation 351

6. You are assessing a patient preoperatively for surgery using the Karnofsky performance score as part of the FACES scoring system, for which the patient receives a point score of 2. **What does this mean with regards to the patient's current health?**
   D. The patient is very ill and needs hospital admission.
   The Karnofsky[2] performance score is a commonly used independent assessment tool that grades a patient's health and functional status using a score of 0 to 100, where 100 is normal health and function without evidence of disease, and where 0 is dead. Scores in between are given in multiples of ten and lower scores indicate poorer health and functional status. This system is often used in other areas of plastic surgery such as for head and neck cancer patients when assessing their fitness for surgery. It is important to note that the scoring differs as an independent assessment tool, as compared to when it is incorporated into the FACES scoring system.

   When used as part of the FACES system, patients can receive between 2 to 9 points depending on the patient's Karnofsky score/health status. For example, a patient will receive 9 points if they have a maximum Karnofsky score of 100 and will receive 2 points if they have a Karnofsky score of 20. See Table 43-1, *Essentials of Plastic Surgery,* second edition for further detail. This patient scores very badly and a score of this grade suggests that admission to the hospital is indicated.

MAJOR COMPLICATIONS AFTER FACE TRANSPLANT SURGERY

7. **Which one of the following complications is most common after face transplant surgery?**
   D. Acute graft rejection
   To date, every face transplant patient with follow-up of more than 1 year has recorded at least one episode of acute graft rejection. These episodes were clinically apparent as erythema, edema with nodules, or papules and were treated satisfactorily by adjustment of immune suppression therapy. No subacute or chronic graft rejection episodes have been reported. Microvascular graft failures have been low (4%) which is consistent with expected autologous free tissue transfer failure rates. As discussed in question 1, there have been two deaths reported in the first follow-up data set. Significant infection rates have been low. Common localized infections include viral or fungal subtypes such as CMV, herpes, and candida. These are generally well treated with medications such as acyclovir or fluconazole, respectively. One of the benefits of face transplant is improved social reintegration and this has been promising in face transplants undertaken so far.

THE PANEL REACTIVE ANTIBODY TEST

8. A patient awaiting face transplant surgery undergoes a panel reactive antibody test as part of their medical clearance. **What specfic information does this test provide?**
   A. A prediction of hyperacute rejection risk
   Panel reactive antibodies are used to determine whether a patient has specific human leukocyte antigen antibodies.[3] A sample of a patient's blood is tested against the lymphocytes of 100 blood donors. The number of donors to which the patient has a reaction is expressed as a percentage (0% to 100%). A high percentage indicates that a patient has a high risk of acute rejection and may have to wait an extended time for a suitable donor (see Chapter 7, *Essentials of Plastic Surgery,* second edition). It does not reflect chronic rejection status or the blood type of the patient. All patients will require antithymocyte globulin preoperatively as part of the depleting agent process, and all patients will have a typical triple therapy maintenance regimen which will include steroids, tacrolimus, and mycophenolate mofetil.

BANFF CLASSIFICATION OF REJECTION

9. A patient who has had face transplant surgery shows some abnormal skin changes in the transplanted area. A biopsy sample shows a dense perivascular infiltrate with mild epidermal and adnexal involvement. *According to the BANFF classification, what grade of rejection is present?*

C. Grade II (moderate rejection)

The Banff classification is used to grade rejection in vascular composite tissue grafts such as face and hand transplants. When evidence of rejection is evident in the skin, small biopsy samples are obtained for analysis.[4,5] The grading system is as follows:

Grade 0: No rejection
Grade I: Mild rejection, seen as mild perivascular infiltrate (lymphocytic)
Grade II: Moderate rejection, seen as moderate to dense perivascular inflammation that can include mild epidermal and adnexal involvement
Grade III: Severe rejection, seen as dense inflammation with epidermal involvement, epithelial apoptosis/necrosis
Grade IV: Necrotizing rejection, seen as necrosis of epidermis and/or other skin elements

This patient has evidence of a grade II reaction and may require alterations to their immunosuppressive regimen. Of historic interest, the Banff conference was first held in Banff, Alberta, Canada in 1991. It is an international meeting to discuss transplant pathology. The twelfth meeting was held in Brazil in 2013.

REFERENCES

1. Siemionow M, Ozturk C. Face transplantation: outcomes, concerns, controversies, and future directions. J Craniofac Surg 23:254-259, 2012.
2. Karnofsky DA, Burchenal JH. The clinical evaluation of chemotherapeutic agents in cancer. In MacLeod CM, ed. Evaluation of Chemotherapeutic Agents. New York: Columbia Univ Press, 1949.
3. U.S. Department of Health and Human Services. Organ Procurement and Transplantation Network. Available at *http://optn.transplant.hrsa.gov/resources/allocationcalculators.asp?index=75*.
4. Cendales LC, Kanitakis J, Schneeberger S, et al. The Banff 2007 working classification of skin-containing composite tissue allograft pathology. Am J Transplant 8:1396-1400, 2008.
5. Solez K. History of the Banff classification of allograft pathology as it approaches its 20th year. Curr Opin Organ Transplant 15:49-51, 2010.

Part IV

Breast

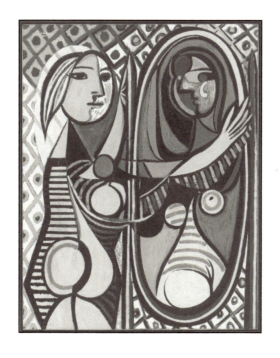

© 2015 Estate of Pablo Picasso / Artists Rights Society (ARS), New York.

44. Breast Anatomy and Embryology

See *Essentials of Plastic Surgery*, second edition, pp. 509-517.

EMBRYOLOGY

1. **Which one of the following statements is correct regarding fetal breast tissue development?**
   A. The milk ridge develops in the third week and extends from the fifth rib to the groin.
   B. The lactiferous ducts develop from cutaneous epithelium beginning in week 8.
   C. Polymastia can occur anywhere along the milk ridge but most commonly occurs on the right at the level of the inframammary crease.
   D. Polythelia is the second most common congenital breast abnormality, occurring in 0.5% to 1% of the population.
   E. The lactiferous ducts develop early in fetal development, but the areolae are rarely present before the seventh month.

DEVELOPMENT

2. **An 18-year-old female presents with concern over delayed breast development. Examination of her breasts shows evidence of low-volume glandular tissue in the subareolar region, with the nipple and breast projecting as a single mound. *According to the Tanner classification, which stage does this represent?***
   A. Stage 1
   B. Stage 2
   C. Stage 3
   D. Stage 4
   E. Stage 5

ANATOMY

3. **Which one of the following statements is correct regarding the anatomy of adult female breasts?**
   A. The breast extends from the third to the sixth rib in the midclavicular line.
   B. The lobule is the functional unit of the breast and is composed of around 18 to 20 acini.
   C. The breast comprises multiple connected lobules drained by approximately 100 lactiferous ducts.
   D. Cooper's ligaments provide breast support and have connections with the deep layer of superficial fascia and parenchyma.
   E. Morgagni's glands are small apocrine glands capable of milk secretion and lubrication.

ARTERIAL SUPPLY

4. **Which one of the following provides a significant arterial supply to the breast parenchyma?**
   A. Lateral thoracic artery
   B. Intercostal perforators
   C. Thoracoacromial artery
   D. Internal mammary artery perforators
   E. All of the above

SENSORY INNERVATION

5. **Which one of the following statements is correct regarding sensory breast innervation?**
   A. The dermatomal distribution of the breasts is T1-5.
   B. Nipple-areolar sensation is most commonly provided by the sixth medial intercostal nerve.
   C. Supraclavicular nerves from the lower fibers of the cervical plexus contribute to innervation of the lower medial portion of the breast.
   D. Breast sensitivity is unrelated to breast size.
   E. Sensory breast innervation is mainly provided by the anterolateral and anteromedial intercostal nerves.

WÜRINGER'S SEPTUM

6. **Which one of the following statements is correct regarding Würinger's septum?**
   A. The septum carries the sensory nerve supply to the nipple.
   B. The septum carries the arterial supply to the nipple.
   C. The septum provides connective tissue support to the breast.
   D. The septum originates from the pectoralis fascia along the fifth rib.
   E. All of the above.

MUSCULATURE OF THE ANTERIOR CHEST WALL

7. **Which one of the following statements is correct regarding muscles of the anterior chest and abdominal wall?**
   A. The pectoralis minor is innervated by the lateral pectoral nerve and inserts on the coronoid process.
   B. The pectoralis major has two heads which insert on the medial side of the intertubercular sulcus.
   C. The serratus anterior originates from the anterior aspects of the first eight ribs and inserts on the medial aspect of the scapula.
   D. The rectus abdominis originates at the seventh to the twelfth costal cartilages and inserts at the pubic line.
   E. The external oblique is innervated by the fourth to tenth intercostal nerves and its key function is to flex the vertebral column.

LYMPHATIC DRAINAGE OF THE BREAST

8. **Which one of the following statements is correct regarding lymphatic drainage of the breast?**
   A. The breast has purely deep lymphatic drainage networks.
   B. All of the breast drains directly into the axillary nodes.
   C. There are three levels of axillary nodes each relating to pectoralis minor.
   D. Lymphatic efferents from the upper outer quadrants drain directly to the supraclavicular nodes.
   E. Rotter's nodes are found deep to pectoralis minor.

BREAST SHAPE AND AESTHETICS

9. Which one of the following statements is correct regarding the normal breast?
A. Close symmetry is common in younger patients.
B. Most fullness should normally be found within the upper pole.
C. A normal notch-to-nipple distance is 28 cm.
D. Ptosis is unrelated to nipple position.
E. The nipple should ideally be level with the midhumeral point.

POLAND'S SYNDROME

10. Which one of the following muscles is always deficient in patients with Poland's syndrome?
A. Pectoralis minor
B. Sternal head of the pectoralis major
C. Latissimus dorsi
D. Serratus anterior
E. Clavicular head of the pectoralis major

COMPLICATIONS AFTER BREAST SURGERY

11. A patient has axillary dissection for carcinoma of the breast and later develops paresthesia in the upper inner arm. *What is the most likely mechanism underlying the pathology of this symptom?*
A. Transection of the medial brachial nerve
B. Transection of the medial antebrachial nerve
C. Transection of the intercostobrachial nerve
D. Development of a compressive seroma
E. Development of a compressive hematoma

Answers

EMBRYOLOGY

1. **Which one of the following statements is correct regarding fetal breast tissue development?**
   B. The lactiferous ducts develop from cutaneous epithelium beginning in week 8.
   The milk ridge extends from the axilla to the groin and develops in week 6 (not week 3). Polymastia (supernumerary breasts) can occur anywhere along the milk ridge but is most common on the left below the inframammary crease. Polythelia (supernumerary nipples) is the most common congenital breast abnormality and occurs in 2% of the population. The lactiferous ducts are modified sweat glands. Toward the end of embryonic development, the acini develop around these glands, creating a mammary pit. The areolae are usually formed by month 5.

DEVELOPMENT

2. An 18-year-old female presents with concern over delayed breast development. Examination of her breasts shows evidence of low-volume glandular tissue in the subareolar region, with the nipple and breast projecting as a single mound. *According to the Tanner classification,[1] which stage does this represent?*
   B. Stage 2
   Tanner described five stages of breast development. Stage 1 is characterized by preadolescent elevation of the nipple without palpable glandular tissue or areolar pigmentation. In stage 5, adolescent breast development is complete, with a smooth contour and no projection of the areola and nipple. The case described represents stage 2, which normally occurs at approximately 10 to 12 years of age. Tanner's stages of breast development are as follows:
   Stage 1: Preadolescent elevation of the nipple is present with no palpable glandular tissue or areolar pigmentation.
   Stage 2: Glandular tissue is present in the subareolar region, and the nipple and breast project as a single mound.
   Stage 3: Glandular tissue is increased and the breast and nipple are enlarged, but the nipple and breast contour remains in a single plane.
   Stage 4: The areolae are enlarged and areolar pigmentation increased, and the nipple and areola form a secondary mound above the level of the breast.
   Stage 5: Adolescent development is complete, with smooth contour and no projection of areola and nipple.

ANATOMY

3. **Which one of the following statements is correct regarding the anatomy of adult female breasts?**
   D. Cooper's ligaments provide breast support and have connections with the deep layer of superficial fascia and parenchyma.
   The adult breast extends from the second to the seventh rib in the midclavicular line. It is composed of multiple lobules consisting of hundreds of acini. The lobules are connected and drained by 16 to 24 lactiferous ducts. Montgomery's glands are large glands that are capable of secreting milk and help to lubricate the nipple during lactation. They represent an intermediate

stage between sweat and mammary glands. Morgagni's tubercles are located near the periphery of the areola and represent the openings of Montgomery's glands.

ARTERIAL SUPPLY

4. Which one of the following provides a significant arterial supply to the breast parenchyma?

E. All of the above

Breast parenchyma is supplied by the internal mammary and intercostal perforators medially and by the lateral thoracic, thoracoacromial, thoracodorsal and intercostal perforators laterally (see Fig. 44-1, *Essentials of Plastic Surgery*, second edition). Its rich blood supply is responsible for maintaining its viability during reconstruction or recontouring surgery.

SENSORY INNERVATION

5. Which of the following statements is correct regarding sensory breast innervation?

E. Sensory breast innervation is mainly provided by the anterolateral and anteromedial intercostal nerves.

The dermatomal distribution of the breast is T3-6 (not T1-5) from the intercostal nerves (see Fig. 44-2, *Essentials of Plastic Surgery*, second edition). Nipple-areolar sensation is most commonly provided by the fourth anterolateral intercostal nerve, although it is supplied by the third or fifth nerves in some cases. Supraclavicular nerves (C3 and C4) contribute to innervation of the upper lateral portion (not the lower medial portion). Breast sensitivity is apparently related to breast size, with studies showing increased sensitivity in females with smaller breasts. Sensation has been shown to improve after breast reduction surgery in patients with initially large breasts.[2]

WÜRINGER'S SEPTUM

6. Which one of the following statements is correct regarding Würinger's septum?

E. All of the above.

Würinger et al[3] undertook anatomic dissections and arterial injection studies on female breasts. They found that there is a connective tissue suspensory system of the breast which acts as an internal brassiere. Within the horizontal part of the suspensory system they identified a septum passing from the pectoral fascia along the fifth rib which is now referred to as *Würinger's septum*. Within this septum is the neurovascular supply to the nipple areola complex. The anatomic nature of the septum means that laterally based breast pedicles are reliable and have a high chance of maintaining sensation following breast surgery (see Chapter 48, *Essentials of Plastic Surgery*, second edition).

MUSCULATURE OF THE ANTERIOR CHEST WALL

7. Which one of the following statements is correct regarding muscles of the anterior chest and abdominal wall?

C. Serratus anterior originates from the anterior aspects of the first eight ribs and inserts on the medial aspect of the scapula.

Serratus anterior plays an important role in stabilization of the scapula against the chest wall. It receives blood supply through the lateral thoracic artery and branches of the thoracodorsal artery. It is innervated by the long thoracic nerve C6-7, and when this nerve is damaged a winged scapula will occur.

The pectoralis minor is innervated by the medial (not the lateral) pectoral nerve and is so named because it originates from the medial cord of the brachial plexus (C8 and T1). It originates from the third to sixth ribs and inserts onto the coronoid process. Its function is to draw the scapula downward and forward. Blood supply to the pectoralis minor is from the pectoral branch of thoracoacromial, lateral thoracic, and a direct branch of from the axillary artery.

The pectoralis major originates from the medial clavicle, sternum, second to sixth ribs, external oblique, and rectus abdominis fascia. It inserts on the intertubercular groove of the humerus laterally (not medially). The latissimus dorsi inserts between the pectoralis and teres major muscles. (It is sometimes described as the "lady between two majors.") The pectoralis major functions to adduct and medially rotate the arm. Innervation is from the medial and lateral pectoral nerves.

The rectus abdominis flexes the vertebral column and tenses the abdominal wall. Innervation is from the seventh to twelfth intercostals. It originates from the pubic line and inserts on the third to seventh (not the seventh to twelfth) costal cartilages. External oblique originates from the lower anterior and lateral ribs, inserting at the iliac crest and medial abdominal fascial aponeurosis. Although it may assist in flexion of the vertebral column, a key role is compression of abdominal contents. It receives innervation from the seventh to twelfth intercostal nerves (not the forth to tenth).

LYMPHATIC DRAINAGE OF THE BREAST

8. Which one of the following statements is correct regarding lymphatic drainage of the breast?

C. There are three levels of axillary nodes, each relating to pectoralis minor.

The axillary lymph nodes are named according to their relationship with the pectoralis minor. Level 1 is lateral to, level 2 is behind, and level 3 is medial to the pectoralis minor, respectively. The breast has an extensive network of superficial and deep lymphatic drainage. Although most of the breast drains into the axillary nodes, not all areas do so. For example, medial drainage follows the internal mammary perforators and drains to the parasternal nodes. Lymphatic drainage from the outer upper quadrant may pass directly to the subscapular nodes. Rotter's nodes are found between the pectoralis major and minor. They are named after the German surgeon, Josef Rotter[4] (1857-1924), who described them in the late nineteenth century, and they may be involved in the metastatic spread of breast cancer.

BREAST SHAPE AND AESTHETICS

9. Which one of the following statements is correct regarding the normal breast?

E. The nipple should ideally be level with the midhumeral point

Although there are a number of "typical" measurements for the "normal" breast, there is actually significant variation between individuals. Some of the "typical" measurements are in keeping with the "ideal" or most aesthetic breast appearance. For example, the height of the nipple should ideally be level with the midhumeral point. This also usually matches with the level of the IMF and a distance of around 19 to 21 cm from the sternal notch (although this does also depend on the patient's height and breast size). This information is useful when planning breast reduction and mastopexy techniques, as it provides a guide as to where to resite the nipple areola complex (see Fig. 44-5, *Essentials of Plastic Surgery,* second edition). The normal breast should have a teardrop shape when viewed from the side and this is due to greater fullness in the lower pole. The breast is tethered at the IMF so naturally a degree of glandular ptosis occurs where the breast soft tissues fall to sit just below this line. The nipple should still remain above the IMF level in the ideal breast. Therefore, while a minimal amount of glandular ptosis is normal and aesthetically pleasing, more significant amounts are not. Degrees of true ptosis are described by the relationship of the nipple to the IMF and breast parenchyma. This is discussed further in Chapter 46. Few women have symmetrical breasts at any age and it is important to identify this before performing breast surgery, as the asymmetry may remain or even be exaggerated after

Chapter 44 ▪ Breast Anatomy and Embryology   361

surgery. For example, when the nipple is lateralized on the breast mound, augmentation will make this more obvious.

POLAND'S SYNDROME

10. Which one of the following muscles is always deficient in patients with Poland's syndrome?
 B. Sternal head of the pectoralis major
 Poland's syndrome is a disorder where affected individuals are born with missing or incompletely formed elements of the upper limb and chest on one side. It occurs in 1:30,000 births with no specific gender preference. The right side is affected twice as often as the left. The current theory is that there is in utero compression of the subclavian artery which causes ischemia and hypoplastic development of key chest and limb structures. The main findings include absence of the sternal head of pectoralis major muscle, absence of the costal cartilages, hypoplasia of the breast and nipple areolar complex, deficiency of subcutaneous fat and axillary hair, and syndactyly or hypoplasia of the upper limb. Although it can cause a variety of muscle abnormalities such as those listed, a consistent feature is absence of the sternal portion of the pectoralis major.

COMPLICATIONS AFTER BREAST SURGERY

11. A patient has axillary dissection for carcinoma of the breast and develops paresthesia in the upper inner arm. What is the most likely mechanism underlying the pathology of this symptom?
 C. Transection of the intercostobrachial nerve
 The medial arm is supplied by the medial brachial and intercostobrachial nerves from T1-2. The intercostobrachial nerve usually joins with the medial brachial nerve. The medial antebrachial nerve supplies the anterior surfaces of the arm and anteromedial forearm. Transection of any of these can result in paresthesia to the arm; however, the most likely cause is transection of the intercostobrachial nerve. Although a postoperative seroma or hematoma can cause paresthesia in the upper limb, it can also directly irritate the brachial plexus and lead to a combined motor and sensory pathology. Other causes of postoperative upper limb dysfunction include nerve stretch or compression from patient positioning.

REFERENCES

1. Tanner JM, ed. Growth at Adolescence. Oxford: Blackwell Scientific, 1962.
2. DelVecchio C, Caloca J Jr, Caloca J, et al. Evaluation of breast sensibility using dermatomal somatosensory evoked potentials. Plast Reconstr Surg 113:1975-1983, 2004.
3. Würinger E. Mader N, Posch E, et al. Nerve and vessel supplying ligamentous suspension of the mammary gland. Plast Reconstr Surg 101:1486-1493, 1998.
4. Vrdoljak DV, Ramljak V, Muzina D, et al. Analysis of metastatic involvement of interpectoral (Rotter's) lymph nodes related to tumor location, size, grade and hormone receptor status in breast cancer. Tumori 91:177-181, 2005.

45. Breast Augmentation

See *Essentials of Plastic Surgery*, second edition, pp. 518-537.

BACKGROUND TO BREAST AUGMENTATION

1. *Which one of the following statements is correct regarding breast augmentation?*
   A. The FDA placed a moratorium on the use of silicone breast implants in 2001.
   B. There is a proven link between silicone implants and systemic autoimmune disease.
   C. There are five generations of silicone implant, if texturing, gel type, and shape are considered.
   D. Saline-filled implants remain the gold standard, because they require a smaller incision and more closely maintain body temperature.
   E. In the United States, silicone implants do not currently have FDA approval for primary breast augmentation.

PATIENT EVALUATION FOR BREAST AUGMENTATION

2. *Which one of the following is not always required during the assessment of patients requesting breast augmentation?*
   A. Assessment of psychological stability and personal motivation for implants
   B. Recent mammograms
   C. Identification of chest wall and vertebral deformities
   D. Measurement of breast base width, notch-to-nipple, and nipple-to-IMF distances
   E. Assessment of skin elasticity and upper/lower pole soft tissue cover

INCISION CHOICE FOR BREAST AUGMENTATION

3. *When choosing the incision site for breast augmentation, which one of the following statements is correct?*
   A. The IMF approach is often well hidden and should be placed at the IMF centered on the NAC.
   B. The transumbilical approach is unsuitable for saline implants.
   C. The periareolar approach is best achieved with direct parenchymal dissection.
   D. The transaxillary approach avoids a scar but risks sensory nerve damage to the arm.
   E. Endoscopic approaches are usually limited to round saline implants.

PLACEMENT OF BREAST IMPLANTS

4. You are deciding whether to place breast implants in a subglandular or submuscular plane in a young, slim fitness coach. **Which one of the following is correct regarding implant placement relevant to this patient?**
   A. Nipple sensation is equally likely to be preserved with submuscular or subglandular implant placement.
   B. Mammography and breast cancer diagnosis are similarly affected, irrespective of the chosen site.
   C. A submuscular site can result in "dancing breasts" that may be unacceptable for this patient.
   D. Capsular contraction rates are unaffected by the choice of implant site.
   E. A subglandular implant will provide a better contour, less prone to palpable implant edges.

DUAL PLANE BREAST IMPLANT PLACEMENT

5. **Which one of the following statements is correct regarding dual plane augmentation?**
   A. By definition, dual plane involves the creation of separate subglandular and submuscular pockets.
   B. Dual plane II involves dissection of a subglandular pocket to the top of the NAC.
   C. Dual plane I is used for breasts in which all of the breast is above the IMF.
   D. Dual plane techniques are used to reduce inferolateral displacement of the implant.
   E. Dual plane III involves dissection of the breast from the pectoralis fascia up to the upper pole limit.

THE BAKER CLASSIFICATION

6. A patient has capsular contracture on both sides. On the left, the implant is painful. On the right, the patient is unaware of any changes. **What classification of contraction does she have?**
   A. Baker IV left, Baker III right
   B. Baker II left, Baker III right
   C. Baker II left, Baker IV right
   D. Baker IV left, Baker II right
   E. Baker IV left, Baker I right

CAPSULAR CONTRACTURE

7. **Which one of the following has traditionally been linked to an increased rate of capsular contraction following primary breast augmentation?**
   A. Use of a polyurethane implant
   B. Implant placement in a submuscular plane.
   C. Use of a textured implant
   D. Use of a silicone-filled implant
   E. Use of a saline-filled implant

8. You have a patient with a capsular contracture after revision augmentation and are explaining to her the biofilm theory relating to capsular contracture. **Which one of the following organisms is most likely to be implicated in this theory?**
   A. Staphylococcus aureus
   B. Streptococcus pyogenese
   C. Staphylococcus saprophyticus
   D. Staphylococcus epidermidis
   E. Streptococcus viridans

IMAGING AND CLINICAL ASSESSMENT IN BREAST AUGMENTATION

9. For each of the following, select the most likely option from the list below. (Each option may be used once, more than once, or not at all.)
   A. A sign of implant rupture observed on MRI
   B. A mammogram view used in patients with breast implants
   C. A type of double-bubble deformity in which the implant remains above the breast mound

   Options:
   a. Stepladder sign
   b. Collis sign
   c. Waterfall
   d. Snowstorm
   e. Eklund view
   f. Dortmund view
   g. Valley view
   h. Bull's-eye view
   i. Linguine sign

COUNSELING PATIENTS FOR BREAST AUGMENTATION

10. Which one of the following represents the greatest risk to a patient undergoing primary subglandular breast augmentation with a silicone form stable implant?
    A. Implant rupture
    B. Altered nipple sensation
    C. Postoperative infection
    D. Anaplastic lymphoma
    E. Postoperative hematoma

SELECTION OF BREAST IMPLANTS FOR COSMETIC AUGMENTATION

11. A slim 30-year-old woman is seen in the outpatient department; she is considering breast augmentation. Examination shows she has good breast symmetry and mild (grade I) ptosis, with nipple-to-notch distances of 26 cm. There are no chest wall deformities evident, and tissue quality is good. *What is the next key step in selection of the optimal implant for this patient?*
    A. Place trial breast sizers within the bra
    B. Measure the nipple to midline distances
    C. Create computer-generated images
    D. Assess the superior pole tissue thickness
    E. Measure breast base width and height

Answers

BACKGROUND TO BREAST AUGMENTATION

1. **Which one of the following statements is correct regarding breast augmentation?**
   C. There are five generations of silicone implant, if texturing, gel type, and shape are considered.

   There are five generations of breast implants. The first generation, which appeared in the 1960s, had a thick shell and thick filler with a Dacron patch to help secure it. The second generation appeared in the 1970s and had a thin shell and a less viscous filler. In the 1980s the third generation implants were released, and these reverted back to a thicker silicone shell with the addition of a barrier coating. Fourth and fifth generation implants represent refined third generation implants with textured shells and cohesive or form stable gel fillers. They are available in anatomic or round shapes. Cohesive gel implants represent the current gold standard, because they are more natural in feel, ripple less, and retain their integrity following rupture.

   Breast augmentation is one of the most common cosmetic procedures, and in 1992 (not 2001) a moratorium was placed on their use by the FDA over safety concerns with silicone implants.[1] This has since been retracted, and a number of silicone prostheses are approved for use in the United States, both for primary augmentation and reconstruction. There is no proven link between silicone implant use and systemic autoimmune disease. However, there is some evidence suggesting a link with anaplastic large cell lymphoma and breast augmentation in a very small number of patients. This is not specific to silicone implants, and further research is needed to fully understand and confirm this proposed link.

PATIENT EVALUATION FOR BREAST AUGMENTATION

2. **Which one of the following is not always required during the assessment of patients requesting breast augmentation?**
   B. Recent mammograms

   Although assessment of a patient's status for breast cancer is important, mammograms are not routinely required. A general rule of thumb is to arrange a mammogram in patients over the age of 40 or those with a personal or family history of breast cancer. Assessment of the other parameters is necessary to optimize patient outcomes for implant selection and placement.

INCISION CHOICE FOR BREAST AUGMENTATION

3. **When choosing the incision site for breast augmentation, which one of the following statements is correct?**
   E. Endoscopic approaches are usually limited to round saline implants.

   There are four approaches to breast augmentation: inframammary, transaxillary, periareolar, and transumbilical. Placement of silicone implants is usually limited to either periareolar or IMF approaches. An IMF approach is most commonly used and allows good access with a scar usually hidden by natural ptosis within a well-defined IMF. The scar should be slightly lateral to the NAC, not in line with it, to minimize visibility medially (1 cm medial and 4 cm lateral). Tissue recruitment from the chest wall may occur during augmentation, and this must be considered when choosing the incision height to avoid placing the scar too high on the final augmented breast.

The periareolar approach can be performed with either direct parenchymal dissection or using a stair-step approach that involves dissection in a subcutaneous plane to the inferior breast before undermining the gland to create the implant pocket. The stair-step approach is preferable, since it avoids the need to breach the parenchyma, which could lead to potential damage to the ducts.

The transaxillary approach does not completely avoid a scar; it just avoids one on the breast mound. It may be performed endoscopically with round implants in either a subglandular or submuscular plane. The transumbilical approach is only suitable for saline implants.

PLACEMENT OF BREAST IMPLANTS

4. You are deciding whether to place breast implants in a subglandular or submuscular plane in a young, slim fitness coach. **Which one of the following is correct regarding implant placement relevant to this patient?**
   C. A submuscular site can result in "dancing breasts" that may be unacceptable for this patient.
   Placement of the implant under the pectoralis major can result in movement of the implant during activity. This is called "dancing breasts" and may be a major problem for patients involved in athletic activities, such as this patient. Nipple sensation is usually preserved following breast augmentation but is more likely to be preserved with submuscular placement, because the fourth intercostal nerve runs within the pectoralis fascia. Standard mammography may be affected by placement of subglandular breast implants, so it is important for patients to inform the radiographer in advance so that screening views may be adapted. Despite this, there is no evidence to suggest breast cancer diagnosis is delayed following breast implant placement in either plane. Capsular contracture rates are traditionally lower with submuscular implant placement.[2] Given that she is thin, however, this patient may benefit from the increased soft tissue coverage that a submuscular site offers. This usually depends on the upper pole soft tissue cover, with more than 2 cm usually required on a pinch test to proceed with subglandular implants.

DUAL PLANE BREAST IMPLANT PLACEMENT

5. **Which one of the following statements is correct regarding dual plane augmentation?**
   C. Dual plane I is used for breasts in which all of the breast is above the IMF.
   Despite its name, dual plane does not always involve dissection of two separate planes, one subglandular and one subpectoral. Only dual plane II and III involve dissection of both pockets. The rationale for using a dual plane technique is to allow the implant to fill the lower pole and avoid the pectoralis muscle, forcing the implant in a superolateral direction.

   The dual plane I technique releases the lower border of the pectoralis major at the IMF and continues with a subpectoral dissection. This is used to for most typical breasts. The criteria include the following: all of the breast is above the IMF, there is a tight attachment of parenchyma to the pectoralis, and the lower pole is minimally stretched.

   Dual plane II and III are used for more ptotic breasts, where there is breast tissue below the IMF and the lower pole is therefore stretched. Dual plane III is also advocated for a constricted breast. The difference between II and III is the extent of dissection of the subglandular pocket. In dual plane II this is continued to the lower border of the areola, and in III this is continued to the top of the areola (not the full extent of the superior pole).

THE BAKER CLASSIFICATION

6. A patient has capsular contracture on both sides. On the left, the implant is painful. On the right, the patient is unaware of any changes. ***What classification of contraction does she have?***
D. Baker IV left, Baker II right
   The Baker classification has four grades, I through IV. A grade I is a soft breast with no evidence of capsule contraction. A grade II breast has a palpable, firm capsule that is not visible; usually only the clinician would notice and diagnose a grade II. A patient is likely to notice grades III and IV. In both grades the breast will have an altered appearance and feel firm. The key difference between grades III and IV is the presence or absence of pain, with IV being painful.

CAPSULAR CONTRACTURE

7. ***Which one of the following has traditionally been linked to an increased rate of capsular contraction following primary breast augmentation?***
D. Use of a silicone-filled implant
   Traditional rates of capsular contracture before the 1992 FDA ban ranged from around 10% to almost 60%, depending on the type of implant used and its anatomic placement. Silicone implants were associated with much higher contracture rates than either saline or polyurethane. Smooth implants were associated with particularly high rates of capsular contracture and this was the reason for implants subsequently being textured. Placement of the implant in the subpectoral plane was also shown to reduce capsular contracture rates. Most recently collected data show less variation between the factors described above, and the most important factor appears to be the setting in which the implant is used. The rates of capsular contracture are lowest in primary breast augmentation, but are higher in both revision augmentation and reconstruction settings (see Box 45-2, *Essentials of Plastic Surgery,* second edition).

8. You have a patient with a capsular contracture after revision augmentation and are explaining to her the biofilm theory relating to capsular contracture. ***Which one of the following organisms is most likely to be implicated in this theory?***
D. Staphylococcus epidermidis
   The biofilm theory is currently the single most well-accepted theory for development of capsular contracture. There is a proposed correlation between subclinical infection and subsequent development of a biofilm, although the precise causal relationship has not been shown. As a single organism, staphylococcus epidermidis is the most commonly implicated organism, but other types of bacteria may also be implicated and a polymicrobial cause is also likely.
   Streptococcus pyogenes is a gram-positive bacterium that is the cause of severe group A streptococcal infections. Staphylococcus saprophyticus is a gram-positive, coagulase-negative facultative species that is a common cause of urinary tract infections. Streptococcus viridans is a commensural of the gastrointestinal and genitourinary tracts that can cause severe infections in immune-compromised patients. Staphylococcus aureus is a bacterium that commonly colonizes human skin and mucosa without causing any problems. It can be implicated in severe soft tissue infections and also have a role in capsular contracture formation.

IMAGING AND CLINICAL ASSESSMENT IN BREAST AUGMENTATION

9. For the following descriptions, the best options are as follows:
   A. A sign of implant rupture observed on MRI
      i. Linguine sign
   B. A mammogram view used in patients with breast implants
      e. Eklund view
   C. A type of double-bubble deformity in which the implant remains above the breast mound
      c. Waterfall

   Ultrasonography can demonstrate implant rupture with two commonly described phenomena: the snowstorm and stepladder signs. The snowstorm sign is seen most commonly in conjunction with an extracapsular rupture from small amounts of free silicone mixing with the surrounding breast tissue. The stepladder sign is seen in association with an intracapsular rupture. It is observed as multiple curvilinear low signal intensity lines within a high signal intensity silicone gel. The lines represent the collapsed implant shell floating in the silicone gel. Magnetic resonance imaging is the gold standard for assessment of implant rupture. The linguine sign is seen on MRI when intracapsular rupture is present; it is analogous to the stepladder sign on ultrasound.

   Achieving adequate mammographic views is more challenging when there are breast implants in place, and the Eklund view is a technique used to displace the implant from the breast. Posterosuperior displacement of the implants is performed with simultaneous anterior traction on the implant.

   The double-bubble deformity occurs when the breast and implant separate to give the appearance of two distinct overlapping mounds. A double-bubble deformity can occur either from the implant displacing inferiorly, leaving breast tissue superiorly, or it can occur with the implant remaining superior and the breast tissue sliding off the implant inferiorly.

   These deformities are classified as A if the implant is "Above" the breast or B if the implant is "Below" the breast. A type A double-bubble can occur when a total submuscular plane is used, because the implant is then held abnormally high on the chest wall, leaving a loose parenchyma to slide inferiorly. This is called a *waterfall deformity*. Type B can occur with overdissection of the IMF, which allows the implant to slide into a lower pocket, resulting in the appearance of two separate folds.

COUNSELING PATIENTS FOR BREAST AUGMENTATION

10. Which one of the following represents the greatest risk to a patient undergoing primary subglandular breast augmentation with a silicone form stable implant?
    B. Altered nipple sensation

    The greatest risk for a patient undergoing primary breast augmentation in this case is alteration of nipple sensation. Permanent sensory change occurs in approximately 15% of patients. The risk of implant rupture is low (probably less than 1% based on most recent studies, although MRI confirmed rupture has been higher [7%] in both Mentor and Allergan studies). Both postoperative infection and hematoma should be discussed with the patient but are low risk (less than 1%). Anaplastic large cell lymphoma links with breast augmentation have received recent press coverage. However, there are approximately 170 cases[3] reported worldwide and the likely risk is estimated at 1:200,000 (see Box 45-1, *Essentials of Plastic Surgery*, second edition, for the trial summaries). There may be a link with texturing and anaplastic large cell lymphoma in this cohort of patients but further information is still awaited. Given the evidence it is advisable to discuss this risk with patients preoperatively in spite of the very low potential risks. When anaplastic large cell lymphoma does occur in patients after breast augmentation, a common presentation is that of a delayed seroma. In such cases it is important to sample the fluid and send it for specific lymphoma analysis.

SELECTION OF BREAST IMPLANTS FOR COSMETIC AUGMENTATION

11. A slim 30-year-old woman is seen in the outpatient department; she is considering breast augmentation. Examination shows she has good breast symmetry and mild (grade I) ptosis, with nipple-to-notch distances of 26 cm. There are no chest wall deformities evident, and tissue quality is good. *What is the next key step in selection of the optimal implant for this patient?*
    E. **Measure breast base width and height**
    There are two key steps now to decide what implant size should be used. The first is to measure breast base width and height; this will enable the surgeon to select an appropriate sized implant for this patient's current breast and frame size. The next step is to confirm what appearance the patient wishes to achieve and how much bigger she wishes her breasts to be. To achieve this, sizers placed in a bra may be helpful. Alternatively, the use of computer-generated images may be helpful. Once this information is available, the appropriate implant sizes can be selected.

REFERENCES

1. US Food and Drug Administration. Medical devices: breast implants. Available at *www.fda.gov/medicaldevices/productsandmedicalProcedures/ImplantsandProsthetics/BreastImplants*.
2. Available at *http://www.mhra.gov.uk/home/groups/dts-bi/documents/websiteresources/con2022634.pdf*.
3. Brody GS, Deapen D, Taylor CR, et al. Anaplastic large cell lymphoma occurring in women with breast implants: analysis of 173 cases. Plast Reconstr Surg 135:695-705, 2015.

46. Mastopexy

See *Essentials of Plastic Surgery*, second edition, pp. 538-551.

BREAST PTOSIS

1. You are in clinic and see a number of women with concerns about their breast appearance. *For each of the following scenarios, select the correct type of ptosis present on clinical examination. (Each option may be used once, more than once, or not at all.)*
   A. A patient presents with a nipple-areolar complex (NAC) at the level of the IMF, with the majority of the breast below this.
   B. A patient has a NAC and most of the glandular breast tissue above the IMF.
   C. A patient presents with her nipple below the IMF at the inferiormost part of the breast.

   Options:
   a. Grade II
   b. Grade III
   c. Grade IV
   d. Pseudoptosis
   e. Constricted breast
   f. Normal (no ptosis present)

CAUSES OF BREAST PTOSIS

2. A 45-year-old mother of two is seen in the office concerning her breast ptosis. *Which one of the following is not a factor in the development of this condition?*
   A. Loss of skin elasticity with increasing age
   B. Decreased breast parenchyma volume
   C. Effects of pregnancy on breast tissue
   D. Attenuation of fibrous attachments between superficial and deep breast fascia
   E. Alterations in the structural integrity of the inframammary fold

TUBEROUS BREAST DEFORMITY

3. *Which one of the following is a typical feature of the tuberous breast?*
   A. A small areola
   B. Absence of the inframammary fold
   C. Increased breast volume
   D. Herniation of parenchymal tissue
   E. Broad breast base

Chapter 46 ■ Mastopexy 371

SURGICAL MANAGEMENT OF THE TUBEROUS BREAST
4. A 17-year-old girl presents with a unilateral tuberous breast deformity. There is severe lower pole skin deficiency and a two-cup size volume difference compared with the contralateral side. The nipple-areolar complex is oversized and the nipple height is slightly lower than on the contralateral side. She prefers the volume and shape of her normal, larger breast. **What is the best initial surgical management for this patient's tuberous breast?**
   A. Periareolar mastopexy with immediate permanent implant
   B. Periareolar mastopexy and fat transfer to the lower pole
   C. Vertical scar mastopexy with contralateral reduction
   D. Inferior pole scoring and insertion of a tissue expander
   E. Periareolar mastopexy with second-stage implant insertion

MASTOPEXY TECHNIQUES
5. *When considering different techniques used for mastopexy, which one of the following is correct?*
   A. Lejour, Lassus, and Hall-Findlay techniques all require approximation of the breast parenchymal pillars inferiorly.
   B. Benelli described the periareolar round block technique with polydiaxone periareolar sutures.
   C. Lassus described a vertical mastopexy with undermining.
   D. Hammond is associated with a short scar technique using a lateral pedicle.
   E. Lejour and Hall-Findlay techniques use the same pedicle.

CLINICAL SCENARIOS IN BREAST ABNORMALITIES
6. *For each of the following clinical scenarios, select the most suitable surgical procedure. (Each answer may be used once, more than once, or not at all.)*
   A. A 35-year-old patient has bilateral pseudoptosis after removal of 200 cc implants. She still has adequate breast volume and satisfactory nipple position.
   B. After significant weight loss, a 50-year-old patient has bilateral grade III ptosis with a nipple-to-notch distance of 32 cm, a large skin excess, and deficient breast volume. She is a nonsmoker, wears an A-cup bra, and wishes to improve both the shape and volume of her breasts.
   C. A 30-year-old patient has breast asymmetry with a notch-to-nipple distance of 28 cm (left) and 24 cm (right). She has adequate breast volume and good quality skin and soft tissues.

Options:
a. Vertical scar mastopexy
b. Periareolar mastopexy
c. Wise pattern mastopexy
d. Inframammary fold wedge excision
e. Single-stage periareolar augmentation-mastopexy
f. Two-stage Wise pattern augmentation-mastopexy
g. Two-stage vertical scar augmentation-mastopexy

OUTCOMES FOLLOWING MASTOPEXY

7. *Which one of the following is correct regarding outcomes after mastopexy?*
   A. When using a vertical scar technique, nipple-areolar elevation is not well maintained over time.
   B. In the long term, breast projection and superior pole fullness are significantly improved, especially when fascial sutures are used.
   C. The inverted-T technique has not demonstrated increased rates of "bottoming out" despite historical concerns.
   D. Periareolar techniques have shown the highest rates of surgeon dissatisfaction among board-certified plastic surgeons.
   E. Overelevation of the nipple is an uncommon finding at long-term follow-up.

MASTOPEXY FOLLOWING MASSIVE WEIGHT LOSS

8. You see a massive-weight-loss patient in clinic requesting breast reshaping surgery. On examination, the patient has severe ptosis with notch-to-nipple distances of 38 cm. She also has underfilled breasts with loss of central breast volume. Severe lateral rolls pass to the posterior axillary line on both sides. In the clinical notes, you record the breast appearance as grade III, according to the Rubin scale. *Which one of the following would be the most appropriate technique to improve breast shape and appearance in this case?*
   A. Vertical scar mastopexy alone
   B. Vertical scar augmentation-mastopexy
   C. Wise pattern mastopexy alone
   D. Wise pattern augmentation-mastopexy
   E. Wise pattern autoaugmentation-mastopexy

Answers

BREAST PTOSIS
1. For the following scenarios, the best options are as follows:
   A. A patient presents with a nipple-areolar complex (NAC) at the level of the IMF, with the majority of the breast below this.
      d. Pseudoptosis
   B. A patient has a NAC and most of the glandular breast tissue above the IMF.
      f. Normal (no ptosis present)
   C. A patient presents with her nipple below the IMF at the inferiormost part of the breast.
      b. Grade III ptosis

   Ptosis derives from the Greek, meaning "falling." The term is used to describe the descent of the breast parenchyma that traditionally occurs with advancing age and various physiologic changes. Regnault classified breast ptosis in 1976:
   - **Grade I:** Mild ptosis; the NAC lies at the level of the IMF.
   - **Grade II:** Moderate ptosis; the NAC lies below the IMF but remains above the most dependent part of the breast parenchyma.
   - **Grade III:** Severe ptosis; the NAC lies well below the IMF and is the most dependent part of the breast on the inferior aspect.

   Pseudoptosis is also called *glandular ptosis* and is present when the NAC is above or at the level of the IMF, but the bulk of the breast parenchyma has descended below the level of the fold. This can occur following breast reduction surgery, particularly with inferior pedicle Wise pattern techniques, and is sometimes described as "bottoming out." In a normal breast, the NAC and the majority of breast tissue should lie above the IMF (Fig. 46-1).

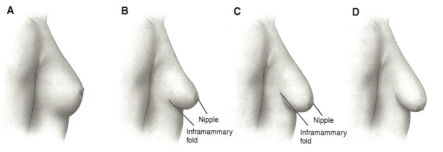

Fig. 46-1 Regnault classification of breast ptosis. **A,** Pseudoptosis. **B,** Grade I ptosis. **C,** Grade II ptosis. **D,** Grade III ptosis.

CAUSES OF BREAST PTOSIS

2. **A 45-year-old mother of two is seen in the office concerning her breast ptosis. Which one of the following is not a factor in the development of this condition?**
    E. Alterations in the structural integrity of the inframammary fold
    A number of factors are likely to be responsible for the development of breast ptosis. Changes in breast volume or composition following pregnancy, weight fluctuations, and menopause are all implicated. Changes in skin elasticity with age will affect the development of ptosis, and smoking is likely to exacerbate these changes.
    The breast parenchyma is covered by fascia split into two layers. The superficial component passes between the breast and the dermis; the deep component passes between breast and pectoralis major fascia. Cooper's ligaments are fibrous attachments that pass between these two fascial layers to provide support to the breast. Attenuation of Cooper's ligaments is also thought to be responsible for breast ptosis, although some authorities disagree with this theory.
    The appearance of breast ptosis is influenced by the adherence of the lower border of the breast tissue at the IMF that secures the lower pole in place and allows the breasts to "fall" or sag over it. Changes at the IMF itself are not responsible for ptosis.

TUBEROUS BREAST DEFORMITY

3. **Which one of the following is a typical feature of the tuberous breast?**
    D. Herniation of parenchymal tissue
    Tuberous breast deformity represents a spectrum of deformity, but typically includes the following features[1]:
    Constricted or narrowed breast base
    High inframammary fold (as opposed to absence of a fold)
    Breast herniation through the areola, leading to large areolae
    Deficiency of breast volume

    Tuberous breast may also be classified using the von Heimburg system which was described in 1996 and has four subtypes based on the degree of hypoplasia and the size of the skin envelope:[2]
    Type I: Hypoplasia of the lower medial quadrant
    Type II: Hypoplasia of the lower medial and lateral quadrants with adequate subareolar skin
    Type III: Hypoplasia of the lower medial and lateral quadrants with deficient subareolar skin
    Type IV: Severe breast constriction. Minimal breast base

    Grolleau proposed another classification system in 1999 reducing the number of subtypes to three based on the degree of hypoplasia of the breast:[3]
    Type I: Hypoplasia of the medial quadrant
    Type II: Hypoplasia of the medial and lateral quadrants
    Type III: Hypoplasia of all four quadrants

    These classification systems can be useful to describe the tuberous breast in medical documentation and also to help guide the most suitable treatment option when planning surgery.

SURGICAL MANAGEMENT OF THE TUBEROUS BREAST

4. A 17-year-old girl presents with a unilateral tuberous breast deformity. There is severe lower pole skin deficiency and a two-cup size volume difference compared with the contralateral side. The nipple-areolar complex is oversized and nipple height is slightly lower than on the contralateral side. She prefers the volume and shape of her normal, larger breast. *What is the best initial surgical management for this patient's tuberous breast?*

   D. Inferior pole scoring and insertion of a tissue expander

   Patients with tuberous breast, as in this case, commonly have significant breast asymmetry. Treatment should address both the lower pole skin deficiency and the volume deficiency. It should also lower the IMF, resite the NAC, and reduce the areola diameter as required. This is usually achieved with a combination of techniques including periareolar or vertical scar mastopexy, inferior pole scoring, and tissue expansion followed by augmentation procedures.

   Given the number of issues that need to be addressed, a staged approach is justified in this case. In the first stage, the lower pole can be expanded by radial release of the constricted tissues, lowering of the IMF, and placement of a breast expander. Once the expansion and volume have been corrected, either a periareolar or vertical scar approach can be taken to reduce the size of the nipple-areolar complex and reposition it on the breast mound. Some surgeons may prefer to incorporate the mastopexy into the first procedure, however options A, B, and E would still be incorrect, because neither a permanent implant nor a fat transfer would be adequate without tissue expansion. In some cases, a contralateral reduction is warranted, but in this case the patient is happy with the larger breast so this should be left alone.

MASTOPEXY TECHNIQUES

5. *When considering different techniques used for mastopexy, which one of the following is correct?*

   A. Lejour, Lassus, and Hall-Findlay techniques all require approximation of the breast parenchymal pillars inferiorly.

   The choice of mastopexy technique depends on the degree of ptosis, surgeon's preference, and patient factors.[4] The Lejour, Lassus, and Hall-Findlay techniques use a vertical scar and approximation of the medial and lateral breast pillars to cone the breast, thereby increasing projection. Differences in the techniques are that wide undermining is performed in both the Lejour and Hall-Findlay techniques, whereas no undermining is performed in the Lassus technique. Lejour and Hall-Findlay may also combine liposuction. Lejour uses a superior pedicle, whereas Hall-Findlay uses a medial pedicle. Hammond's technique is a short scar, periareolar, inferior pedicle procedure (rather than lateral pedicle). Benelli described the purse-string suture using a permanent suture and not a long-acting resorbable suture like polydiaxone.

CLINICAL SCENARIOS IN BREAST ABNORMALITIES

6. *For the following scenarios, the best options are as follows:*
   A. *A 35-year-old patient has bilateral pseudoptosis after removal of 200 cc implants. She still has adequate breast volume and satisfactory nipple position.*
      d. **Inframammary fold wedge excision**
         In the first case, the nipple height is acceptable, so a standard mastopexy technique is not required. The pseudoptosis is caused by bottoming out of the breast and may be corrected by performing a transverse wedge excision in the IMF. Rohrich et al[4] have described technique selection for breast contouring at the time of breast implant removal that is based on ptosis type and NAC size and location.
   B. *After significant weight loss, a 50-year-old patient has bilateral grade III ptosis with a notch-to-nipple distance of 32 cm, a large skin excess, and deficient breast volume. She is a nonsmoker, wears an A-cup bra, and wishes to improve both the shape and volume of her breasts.*
      f. **Two-stage Wise pattern augmentation-mastopexy**
         After significant weight loss, patients commonly have empty, ptotic breasts that require volume replacement with a prosthesis and mastopexy to reduce skin volume and to raise the NAC. There is debate whether to do this as a single or a multistaged technique, because augmentation and mastopexy techniques work against one another. Achieving satisfactory results in a single stage is challenging. Given the amount of skin excess in such patients, a periareolar or vertical scar approach is less likely to be suitable. The volume of skin excess in this patient indicates that she would require an inverted-T skin pattern.
   C. *A 30-year-old patient has breast asymmetry with a notch-to-nipple distance of 28 cm (left) and 24 cm (right). She has adequate breast volume and good quality skin and soft tissues.*
      a. **Vertical scar mastopexy**
         This woman has mild to moderate ptosis, and this may be treated with a vertical scar technique. A Benelli periareolar technique could potentially be used, but a simple periareolar technique is usually useful only in patients with mild ptosis.

OUTCOMES FOLLOWING MASTOPEXY

7. *Which one of the following is correct regarding outcomes after mastopexy?*
   D. **Periareolar techniques have shown the highest rates of surgeon dissatisfaction among board-certified plastic surgeons.**
      A survey of board-certified plastic surgeons found that periareolar techniques had the highest rate of surgeon dissatisfaction and the highest rate of revision.[5] Although most popular, the inverted-T group reported a significantly greater frequency of bottoming out ($p = 0.043$) and excess scarring along the inframammary fold ($p = 0.001$), compared with the short scar and periareolar groups.

      A review of 1700 vertical scar procedures showed that the NAC was 1.3 cm higher at day 5 after surgery and remained 1 cm higher 4 years after surgery compared with preoperative measurements, suggesting that elevation of the nipple is well maintained over time.[6]

      A review of 82 publications on mastopexy and reduction, including the most popular techniques, showed that neither breast projection or upper pole projection were increased significantly.[7] Methods to increase upper pole fullness or projection, such as fascial sutures and autoaugmentation, generally did not maintain shape in the long term. Nipple overelevation was observed in around 40% of patients.

MASTOPEXY FOLLOWING MASSIVE WEIGHT LOSS

8. You see a massive-weight-loss patient in clinic requesting breast reshaping surgery. On examination, the patient has severe ptosis with notch-to-nipple distances of 38 cm. She also has underfilled breasts with loss of central breast volume. Severe lateral rolls pass to the posterior axillary line on both sides. In the clinical notes, you record the breast appearance as grade III, according to the Rubin scale. **Which one of the following would be the most appropriate technique to improve breast shape and appearance in this case?**

E. Wise pattern autoaugmentation-mastopexy

Rubin has classified the severity of the breast deformity following massive weight loss into three grades:

Grade I: Ptosis grade I or II or severe macromastia
Grade II: Ptosis grade III, moderate volume loss or constricted breast
Grade III: Severe lateral roll and or severe volume loss with loose skin

The grading has clinical relevance as it can guide surgical management of these patients.

In this grade III case, a Wise pattern approach with long scars is required to address the skin excess. Implant augmentation is best avoided providing the existing volume can create a reasonable result. In such cases a dermal suspension autoaugmentation procedure can be undertaken. This is based on a Wise pattern technique and uses deepithelialized tissue from the lateral roll and inferomedial breast to autoaugment the breast volume by anchoring the flaps to the anterior chest wall around a degloved breast mound (see Figs. 46-6 through 46-9, *Essentials of Plastic Surgery,* second edition).

Less severe grades I and II may be effectively managed with either vertical scar or Wise pattern skin approaches and will often need additional volume from prosthetic implant placement either as single- or two-stage procedures.

REFERENCES

1. Rees TD, Aston SJ. The tuberous breast. Clin Plast Surg 3:339-347, 1976.
2. von Heimburg D, Exner K, Kruft S, et al. The tuberous breast deformity: classification and treatment. Br J Plast Surg 49:339-445, 1996.
3. Grolleau JL, Lanfrey E, Lavigne B, et al. Breast base anomalies: treatment strategy for tuberous breasts, minor deformities, and asymmetry. Plast Reconstr Surg 104:2040-2048, 1999.
4. Rohrich RJ, Beran SJ, Restifo RJ, et al. Aesthetic management of the breast following explantation: evaluation and mastopexy options. Plast Reconstr Surg 101:827-837, 1998.
5. Rohrich RJ, Gosman AA, Brown SA, et al. Mastopexy preferences: a survey of board-certified plastic surgeons. Plast Reconstr Surg 118:1631-1638, 2006.
6. Ahmad J, Lista F. Vertical scar reduction mammaplasty: the fate of nipple-areola complex position and inferior pole length. Plast Reconstr Surg 121:1084-1091, 2008.
7. Swanson E. A retrospective photometric study of 82 published reports of mastopexy and breast reduction. Plast Reconstr Surg 128:1282-1301, 2011.

47. Augmentation-Mastopexy

See *Essentials of Plastic Surgery*, second edition, pp. 552-557.

GENERAL PRINCIPLES

1. **Which one of the following statements is correct regarding augmentation-mastopexy?**
   A. Most patients with breast skin excess and volume deficiency require augmentation-mastopexy.
   B. It is safer and more cost effective to perform augmentation-mastopexy in a single stage.
   C. Results using two-stage augmentation-mastopexy are usually more predictable.
   D. In spite of high revision rates, levels of malpractice claims following surgery are low.
   E. When staging augmentation-mastopexy, the augmentation should be performed first.

SELECTION OF BREAST REJUVENATION PROCEDURES

2. A patient presents after two pregnancies, because she is considering augmentation-mastopexy. On examination she has ptotic, underfilled symmetrical breasts. The distance from her sternal notch-to-nipple–areola complex (NAC) measures 30 cm on both sides. Her anterior skin stretch measurement is 5 cm at the NAC, with an IMF-to-NAC distance of 12 cm on stretch. You anticipate an excision of 7 cm of skin to adequately uplift her breasts. **Which one of the following is the best option for this patient?**
   A. Breast augmentation alone
   B. Staged augmentation-mastopexy
   C. Mastopexy alone
   D. Single-stage augmentation-mastopexy
   E. Staged autoaugmentation-mastopexy

CONTRAINDICATIONS TO SINGLE-STAGE AUGMENTATION-MASTOPEXY

3. A patient is referred for a second opinion regarding a single-stage augmentation-mastopexy. **Which one of the following may represent a contraindication to this surgery?**
   A. Tuberous breast deformity
   B. Significant breast asymmetry
   C. A large vertical skin excess
   D. Less than 2 cm of breast tissue below the IMF
   E. All of the above

SELECTION OF A SKIN INCISION FOR AUGMENTATION-MASTOPEXY

4. You assess a patient with moderate ptosis for augmentation-mastopexy. Her nipples are sited 4 cm below her IMF, and there is moderate horizontal, but minimal vertical skin excess. *Which one of the following skin markings is best suited to this patient?*
   A. Short inverted-T scar
   B. Full Wise pattern scar
   C. Vertical scar
   D. Horizontal scar
   E. Periareolar scar

REOPERATION RATES AFTER AUGMENTATION-MASTOPEXY

5. You plan a single-stage augmentation-mastopexy for a 40-year-old woman. *What is the approximate risk of revision surgery?*
   A. Less than 1%
   B. 5%
   C. 10%
   D. 20%
   E. 33%

Answers

GENERAL PRINCIPLES

1. **Which one of the following statements is correct regarding augmentation-mastopexy?**

   C. Results using two-stage augmentation-mastopexy are usually more predictable.

   Augmentation-mastopexy can be undertaken as a single-stage procedure, but a two-stage approach is generally thought to be more predictable. Many patients with combined breast volume deficiency and skin excess can be managed successfully with either augmentation or mastopexy alone. Augmentation-mastopexy is only required for patients who require additional breast volume and have skin excess that cannot be compensated for by augmentation or mastopexy alone. It may be more cost effective in the short term to undertake augmentation-mastopexy in a single stage, but the long-term costs as a result of high revision rates, can offset this.

   It is not necessarily safer to undertake a single rather than a two-stage procedure, although the number of general anesthetic procedures will be reduced. Augmentation-mastopexy techniques are associated with high revision rates of up to one in five, although this may be reduced to less than 1 in 10 by staging the procedure.

   Augmentation-mastopexy is one of the most common causes for malpractice claims. It represents a real challenge for the surgeon who has to balance the two opposing factors; skin excess, and volume deficiency with augmentation and mastopexy techniques, essentially working against one another.

   The order of augmentation-mastopexy will be guided by the clinical situation and either stage may be undertaken first. In general, if the primary goal is ptosis correction, then the mastopexy should be performed first. If the primary goal is to improve projection or upper pole fullness, then the implant should be placed first.[1]

SELECTION OF BREAST REJUVENATION PROCEDURES

2. A patient presents after two pregnancies, because she is considering augmentation-mastopexy. On examination she has ptotic, underfilled symmetrical breasts. The distance from her sternal notch-to-nipple–areola complex (NAC) measures 30 cm on both sides. Her anterior skin stretch measurement is 5 cm at the NAC, with an IMF-to-NAC distance of 12 cm on stretch. You anticipate an excision of 7 cm of skin to adequately uplift her breasts. **Which one of the following is the best option for this patient?**

   B. Staged augmentation-mastopexy

   Lee et al[1] have developed an algorithm to guide selection of augmentation-mastopexy procedures (see Figs. 47-3 and 47-4, *Essentials of Plastic Surgery,* second edition). They consider the following three key measurements to be important factors:

   NAC anterior skin stretch
   NAC-to-IMF vertical skin stretch
   Vertical skin and parenchymal excess

   Skin stretch refers to nipple excursion on light anterior traction and provides information on the laxity in the AP plane. Nipple-to-IMF distance on maximal stretch provides information on the laxity in the vertical dimension. *Vertical excess* is the anticipated excess skin/parenchyma to be

resected. A two-stage augmentation-mastopexy procedure is advocated for this patient because of her large skin excess.

CONTRAINDICATIONS TO SINGLE-STAGE AUGMENTATION-MASTOPEXY

3. A patient is referred for a second opinion regarding a single-stage augmentation-mastopexy. *Which one of the following may represent a contraindication to this surgery?*

E. All of the above

The contraindications to single-stage augmentation-mastopexy are a tuberous breast deformity, significant asymmetry, a large amount of vertical skin excess, and mild ptosis/pseudoptosis (because a mastopexy may not be required). The presence of less than 2 cm of breast tissue below the IMF suggests minimal ptosis or pseudoptosis. An anterior skin stretch of less than 4 cm should be treated with augmentation alone, whereas a distance of 6 cm is an indication for augmentation-mastopexy, although it is not specific to either a single-stage or two-stage procedure.

SELECTION OF A SKIN INCISION FOR AUGMENTATION-MASTOPEXY

4. You assess a patient with moderate ptosis for augmentation-mastopexy. Her nipples are 4 cm below her IMF, and there is moderate horizontal, but minimal vertical skin excess. *Which one of the following skin markings is best suited to this patient?*

C. Vertical scar

Selection of a skin pattern for an augmentation-mastopexy depends on the anticipated amount of skin excess after augmentation. The guidelines for selection are as follows:
  A periareolar pattern is recommended for patients with minimal ptosis.
    The nipple is less than 2 cm below the IMF *and*
    The NAC is at or above the breast border (and does not point inferiorly) *and*
    No more than 3 or 4 cm of associated breast ptosis is present.
  A vertical pattern is recommended for patients with moderate ptosis.
    The nipple is greater than 2 cm below the IMF *and*
    Horizontal skin excess and minimal vertical skin excess are present.
  A Wise pattern is recommended for patients with severe ptosis.
    The nipple is greater than 2 cm below the IMF *and*
    Both vertical and horizontal skin excess are present.
As this patient has horizontal skin excess without vertical skin excess in the presence of moderate ptosis, she could be managed with a vertical scar approach, according to these guidelines. The use of a short T-scar can be useful when undertaking a vertical scar technique if it is found that there remains an excess of skin which is difficult to absorb in the vertical scar alone.[2,3]

REOPERATION RATES AFTER AUGMENTATION-MASTOPEXY

5. You plan a single-stage augmentation-mastopexy for a 40-year-old woman. *What is the approximate risk of revision surgery?*

D. 20%

Recent data from Lee et al[1] show similarly low rates of approximately 7% for either the single-stage or the two-stage procedure. The authors applied their algorithm to determine the appropriate augmentation-mastopexy procedure for each patient (see Fig. 47-1, *Essentials of Plastic Surgery*, second edition)). However, two other recent large series have published reoperation rates of 15% to 20% for single-stage procedures.[4,5] Therefore it is prudent to counsel patients to expect this level of risk, from a conservative standpoint.

REFERENCES

1. Lee MR, Unger JG, Adams WP Jr. The tissue-based triad: a process approach to augmentation mastopexy. Plast Reconstr Surg 134:215-225, 2014.
2. Davison SP, Spear SL. Simultaneous breast augmentation with periareolar mastopexy. Semin Plast Surg 18:189-201, 2004.
3. Kirwan L. A classification and algorithm for treatment of breast ptosis. Aesthet Surg J 22:355-363, 2002.
4. Stevens WG, Freeman ME, Stoker DA, et al. One-stage mastopexy with breast augmentation: a review of 321 patients. Plast Reconstr Surg 120:1674-1679, 2007.
5. Calobrace MB, Herdt DR, Cothron KJ. Simultaneous augmentation/mastopexy: a retrospective 5-year review of 332 consecutive cases. Plast Reconstr Surg 131:145-156, 2013.

48. Breast Reduction

See *Essentials of Plastic Surgery*, second edition, pp. 558-572.

IDEAL BREAST AESTHETIC MEASUREMENTS

1. **Which one of the following is a characteristic of an ideal breast, as described by Penn in his 1955 study?**
   A. The notch-to-nipple distance is equivalent to the internipple distance.
   B. The base width is 11 to 12 cm.
   C. The notch-to-nipple distance is 24 cm.
   D. The nipple-to-inframammary fold (IMF) distance is 4 cm.
   E. The areolar diameter is 5 cm.

AESTHETICS OF THE NORMAL BREAST

2. **In general, when marking the new nipple position for a bilateral breast reduction, where should the nipple be vertically positioned?**
   A. A distance of 26 cm from the sternal notch
   B. A distance of 8 cm from the inframammary fold
   C. Level with the humerus proximal one-third to two-third junction
   D. At Pitanguy's point on the anterior breast
   E. At a distance of 20 cm from the midclavicular point

PATHOPHYSIOLOGY OF HYPERMASTIA

3. **Which one of the following statements is thought to occur in patients with hypermastia?**
   A. An increase in the level of circulating estrogens
   B. An increase in the number of estrogen receptors
   C. Volume increases that predominate in glandular tissue
   D. An imbalance between estrogen and progesterone production
   E. An altered response to circulating estrogens

JUVENILE VIRGINAL HYPERTROPHY OF THE BREAST

4. You see a 12-year-old girl in clinic who has developed excessively large breasts over the past twelve months. Examination shows her to be of slim build with symmetrical breasts that have an estimated volume in excess of 2000 g per side. **Which one of the following is correct?**
   A. The condition is likely to regress once puberty stops.
   B. Medical management is the first-line therapy.
   C. Following surgical resection, recurrence does not occur.
   D. Blood tests are likely to show an abnormal sex hormone profile.
   E. Symptoms are likely to have developed just after her first menstrual period.

SUCTION LIPECTOMY

5. In which one of the following settings might suction lipectomy represent a reasonable alternative to standard breast reduction techniques in the management of hypermastia?
A. In young patients with large, dense nonptotic breasts
B. In young, slim patients with mild ptosis wanting to breast-feed
C. In older patients with soft, heavy breasts and less concern for cosmesis
D. In patients of any age where only small volumes (<250 mls) need to be removed
E. None of the above, as it should only be used in conjunction with an excisional technique

PEDICLE DESIGNS IN BREAST REDUCTION

6. All young patients undergoing breast reduction must be warned of the potential risks associated with breast-feeding and loss of nipple sensation following surgery. The effects of these are related to pedicle design. **Which one of the following pedicles should be particularly avoided in young patients who hope to breast-feed and maintain nipple sensation following their breast reduction?**
A. Central pedicle
B. Inferior pedicle
C. Superior pedicle
D. Superomedial pedicle
E. Lateral pedicle

7. Which one of the following pedicle designs best allows for preservation of Würinger's septum and may subsequently lead to improved vascular supply and sensory innervation to the nipple?
A. Medial pedicle
B. Inferior pedicle
C. Superior pedicle
D. Superomedial pedicle
E. Lateral pedicle

SKIN PATTERN EXCISION IN BREAST REDUCTION

8. Which one of the following statements is correct regarding breast reduction techniques?
A. A Wise pattern relies on parenchyma to shape and hold the skin.
B. Inverted-T and vertical scar techniques invariably require subsequent dog-ear excision.
C. Free nipple grafts do not preserve nipple sensation, but lactation is usually possible.
D. Vertical scar techniques rely on skin to shape and hold the breast.
E. Periareolar patterns are not usually useful for breast reduction cases and can stretch the NAC.

MARKINGS FOR INVERTED-T BREAST REDUCTION

9. Which one of the following statements is correct when marking a patient for an inverted-T breast reduction?
A. The breast meridian will determine the vertical nipple position.
B. The vertical limbs should be 5 cm long to minimize bottoming out.
C. The NAC cut-out should be designed slightly larger than the areolar diameter.
D. In heavy pendulous breasts the nipple should be marked slightly lower.
E. The horizontal lines joining the vertical limbs and IMF should be straight.

INFILTRATION FOR BREAST REDUCTION

10. You are planning a bilateral breast reduction procedure and have decided to inject the breast tissue with an infiltration of a solution that contains dilute epinephrine and local anesthetic. *Based on evidence from multiple studies, which one of the following has consistently been demonstrated to be significantly reduced by this strategy?*
    - A. Operating duration
    - B. Hospital stay
    - C. Postoperative pain at 9 hours
    - D. Intraoperative blood loss
    - E. Skin flap viability

PROBLEMS WITH PERFUSION OF THE NAC

11. You are using an inverted-T pattern with an inferior pedicle to perform a bilateral breast reduction in a 37-year-old woman. You have satisfactorily reduced the first side and are in the process of elevating the pedicle on the second side when your resident points out that the nipple appears severely compromised. *What is your next step in management of this patient?*
    - A. Continue with the procedure as planned.
    - B. Temporarily stop the procedure, assess temperature, urine output, and blood pressure.
    - C. Apply topical nitroglycerin.
    - D. Convert to a free nipple graft on that side.
    - E. Confirm that the pedicle is not kinked, then resect more tissue from the pedicle to decrease bulk and oxygen requirements.

EVIDENCE IN BREAST REDUCTION

12. You are trying to evaluate evidence to guide your practice in breast reduction surgery. *Which one of the following is correct?*
    - A. A correlation exists between increasing excision volume and greater symptom relief.
    - B. The use of drains in breast reduction surgery is unproven to decrease hematomas.
    - C. Most patients with hypermastia seek treatment for purely cosmetic reasons.
    - D. The symptoms of hypermastia are much less severe than with chronic medical conditions.
    - E. Patients with a BMI greater than 25 have more severe functional symptoms.

Answers

IDEAL BREAST AESTHETIC MEASUREMENTS

1. Which one of the following is a characteristic of the ideal breast, as described by Penn in his 1955 study?

A. A notch-to-nipple distance is equivalent to internipple distance.

Penn[1] studied breast aesthetics in the 1950s. He reviewed a number of females and concluded that certain measurements provided an aesthetically pleasing breast. In Penn's ideal breast measurements, the sternal notch-to-nipple distance was 21 cm and was equivalent to the internipple distance. The vertical nipple-to-IMF distance was 7 cm. Breast base width was not described. A normal nipple-areolar complex is between 3.8 and 4.5 cm but there is significant variation. A clear understanding of normal breast aesthetics is vital for performing corrective breast surgery (Fig. 48-1).

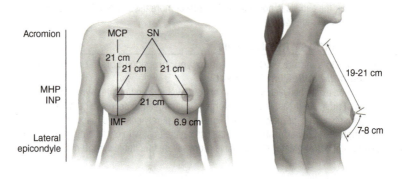

Fig. 48-1 Ideal breast measurements. (*IMF,* Inframammary fold; *INP,* ideal nipple plane; *MCP,* midclavicular point; *MHP,* midhumeral plane; *SN,* sternal notch.)

AESTHETICS OF THE NORMAL BREAST

2. In general, when marking the new nipple position for a bilateral breast reduction, where should the nipple be vertically positioned?

D. At Pitanguy's point on the anterior breast

As discussed in question 1, classic Penn numbers for nipple position are 21 cm from the sternal notch-to-nipple and a nipple-to-IMF distance of approximately 7 cm.

When marking up a patient for bilateral breast reduction, there are three useful guides to vertical nipple placement: the IMF, the distance from the sternal notch, and the midhumeral point when arms are placed by the patient's side. The point at which the IMF level is transposed to the anterior breast is known as Pitanguy's point and is a reliable guide to ideal nipple position in most patients. A range of distances (21 to 24 cm) from the sternal notch-to-nipple are generally applicable, but 26 cm would be too low in most cases. Many surgeons will use all three measurements/landmarks to guide their decision-making.

PATHOPHYSIOLOGY OF HYPERMASTIA

3. Which one of the following statements is thought to occur in patients with hypermastia?

E. An altered response to circulating estrogens

In most patients with hypermastia, there are both normal estrogen levels and receptor number, which suggests that the abnormal excessive breast growth may be the result of an altered response to normal circulating estrogens. The main increase in breast volume is observed in fibrous and fatty tissue rather than within glandular tissue.[2]

JUVENILE VIRGINAL HYPERTROPHY OF THE BREAST

4. You see a 12-year-old girl in clinic who has developed excessively large breasts over the past twelve months. Examination shows her to be of slim build with symmetrical breasts that have an estimated volume in excess of 2000 g per side. Which one of the following is correct?

E. Symptoms are likely to have developed just after her first menstrual period.

Juvenile virginal hypertrophy of the breast (Gigantomastia) has an unknown etiology and patients usually have a normal endocrine profile. Onset occurs shortly after the girl's first menstruation with excessive growth of both breasts. Surgical management with breast reduction is the mainstay of treatment with at least 1800 g typically removed. There is a risk of recurrence following resection and this is particularly high during pregnancy. Regression is rare without intervention.

SUCTION LIPECTOMY

5. In which one of the following settings might suction lipectomy represent a reasonable alternative to standard breast reduction techniques in the management of hypermastia?

C. In older patients with soft, heavy breasts and less concern for cosmesis

Suction lipectomy has limited indications for use as a stand-alone technique in breast reduction. It is more commonly used in conjunction with an excisional technique to shape specific areas of the breast. When used independently as a reduction technique it is best reserved for older patients with large, heavy breasts as they tend to have a higher proportion of fat within the breast that can be removed with liposuction. Suction lipectomy is less effective in younger patients as they have more parenchyma and less fatty tissue. This is particularly true in slimmer patients. Advantages of lipectomy over excisional techniques include reduced scarring, and preservation of nipple innervations and lactation. However it is less effective at correcting ptosis and can lead to a flatter breast shape. Suction lipectomy has been used successfully to treat macromastia in certain patient groups and this was not limited to small volume reduction. For example, in a series published by Courtiss[3] volumes of up to 835 cc was removed from each breast, and in a study by Gray[4] up to 2250 cc was removed with good outcomes and no reported complications.

PEDICLE DESIGNS IN BREAST REDUCTION

6. All young patients undergoing breast reduction must be warned of the potential risks associated with breast-feeding and loss of nipple sensation following surgery. The effects of these are related to pedicle design. Which one of the following pedicles should be particularly avoided in young patients who hope to breast-feed and maintain nipple sensation following their breast reduction?

C. Superior pedicle

With all pedicle designs there is a risk of poor breast-feeding potential and altered sensation, but the superior pedicle is particularly poor because the nipple-areola complex (NAC) is based on dermal rather than dermoglandular tissue. The perceived benefit of this technique is that ptosis may be reduced and projection improved because of inferior tissue excision. The inferior pedicle and central mound are reasonable choices for maintenance of sensation and breast-feeding potential. Around three quarters of patients with inferior pedicle reductions will secrete postpartum milk.[5]

7. **Which one of the following pedicle designs best allows for preservation of Würinger's septum and may subsequently lead to improved vascular supply and sensory innervations to the nipple?**
   E. **Lateral pedicle**
   Würinger's septum (also described in Chapter 44) is part of a brassiere-like connective tissue suspensory system of the breast. It is a horizontal septum originating from the pectoral fascia along the fifth rib and merges with lateral and medial vertical ligaments. Within it are branches of the thoracoacromial, lateral thoracic, and fourth to sixth intercostal arteries. It also carries the main contributory nerve to the nipple (fourth intercostal). The lateral pedicle is most likely to maintain this septum although the central mound should also do so with careful dissection (see Fig. 48-7, *Essentials of Plastic Surgery,* second edition).

SKIN PATTERN EXCISION IN BREAST REDUCTION

8. **Which one of the following statements is correct regarding breast reduction techniques?**
   E. **Periareolar patterns are not usually useful for breast reduction cases and can stretch the NAC.**
   An inverted-T or Wise pattern relies on the skin to act as an external brassiere and support the breast. This can lead to bottoming out in the long term. For this reason it receives criticism from proponents of the vertical scar techniques, which aim to reshape the breast and provide support from within using parenchymal pillar sutures. Skin is then redraped over the top. As discussed in question 6, the ability to lactate after breast reduction is highly variable and seems to be affected by pedicle selection. Two issues require consideration: Is any amount of lactation possible, and is the volume adequate to successfully breast-feed? In theory, the ducts can recannulate after free nipple grafts, but the likelihood of successful lactation is negligible. Although periareolar approaches can be used for small mastopexy cases, their use for reduction mammaplasty is limited to very small reductions.

MARKINGS FOR INVERTED-T BREAST REDUCTION

9. **Which one of the following statements is correct when marking a patient for an inverted-T breast reduction?**
   D. **In heavy pendulous breasts the nipple should be marked slightly lower.**
   When marking a breast for an inverted-T scar technique in breast reduction, the nipple is usually placed at the level of the IMF, which equates to Pitanguy's line (see question 2). However, in heavy pendulous breasts it is wise to lower the nipple slightly to avoid overcorrection with the nipple ending up too high postoperatively. This is because once the weight of the breast parenchyma has been reduced, the elastic recoil of the skin will tend to lift the NAC above the estimated level. Correction of the high riding nipple is difficult following uplift procedures and will create scars above the NAC. The breast meridian will provide a guide for the horizontal, rather than vertical placement of the nipple. The vertical limbs should be 7 to 8 cm and are left this short to minimize bottoming out of the breast postoperatively. If they are too short however, there will be excessive skin tension during closure that can lead to wound dehiscence. The cut-out for the NAC should be slightly smaller than the NAC to minimize postoperative stretch. The vertical limbs of a breast

reduction are straight but the horizontal limbs should be curvilinear with a lazy S-pattern, as this helps to reduce the medial and lateral dog ears, while maintaining adequate skin at the T-junction. The use of curvilinear limbs on the lateral skin flaps increases the wound edge length on this side which can help any length discrepancy which exists compared with the IMF wound edge.

INFILTRATION FOR BREAST REDUCTION

10. You are planning a bilateral breast reduction procedure and have decided to inject the breast tissue with infiltration of a solution that contains dilute epinephrine and local anesthetic. **Based on evidence from multiple studies, which one of the following has consistently been demonstrated to be significantly reduced by this strategy?**
    D. Intraoperative blood loss
    Multiple studies have shown that infiltration with a solution of dilute epinephrine for breast reduction can significantly decrease intraoperative blood loss.[6-10] This seems to be a fairly consistent finding across multiple studies and represents the major reproducible benefit of performing such a technique.

    Solutions that contain a local anesthetic have been shown to decrease postoperative pain in some studies. However, this was true only during the very early postoperative period. This is expected, because the effects of local anesthetic agents are short lived. Some studies have shown decreased operating time, presumably attributable to a blood-free operating field, whereas others have shown reduced postoperative drainage, but these results have not been consistent across the studies. Hospital stay at times trended toward shorter time periods, but they were not significantly different.

PROBLEMS WITH PERFUSION OF THE NAC

11. You are using an inverted-T pattern with an inferior pedicle to perform a bilateral breast reduction in a 37-year-old woman. You have satisfactorily reduced the first side and are in the process of elevating the pedicle on the second side when your resident points out that the nipple appears severely compromised. **What is your next step in management of this patient?**
    B. Temporarily stop the procedure, assess temperature, urine output, and blood pressure.
    The NAC can become compromised during or after a breast reduction procedure. This can result from poor arterial inflow leading to a pale nipple with no red bleeding evident or from venous congestion leading to a purple-colored nipple. Management of a compromised nipple is dependent on the likely cause and timing of the problem. Several key factors need to be confirmed. Patients should be warm and well perfused, with adequate blood pressure and urine output. The pedicle should be examined for signs of damage or kinking. Cessation of the procedure for a short time is advocated to assess these parameters and to allow the pedicle vasculature to recover from possible spasm. Local anesthetic infiltration with epinephrine may be contributing to an arterial inflow problem. If a patient is cardiovascularly optimized and the nipple continues to appear nonviable, then conversion to a free nipple graft may be sensible providing that all other factors have been addressed. If the compromise occurs during closure, or begins postoperatively, then it may be due to localized swelling causing vessel compression. Intraoperatively the sutures can be removed to see if the nipple appearance improves. If so, loose closure may be indicated. If the compromise occurs postoperatively, it may be necessary to return to surgery, for example, to evacuate a hematoma (and reduce compression), to check for pedicle compression, or to convert to a free nipple graft.

    Nitroglycerine is a potent topical vasodilator that increases local blood flow by dilating arteries and veins. While application of a topical nitroglycerine patch or ointment to the compromised nipple might be tempting, if the cause of inadequate perfusion is compromise of the pedicle for which the nipple is an indicator, then this will not be helped because the vascularity of the deeper tissues will not be affected.

EVIDENCE IN BREAST REDUCTION
12. You are trying to evaluate evidence to guide your practice in breast reduction surgery. **Which one of the following is correct?**
    B. The use of drains in breast reduction surgery is unproven to decrease hematomas.
    A number of studies have confirmed that there is no benefit in using drains in breast reduction patients with regard to hematoma rates.[11,12,13] A randomized controlled study by Collis et al[14] compared the use of drains in reduction mammaplasty with no drains in 150 patients and showed no difference in hematoma rates when a drain was or was not used. The incidence of wound healing or other complication was also unaffected by drain use.

    The American Society of Plastic Surgeons (ASPS) have published evidence-based guidelines[15,16] on breast reduction and concluded that there is no correlation between volume excision and symptom relief. Most patients seek breast reduction surgery for functional reasons, although cosmesis is often a secondary concern also identified.[17] The functional symptoms of hyperamastia are reported to be a comparable severity to those of a patient with a chronic medical condition, but there is no evidence to show that patients with a higher BMI (>25) have more severe symptoms. Reduction weights greater than 800 g are associated with higher rates of complications including fat necrosis, wound dehiscence, delayed wound healing, seroma and hematoma.

REFERENCES
1. Penn J. Breast reduction. Br J Plast Surg 7:357-371, 1955.
2. Jabs AD. Mammary hypertrophy is not associated with increased estrogen receptors. Plast Reconstr Surg 86:64-66, 1990.
3. Courtiss EH. Reduction mammoplasty by suction alone. Plast Reconstr Surg 92:1276-1284, 1993.
4. Gray, LN. Liposuction breast reduction. Aesthetic Plast Surg 22:159-162, 1998
5. Schlenz I, Rigel S, Schemper M, et al. Alteration of nipple and areola sensitivity by reduction mammaplasty: a prospective comparison of five techniques. Plast Reconstr Surg 115:743-751; discussion 752-754, 2005.
6. Soueid A, Nawinne M, Khan H. Randomized clinical trial on the effects of the use of diluted adrenaline solution in reduction mammaplasty: same patient, same technique, same surgeon. Plast Reconstr Surg 121:30e-33e, 2008.
7. Thomas SS, Srivastava S, Nancarrow JD, et al. Dilute adrenaline infiltration and reduced blood loss in reduction mammaplasty. Ann Plast Surg 43:127-131, 1999.
8. Rosaeg OP, Bell M, Cicutti NJ, et al. Pre-incision infiltration with lidocaine reduces pain and opioid consumption after reduction mammoplasty. Reg Anesth Pain Med 23:575-579, 1998.
9. Wilmink H, Spauwen PH, Hartman EH, et al. Preoperative injection using a diluted anesthetic/adrenaline solution significantly reduces blood loss in reduction mammaplasty. Plast Reconstr Surg 102:373-376, 1998.
10. Samdal F, Serra M, Skolleborg KC. The effects of infiltration with adrenaline on blood loss during reduction mammaplasty: an early survey. Scand J Plast Reconstr Hand Surg 26:211-215, 1992.
11. Wrye SW, Banducci DR, Mackay D, et al. Routine drainage is not required in reduction mammaplasty. Plast Reconstr Surg 111:113-117, 2003.
12. Corion LU, Smeulders MJ, van Zuijlen PP, et al. Draining after breast reduction: a randomized controlled inter-patient study. J Plast Reconstr Aesthet Surg 62:865-868, 2009.

13. Matarasso A, Wallach SG, Rankin M. Reevaluating the need for routine drainage in reduction mammaplasty. Plast Reconstr Surg 102:1917-1921, 1998
14. Collis N, McGuiness CM, Batchelor AG. Drainage in breast reduction surgery: a prospective randomised intra-patient trail. Br J Plast Surg 58:286-289, 2005.
15. American Society of Plastic Surgeons. Evidence-based clinical practice guideline: reduction mammaplasty. Available at *www.plasticsurgery.org/Documents/medical-professionals/health-policy/evidence-practice/Reduction%20Mammaplasty_%20Evidence%20Based%20Guidelines_v5.pdf.*
16. American Society of Plastic Surgeons. Reduction mammaplasty: ASPS recommended insurance coverage criteria for third-party payers. Available at *www.plasticsurgery.org/Documents/medical-professionals/health-policy/insurance/Reduction_Mammaplasty_Coverage_Criteria.pdf.*
17. Schnur PL, Hoehn JG, Ilsturp DM, et al. Reduction mammaplasty: cosmetic or reconstructive procedure? Ann Plast Surg 27:232-237, 1991.

49. Gynecomastia

See *Essentials of Plastic Surgery*, second edition, pp. 573-579.

GENERAL ASPECTS OF GYNECOMASTIA
1. **Which one of the following is correct regarding gynecomastia?**
   A. Gynecomastia is either a physiologic or pathologic condition.
   B. Less than 1 in 10 males experience it during their lifetime.
   C. Up to a half of cases are bilateral.
   D. Adolescent males are very commonly affected.
   E. It is associated with an increased risk of breast cancer.

GENERAL CAUSES OF GYNECOMASTIA
2. **What is the most common cause of gynecomastia?**
   A. Pubertal circulating hormone excess
   B. Use of anabolic steroids
   C. Testicular tumors
   D. Liver cirrhosis
   E. Idiopathic cause

PHARMACOLOGIC CAUSES OF GYNECOMASTIA
3. It is vital to review prescription and nonprescription drugs of patients with gynecomastia. **Which one of the following is not usually expected to cause gynecomastia?**
   A. Marijuana
   B. Spironolactone
   C. Cimetidine
   D. Simvastatin
   E. Anabolic steroids

PREOPERATIVE WORKUP
4. **When assessing a patient in clinic with gynecomastia, which one of the following is correct?**
   A. There is no need to differentiate between excess glandular and adipose tissue.
   B. Testicular examination and an ultrasound scan should be performed in every case.
   C. Blood tests for beta HCG, FSH, LH, and testosterone are rarely required.
   D. A tall, lanky patient with an abnormal testicular examination may require genetic testing.
   E. The neck and abdomen do not routinely need to be examined.

BREAST CANCER IN MALES

5. A 55-year-old man presents with a 3-month history of unilateral gynecomastia. Examination reveals mild glandular gynecomastia, according to the Simon classification, with no evidence of testicular abnormality or axillary lymphadenopathy. He takes nifedipine and aspirin and no other medications. His older sister had a mastectomy for right-sided breast cancer at age 70 and continues to do well. **Which one of the following statements is correct regarding the patient?**
   A. His risk of developing breast cancer is typically one twentieth that of his sister.
   B. None of his medications are likely to account for gynecomastia.
   C. His age is the most common age for a diagnosis of male breast cancer.
   D. Mammography is the best clinical investigation to exclude malignancy.
   E. His risk of malignancy is unaffected by his sister's previous disease.

CLASSIFICATION AND STAGING

6. **What is the most clinically relevant aspect of the various staging systems for gynecomastia?**
   A. They allow data collection for comparative research.
   B. They enable doctors to communicate about the nature of the patient's disease.
   C. They inform the patient of their likely long-term outcome.
   D. They guide the surgical decision-making process.
   E. They provide information on the likely risk of recurrence.

MANAGEMENT OF GYNECOMASTIA

7. **Which one of the following statements is correct regarding management of gynecomastia?**
   A. Idiopathic gynecomastia regresses spontaneously within 3 months of enlargement.
   B. Tamoxifen or testosterone may be useful for lumpy gynecomastia.
   C. Idiopathic gynecomastia present for longer than 1 year is unlikely to fully regress.
   D. Surgical treatments include liposuction and excisional techniques that preserve the inframammary fold.
   E. Excisional techniques have generally better outcomes than liposuction techniques.

8. A 20-year-old man presents with unilateral idiopathic gynecomastia. On examination he has moderate breast enlargement with palpable glandular and fatty breast tissue. Skin quality is good with modest excess. **Which one of the following is correct?**
   A. His condition would be best suited to ultrasound-assisted liposuction.
   B. He would be likely to require concurrent surgical resection.
   C. Postoperative bruising is worse when using ultrasound-assisted liposuction versus suction-assisted liposuction.
   D. Incision sites for liposuction should be placed symmetrically at the inframammary fold.
   E. Postoperative use of compression garments is not normally required.

9. You consult a 40-year-old patient with a 1-year history of idiopathic bilateral gynecomastia. Examination reveals large symmetrical breasts with more than 500 g of excess fibrofatty tissue and significant skin excess on each side. The nipple-to-IMF distance is 30 cm and the nipple is situated below the inframammary fold. **Which one of the following surgical options is most likely to provide the best aesthetic result?**
   A. Single-stage liposuction only
   B. Single-stage surgical excision only
   C. Single-stage liposuction with surgical excision
   D. Staged liposuction, then surgical excision
   E. Staged surgical excision, then liposuction

Answers

GENERAL ASPECTS OF GYNECOMASTIA
1. Which one of the following is correct regarding gynecomastia?
D. Adolescent males are very commonly affected.

Gynecomastia may be physiologic, pathologic, or pharmacologic, and most males have it to some degree during their lives. Three quarters (not half) of cases are bilateral. Two thirds of males have it during puberty. No evidence suggests an increased risk of breast cancer in association with gynecomastia in the general population.

GENERAL CAUSES OF GYNECOMASTIA
2. What is the most common cause of gynecomastia?
E. Idiopathic cause

All the options presented are potential causes of gynecomastia, but most cases have no obvious precipitating cause. A thorough history should be obtained and an examination performed to exclude a potentially treatable cause before surgical management begins. Once this has been established, decisions can be made regarding the choice of surgical intervention.

PHARMACOLOGIC CAUSES OF GYNECOMASTIA
3. It is vital to review prescription and nonprescription drugs of patients with gynecomastia. **Which one of the following is not usually expected to cause gynecomastia?**
D. Simvastatin

Numerous medications are known to cause gynecomastia (see Box 49-2, *Essentials of Plastic Surgery,* second edition). This highlights the importance of obtaining a thorough medical history during assessment of these patients. Reversible causes can be established and managed accordingly. Whether or not statins can cause gynecomastia has been debated. This was discussed in the New England Journal of Medicine in 2007.[1,2] The available evidence linking statins to gynecomastia was based on case reports only and involved pravastatin and atorvastatin rather than simvastatin. Overall, the evidence was weak. Simvastatin is unlikely to be a significant factor in gynecomastia.

PREOPERATIVE WORKUP
4. When assessing a patient in clinic with gynecomastia, **which one of the following is correct?**
D. A tall, lanky patient with an abnormal testicular examination may require genetic testing.

Young, lanky patients with gynecomastia and abnormal testicular development may have the chromosomal abnormality 47XXY. This condition is known as Klinefelter's syndrome[3] following its description in 1942. It is also associated with other feminizing features such as a lack of male hair distribution. Patients are likely to be infertile and have an increased risk of developing breast cancer (greater than 60 times). Further confirmation of the diagnosis is required.

A thorough breast examination can help to differentiate between glandular and adipose tissue and is important as it can affect the surgical options available for treatment. It also helps to identify or exclude the presence of potential breast malignancy. A routine assessment should also continue with examination of the neck and abdomen to identify thyroid, liver, or other abdominal masses. Examination of the testes is routine but further imaging, such as ultrasound is only required if pathology is suspected. It is standard practice to obtain a set of baseline blood tests to assess the hormone profile in cases of gynecomastia, if this has not already been completed by the referring physician.[4,5]

BREAST CANCER IN MALES

5. A 55-year-old man presents with a 3-month history of unilateral gynecomastia. Examination reveals mild glandular gynecomastia, according to the Simon classification,[6] with no evidence of testicular abnormality or axillary lymphadenopathy. He takes nifedipine and aspirin and no other medications. His older sister had a mastectomy for right-sided breast cancer at age 70 and continues to do well. **Which one of the following statements is correct regarding the patient?**
   D. Mammography is the best clinical investigation to exclude malignancy.
   Male breast cancer accounts for only 1% of all breast cancer (not 5%). Therefore the risk for a male is usually only one hundredth that of a female patient. The risk increases if a female family member is diagnosed with breast cancer. The most common age at diagnosis in males is around 65 years of age. Although nifedipine may be a cause of gynecomastia, new-onset unilateral disease requires exclusion of malignancy. Mammography is the best modality, with a 90% sensitivity and specificity for distinguishing between benign and malignant lesions.

CLASSIFICATION AND STAGING

6. **What is the most clinically relevant aspect of the various staging systems for gynecomastia?**
   D. They guide the surgical decision-making process.
   They key purpose of each of the classification systems for gynecomastia is that they help to guide the surgical decision-making process. This is true for both the Rohrich[7] and Simon[6] classifications as they focus on the composition and volume of the glandular/fatty breast constituents and the quality and volume of the skin. Higher grades correlate to more severe gynecomastia which often involves skin excess. Where there is an isolated volume excess or where the skin excess is mild, then no skin resection is required. Conversely where there is a significant excess of skin and breast tissue then both will have to be removed. In general, having classification systems also helps clinicians communicate with one another and can be useful for research and projecting outcomes, but these are less important in clinical practice within gynecomastia.

MANAGEMENT OF GYNECOMASTIA

7. **Which one of the following statements is correct regarding management of gynecomastia?**
   C. Idiopathic gynecomastia present for longer than 1 year is unlikely to fully regress.
   Idiopathic gynecomastia often regresses between 3 and 18 months. Once it has been present for longer than a year, it is unlikely to completely regress because of tissue fibrosis. Although tamoxifen is useful for lump-type gynecomastia, testosterone appears to have a limited benefit. Surgical treatments, especially liposuction, should cause disruption of the inframammary fold, which reduces the feminine appearance of the breast. In general, UAL is the best treatment particularly for grade 1 and 2a (Simon classification).[6] Grade 2b and 3 may also be satisfactorily managed with liposuction but can require skin or breast tissue excision. The key benefit of liposuction is reduced scarring. Other complications can be reduced.

8. A 20-year-old man presents with unilateral idiopathic gynecomastia. On examination he has moderate breast enlargement with palpable glandular and fatty breast tissue. Skin quality is good with modest excess. **Which one of the following is correct?**
   A. **His condition would be best suited to ultrasound-assisted liposuction.**
      This patient has a moderate excess of both fatty and glandular tissue to the breast with a mild skin excess. He is ideally suited to ultrasound-assisted liposuction (UAL), rather than suction-assisted liposuction, as this has shown good results in treating gynecomastia. Given his age and skin quality he should not require skin excision or concurrent glandular tissue excision. UAL is associated with reduced bleeding and bruising and radiographic dye studies have shown significantly less vascular disruption with UAL than with traditional techniques. The incision sites should be placed away from the inframammary fold in order to achieve adequate cross-hatching across the fold and into the glandular tissue. Compression garments are uniformly recommended following this procedure. Duration is usually 4 to 6 weeks.[7,8]

9. You consult a 40-year-old patient with a 1-year history of idiopathic bilateral gynecomastia. Examination reveals large symmetrical breasts with more than 500 g of excess fibrofatty tissue and significant skin excess on each side. The nipple-to-IMF distance is 30 cm and the nipple is situated below the inframammary fold. **Which one of the following surgical options is most likely to provide the best aesthetic result?**
   D. **Staged liposuction, then surgical excision**
      This man has a combination of significant skin and glandular excess giving a feminine appearance to the breasts. This condition cannot be treated adequately with liposuction alone. Proceeding with liposuction first as part of a two-stage process is beneficial because it can reduce the breast volume significantly and allow for skin shrinkage prior to surgical excision. The subsequent scarring incurred during the second stage should be reduced by adopting this approach. In a large study by Rohrich et al,[8] most patients with a similar degree of gynecomastia to the patient described were initially treated with ultrasound-assisted liposuction and went on to have a second-stage excision at 6 to 9 months; once skin retraction had taken place.

REFERENCES

1. Braunstein GD. Gynecomastia. N Engl J Med 357:1229-1237, 2007.
2. Westenend PJ, Storm R, Oostenbrock RJ. Gynecomastia. N Engl J Med 357:2636-2637, 2007.
3. Klinefelter HF Jr, Reifenstein EC Jr, Albright F. Syndrome characterized by gynecomastia aspermatogenesis without a-Leydigism and increased excretion of follicle-stimulating hormone. J Clin Endocr Metabl 2:615-624, 1942.
4. Klinefelter syndrome: a cohort study. J Natl Cancer Inst 97:1204-1210, 2005.
5. Brinton LA. Breast cancer risk among patients with Klinefelter syndrome. Acta Paediatr 100:814-818, 2011.
6. Simon BB, Hoffman S, Kahn S. Classification and surgical correction of gynecomastia. Plast Reconstr Surg 51:48-52, 1973.
7. Rohrich RJ, Ha RY, Kenkel JM, et al. Classification and management of gynecomastia: defining the role of ultrasound-assisted liposuction. Plast Reconstr Surg 111:909-923, 2003.
8. Gingrass MK, Shermak MA. The treatment of gynecomastia with ultrasound-assisted lipoplasty. Perspect Plast Surg 12:101-106, 1999.

50. Breast Cancer and Reconstruction

See *Essentials of Plastic Surgery*, second edition, pp. 580-592.

BREAST CANCER STATISTICS

1. For each of the following statements, select the best option. (Each option may be used once, more than once, or not at all.)
   A. This is the lifetime risk for a woman to develop breast cancer.
   B. This is the percentage of female breast cancer cases that are sporadic.
   C. This is the lifetime risk of breast cancer development in female patients who are BRCA1 or BRCA2 positive.

   Options:
   a. 1%
   b. 12%
   c. 25%
   d. 40%
   e. 65%
   f. 80%
   g. 95%

RISK FACTORS FOR BREAST CANCER

2. A woman is seen in clinic wishing to assess her risk for development of breast cancer. A medical history is obtained. She had an early menarche at age 11, but has never had any children. She is the wife of a successful businessman and drinks over the recommended daily amount of alcohol. Her mother and sister have both developed breast cancer within the past five years. **Which one of the following factors is most significant with respect to elevation of her risk status?**
   A. Social status
   B. Alcohol consumption
   C. Nulliparity
   D. Early menarche
   E. Family history

TNM STAGING OF BREAST TUMORS

3. For each of the following clinical scenarios, select the correct staging according to the TNM classification system. (Each option may be used once, more than once, or not at all.)
   A. A patient has a 2.5 cm tumor, six positive axillary nodes, and no distant spread.
   B. A patient has a 1 cm tumor, nodes not assessed, and no distant spread.
   C. A patient has a 1 cm tumor invading the chest wall and three axillary nodes and evidence of bone metastases on chest radiographs.

Options:
a. T1N0M0
b. T1NXM0
c. T2N2M0
d. T2N0M0
e. T2NXM0
f. T3N1M1
g. T4N1M1
h. T4N2M1

BREAST CONSERVATION THERAPY

4. Which one of the following represents a contraindication to breast conservation therapy?
   A. Previous breast irradiation
   B. Tumors larger than 3 cm diameter
   C. Unifocal disease
   D. Ductal carcinoma in situ
   E. Tumors in large fatty breasts

TREATMENT AND PROGNOSIS IN BREAST CANCER

5. In a female patient with a primary T2N0M0 breast cancer, **which one of the following is correct?**
   A. Her overall survival is unaffected whether breast conservation surgery or mastectomy is performed.
   B. Her risk of local recurrence is unaffected by whether breast conservation surgery or mastectomy is performed.
   C. Postoperative radiotherapy is required irrespective of whether breast conservation surgery or mastectomy is performed.
   D. She has a 95% chance of being alive at five years given her disease stage.
   E. Sentinel lymph node biopsy for this patient has only 65% sensitivity and specificity for breast cancer.

TYPES OF MASTECTOMY

6. A patient is referred to clinic for delayed reconstruction following a modified radical mastectomy for breast cancer. **Which one of the following anatomic structures will have been completely preserved?**
   A. Nipple areolar complex
   B. Breast skin
   C. Axillary nodes
   D. Pectoralis major
   E. Breast parenchyma

IMPLANT-BASED BREAST RECONSTRUCTION

7. Which one of the following statements is correct regarding implant-based versus autologous reconstruction techniques?
A. They are less commonly performed.
B. They provide long-term cost benefits.
C. They result in fewer long-term complications.
D. It is harder to match with a natural breast.
E. They are less likely to require revision surgery.

THE LATISSIMUS DORSI FLAP

8. Which one of the following statements is correct regarding breast reconstruction with the latissimus dorsi (LD) flap?
A. The vascular supply arises from the thoracoacromial vessels and intercostal perforators.
B. In most patients, it avoids the requirement for a prosthetic implant.
C. Seroma rates of up to 35% are commonly observed postoperatively.
D. Many patients incur significant permanent functional loss on the ipsilateral shoulder.
E. Donor site seroma rates are significantly reduced by placement of progressive tension sutures.

PEDICLED TRAM FLAP FOR BREAST RECONSTRUCTION

9. Which one of the following is correct regarding the pedicled transverse rectus abdominis myocutaneous (TRAM) flap?
A. Holm et al modified the nomenclature of Hartrampfs original four perfusion zones by switching zones two and four.
B. Delay of a pedicled TRAM flap for 3 weeks before transfer is optimal.
C. A pedicled TRAM flap has a decreased rate of fat necrosis, compared with a free TRAM flap.
D. A pedicled TRAM flap may still require a microvascular anastomoses to remain viable.
E. Delay of a pedicled TRAM flap involves a preliminary stage to divide the deep superior epigastric artery.

RECIPIENT VESSELS IN FREE FLAP BREAST RECONSTRUCTION

10. Which one of the following represents a disadvantage of using the internal mammary vessels when performing breast reconstruction with a free TRAM flap?
A. There is a high risk of pneumothorax.
B. There is commonly a vessel size mismatch.
C. The internal mammary vein is often absent.
D. The operating field is mobile during the anastomosis.
E. The flap pedicle often has insufficient length.

11. While performing free tissue transfer for breast reconstruction, you have been trying for an extended period of time to achieve a satisfactory venous anastomosis with the internal mammary vein but are unsuccessful. The arterial anastomosis is running well and you do not wish to redo it. *Which one of the following vessels can be used as an alternative venous outflow source in this situation without preparing a vessel graft or resiting the artery?*
A. The lateral thoracic vein
B. The axillary vein
C. The thoracodorsal vein
D. The cephalic vein
E. The internal jugular vein

Chapter 50 ▪ Breast Cancer and Reconstruction   401

FREE TRAM FLAP RECONSTRUCTION

12. You are supervising a senior resident as they raise a free TRAM flap. **What is the main reason to encourage them to dissect the superficial epigastric vein during this procedure?**
    A. To perform the primary venous anastomosis of the flap.
    B. As backup in case a vein graft is subsequently required.
    C. To develop their skills in vessel dissection in a relaxed setting.
    D. In case the flap turns out to have a dominant superficial drainage.
    E. To minimize the risk of hematoma in the groin.

13. **Which one of the following is true of free TRAM flaps?**
    A. Even muscle sparing TRAMs sacrifice the medial part of the rectus muscle.
    B. Zones I and III are based on the same side as the deep inferior epigastric vessels.
    C. A fascial sparing TRAM is the same as a DIEP flap.
    D. The most common complication of a free TRAM flap is total flap loss.
    E. It is always better to sacrifice more muscle rather than risk flap viability.

SELECTION OF BREAST RECONSTRUCTION TECHNIQUE

14. A 40-year-old woman is to have bilateral prophylactic mastectomies as she is BRCA positive. A skin-sparing approach is planned with preservation of the nipple-areola complex. She is otherwise fit and well and is a nonsmoker. On examination she has small breasts; estimated volume is 300 cc with good skin quality. Her BMI is 21 and she wishes to moderately increase her breast size. **Which one of the following is the most suitable reconstructive option for this patient?**
    A. Implants only
    B. Implants and deepithelialized inferiorly based skin flaps
    C. Implants and acellular dermal matrix
    D. Pedicled TRAM flaps
    E. Pedicled musculocutaneous LD flaps with implants

Answers

BREAST CANCER STATISTICS
1. *For the following scenarios, the best options are as follows:*
   A. *This is the lifetime risk for a woman to develop breast cancer.*
      b. 12%
   B. *This is the percentage of female breast cancer cases that are sporadic.*
      f. 80%
   C. *This is the lifetime risk of breast cancer development in female patients who are BRCA1 or BRCA2 positive.*
      e. 65%

   Breast cancer is the most common cancer in females (not including nonmelanoma skin cancers), with a lifetime risk of 1 in 8 or 12%. It is the second most common cause of cancer deaths in females (after lung cancer) and is most commonly sporadic (80% of cases). Approximately 15% of cases are familial. Patients who are *BRCA* positive represent only a small proportion (5%) of all breast cancer patients. However, this patient group has a significantly increased risk of developing breast cancer (estimated at 65%). As discussed in Chapter 49, male breast cancer is much less common and represents approximately 1% of all breast cancer cases with a lifetime risk of 1 in 1000.

RISK FACTORS FOR BREAST CANCER
2. A woman is seen in clinic wishing to assess her risk for development of breast cancer. A medical history is obtained. She had an early menarche at age 11, but has never had any children. She is the wife of a successful businessman and drinks over the recommended daily amount of alcohol. Her mother and sister have both developed breast cancer within the past five years. **Which one of the following factors is most significant with respect to elevation of her risk status?**
   E. Family history

   This patient has a number of risk factors for development of breast cancer. The most significant of these is her family history, having two first-degree relatives affected. Risk of developing breast cancer is generally stratified into three groups: strong, moderate, and low.

   Strong risk factors include age over 65, BRCA positive status, biopsy confirmed atypical hyperplasia, and a personal history of breast cancer; none of which this patient has. Moderate risk factors include two first-degree relatives with breast cancer, high endogenous estrogen, high dose radiation to the chest, and high postmenopausal bone density; one of which this patient has. Low-risk elevators include high alcohol consumption, early menarche, late menopause, nulliparity, late age at first pregnancy (<30), HRT, obesity, and high socioeconomic status; a number of which this lady has.

Chapter 50 ■ Breast Cancer and Reconstruction   403

TNM STAGING OF BREAST TUMORS
3. For the following scenarios, the best options are as follows:
   A. A patient has a 2.5 cm tumor, six positive axillary nodes, and no distant spread.
      c. **T2N2M0**
   B. A patient has a 1 cm tumor, nodes not assessed, and no distant spread.
      b. **T1NXM0**
   C. A patient has a 1 cm tumor invading the chest wall and three axillary nodes, and evidence of bone metastases on chest radiographs.
      g. **T4N1M1**

   The American Joint Committee on Cancer system for staging breast cancers is as follows:
   Primary Tumor (T)
      TX: Cannot be assessed
      T0: No evidence of tumor
      Tis: Carcinoma in situ
      T1: Smaller than 2 cm
      T2: 2 to 5 cm
      T3: Larger than 5 cm
      T4: Any size and invades chest wall or skin (includes inflammatory breast cancer)
   Lymph Nodes (N)
      NX: Cannot be assessed
      N0: No evidence of spread
      N1: 1 to 3 axillary nodes
      N2: 4 to 9 axillary nodes or enlarged internal mammary node
      N3: 10 or more axillary plus mammary or supraclavicular nodes
   Metastasis (M)
      MX: Cannot be assessed
      M0: No distant disease
      M1: Metastatic (most commonly bone, lung, brain, and liver)

BREAST CONSERVATION THERAPY
4. Which one of the following represents a contraindication to breast conservation therapy?
   A. **Previous breast irradiation**

   Breast conservation therapy may be considered in patients with small primary tumors including DCIS, particularly in moderate to large breasts. Often the ratio of tumor to breast size is a major factor in the decision-making process and having large fatty breasts can lend itself well to wide local excision with a therapeutic mammoplasty, combined with a symmetrizing reduction performed on the opposite side. This approach relies on the principles of reduction mammoplasty described in Chapter 48, adapted to allow tumor resection with a more cosmetic approach. These are so-called "oncoplastic techniques." The key contraindications to breast conserving therapy are previous breast irradiation, recurrent or multifocal disease, tumors greater than 5 cm in diameter, inflammatory breast disease, and a high tumor size to breast size ratio.

TREATMENT AND PROGNOSIS IN BREAST CANCER

5. In a female patient with a primary T2N0M0 breast cancer, *which one of the following is correct?*
   A. Her overall survival is unaffected whether breast conservation surgery or mastectomy is performed.
   For most small to medium breast cancers, the survival rates are equivalent for breast conservation surgery or mastectomy. Breast conservation surgery is sometimes described as a lumpectomy or partial mastectomy and involves removal of the tumor with the surrounding portion of the breast. In almost all cases, postoperative radiotherapy is given. In contrast, patients who opt for a mastectomy do not usually require radiotherapy unless the tumor is particularly aggressive. While the overall survival does not differ between the two treatment modalities, the risk of local recurrence does, with breast conservation patients more likely to develop a recurrence. Most patients have to weigh the risks and benefits involved with respect to either complete mastectomy or breast conservation surgery and radiotherapy.

   With stage IIa disease, five-year survival is only expected to be around 80%. Only patients with in situ disease (stage 0) can expect a 95%, 5-year survival. Sentinel lymph node biopsy is routine in breast cancer because it has a high sensitivity and specificity (92% and 100%, respectively).[1]

TYPES OF MASTECTOMY

6. A patient is referred to clinic for delayed reconstruction following a modified radical mastectomy for breast cancer. *Which one of the following anatomic structures will have been completely preserved?*
   D. Pectoralis major
   This patient would have their pectoralis major muscle preserved. A simple mastectomy involves removal of the nipple-areola complex, breast parenchyma, and some of the breast skin in an ellipse around the nipple, but the axilla is spared. A radical mastectomy combines a simple mastectomy with axillary clearance and removal of pectoralis major. A modified radical mastectomy, as described in this case, involves a simple mastectomy and an axillary clearance with preservation of the chest wall musculature. Other, less invasive mastectomy procedures include nipple-sparing, areola-sparing, or skin-sparing techniques, which are generally performed as prophylactic risk-reducing procedures in the absence of proven disease.

IMPLANT-BASED BREAST RECONSTRUCTION

7. *Which one of the following statements is correct regarding implant-based versus autologous reconstruction techniques?*
   D. It is harder to match with a natural breast.
   Implant-based reconstruction is the most common form of reconstruction in the U.S. and it carries with it a number of advantages over autologous techniques. These include a lower initial cost, reduced OR time, reduced hospital stay, avoidance of a donor scar, and in most cases, the technique is technically simpler. In the longer term, many of the advantages may be lost because the need for subsequent revision is increased as a result of complications such as capsular contracture and implant rupture. In addition, it is difficult to achieve symmetry in unilateral reconstruction as the soft tissue characteristics of a natural breast cannot be recreated and natural ptosis does not develop over time. This is a key point to highlight to patients undergoing unilateral reconstruction to ensure they are well informed preoperatively and have realistic expectations for surgery. A technique that may help both the appearance and feel of an implant reconstruction is fat transfer, as this alters the ratio of autologous to implant volume (see Chapter 89).

THE LATISSIMUS DORSI FLAP

8. Which one of the following statements is correct regarding breast reconstruction with the latissimus dorsi (LD) flap?

E. Donor site seroma rates are significantly reduced by placement of progressive tension sutures.

The latissimus dorsi flap can be useful for reconstruction of the breast, but it carries a high risk of seroma formation at the donor site. This is estimated to be as high as 80% in some series.[2] The use of progressive tension sutures has been shown to significantly reduce seroma formation, as this reduces the effective size of the dissected subcutaneous pocket with quilting.[3] The vascular supply is from the thoracodorsal artery (not the thoracoacromial) as well as the posterior intercostal and lumbar perforators. This makes it a type V flap according to the Mathes and Nahai classification.[4] Innervation is from the thoracodorsal nerve, which originates from the posterior cord of the brachial plexus and many surgeons divide this during flap harvest to stop unwanted postoperative contractions. It can usually be identified close to the pedicle in the axilla and its identification confirmed with gentle compression using forceps. This illicits a contraction in the muscle. Most patients still require a breast prosthesis when using this flap. The extended LD can be useful for obtaining more soft tissue cover in breast reconstruction, as this includes adipose tissue above and below the muscle, but even this can only be used without an implant in small to medium or partial reconstructions. Larger breasts will always require a supplementary implant. Very few patients experience problems with shoulder function after using this flap, although those involved in physical activities such as climbing or swimming may be affected.

A benefit of using an LD and implant versus implant alone is the effect on capsular contracture formation which appears to be reduced. Pinsolle et al[5] undertook a retrospective study of 266 immediate breast reconstructions over a 12-year period. Of these, 61% were reconstructed with an LD myocutaneous flap and implant. Capsular contractures were less frequent when the LD was used. In spite of the benefits of using this flap, it is generally kept as a lifeboat for when other forms of reconstruction, such as implants or free TRAM/DIEP, fail.

PEDICLED TRAM FLAP FOR BREAST RECONSTRUCTION

9. Which one of the following is correct regarding the pedicled transverse rectus abdominis myocutaneous (TRAM) flap?

D. A pedicled TRAM flap may still require a microvascular anastomoses to remain viable.

A pedicled TRAM flap does not always avoid the use of microvascular surgery, as it may be necessary to supercharge it by anastomosing the deep inferior epigastric vessels into the thoracodorsal vessels. For this reason the deep inferior artery and vein should be carefully dissected with preservation of length.

The pedicled TRAM flap has an increased (not decreased) rate of fat necrosis compared with the free TRAM. This is because the inferior epigastric vessels are likely to represent the dominant blood supply. It is best to delay the pedicled TRAM flap by division of the deep inferior epigastric (not deep superior) vessels one to two weeks (not three) before it is transposed. Delay is the surgical interruption of a portion of the blood supply to a flap at a preliminary stage before final transfer. Delay is thought to work by opening up choke vessels within the flap secondary to local tissue ischemia. This is discussed further in Chapter 4.

Hartrampf[6] described four perfusion zones with respect to the anterior abdominal wall and the pedicled TRAM.

    I: Ipsilateral to pedicle overlying rectus muscle
    II: Contralateral to pedicle overlying contralateral rectus muscle
    III: Ipsilateral to pedicle, lateral to the rectus muscle
    IV: Contralateral to pedicle, lateral to the contralateral rectus muscle

In his original description described above, Hartrampf had zones I and II on opposite sides of the midline. Holm[7] subsequently undertook intraoperative perfusion studies and showed that perfusion in Hartrampf's original zone III was superior to that of zone II and so recommended that these two zones were renamed.

RECIPIENT VESSELS IN FREE FLAP BREAST RECONSTRUCTION

10. **Which one of the following represents a disadvantage of using the internal mammary vessels when performing breast reconstruction with a free TRAM flap?**
    D. The operating field is mobile during the anastomosis.
    One particular challenge of performing a free flap anastomosis to the internal mammary vessels is that respiration causes the operating field to move. This can interfere with the focus of the microscope and makes the process significantly more difficult. It is important to communicate with the anesthesiologist so that the effects of ventilation on the operative field can be minimized. This may be achieved by using high-volume, low-rate settings on the ventilator. The other challenges of using the internal mammary vessels are that access can be difficult, especially in patients after radiation. Access generally requires removal of a section of rib cartilage and careful dissection of the vessels just superficial to pleura. Although the risk is only small, it is possible to cause a pneumothorax while doing this part of the procedure. The vessels are usually well matched for size to the deep inferior epigastric pedicle and are consistently present in most patients. However, the vessels may be thin walled and friable, especially following radiotherapy. They are rarely absent but may be smaller on the left than the right. The inferior epigastric pedicle does have sufficient length to comfortably reach this area for anastomosis.

11. While performing free tissue transfer for breast reconstruction, you have been trying for an extended period of time to achieve a satisfactory venous anastomosis with the internal mammary vein but are unsuccessful. The arterial anastomosis is running well and you do not wish to redo it. **Which one of the following vessels can be used as an alternative venous outflow source in this situation without preparing a vessel graft or resiting the artery?**
    D. The cephalic vein
    There are two main options available in this situation that will avoid both reanastamosing the artery and utilizing a vein graft. The first of these is a cephalic turndown, where the cephalic vein is elevated from distal to proximal in the upper arm into the deltopectoral groove. It is then transposed medially to allow direct venous anastomosis. The second option (not listed) is to dissect the external jugular vein (not the internal) in the neck from cranial to caudal and pass the vessel from the neck into the zone where the arterial anastomosis is sited. The other options would each require a vein graft to adequately reach the TRAM flap pedicle.

FREE TRAM FLAP RECONSTRUCTION

12. You are supervising a senior resident as they raise a free TRAM flap. **What is the main reason to encourage them to dissect the superficial epigastric vein during this procedure?**
    D. In case the flap turns out to have a dominant superficial drainage.
    The reason for dissecting and preserving length of the superficial inferior epigastric vessels is that some abdominal flaps are heavily reliant on this system for venous outflow. In some cases, the superficial system is the dominant system. This may display as a grossly congested flap following completion of satisfactory anastomoses at the recipient site. In such cases, it can be helpful to perform a second venous anastomosis to one of the lateral chest wall or axillary vessels in order to generate satisfactory venous outflow and maintain flap viability. The

primary anastomosis for a typical TRAM flap is the deep inferior epigastric vein. If the vein graft is required, then this can be harvested at the necessary time. Practicing dissection skills on vessels not primarily used in a reconstruction can be a useful training exercise but should not compromise patient safety or unnecessarily extend the operating duration.

13. Which one of the following is true of free TRAM flaps?
E. It is always better to sacrifice more muscle rather than risk flap viability.
The most important objective when performing a free TRAM is to safely transfer the skin and soft tissues of the anterior abdominal wall to the chest in order to reconstruct a breast mound. Although preservation of muscle and fascia are important and should be maximized during surgery, this should not be done with risk of compromise to the flap. TRAM flaps can use the full width of the muscle or can spare muscle. The classification for muscle-sparing TRAMs has four categories: MS-0 to MS-3, where 0 = no muscle spared, 1 = lateral muscle spared, 2 = medial and lateral muscle spared, and 3 = all muscle spared.[8] They can also be fascia-sparing but this is not the same as a DIEP, which spares muscle and involves taking a small cuff of fascia around the perforating vessels. The most common complication following a free TRAM flap is a noninfectious wound complication. This may be as high as 40% but generally resolves without intervention. Total flap loss is expected to be less than 5% based on the results from large series. The vascular zones within a free TRAM flap have I and II on the same side as the deep inferior epigastric vessels being harvested. Zones III and IV are on the contralateral side (see Fig. 50-2, *Essentials of Plastic Surgery*, second edition.). It is advisable therefore to orientate the flap on the chest so as to place these zones medially and discard zone IV. This means that the less well-perfused zone(s) will be lateral, and if the lateral flap does not survive further reconstruction in this area is more straightforward.

SELECTION OF BREAST RECONSTRUCTION TECHNIQUE

14. A 40-year-old woman is to have bilateral prophylactic mastectomies as she is BRCA positive. A skin-sparing approach is planned with preservation of the nipple-areolar complex. She is otherwise fit and well and is a nonsmoker. On examination she has small breasts; estimated volume is 300 cc with good skin quality. Her BMI is 21 and she wishes to moderately increase her breast size. **Which one of the following is the most suitable reconstructive option for this patient?**
C. Implants and acellular dermal matrix
The simplest approach to reconstruction for this patient is to utilize an implant-based technique. As she is disease free, her skin envelope is maintained and no postoperative radiotherapy will be needed. These factors support the use of a prosthetic device. It is important to provide complete soft tissue cover for the implants as the skin flaps will be thin in this patient. For such cases, the use of dermal matrix has become popular. Superiorly the implant/expander can be covered by the pectoralis major muscle and serratus anterior. Inferiorly the dermal matrix can cover the implant from the inframammary fold to the pectoralis muscle. In larger breasted patients, the use of a deepithelialized inferior skin flap is favored to provide additional implant cover without a dermal matrix. This patient does not have sufficient breast tissue for this approach. To use bilateral pedicled TRAM flaps in this patient would be a poor choice, particularly given her age, because of the morbidity associated with sacrifice of both rectus muscles. In addition, given her BMI it is unlikely she will have sufficient tissue for autologous reconstruction. Bilateral LD flaps could be used to provide additional implant cover but there is no need for harvesting skin as the native breast skin is preserved. Use of LD muscle flaps would also involve significant back scarring, which can be avoided by using an implant and matrix combination.

REFERENCES

1. Edge SB, Byrd Dr, Compton CC, et al, eds. AJCC Cancer Staging Manual, ed 7. New York: Springer, 2009.
2. Delay E, Gounot N, Bouillot A, et al. Autologous latissimus breast reconstruction: a 3-year clinical experience with 100 patients. Plast Reconstr Surg 102:1461, 1998.
3. Rios JL, Pollock T, Adams WP. Progressive tension sutures to prevent seroma formation after latissimus dorsi harvest. Plast Reconstr Surg 112:1779, 2003.
4. Mathes SJ, Nahai F. Classification of the vascular anatomy of muscles: experimental and clinical correlation. Plast Reconstr Surg 67:177-187, 1981.
5. Pinsolle V, Grinfeder C, Mathoulin-Pelissier S, et al. Complications analysis of 266 immediate breast reconstructions. J Plast Reconstr Aesthet Surg 59:1017-1024, 2006.
6. Hartrampf CR, Scheflan M, Black PW. Breast reconstruction with a transverse abdominal island flap. Plast Reconstr Surg 69:216-225, 1982.
7. Holm C, Mayr M, Höfter E, et al. Perfusion zones of the DIEP flap revisited: a clinical study. Plast Reconstr Surg 117:37-43, 2006.
8. Nahabedian MY, Dooley W, Singh N, et al. Contour abnormalities of the abdomen after breast reconstruction with abdominal flaps: the role of muscle preservation. Plast Reconstr Surg 109:91, 2002.

51. Nipple-Areolar Reconstruction

See *Essentials of Plastic Surgery*, second edition, pp. 593-604.

NIPPLE RECONSTRUCTION
1. **Which one of the following statements is correct regarding nipple reconstruction?**
   A. It is ideally performed at the same time as breast mound reconstruction.
   B. There is a single gold standard technique that has been uniformly adopted by surgeons.
   C. It is usually performed as an inpatient procedure under general anesthesia.
   D. Patient downtime is usually 2 to 3 weeks following nipple reconstruction.
   E. It correlates highly with enhanced patient satisfaction following breast reconstruction.

NIPPLE POSITIONING
2. **Which one of the following statements is correct regarding markings for a C-V flap nipple reconstruction?**
   A. The patient should be marked when lying supine on the OR table.
   B. The surgeon should independently select the new nipple position
   C. The nipple must overlie the point of maximal breast projection.
   D. Accurate anatomic placement is less important than achieving symmetry.
   E. The V flaps must be oriented transversely, with the base of the C flap inferior.

NIPPLE RECONSTRUCTION TECHNIQUES
3. **For each of the following descriptions, select the most likely nipple reconstruction type. (Each answer may be used once, more than once, or not at all.)**
   A. This technique uses a central dermal/fat flap with bilateral partial or full-thickness wings and traditionally uses a full-thickness skin graft for closure.
   B. This technique involves a pull-out flap that is folded over on itself and the donor site is closed directly with a purse-string suture.
   C. This technique uses three triangular flaps and one vertical cutaneous/fat flap with two bilateral, full-thickness skin arms oriented at 90-degree angles. No skin graft is required.

   Options:
   a. Star flap
   b. Fishtail flap
   c. Bell flap
   d. S flap
   e. Skate flap
   f. C-V flap
   g. Modified skate flap

LONG-TERM PROBLEMS WITH NIPPLE RECONSTRUCTION

4. Which one of the following is the most significant long-term challenge of nipple reconstruction with local flap techniques?
   A. Fading of the areola
   B. Scar stretch
   C. Maintaining projection
   D. Patient satisfaction
   E. Hypertrophic scarring

LOSS OF PROJECTION AFTER NIPPLE RECONSTRUCTION

5. You are consenting a patient for nipple reconstruction using a local skin flap technique. *What is the expected approximate projection loss 2 years after nipple reconstruction?*
   A. 5%
   B. 15%
   C. 25%
   D. 35%
   E. 50%

FLAP DESIGN FOR NIPPLE RECONSTRUCTION

6. When designing a C-V flap for nipple reconstruction, which one of the following dimensions will dictate the initial nipple projection?
   A. Width of the C component
   B. Length of the C component
   C. Width of the V component
   D. Length of the V component
   E. Depth of the V component

INVERTED NIPPLES

7. What is the most common cause of nipple inversion?
   A. Acute mastitis
   B. Chronic mastitis
   C. Breast carcinoma
   D. Paget's disease
   E. Congenital

8. What is the key feature to consider when grading nipple inversion?
   A. The underlying cause
   B. The chronicity
   C. The ability to successfully breast-feed
   D. The ability to manually correct the inversion
   E. The projection compared with the opposite side

Answers

NIPPLE RECONSTRUCTION

1. **Which one of the following statements is correct regarding nipple reconstruction?**
   E. It correlates highly with enhanced patient satisfaction following breast reconstruction.

   Nipple-areolar reconstruction is undertaken to complete a breast reconstruction such that it looks more like a natural looking breast. Retrospective analyses have shown that patient satisfaction with their breast reconstruction highly correlates with the presence of a nipple and areola.[1] It is best to wait a few months following breast mound reconstruction before reconstructing the nipple, irrespective of the original breast mound reconstructive technique, as this allows the breast tissue to stabilize and develop a more natural ptosis. Performing the nipple reconstruction early increases the risk of incorrect placement.

   Unfortunately there is no gold standard technique for consistently producing the ideal nipple and many different techniques are, therefore, in use. Such techniques include local flaps and nipple sharing, each of which is simple and can be undertaken with local anesthetic as an outpatient procedure. The downtime is very short and most patients can return to normal activities the following day.

NIPPLE POSITIONING

2. **Which one of the following statements is correct regarding markings for a C-V flap nipple reconstruction?**
   D. Accurate anatomic placement is less important than achieving symmetry.

   A key goal of nipple reconstruction is to achieve symmetry between the two breasts and for this reason the new nipple may need to be placed in a nonanatomic position. Ideally the nipple will be sited at the point of maximal projection (or convexity), but this is not always possible when considering symmetry.

   Nipple position is an important contributor to the final result of breast reconstruction and the patient should be involved in the decision-making process, because this improves patient satisfaction. Patients should be marked standing straight with the shoulders relaxed, in the presence of a chaperone. The orientation of the C-V flap will depend on the orientation of scars on the breast mound rather than be limited to a set transverse design.

NIPPLE RECONSTRUCTION TECHNIQUES

3. *For each of the following descriptions, the most likely reconstruction type is as follows:*
   A. *This technique uses a central dermal/fat flap with bilateral partial or full-thickness wings and traditionally uses a full-thickness skin graft for closure.*
      e. **Skate flap**
   B. *This technique involves a pull-out flap that is folded over on itself and the donor site is closed directly with a purse-string suture.*
      c. **Bell flap**
   C. *This technique uses three triangular flaps and one vertical cutaneous/fat flap with two bilateral, full-thickness skin arms oriented at 90-degree angles. No skin graft is required.*
      a. **Star flap**

   There are a range of different local flap techniques used in nipple reconstruction and many of these are described and illustrated in *Essentials of Plastic Surgery*, second edition. The skate flap is a popular and traditional flap that uses local flaps and a skin graft to provide predictable, versatile nipple reconstruction (Fig. 51-1)

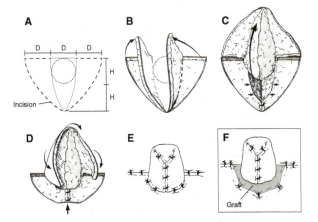

Fig. 51-1 **A-C,** Skate flap with primary closure of donor site. **D-F,** With skin graft.

Chapter 51 ▪ Nipple-Areolar Reconstruction

The Bell flap is useful for reconstructing a nipple that requires little projection and involves a local flap without skin grafting (Fig. 51-2).

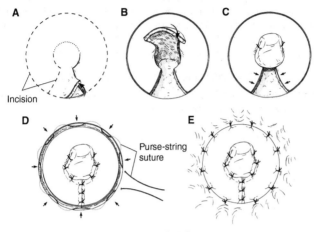

Fig. 51-2 Bell flap.

The star flap is a derivative of the skate flap that avoids the use of a skin graft. It is simple to create but tends not to provide much projection (Fig. 51-3).

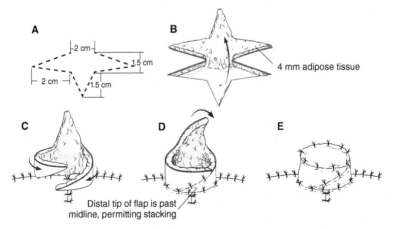

Fig. 51-3 Star flap.

The fishtail flap is a modification of the C-V flap where the V flaps are angulated to be less than 180 degrees from one another (see Fig. 51-5, *Essentials of Plastic Surgery,* second edition). The S flap uses two adjacent flaps in conjunction with a full-thickness skin graft and is useful in areas where a scar crosses the proposed location for the nipple (see Fig. 51-10, *Essentials of Plastic Surgery,* second edition). The modified skate flap avoids skin grafting by using local flaps to achieve direct closure (see Fig. 51-4, *Essentials of Plastic Surgery,* second edition).

For further reading, see also the review article by Farhadi et al.[2]

LONG-TERM PROBLEMS WITH NIPPLE RECONSTRUCTION

4. **Which one of the following is the most significant long-term challenge of nipple reconstruction with local flap techniques?**
   C. **Maintaining projection**

   The main problem with local flap nipple reconstruction techniques is a lack of long-term projection. Areolar fading occurs after tattooing but can easily be touched up in clinic. Patient satisfaction is a very important goal of nipple reconstruction, and patients are generally very satisfied after this procedure. Some studies suggest that the principle determinant of patient dissatisfaction with nipple reconstruction is excessive flattening.[3] However this is not uniformly the case, and patients have been shown to have high levels of satisfaction even where nipple projection is not well maintained.[4] Scar stretch can be a problem as scars do not reliably accept tattoo pigments, but hypertrophic scarring is uncommon and may be treated with conservative measures such as massage, silicone therapy, and steroid injection.

LOSS OF PROJECTION AFTER NIPPLE RECONSTRUCTION

5. You are consenting a patient for nipple reconstruction using a local skin flap technique. **What is the expected approximate projection loss 2 years after nipple reconstruction?**
   E. **50%**

   Loss of nipple projection will depend on several factors such as flap design and tissue quality. Reports of projection loss vary within the literature and range from 43% to 71% when C-V–type skin flaps are used. Banducci et al[5] reported a decrease of 71% at 3 years using a modified star flap. Shestak et al[6] observed a 50% to 70% reduction at 2 years with local flaps (including star, skate, and bell flaps). Attempts to improve projection include placing auricular cartilage or AlloDerm within the nipple construct and these have reported varied results. Jones and Erdmann[4] found a 67% reduction at 2 years even when cartilage grafts were placed inside the construct.

   The dressings placed around the nipple reconstruction may affect the reconstruction and compression should be avoided. This is usually achieved by placing a donut-shaped dressing around the nipple and avoiding direct pressure from garments.

FLAP DESIGN FOR NIPPLE RECONSTRUCTION

6. **When designing a C-V flap for nipple reconstruction, which one of the following dimensions will dictate the initial nipple projection?**
   C. **Width of the V component**

   The C-V flap has evolved from the skate flap and preoperative markings are shown in Fig. 51-5, *Essentials of Plastic Surgery,* second edition. It comprises of a central C flap with bilateral V flaps. The V flaps wrap around to form a cylinder-shaped construct which creates the walls of the nipple papule and the C component then forms the construct lid. The main factor that will dictate the initial nipple projection will therefore be the width of the V flaps. The length and depth of the V flaps will dictate how wide or bulky the papule is. It is advisable to oversize the flaps to allow

for subsequent shrinkage, as discussed in question 5. A rule of thumb is to create a nipple that starts off twice the desired final height.

INVERTED NIPPLES

7. What is the most common cause of nipple inversion?
E. Congenital

Nipple inversion is relatively common and affects one in ten women of child-bearing age. It is usually bilateral and many cases are as a result of chronic mastitis, but the most common cause is congenital. Other important causes include breast cancer and Paget's disease of the nipple and these must be diagnosed and treated early. Inversion results from relative shortness of the lactiferous ducts that tether the nipple and prevent normal projection, and a paucity of normal dense collagenous tissue surrounding the ducts.[7]

8. What is the key feature to consider when grading nipple inversion?
D. The ability to manually correct the inversion

Evaluation of patients with inverted nipples involves an assessment of whether the inversion can be manually corrected and whether it maintains correction following release of traction. This is important as it provides information on the severity and guides surgical management. The classification system by Han and Hong[8] formally grades the severity of nipple inversion based on the findings of this assessment:

   Grade I: Nipple can be easily pulled out manually and maintains projection without traction.
   Grade II: Nipple can be pulled out manually but with less ease than grade I and tends to retract.
   Grade III: Nipple is inverted, difficult to pull out manually, and promptly retracts.

Surgical management involves release of the pathologic bands with or without release of the lactiferous ducts and creation of tightness at the neck of the inverted nipple using a purse-string suture. Additional bulk may also be added beneath the nipple using cartilage or adjacent dermal fat flaps providing that full release has been undertaken.

REFERENCES

1. Wellisch DK, Schain WS, Noone RB, et al. The psychological contribution of nipple addition in breast reconstruction. Plast Reconstr Surg 80:699-704, 1987.
2. Farhadi J, Maksvytyte GK, Schaefer DJ, et al. Reconstruction of the nipple-areola complex: an update. J Plast Reconstr Aesthet Surg 59:40-53, 2006.
3. Jabor MA, Shayni M, Collins DR, et al. Nipple-areolar reconstruction: satisfaction and clinical determinants. Plast Reconstr Surg 110:457-463, 2002.
4. Jones AP, Erdmann M. Projection and patient satisfaction using the "Hamburger" nipple reconstruction technique. J Plast Reconstr Aesthet Surg 65:207-212, 2012.
5. Banducci DR, Le TK, Hughes KC. Long-term follow-up of a modified Anton-Hartrampf nipple reconstruction. Ann Plast Surg 43:467-469; discussion 469-470, 1999.
6. Shestak KC, Gabriel A, Landecker A, et al. Assessment of long-term nipple projection: a comparison of three techniques. Plast Reconstr Surg 110:780-786, 2002.
7. Schwager RG, Smith JW, Gray GF, et al. Inversion of the human female nipple, with a simple method of treatment. Plast Reconstr Surg 54:564-569, 1974.
8. Han S, Hong YG. The inverted nipple: its grading and surgical correction. Plast Reconstr Surg 104:389-395, 1999.

Part V

Trunk and Lower Extremity

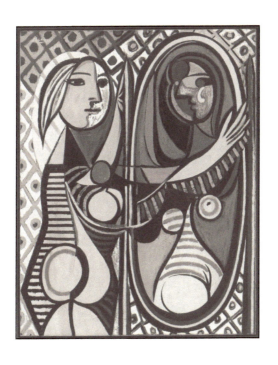

© 2015 Estate of Pablo Picasso / Artists Rights Society (ARS), New York.

52. Chest Wall Reconstruction

See *Essentials of Plastic Surgery*, second edition, pp. 607-618.

ANATOMY OF THE CHEST WALL

1. **Which one of the following statements is correct regarding the anatomy of the chest wall?**
   A. The visceral and parietal pleura have identical embryologic origins.
   B. Of the twelve paired ribs, up to eight directly articulate with the sternum.
   C. The sternum has three distinct components in all patient groups.
   D. Neurovascular bundles lie at the inferior margin of the ribs, between the external and internal intercostal muscles.
   E. The internal mammary vessels usually bifurcate at the level of the fifth interspace.

MUSCLES OF RESPIRATION

2. **Select the muscle being described in each of the following statements. (Each answer may be used once, more than once, or not at all.)**
   A. This primary muscle of respiration is supplied by the thoracic nerves.
   B. This secondary muscle of respiration is found within the neck and supplied by the spinal accessory nerve.
   C. This muscle of the thorax can aid respiration in times of respiratory distress and is supplied by C5-7 only.

   Options:
   a. Serratus anterior
   b. Diaphragm
   c. Scalenus medius
   d. Sternocleidomastoid
   e. Levatores costarum
   f. Internal intercostal
   g. Pectoralis minor
   h. Trapezius

RECONSTRUCTION OF CHEST WALL DEFECTS

3. **Which one of the following statements is correct regarding the causes and management of chest wall defects?**
   A. Sternal defects are usually classified according to the site and size of the soft tissue defect.
   B. The thoracic skeleton should usually be reconstructed if more than two ribs are resected.
   C. The omentum may be used to reconstruct the chest wall and is supplied by the superior epigastric vessels.
   D. Some large skeletal defects may not need reconstruction if they are posterior or at sites of previous radiotherapy.
   E. The Eloesser flap is used to treat bronchopleural fistula in preference to thoracoplasty.

CLASSIFICATION OF STERNOTOMY DEFECTS

4. Which one of the following is a key component of the Pairolero classification for sternal defects?
   A. Defect location
   B. Defect size
   C. Chronicity of wound
   D. Underlying cause of defect
   E. Volume of bone loss

SOFT TISSUE RECONSTRUCTION OF THE CHEST WALL

5. For each of the following clinical scenarios, select the most appropriate soft tissue reconstructive option. (Each option may be used once, more than once, or not at all.)
   A. A 68-year-old man with right-sided Poland's syndrome is referred 4 weeks after coronary bypass surgery. He has a 10 by 5 cm dehisced midline sternotomy wound passing from the inferior xiphisternum to the fifth intercostal space. His left internal mammary artery was harvested as a graft. The wound is clean, with negative results of bone biopsy and swab analyses.
   B. A 65-year-old patient presents with a history of left-sided thoracotomy for excision of a lung tumor. He is referred by the cardiothoracic team following an infection after open cardiac valve replacement. He has an 8 by 4 cm defect over the left upper third of his sternum, with sternal loss and exposed mediastinum. The right internal mammary vessels are preserved on arteriography.
   C. A slim, 47-year-old woman has a 20 by 15 cm defect of her anterior chest wall after resection of a recurrent sarcoma. Her left pectoralis major and minor were resected, along with large portions of ribs three through seven. Her first reconstruction involved a pedicled latissimus dorsi flap from the left side. Her past surgical history also includes an open cholecystectomy.

Options:
a. Left pectoralis major turnover
b. Right pectoralis major turnover
c. Right pectoralis major advancement
d. Left vertical rectus abdominis myocutaneous flap
e. Right vertical rectus abdominis myocutaneous flap
f. Pedicled omental flap
g. Left pedicled latissimus dorsi myocutaneous flap

POLAND'S SYNDROME

6. Which one of the following statements is correct regarding Poland's syndrome?
   A. Incidence is 1:500,000 live births.
   B. The left side is most commonly affected.
   C. It can occur after subclavian artery compression during the second trimester.
   D. Facial weakness and a squint are sometimes also evident.
   E. The clavicular head of the pectoralis major is normally absent.

KEY FINDINGS IN POLAND'S SYNDROME

7. Which one of the following is a less common finding in patients with Poland's syndrome?
A. Absence of the sternal head of pectoralis major
B. Breast hypoplasia that may affect the NAC
C. Absence of pectoralis minor
D. Deficiency of subcutaneous fat and axillary hair
E. Hypoplasia of ipsilateral extremity with syndactyly

PECTUS EXCAVATUM

8. A 4-year-old boy is brought to your clinic with a moderate pectus excavatum. Which one of the following statements is correct regarding this diagnosis?
A. This is also called *pigeon chest* and results from excessive growth of the lower costal cartilages.
B. This is less common than pectus carinatum and has an equal sex distribution.
C. His sternum will have a tendency to rotate if costal growth is mismatched and untreated.
D. His abnormality should improve with increasing age but will never fully resolve.
E. Surgery should be delayed until growth is complete.

PECTUS CARINATUM

9. A teenage girl presents with concerns about her overly prominent sternum, which she would like to have altered. Which one of the following statements is correct regarding pectus carinatum?
A. It is characterized by an anterior protrusion of the sternum and costal cartilages, commonly causing respiratory difficulties.
B. Females are most commonly affected and most have a positive family history.
C. Surgical correction specifically relies on the Ravitch technique.
D. The most common site of protrusion is the manubrium, with depression of the sternal body.
E. One defect subtype is commonly seen in conjunction with Poland's syndrome.

Answers

ANATOMY OF THE CHEST WALL
1. **Which one of the following statements is correct regarding the anatomy of the chest wall?**
   B. Of the twelve paired ribs, up to eight directly articulate with the sternum.
   There are twelve paired ribs, seven or eight of which are true ribs and articulate directly with the sternum. The first rib articulates with the T1 vertebra only and does not contact C7. The remaining true ribs articulate with their corresponding vertebra and the one above. False ribs articulate with the costal cartilages and the vertebra. The two floating ribs articulate only with their vertebral bodies.

   The parietal and visceral pleura have separate embryologic origins, including vascular, lymphatic, and neural supply.

   By the start of the fifth decade, the xiphoid has usually ossified and united with the body of the sternum so it is no longer a three-part construct. The neurovascular bundles are found between the internal and innermost intercostals (not the external and internal). They are arranged as vein, artery, and nerve in descending order.

   The internal mammary artery arises from the first part of the subclavian artery passing 1 cm lateral to the sternum. The internal mammary vessels are highly relevant to chest wall reconstruction because they supply commonly used flaps such as the rectus abdominus and pectoralis major muscles. Furthermore they may be sacrificed during cardiac procedures such as coronary bypass grafting or major chest wall resections. The internal mammary vessels are also relevant to free tissue transfer to the chest wall such as for anastomoses in breast reconstruction. Knowledge of their anatomy is therefore important. When using these vessels for free tissue transfer, the third intercostal space or higher is often used for access, because the veins get progressively smaller distally and usually bifurcate at or distal to this point. The veins and artery are usually a good caliber at this level.

MUSCLES OF RESPIRATION
2. **For the following scenarios, the best options are as follows:**
   A. This primary muscle of respiration is supplied by the thoracic nerves.
      f. Internal intercostal
   B. This secondary muscle of respiration is found within the neck and supplied by the spinal accessory nerve.
      d. Sternocleidomastoid
   C. This muscle of the thorax can aid respiration in times of respiratory distress and is supplied by C5-7 only.
      a. Serratus anterior
         Muscles involved in respiration can be classified in three groups: primary, secondary, and accessory (used in times of respiratory distress).[1] Primary muscles are the diaphragm and

intercostals, which are supplied by the phrenic nerve and intercostal nerves, respectively. The intercostal nerves are formed by the anterior divisions of the T1-11 thoracic nerves.

Secondary muscles of respiration are the sternocleidomastoid, serratus posterior, and levatores costarum. The innervation of these muscles is the spinal accessory for the sternocleidomastoid, T9-12 intercostal nerves for the serratus posterior, and the lateral divisions of the posterior primary rami of the corresponding spinal nerves for the levatores costarum.

Accessory muscles of respiration include the serratus anterior, supplied by the long thoracic nerve (C5-7), and the pectoralis major, supplied by medial and lateral pectoral nerves (C5-7 and C8, T1, respectively). The scalenes can also contribute to respiration. They are supplied by C4-6.

RECONSTRUCTION OF CHEST WALL DEFECTS

3. **Which one of the following statements is correct regarding the causes and management of chest wall defects?**
   D. Some large skeletal defects may not need reconstruction if they are posterior or at sites of previous radiotherapy.

   Decisions regarding reconstruction of the thoracic skeleton will be made on an individual patient basis depending on baseline respiratory function and the impact of the defect on respiratory function; however, the usual guidelines for reconstruction of the thoracic skeleton are:
   1. Defects where four contiguous ribs have been removed
   2. Defects larger than 5 cm in diameter

   But these indications will differ as follows:
   1. Previous radiation treatment stiffens the chest wall so larger defects may be tolerated without reconstruction.
   2. Posterior defects are better tolerated without reconstruction given the support of the bony scapula and musculature.
   3. Patients with poor respiratory reserve such as COPD will tolerate defects less well and may benefit from reconstruction of smaller defects.

   Sternal defects can be classified by using either the Pairolero and Arnold[2] or Starzynski et al[3] classifications. These are significantly different to one another, although each has the same number of grades/types. The Starzynski classification is based on the anatomic structures missing, as well as the physiological deficit incurred. The Pairolero classification is based on chronicity and the presence or absence of infection.

   The omental flap is a useful option for chest wall reconstruction and receives blood supply from the gastroepiploic vessels, not the superior epigastric vessels. The Eloesser flap is an inferiorly based U-shaped flap from the posterior chest wall that is turned into the thoracic cavity to facilitate passive drainage of empyema. It does not address bronchopleural fistula. Thoracoplasty treats both bronchopleural fistula and empyema in a single surgery, but results in rib cage deformity and interferes with upper limb function.

CLASSIFICATION OF STERNOTOMY DEFECTS

4. Which one of the following is a key component of the Pairolero classification for sternal defects?

C. Chronicity of wound

Pairolero and Arnold[2] described a classification for sternotomy wounds in 1986. The classification is based on the timing of the defect relative to surgery (early, intermediate, or late) and the presence or absence of active infection as evidenced by cellulitis, positive swabs, or osteomyelitis. They described treatment according to the subtype as follows:

Type 1: Serosanguineous drainage within the first 3 days of surgery
No active infection
Treatment: Reexploration, debridement, and closure of the defect directly
Type 2: Purulent discharge within the first 3 weeks of surgery
Active infection evident
Treatment: Exploration, debridement, and coverage of the defect with a soft tissue flap
Type 3: Chronically infected wound months or years after surgery

The other factors listed do not form part of the Pairolero description. This classification system is often discussed in the setting of clinical viva scenarios in plastic surgery.

SOFT TISSUE RECONSTRUCTION OF THE CHEST WALL

5. For the following scenarios, the best options are as follows:

A. A 68-year-old man with right-sided Poland's syndrome is referred 4 weeks after coronary bypass surgery. He has a 10 by 5 cm dehisced midline sternotomy wound passing from the inferior xiphisternum to the fifth intercostal space. His left internal mammary artery was harvested as a graft. The wound is clean, with negative results of bone biopsy and swab analyses.

e. Right vertical rectus abdominis myocutaneous flap

This patient probably requires reconstruction with a right vertical rectus abdominis myocutaneous flap. This is the most appropriate option, because it provides good soft tissue cover with robust skin. The internal mammary vessels supplying the flap are intact, whereas they are not on the other side. The defect is probably too low for a left pectoralis major reconstruction and the diagnosis of Poland's syndrome suggests this muscle is not available for harvest on the right-hand side. The omental flap would also provide useful cover but a skin graft would also be required and the abdominal cavity would have to be opened. A left latissimus dorsi myocutaneous flap could be used. A disadvantage would be a need to turn the patient intraoperatively. Achieving adequate reach would likely require detachment at the humeral insertion and division of the thoracodorsal nerve.

B. A 65-year-old patient presents with a history of left-sided thoracotomy for excision of a lung tumor. He is referred by the cardiothoracic team following an infection after open cardiac valve replacement. He has an 8 by 4 cm defect over the left upper third of his sternum, with sternal loss and exposed mediastinum. The right internal mammary vessels are preserved on arteriography.

b. Right pectoralis major turnover

This patient has a proximal left-sided defect that is relatively small, and the contralateral internal mammary is preserved. Therefore a right pectoralis major turnover flap combined with a split-skin graft is a suitable option. A pedicled ipsilateral latissimus dorsi is usually an option if reach is sufficient. However, it is not available on the ipsilateral side in this patient because of the previous thoracotomy.

C. *A slim, 47-year-old woman has a 20 by 15 cm defect of her anterior chest wall after resection of a recurrent sarcoma. Her left pectoralis major and minor were resected, along with large portions of ribs three through seven. Her first reconstruction involved a pedicled latissimus dorsi flap from the left side. Her past surgical history also includes an open cholecystectomy.*

   f. Pedicled omental flap

      This patient has no remaining local muscle flap options to reconstruct a defect of this size. In this case an omental flap would represent the best choice from the options listed. Omental flaps are traditionally used more often than free tissue transfers to reconstruct extensive chest wall defects. If a free muscle transfer was used in this case, a free contralateral latissimus dorsi would be a reasonable choice. She is not a good candidate for reconstruction with a right vertical rectus flap because of the previous cholecystectomy incision.

POLAND'S SYNDROME

6. *Which one of the following statements is correct regarding Poland's syndrome?*

   D. Facial weakness and a squint are sometimes also evident.

      Poland's syndrome is a congenital condition in which there are a number of upper limb and chest wall abnormalities. It occurs in approximately 1:30,000 births and affects males and females equally. The right side is affected more often than the left side by a ratio 2:1. It is postulated that the subclavian vessels are compressed in the first (not second) trimester. A consistent finding is the absence of the sternal head (not the clavicular head) of the pectoralis major. Although rare, Poland's syndrome can be associated with Möbius syndrome and therefore with the absence of cranial nerves VI and VII. Patients with Poland's syndrome are often seen by plastic surgeons with regard to reconstruction of both the upper limb and chest/breast deformities.

KEY FINDINGS IN POLAND'S SYNDROME

7. *Which one of the following is a less common finding in patients with Poland's syndrome?*

   C. Absence of pectoralis minor

      As discussed in question 6, Poland's syndrome represents a spectrum of abnormalities affecting the ipsilateral chest wall and upper limb. Common key findings include the following:

         Absence of the sternal head of the pectoralis major
         Absence of costal cartilages
         Hypoplasia of breast tissue, including the nipple-areola complex
         Deficiency of subcutaneous fat and axillary hair
         Syndactyly or hypoplasia of the ipsilateral extremity

      Additional features that occur less commonly include the following:

         Absence of the pectoralis minor
         Shortening of the forearm
         Deformity of chest wall muscles, including the serratus, latissimus dorsi, and external oblique
         Total absence of anterolateral ribs with herniation of the lung
         Associations with Möbius syndrome
         Symphalangism

      Common surgical procedures for the chest in Poland's patients include latissimus dorsi transfer to reconstruct the pectoralis major deficiency, and breast reconstruction with a variety of implant of autologous techniques. Surgery for the limb may include syndactyly release and occasionally, free toe-to-hand transfer.

PECTUS EXCAVATUM

8. A 4-year-old boy is brought to your clinic with a moderate pectus excavatum. **Which one of the following statements is correct regarding this diagnosis?**
   C. **His sternum will have a tendency to rotate if costal growth is mismatched and untreated.**
   Pectus excavatum is the most common chest wall deformity affecting one in four hundred children and affects males more than females with a ratio of 4:1. It occurs 10 times more frequently than pectus carinatum and is called funnel chest, not pigeon chest. (Pigeon chest refers to pectus carinatum). Funnel chest occurs secondary to excess growth of the lower costal cartilages resulting in a sternal depression. The sternum will rotate if growth is greater on one side. The condition becomes progressively worse with time and continued growth, leaving a cosmetic and sometimes functional deformity. It is treated surgically, relatively early (2 to 5 years of age is recommended) using a Nuss procedure, a sternal turnover, or sternal osteotomies.

PECTUS CARINATUM

9. A teenage girl presents with concerns about her overly prominent sternum, which she would like to have altered. **Which one of the following statements is correct regarding pectus carinatum?**
   E. **One defect subtype is commonly seen in conjunction with Poland's syndrome.**
   Pectus carinatum (pigeon chest) is characterized by anterior protrusion of the sternum but rarely causes physiologic symptoms. It affects males more than females (4:1 ratio), and a positive family history is present in a third of cases. Three subtypes are recognized: chondrogladiolar (most common), pouter pigeon chest, and lateral depression of the ribs. The latter is commonly associated with Poland's syndrome. Pouter pigeon chest is least common and involves protrusion of the manubrium and depression of the sternal body. Chondrogladiolar is most common and involves anterior displacement of the sternal body and symmetrical concavity of costal cartilages. Several surgical options are available, including repositioning of the sternum, excision of costal cartilages, and the use of strut techniques such as the Ravitch procedure. This technique is, however, not absolutely required and is not totally specific to pectus carinatum.

REFERENCES

1. Standring S, ed. Gray's Anatomy: The Anatomical Basis of Clinical Practice, Expert Consult, ed 40. Philadelphia: Churchill Livingstone Elsevier, 2008. Available at *http://www.graysanatomyonline.com/*.
2. Pairolero PC, Arnold PG. Management of infected median sternotomy wounds. Ann Thorac Surg 42:1-2, 1986.
3. Starzynski TE, Snyderman RK, Beattie EJ Jr. Problems of major chest wall reconstruction. Plast Reconstr Surg 44:525-535, 1969.

53. Abdominal Wall Reconstruction

See *Essentials of Plastic Surgery*, second edition, pp. 619-631.

ANATOMY OF THE ANTERIOR ABDOMINAL WALL

1. **Which one of the following statements is correct regarding the structure of the anterior abdominal wall?**
   A. The anterior axillary line represents the lateral border of the anterior abdominal wall.
   B. Below the arcuate line the rectus sheath contains only transversalis fascia.
   C. The pyramidalis is a functionally important triangular muscle that tenses the linea alba.
   D. The arcuate line is found below the level of the anterior superior iliac spines.
   E. The anterior rectus sheath comprises the external and internal oblique aponeuroses.

GRADING OF HERNIA DEFECTS

2. In 2010 the Ventral Hernia Working Group (VHWG) published guidelines for the management of ventral abdominal wall hernias. **Which one of the following is a key component of this system?**
   A. Hernia size
   B. Hernia site
   C. Method of repair
   D. Functional impairment
   E. Infection

3. The VHWG classification system was revised by Kanters et al. **What was the main improvement compared to the previous grading system?**
   A. It was formally validated.
   B. The number of grades were increased.
   C. The grades were determined based on method of repair.
   D. The grades were based on hernia size.
   E. Repair material choice affected the grading system.

PRINCIPLES OF REPAIR

4. **Which one of the following statements is true when reconstructing abdominal wall defects?**
   A. Blood sugar levels should ideally be less than 110 mg/dl.
   B. Smoking must be stopped 3 months before reconstruction.
   C. Repairs should always be reinforced using acellular dermal matrix.
   D. Debridement and repair must be performed in separate stages.
   E. Reinforcing materials should be avoided in previous fistulation sites.

ADJUNCTS TO CLOSURE OF ABDOMINAL WALL DEFECTS

5. **Which one of the following statements is correct regarding techniques for abdominal wall reconstruction?**
   A. Heavyweight small-pore polypropylene is an absorbable mesh with poor resistance to bacterial contamination that demonstrates low extrusion rates.
   B. Gore-Tex sheet is manufactured from expanded polytetrafluoroethylene (ePTFE) and can facilitate fluid egress and fibrous ingrowth in abdominal wounds.
   C. Tissue expanders in the abdominal region should always be placed in the subcutaneous plane.
   D. Polyglycolic acid is useful as temporary support in abdominal wall defects but may lead to hernia formation in the longer term.
   E. AlloDerm (LifeCell, Branchburg, NJ) is a freeze-dried porcine acellular dermis that is stronger than fascia lata.

ALLOPLASTIC COMPOSITE MATERIALS

6. **What is the main proposed benefit of using newer composite or barrier-coated prosthetic materials for abdominal wall repair, as compared to traditional alloplastic materials?**
   A. They provide a financial cost savings.
   B. They completely resorb, leaving less foreign body material.
   C. They provide far better tissue integration.
   D. They may reduce formation of tissue adhesions.
   E. They negate the need for omental bowel cover.

BIOPROSTHETIC MATERIALS

7. **Which one of the following statements is correct regarding biologic materials in abdominal wall reconstruction?**
   A. They are recommended for use in all wound types.
   B. They are all crosslinked to control enzymatic degradation.
   C. Hernia recurrence rates are uniformly low following their use.
   D. They are ideal for use in bridging interpositional repairs.
   E. They may be placed directly on the bowel with low adhesion rates.

COMPONENT SEPARATION

8. You are planning a component separation on a patient with an anterior abdominal wall defect. **Which one of the following statements is correct regarding this procedure?**
   A. Ramirez et al originally described this procedure as purely anatomic.
   B. Abdominal wall closure is significantly enhanced when the rectus abdominis is advanced with the external oblique.
   C. The key plane of dissection is between the internal oblique and transversus abdominis.
   D. The main neurovascular structures supplying the abdominal wall are found between the internal and external oblique muscles.
   E. Release of the rectus from its posterior sheath can increase advancement by an additional 2 cm at all levels.

9. *According to the original study by Ramirez et al, how much advancement can be achieved at the waist after a bilateral component separation?*
   A. 6 cm
   B. 10 cm
   C. 20 cm
   D. 24 cm
   E. 30 cm

APPROACHES TO ABDOMINAL WALL REPAIR

10. You have just completed a free tissue transfer for breast reconstruction using a muscle-sparing transverse rectus abdominis myocutaneous (TRAM) flap instead of the planned deep inferior epigastric perforator (DIEP) flap. A 5 by 8 cm fascial defect of the anterior rectus sheath is present. *How should this defect be reconstructed?*
    A. Direct fascial repair alone
    B. Onlay graft with acellular dermal matrix
    C. Inlay repair with polyglactin mesh
    D. Inlay repair with polypropylene mesh
    E. Component separation

MANAGEMENT OF ABDOMINAL WALL HERNIAS

11. A 50-year-old woman has a large, chronic rectus sheath hernia following emergency paramedian laparotomy for bowel perforation. The initial abdominal wall repair took months to heal after partial dehiscence occurred. She has a 5 by 10 cm abdominal wall hernia to the left of the midline and is concerned about function, cosmesis, and discomfort. *Which one of the following is the most appropriate option for management of this patient?*
    A. Lifestyle modification
    B. Direct repair of the hernia with permanent mesh
    C. Direct repair of the hernia with acellular dermal matrix
    D. Component separation with permanent mesh
    E. Component separation with acellular dermal matrix

430   Part V ▪ Trunk and Lower Extremity

Answers

ANATOMY OF THE ANTERIOR ABDOMINAL WALL
1. **Which one of the following statements is correct regarding the structure of the anterior abdominal wall?**
   E. The anterior rectus sheath comprises the external and internal oblique aponeuroses.
   The anterior rectus sheath comprises the external oblique aponeurosis and the anterior leaf of the internal oblique aponeurosis throughout its length. The arcuate line is found at the level of the anterior superior iliac spines and above this. Above the arcuate line, the posterior leaf of the internal oblique aponeurosis forms the posterior sheath, along with the transversus abdominis and transversalis fascia. Below the arcuate line, the posterior sheath consists of only transversalis fascia, and everything else is anterior to the rectus abdominis. This is why patients are at increased risk of developing iatrogenic hernias of the lower abdomen following laparotomy or free TRAM harvest.
   The lateral border of the anterior abdominal wall is the midaxillary line (not the anterior axillary line). The superior border is the xiphisternum and the seventh to twelfth costal cartilages. The inferior border is the pubic tubercle and inguinal ligament. The paired pyramidalis muscles are small triangular structures sited between the rectus abdominis and the posterior surface of the rectus sheath. They are functionally unimportant and often absent. It has been postulated that they serve to tense the linea alba.[1]

GRADING OF HERNIA DEFECTS
2. **In 2010 the Ventral Hernia Working Group (VHWG) published guidelines for the management of ventral abdominal wall hernias. Which one of the following is a key component of this system?**
   E. Infection
   The Ventral Hernia Working Group[2] (VHWG) has described a four-grade system for classifying hernias. The intention of this system was to improve risk stratification for patients with ventral wall hernia. The key factor within this system is either the presence or absence of infection or the risk of its subsequent development. *Grade 1* represents a low-risk hernia without infection or wound contamination. *Grade 2* represents a hernia without active infection but with an increased systemic risk of infection such as smoking, diabetes, or obesity. *Grade 3* refers to a potentially contaminated hernia, as seen in patients with a stoma or previous infection. *Grade 4* is an actively infected hernia. This classification system does not refer to hernia size, specific location, method of repair, or functional impairment.

3. **The VHWG classification system was revised by Kanters et al. What was the main improvement compared to the previous grading system?**
   A. It was formally validated
   The revised classification system proposed by Kanters et al[3] followed a review of a group of 299 patients who had undergone ventral wall hernia repair. The study was undertaken to evaluate the accuracy of the original classification in predicting surgical site occurrence after open ventral hernia repair. Following the study, the authors concluded that modification of the original VHWG classification system to three grades instead of four, with redistribution of patients from the original grades, significantly improves the accuracy of predicting surgical site occurrence.[2] Using

Chapter 53 ■ Abdominal Wall Reconstruction   431

the revised system, patients are stratified according to their comorbidities, their prior history of wound infection, and their CDC wound contamination status. The Kanters classification is currently the only formally validated system for ventral hernia repair. The grade of abdominal wall hernia using this system helps guide the nature of the surgical repair..

PRINCIPLES OF REPAIR

4. Which one of the following statements is true when reconstructing abdominal wall defects?
   A. Blood sugar levels should ideally be less than 110 mg/dl.

   Principles in repair of abdominal wall hernias include patient optimization, preparation of the wound, and appropriate surgical techniques. Blood sugar levels should be less than 110 mg/dl and smoking cessation must be complete at least 4 weeks before surgery to optimize postoperative healing. The wound must be adequately debrided and may require serial procedures before reconstruction. However, the two procedures do not always need to be staged. Repairs should always be reinforced and this fact is supported by level A evidence.[2] The repair material will differ according to the grade of ventral wall hernia. Nonabsorbable mesh is preferred in low risk repairs. Fistulas must be adequately addressed prior to reconstruction, but these sites still need reinforcement.

ADJUNCTS TO CLOSURE OF ABDOMINAL WALL DEFECTS

5. Which one of the following statements is correct regarding techniques for abdominal wall reconstruction?
   D. Polyglycolic acid is useful as temporary support in abdominal wall defects but may lead to hernia formation in the longer term.

   Polyglycolic acid and polyglactin 910 are both absorbable materials that can be used as temporary mesh supports in abdominal wall reconstruction. They are not suitable for repairs of areas deficient in fascia, because their lack of permanence can result in hernia formation in the long term. Nonabsorbable polypropylene mesh, such as Marlex is durable and strong with good resistance to bacterial contamination. Gore-Tex sheet is produced with ePTFE, but its use is limited because it does not allow fluid egress or fibrous ingrowth. Tissue expanders can be placed between the internal and external oblique muscles and in the subcutaneous plane. AlloDerm is freeze-dried human cadaver dermis and is not available in the United Kingdom. Furthermore, it tends to stretch over time and may be insufficient to prevent bulging and herniation. Instead, a porcine acellular dermal matrix, which is less prone to stretching and has comparable strength to fascia lata, can be used in many countries.

ALLOPLASTIC COMPOSITE MATERIALS

6. What is the main proposed benefit of using newer composite or barrier-coated prosthetic materials for abdominal wall repair, as compared to traditional alloplastic materials?
   D. They may reduce formation of tissue adhesions.

   There are a number of newer composite prosthetics that combine both absorbable and nonabsorbable materials such as polypropylene and polyglactin, or nonabsorbable and tissue separating barrier materials such as polypropylene and cellulose. Proceed and Supramesh are examples of the latter type and should help maintain tissue separation and adhesion formation. The benefits of materials such as Vypro and Ultrapro, which contain a combination of absorbable and nonabsorbable alloplastic material, are that handling and initial strength may be improved while reducing the amount of foreign body present in the longer term. None of these materials contain purely absorbable material and will not completely resorb, and tissue integration differs between materials, but will never match that of normal tissue. A caveat with these materials is that they tend to be more expensive than traditional prosthetics. Although these newer materials should reduce bowel adhesions, it is still advisable to cover the bowel with omentum to separate the bowel from the mesh.

BIOPROSTHETIC MATERIALS

7. Which one of the following statements is correct regarding biologic materials in abdominal wall reconstruction?

E. They may be placed directly on the bowel with low adhesion rates.

There are a variety of acellular dermal matrices (ADM) in use. They are either bovine, porcine, or human in origin. They are expensive compared with alloplastic materials and their use should be targeted to contaminated wounds in which prosthetic mesh must be avoided. Permacol is an example of a crosslinked porcine ADM. Cross-linking will help to control enzymatic degradation of the graft, but it tends to make the product behave more like a synthetic with less tissue integration. The vast majority of ADMs such as Surgimend, AlloDerm, XenMatrix, and Strattice are not crosslinked. Hernia recurrence rates are highly variable when using ADMs[4] and the highest rates are when used as a bridging technique. A major benefit of their use is that they produce few visceral adhesions compared with prosthetics and may be placed directly onto the bowel.

COMPONENT SEPARATION

8. You are planning a component separation on a patient with an anterior abdominal wall defect. *Which one of the following statements is correct regarding this procedure?*

E. Release of the rectus from its posterior sheath can increase advancement by an additional 2 cm at all levels.

In 1990 Ramirez et al[5] published results of a clinical and anatomic study to determine whether separation of the components of the abdominal wall musculature allows increased mobilization of each to close large abdominal wall defects. They dissected 10 cadavers and found that the external and internal oblique muscles could be separated in a relatively avascular plane. This allowed medial advancement of the rectus (once elevated from the posterior sheath) as a composite with the internal oblique (not external oblique) and transversus abdominis muscles. The advancement was far greater than with direct closure of all components as a single composite. The neurovascular structures were identified between the internal oblique and transversus abdominis, and these two structures were tightly adherent to one another.

To perform the procedure, the external oblique aponeurosis is split longitudinally at the linea alba. This plane is developed laterally between the external and internal oblique muscles to the midaxillary line. The posterior rectus sheath is also separated from the rectus via a midline incision to facilitate advancement.

After their anatomic study, Ramirez et al performed the procedure in 11 clinical cases, which were also presented in the paper. Good clinical outcomes were observed in all cases. In four of the patients who had preoperative back pain, this problem resolved after surgery.

Although Ramirez et al are quoted as having originally described the technique, the first description of this concept actually dates back to a paper by Young[6] in 1961 for repair of epigastric hernias.

Chapter 53 ■ Abdominal Wall Reconstruction

9. *According to the original study by Ramirez et al, how much advancement can be achieved at the waist after a bilateral component separation?*
C. 20 cm
   Ramirez et al[5] quoted the following figures for unilateral advancement: 5 cm at the epigastrium, 10 cm at the middle third, and 3 cm in the suprapubic region. These figures are doubled for the bilateral advancement. Although some surgeons report much greater advancement at the midabdomen, they also indicate that advancement of the upper and lower third are difficult to achieve without posterior sheath release or extension over the costal margins.

APPROACHES TO ABDOMINAL WALL REPAIR

10. You have just completed a free tissue transfer for breast reconstruction using a muscle-sparing transverse rectus abdominis myocutaneous (TRAM) flap instead of the planned deep inferior epigastric perforator (DIEP) flap. A 5 by 8 cm fascial defect of the anterior rectus sheath is present. *How should this defect be reconstructed?*
D. Inlay repair with polypropylene mesh
   When a planned DIEP flap requires conversion to a muscle-sparing TRAM flap, a residual fascial defect in the anterior rectus sheath warrants repair. If the defect is small (less than 2 cm wide), direct closure may be possible; otherwise, reinforced closure is required. Although the benefits of mesh over direct repair are debated, Luijendijk et al[7] conducted a large study that showed significantly lower rates of incisional hernia recurrence where mesh repairs were used, compared with direct suture repair only. Wan et al[8] showed similar rates of hernia in patients after a TRAM flap with mesh repair, compared with those who had a DIEP procedure. Without a mesh repair, the rates were higher in the TRAM group.

   Permanent mesh such as polypropylene is probably the best option for this clean, elective surgery. These products are inert, readily available, inexpensive, and provide good long-term strength and support. Inlay mesh repair is in theory biomechanically superior, because the forces acting on it by intraabdominal pressure will push the interface between mesh and abdominal wall firmly together at the areas of overlap. Debate exists over the benefits of underlay versus overlay techniques. However, the VHWG[2] suggested the use of an underlay rather than an overlay in open procedures for abdominal wall repair. Polyglactin 910 is less appropriate, given that it is absorbable and cannot provide long-term support. Acellular dermal matrix has a role in abdominal wound closure, but the benefits in this situation do not support the increased cost. Component separation would not be required for a defect of this nature.

MANAGEMENT OF ABDOMINAL WALL HERNIAS

11. A 50-year-old woman has a large, chronic rectus sheath hernia following emergency paramedian laparotomy for bowel perforation. The initial abdominal wall repair took months to heal after partial dehiscence occurred. She has a 5 by 10 cm abdominal wall hernia to the left of the midline and is concerned about function, cosmesis, and discomfort. *Which one of the following is the most appropriate option for management of this patient?*
E. Component separation with acellular dermal matrix
   This patient has a number of options, including lifestyle modification or revision surgery. The former is unlikely to be acceptable to this patient given her age and lifestyle demands. A key principle in repair of this hernia is to reapproximate and centralize the rectus muscles and for this a component separation should be used. The repair will also need reinforcement with a mesh. In this case a permanent mesh such as polypropylene is best avoided given that this was previously a contaminated wound. A dermal matrix is a better choice.

A further option not listed is a Rives-Stoppa procedure. The Rives-Stoppa technique can be useful in patients with a large ventral hernia. It employs a reinforcing mesh sublay in the retromuscular space between the rectus muscle and the posterior rectus sheath, but it can be limited by the lateral edge of the posterior rectus sheath. Therefore, for larger defects, a larger inlay mesh is sometimes placed behind the rectus sheath but outside of the peritoneum.

REFERENCES

1. Lovering RM, Anderson LD. Architecture and fiber type of the pyramidalis muscle. Anat Sci Int 83:294-297, 2008.
2. Breuing K, Butler CE, Ferzoco S, et al; Ventral Hernia Working Group. Incisional ventral hernias: review of the literature and recommendations regarding the grading and technique of repair. Surgery 148:544-558, 2010.
3. Kanters AE, Krpata DM, Blatnik JA, et al. Modified hernia grading scale to stratify surgical site occurrence after open ventral hernia repairs. J Am Col Surg 215:787-793, 2012.
4. Janis JE, O'Neill AC, Ahmad J, et al. Acellular dermal matrices in abdominal wall reconstruction: a systematic review of the current evidence. Plast Reconstr Surg 130(5 Suppl 2):183S-193S, 2012.
5. Ramirez OM, Ruas E, Dellon AL. "Components separation" method for closure of abdominal-wall defects: an anatomic and clinical study. Plast Reconstr Surg 86:519-526, 1990.
6. Young D. Repair of epigastric incisional hernia. Br J Surg 48:514-516, 1961.
7. Luijendijk RW, Hop WC, van den Tol MP, et al. A comparison of suture repair with mesh repair for incisional hernia. N Engl J Med 10:343:392-398, 2000.
8. Wan DC, Tseng CY, Anderson-Dam J, et al. Inclusion of mesh in donor-site repair of free TRAM and muscle-sparing free TRAM flaps yields rates of abdominal complications comparable to those of DIEP flap reconstruction. Plast Reconstr Surg 126:367-374, 2010.

54. Genitourinary Reconstruction

See *Essentials of Plastic Surgery*, second edition, pp. 632-640.

EMBRYOLOGY OF THE GENITOURINARY SYSTEM

1. **For each of the following structures, select its germinal layer of origin. (Each answer may be used once, more than once, or not at all.)**
   A. The nephric system
   B. Müllerian and wolffian ducts
   C. External genitalia

   Options:
   a. Endoderm
   b. Mesoderm
   c. Ectoderm

2. **During embryonic development of the GU system, which one of the following is true?**
   A. Male and female differentiation begins at the beginning of the second trimester.
   B. The default process for fetal differentiation is development of male external genitalia.
   C. The external genitalia for both sexes develop from the mesonephric ducts.
   D. The interstitial cells of Leydig produce a testosterone analogue that directs male development.
   E. Müllerian inhibiting substance (MIS) activates the Sertoli cells to direct female differentiation.

VAGINAL DEFECTS

3. A young patient is seen in clinic with congenital absence of the vagina. **Which one of the following statements is correct?**
   A. Her condition is caused by the congenital absence of the mesonephric ducts.
   B. She will almost certainly have associated urinary abnormalities.
   C. She will have a nonfunctional uterus, even if it is present.
   D. Her diagnosis is synonymous with Mayer-Rokitansky-Küster-Hauser syndrome.
   E. Her condition is relatively common, affecting 1 in 1000 live births.

MANAGEMENT OF VAGINAL AGENESIS

4. Match each of the following descriptions with the technique for management of vaginal agenesis. (Each answer may be used once, more than once, or not at all.)
   A. This reconstructive technique involves vulvoperineal fasciocutaneous flaps.
   B. This laparoscopic technique for vaginal agenesis correction uses traction sutures and a bead.
   C. This is a nonsurgical technique for vaginal agenesis correction.

   Options:
   a. Frank's technique
   b. McIndoe procedure
   c. Málaga technique
   d. Cordeiro procedure
   e. Rubin's technique
   f. Vecchietti procedure

CLASSIFICATION OF VAGINAL WALL DEFECTS

5. Which one of the following is true of the Cordiero classification for vaginal defects?
   A. Defects are classified by size in cm^2.
   B. Defects are classified by chronicity.
   C. Defects are classified by cause.
   D. Defects are classified by location.
   E. Defects are classified by infection risk.

CLINICAL CASES OF VAGINAL RECONSTRUCTION

6. For each of the following scenarios, select the most appropriate treatment option according to the algorithm proposed by Cordeiro et al. (Each option may be used once, more than once, or not at all.)
   A. A patient with a partial vaginal defect affecting the posterior wall only requires surgical management.
   B. A patient with a circumferential total vaginal defect requires surgical management.
   C. A patient has a partial lateral wall vaginal defect that requires surgical management.

   Options:
   a. Decompressive colpotomy
   b. Split-thickness skin graft and prosthetic
   c. Bilateral gracilis myocutaneous flaps
   d. Rectus abdominis flap
   e. Lotus petal flap
   f. Singapore flap
   g. Rolled rectus abdominis flap

HYPOSPADIAS

7. A young baby with hypospadias is referred to you by the pediatric team. **Which one of the following statements is correct regarding this condition?**
   A. The male urethral meatus is abnormally located dorsally between the corona and perineum.
   B. The incidence ranges from 1:4000 to 1:6000 live births.
   C. Surgical treatment usually begins after the fifth birthday.
   D. The presence of chordee can cause a ventral penile curvature.
   E. It least commonly involves the middle third of the penile shaft.

Chapter 54 ■ Genitourinary Reconstruction

SURGICAL CORRECTION OF HYPOSPADIAS

8. Match each of the following descriptions to the correct technique. (Each answer may be used once, more than once, or not at all.)
   A. A single-stage technique that involves a longitudinal incision through the midline epithelium of the urethral plate, which is subsequently tubularized
   B. A technique which uses local foreskin tissue as an island flap to reconstruct the urethra and ventral surface in a single stage
   C. A technique for distal shaft variants that involves a meatally based turnover skin flap

   Options:
   a. Meatal advancement and glanuloplasty (MAGPI) technique
   b. Urethral advancement
   c. Snodgrass (tubular incised plate [TIP]) technique
   d. Flip-flap technique
   e. Bracka technique (full-thickness graft urethroplasty)
   f. Preputial flap urethroplasty
   g. Cantwell-Ramsey technique
   h. Young technique

EPISPADIAS

9. A new patient with a diagnosis of epispadias is referred to you. **Which one of the following is a key feature occurring with this condition?**
   A. Bladder exstrophy
   B. Absent testes
   C. Undescended testes
   D. Duplication of the urethra
   E. A short, straight penis

PEYRONIE'S DISEASE

10. Which one of the following statements is correct regarding Peyronie's disease?
    A. One in five hundred men aged 40 to 60 years are affected.
    B. Painful erections are the only presenting symptom.
    C. Almost all patients also have Dupuytren's disease.
    D. Surgical treatment involves plication or dermal grafting.
    E. Plication techniques are ideal if the penis is short.

TREATMENT OF PEYRONIE'S DISEASE

11. You are planning surgical correction of a penile curvature caused by Peyronie's disease. **Which one of the following is the abnormal tissue layer?**
    A. Skin
    B. Dartos fascia
    C. Buck's fascia
    D. Tunica albuginea
    E. Corpus cavernosa

FOURNIER'S GANGRENE

12. You are called to the OR by a general surgical colleague to assist with a case of Fournier's gangrene. You jointly debride the perineal and scrotal region until healthy viable tissue remains. **What is the next step in management of this patient?**
    A. Local wound care with topical antibiotics and early reassessment
    B. Split-thickness skin graft reconstruction
    C. Direct closure if possible, with or without undermining
    D. Application of a negative-pressure dressing and early reassessment
    E. Local tissue flap wound closure over drains and minimal dressings to facilitate observation

Answers

EMBRYOLOGY OF THE GENITOURINARY SYSTEM

1. *For the following structures, the best options are as follows:*
   A. *The nephric system*
      b. **Mesoderm**
   B. *Müllerian and wolffian ducts*
      b. **Mesoderm**
   C. *External genitalia*
      c. **Ectoderm**

   Most structures within the genitourinary system arise from the mesoderm. These include the nephric system, the müllerian and wolffian ducts, and the gonads. The ectoderm forms the external genitalia. The endoderm forms the cloaca and membrane.

2. *During embryonic development of the GU system, which one of the following is true?*
   D. **The interstitial cells of Leydig produce a testosterone analogue that directs male development.**

   A developing fetus has the ability to develop into male or female and the default differentiation is female (not male) unless this process is interrupted. Male and female differentiation begins at week 6 in the first (not second) trimester. At this point, all fetuses have the precursors for both male and female differentiation. These are the mesonephric (wolffian) and paramesonephric (müllerian) ducts that develop into male and female reproductive structures, respectively. The differentiation into a male is influenced by müllerian inhibiting substance which is produced by (and not acting on) Sertoli cells. This substance causes paramesonephric duct regression. A testosterone analogue is produced by the interstitial cells of Leydig, which serves to stimulate masculine development of the mesonephric ducts which then form the epididymis, vas deferens, and seminal vesicles. In the absence of MIS, the paramesonephric ducts develop into the upper vagina, fallopian tubes, and uterus.

VAGINAL DEFECTS

3. A young patient is seen in clinic with congenital absence of the vagina. *Which one of the following statements is correct?*
   D. **Her diagnosis is synonymous with Mayer-Rokitanksy-Küster-Hauser syndrome.**

   Mayer-Rokitansky-Küster-Hauser syndrome is a condition of vaginal agenesis. While it is a rare condition, incidence varies from 1:4000 to 1:80,000, it is not caused by a congenital absence of the mesonephric duct. It may be caused by either a defect in the paramesonephric duct or fusion of the urogenital sinus with the paramesonephric duct.

   Associated urinary abnormalities such as ectopy, duplication, and agenesis occur in 25% to 50%, but not all patients. The clinical findings are of two types: a genetic female with or without a functioning uterus and absent vagina, who is otherwise normal; or a genetic female with or without a functioning uterus and absent vagina, who also has associated skeletal, urinary, or digestive system anomalies.

MANAGEMENT OF VAGINAL AGENESIS

4. For the following descriptions, the best options are as follows:
A. This reconstructive technique involves vulvoperineal fasciocutaneous flaps.
   c. Málaga technique
B. This laparoscopic technique for vaginal agenesis correction uses traction sutures and a bead.
   f. Vecchietti procedure
C. This is a nonsurgical technique for vaginal agenesis correction.
   a. Frank's technique

Several reconstructive options are available for vaginal agenesis. Frank's technique is a nonsurgical serial dilation procedure. A Málaga flap uses vulvoperineal fasciocutaneous flaps, whereas a McIndoe procedure involves a skin graft after dissection of a tunnel in the perineum, between the rectum and the bladder. This is associated with subsequent stricture and fistula formation. Vascularized bowel can be used to reconstruct the vagina but is associated with excessive mucus secretion and bleeding during intercourse. Other flaps have been described, including rectus abdominis, gracilis, and pudendal thigh flaps. The Vecchietti procedure is performed laparoscopically and uses traction sutures to help form a neovagina.

Vaginal agenesis can be associated with other anomalies, including imperforate hymen, double vagina, and an introitus obstruction. These can be treated surgically. An imperforate hymen can be treated with perforation and oversewing of the edges. A double vagina can be treated with a transverse incision of the septum. An obstructed introitus can be treated with a vaginoplasty.

CLASSIFICATION OF VAGINAL WALL DEFECTS

5. Which one of the following is true of the Cordiero classification for vaginal defects?
D. Defects are classified by location.

The Cordiero classification[1] considers two main features of the vaginal defect: the location (for example, anterior, posterior, or lateral wall) and the extent of the defect (for example, partial or circumferential defect). The actual size, cause, infection risk, and chronicity are not considered. The classification is as follows (Fig. 54-1):

Type IA: Partial defect involving the anterior or lateral wall
Type IB: Partial defect involving the posterior wall
Type IIA: Circumferential defect involving the upper two thirds
Type IIB: Circumferential total defect

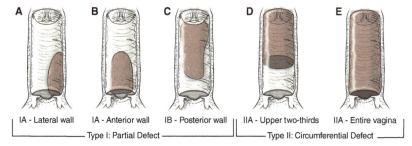

Fig. 54-1 Classification of vaginal defects used to guide reconstruction.

CLINICAL CASES OF VAGINAL RECONSTRUCTION

6. **For each of the following scenarios, select the most appropriate treatment option according to the algorithm proposed by Cordeiro et al.**
   A. A patient with a partial vaginal defect affecting the posterior wall only requires surgical management.
      d. Rectus abdominis flap
   B. A patient with a circumferential total vaginal defect requires surgical management.
      c. Bilateral gracilis myocutaneous flaps
   C. A patient has a partial lateral wall vaginal defect that requires surgical management.
      f. Singapore flap

   Vaginal and vulvar defects most commonly occur following oncologic resection, but may also be secondary to radiation therapy, infection, and trauma. Cordeiro has proposed a treatment algorithm in keeping with the classification system for vaginal wall defects.
   Partial defects (Type I) are either reconstructed with a modified singapore flap, if they are anterior or lateral, and a rectus abdominis flap, if they are posterior. The Singapore flap is a really useful and reliable flap for reconstruction of partial defects of the vagina. It is a fasciocutaneous flap based on the posterior labial arteries. The flap is designed running parallel to the medial thigh crease and raised deep-to-deep fascia from anterior to posterior. The flap can then be tunneled subcutaneously under the labia to be inset into the vaginal vault. The donor defect can be closed directly within the thigh crease with minimal cosmetic consequence. Although not part of the Cordeiro algorithm for partial posterior defects, the modified Singapore flap can be reliably used for these defects too. Circumferential defects can be reconstructed using a rolled rectus abdominis flap, if the upper two thirds are involved, or bilateral gracilis flaps if the defect is total (see Fig. 54-2, *Essentials of Plastic Surgery,* second edition). Alternatively bilateral Singapore type flaps may also be used.

HYPOSPADIAS

7. **A young baby with hypospadias is referred to you by the pediatric team. Which one of the following statements is correct regarding this condition?**
   D. The presence of chordee can cause a ventral penile curvature.

   Hypospadias is a congenital abnormality of the male urogenital tract that occurs in 1:150 to 1:300 males. It involves a proximally based ventral meatus (occurring anywhere between the glans and perineum), a hooded prepuce, and chordee, which may cause a ventral curvature of the penis. Hypospadias can be subdivided based on the meatal position into proximal, middle, or distal third subtypes. Distal are most common (50%), and proximal are least common (20%). Treatment is surgical and is usually performed between 6 and 9 months of age.

SURGICAL CORRECTION OF HYPOSPADIAS

8. **For the following scenarios, the best options are as follows:**
   A. A single-stage technique that involves a longitudinal incision through the midline epithelium of the urethral plate, which is subsequently tubularized
      c. Snodgrass (tubular incised plate [TIP]) technique
   B. A technique which uses local foreskin tissue as an island flap to reconstruct the urethra and ventral surface in a single stage
      f. Preputial flap urethroplasty

C. A technique for distal shaft variants, which involves a meatally based turnover skin flap
   d. Flip-flap technique

   Hypospadias surgery has several goals.[2] They include release of the chordee to straighten the penis, creation of a new urethra, and advancement of the urethral meatus to the correct anatomic position. Correction of these abnormalities should improve both function and cosmesis of the penis. A number of techniques are currently used. The most common are the single-stage TIP procedure popularized by Snodgrass[3] and the two-stage, full-thickness graft technique described by Bracka.[4] The MAGPI technique is indicated for coronal and glanular variants and involves a vertical incision in the transverse mucosal bar distal to the meatal opening, which is closed transversely. A glanuloplasty is achieved by midline approximation of the lateral glans wings. This technique does not treat chordee.

   In the TIP procedure a longitudinal incision is made through the midline epithelium of the urethral plate, extending from the hypospadias meatus to the end of the glans. The plate is then tubularized on itself, and the dorsal prepuce is mobilized and used to cover the urethroplasty.

   Mathieu[5] described the flip-flap technique, which transposes the proximal soft tissues over the urethral defect. Duckett[6] described the preputial flap. This involves an island flap from the prepuce to the ventral surface of the penis that is used as a tube for the urethra.

   The Cantwell-Ramsey, Young, and W-flap techniques are used for the correction of epispadias rather than hypospadias.

EPISPADIAS

9. A new patient with a diagnosis of epispadias is referred to you. *Which one of the following is a key feature occurring with this condition?*
   A. Bladder exstrophy

   Epispadias is a severe congenital anomaly involving the penis, which is typically short, wide, and stubby with clefting and flattening of the glans and a dorsally placed urethral meatus. The penis usually has a dorsal curvature. It usually occurs in conjunction with bladder exstrophy, but the other abnormalities listed are not specifically associated with this condition. Epispadias occurs in 1 in 30,000 males (compared with 1 in 350 for hypospadias). Principles of reconstruction are similar in each condition but with specific techniques described for epispadias.

PEYRONIE'S DISEASE

10. *Which one of the following statements is correct regarding Peyronie's disease?*
    D. Surgical treatment involves plication or dermal grafting.

    Peyronie's disease is a fibroproliferative condition of unknown cause that affects the penile shaft. It results in abnormal curvature and painful erections and affects approximately 1 in 100 men between 40 and 60 years of age. Although plication techniques are regularly used, they tend to leave a 20% reduction in erect length, which can be unacceptable to men whose penis was short preoperatively.

TREATMENT OF PEYRONIE'S DISEASE

11. You are planning surgical correction of a penile curvature caused by Peyronie's disease. *Which one of the following is the abnormal tissue layer?*
    D. Tunica albuginea

    Peyronie's disease is a localized penile disorder of collagen primarily involving the tunica albuginea. The penis has a number of key layers. From superficial to deep, these are the skin,

Dartos fascia, and then Buck's fascia. The tunica albuginea lies deeper still and surrounds each corpus cavernosa which are the erectile components of the penile shaft. The deep arteries lie within this tissue. There are two dorsal veins, one deep to skin and the other deep to the deep fascia (Buck's). The dorsal arteries and nerves are also found in this layer. The urethra is located in the midline and is covered by the corpus spongiosum which is also covered by deep fascia (Buck's). Knowledge of these layers is important in penile surgery and understanding techniques for hypospadias, epispadias, and Peyronie's disease. Ten percent of patients also have Dupuytren's contracture of the palmar fascia, and trials of collagenase therapy have been undertaken as an alternative to surgery in this condition.[7]

FOURNIER'S GANGRENE

12. You are called to the OR by a general surgical colleague to assist with a case of Fournier's gangrene. You jointly debride the perineal and scrotal region until healthy viable tissue remains. *What is the next step in the management of this patient?*

A. Local wound care with topical antibiotics and early reassessment

Fournier's gangrene is a potentially life-threatening, rapidly progressing, soft tissue infection within the spectrum of necrotizing fasciitis. Patients need urgent resuscitation, intravenous antibiotics, and early debridement in the OR, as in this case. Following initial debridement, the wounds should be temporized with simple dressings ± topical antibiotics. Sometimes it is necessary to place the testes in temporary thigh pouches or suture them together to stop retraction. The wounds should then be revisited in the OR within 24 hours, or sooner if the patient remains unwell or has visible spread of continued infection/necrosis. There is no justification for attempting to close the wounds at this stage or apply a negative-pressure dressing. A negative-pressure dressing can, however, be very useful beyond the second assessment to manage wound exudate and reduce the defect size, providing that infection is controlled and a satisfactory seal can be achieved. Reconstruction should only be initiated once the infection has completely resolved. Skin grafts are usually preferred for the lower abdomen and groin rather than attempts at direct closure, with or without local tissue flaps or undermining.

REFERENCES

1. Cordeiro PG, Pusic AL, Disa JJ. A classification system and reconstructive algorithm for acquired vaginal defects. Plast Reconstr Surg 110:1058-1065, 2002.
2. Baskin LS, Ebbers MB. Hypospadias: anatomy, etiology and technique. J Ped Surg 41:463-472, 2006.
3. Snodgrass W. Tubularized, incised plate urethroplasty for distal hypospadias. J Urol 151:464-465, 1994.
4. Bracka A. The role of two-stage repair in modern hypospadiology. Indian J Urol 24:210-218, 2008.
5. Mathieu P. Treatment in a time of the balanic and juxta-balanic hypospadias. J Chir (Paris) 39:481-484, 1932.
6. Duckett WW Jr. Transverse preputial island flap technique for repair of severe hypospadias. Urol Clin North Am 7:423-430, 1980.
7. Jain S, Mavuduru RM, Agarwal SK, et al. Re: clinical efficacy, safety and tolerability of collagenase clostridium histolyticum for the treatment of peyronie disease in 2 large double-blind, randomized, placebo controlled phase 3 studies: M. Gelbard, I. Goldsetin, W.J. Hellstrom, C.G. McMahon, T. Smith, J. Tursi, N. Jones, G.J. Kaufman and C.C. Carson III. J Urol 190:199-207, 2013; J Urol 191:561-563, 2014.

55. Pressure Sores

See *Essentials of Plastic Surgery*, second edition, pp. 641-650.

SITES OF PRESSURE SORE DEVELOPMENT
1. What is the most common anatomic site for development of a pressure sore?
   A. Ischial tuberosity
   B. Greater trochanter
   C. Scalp
   D. Sacrum
   E. Heel

ETIOLOGIC FACTORS
2. Which one of the following is an extrinsic factor in development of pressure sores?
   A. Ischemia
   B. Infection
   C. Malnutrition
   D. Smoking
   E. Moisture

BRADEN SCALE
3. Which one of the following scores indicates the highest risk on the Braden scale?
   A. 0
   B. 3
   C. 6
   D. 9
   E. 12

PRESSURE SORE STAGING
4. A patient has a pressure sore on the left heel measuring 5 cm. It involves full-thickness tissue loss to, but not through, fascia or bone. **What stage is this sore?**
   A. Stage I
   B. Stage II
   C. Stage III
   D. Stage IV
   E. Unstageable

PRESSURE VALUES RECORDED IN PRESSURE SORE STUDIES
5. For each of the following statements, select the pressure that is most likely described. (Each option may be used once, more than once, or not at all.)
   A. The external pressure measured at the ischial tuberosity of a patient who is sitting with feet supported
   B. The normal capillary closing pressure at the arterial end
   C. The maximal external pressure in the heel of a patient who is supine

   Options:
   a. 12 mm Hg
   b. 32 mm Hg
   c. 45 mm Hg
   d. 60 mm Hg
   e. 80 mm Hg
   f. 100 mm Hg

PREVENTION OF PRESSURE SORES

6. **Which one of the following is aimed at treating pressure sores on the basis of Kosiak's principle?**
   A. Meticulous skin care
   B. Care with transfers
   C. Minimization of spasticity
   D. Regular turning
   E. Smoking cessation

ASSESSMENT OF PRESSURE SORES

7. A patient is referred to you with a grade IV pressure sore in the sacral region. The patient has multiple comorbidities and sepsis. Osteomyelitis is suspected. **Which one of the following tests is the benchmark for diagnosis?**
   A. Culture swab
   B. Contrast CT
   C. MRI
   D. Bone biopsy
   E. Plain radiographs

ASSESSMENT OF OSTEOMYELITIS

8. A patient requires imaging for suspected osteomyelitis from a trochanteric pressure sore. **What is the sensitivity of MRI in detecting osteomyelitis?**
   A. 25%
   B. 56%
   C. 68%
   D. 80%
   E. 97%

DAKIN'S SOLUTION

9. You are reviewing a patient who has a trochanteric pressure sore, and the nurse suggests cleaning the wound with Dakin's solution. You have not used this before and decide to research the product before you proceed. **Which one of the following statements is correct regarding Dakin's solution?**
   A. It contains silver sulfadiazine.
   B. It is nontoxic to healthy tissue.
   C. It should be used in undiluted form.
   D. Treatment duration should be limited to 14 days.
   E. It is useful where *Pseudomonas* is suspected.

PRESSURE SORE SURGERY

10. **When performing surgical debridement and reconstruction of grade IV pressure sores, which one of the following should generally be avoided?**
    A. Methylene blue application
    B. Tumescent infiltration
    C. Excision of unaffected bony prominences
    D. Obliteration of dead space
    E. Flap design to allow readvancement

RECURRENCE RATES AFTER PRESSURE SORE RECONSTRUCTION

11. Which one of the following statements is correct regarding recurrence rates after pressure sore reconstruction?
A. Myocutaneous flaps have a higher ulcer recurrence rate than fasciocutaneous flaps.
B. Paraplegic patients have a 30% risk of recurrence at the same site over 18 months.
C. Nonparaplegic patients have a higher rate of recurrence than paraplegic patients.
D. Myocutaneous and fasciocutaneous reconstructions have comparable ulcer recurrence rates in many series.
E. Young posttraumatic paraplegic patients generally heal better than other subgroups.

Answers

SITES OF PRESSURE SORE DEVELOPMENT
1. *What is the most common anatomic site for development of a pressure sore?*
   A. Ischial tuberosity
   The site of pressure sore development will depend on several factors such as patient mobility, positioning, and local anatomy. However, the most common overall site is the ischial tuberosity. This occurs most frequently in wheelchair-bound patients, particularly those with spinal cord injuries and other individuals such as frail, elderly patients who spend long periods of time in a seated position. Other common sites are the sacrum and heels in bed-bound patients laying supine. The greater trochanter is at risk in individuals laying in a lateral position for extended periods. The posterior scalp (occiput) is at risk for patients in intensive care for extended periods due to immobility.

ETIOLOGIC FACTORS
2. *Which one of the following is an extrinsic factor in development of pressure sores?*
   E. Moisture
   Causal factors in the development of pressure sores can be classified as intrinsic or extrinsic. Key extrinsic factors are the forces of shear, friction, and pressure (compression). However, moisture is also an extrinsic factor, and this increases the risk of pressure sore development in incontinent patients. Intrinsic factors include ischemia, infection, sensory loss, vascular disease, and malnutrition. Management of pressure sores is based on treatment of both intrinsic and extrinsic factors.

BRADEN SCALE
3. *Which one of the following scores indicates the highest risk on the Braden scale?*
   C. 6
   A number of scoring systems have been created to assess the risk of developing a pressure sore. The Braden scale is one example. It has subscales, including sensory perception, skin moisture, activity, mobility, nutrition, and local mechanical forces that act on wounds.
   Composite scores range from 6 to 23, with lower scores indicating an increased risk for pressure sore development. Other systems include the Waterlow score, which places patients in different risk strategies (low, medium, and high) based on factors such as BMI, skin type, sex, malnutrition, continence, mobility, and age.[1]
   Although the assessment and scoring of a pressure sore is typically undertaken by the nursing team, understanding the workings of these systems is highly relevant to the surgical team both for delivery of high quality, safe patient care and for the preparation for clinical exams.

PRESSURE SORE STAGING

4. A patient has a pressure sore on the left heel measuring 5 cm. It involves full-thickness tissue loss to, but not through, fascia or bone. *What stage is this sore?*

C. Stage III

Pressure sores are graded into one of four stages according to the National Pressure Ulcer Advisory Panel. Stage I involves nonblanching erythema of intact skin. Stage II is a partial-thickness defect presenting as a blister. Stage III is a full-thickness skin defect, as in this case, that does not go through fascia. Stage IV includes underlying bone, muscle, tendon, or joint capsule. In cases in which full assessment is not possible clinically (e.g., soft tissue cover obscures deeper structures) two alternative grades can be used: unstageable and suspected deep. Pressure sores evolve over time, so they should be repeatedly inspected during the early stages to prevent understaging because of overlooked deep tissue damage, (see Fig. 55-2, *Essentials of Plastic Surgery*, second edition). Assessment of pressure areas is now part of the WHO checklist during surgery, so all surgeons should be regularly involved in this assessment. Being able to reliably assess grade of the pressure sore in the context of a patient's overall health is important with respect to selecting the best management plan for them.

PRESSURE VALUES RECORDED IN PRESSURE SORE STUDIES

5. *For the following scenarios, the best options are as follows:*
   A. *The external pressure measured at the ischial tuberosity of a patient who is sitting with feet supported*
      f. 100 mm Hg
   B. *The normal capillary closing pressure at the arterial end*
      b. 32 mm Hg
   C. *The maximal external pressure in the heel of a patient who is supine*
      c. 45 mm Hg

Capillary blood pressure ranges from 12 mm Hg at the venous end to 32 mm Hg at the arterial end. If external pressure exceeds the capillary opening pressure, then perfusion is reduced. For short time periods, this will have no detrimental effect. However, if it is continued for an extended time, ischemia and tissue damage will occur. An inverse relationship exists between the amount of pressure and the duration required to cause pressure necrosis.

Animal studies have shown that a pressure of 70 mm Hg applied over 2 hours was sufficient to cause pathologic changes in dogs. In a porcine model, pressure of 100 mm Hg for only 10 minutes caused muscle necrosis. Changes in the skin occur later than those in muscle, suggesting that pressure sores begin deep and the skin changes are late signs. Lindan et al[2] performed a landmark study in 1965. They observed pressures of up to 60 mm Hg in the sacral area of humans who were in a supine position (see Fig. 55-1, *Essentials of Plastic Surgery*, second edition). Pressure in the heels, occiput, and buttocks was approximately 40 mm Hg. Measurements of patients in the seated position were greatest at the ischial tuberosities and were in the order of 100 mm Hg. This helps explain the high incidence of ischial pressure sores.

PREVENTION OF PRESSURE SORES

6. Which one of the following is aimed at treating pressure sores on the basis of Kosiak's principle?

D. Regular turning

All of the choices are vital components of prevention and nonsurgical management of pressure sores. However, according to the Kosiak principle, tissues tolerate increased pressure if it is interspersed with pressure-free periods.[3] Seated patients should therefore be lifted every 10 minutes for 10 seconds, and supine patients should be turned every 2 hours.

Kosiak[4] first demonstrated the principle in 1959 by applying varying loads to the trochanters and ischial tuberosities of dogs. He found that high loads for short periods or low loads for long periods caused pressure ulcers. He later used a rat model to show that removal of pressure for short periods of time provided relief and resulted in less tissue damage.[5] Tissues are more susceptible to a constant load as opposed to an intermittent load.

Similarly, Dinsdale[6] showed prevention of injury when pressure was relieved for short durations, for example, 5 minutes of relief from a pressure of more than 400 mm Hg.

ASSESSMENT OF PRESSURE SORES

7. A patient is referred to you with a grade IV pressure sore in the sacral region. The patient has multiple comorbidities and sepsis. Osteomyelitis is suspected. Which one of the following tests is the benchmark for diagnosis?

D. Bone biopsy

The benchmark test for diagnosis of osteomyelitis within a deep pressure area is a positive bone biopsy. However this is not always technically possible unless the patient is in the OR. Routine microbiology swabs from pressure sores will show growth of multiple organisms and interpretation of these results needs to be combined with a clinical evaluation to assess for evidence of local infection. The best noninvasive option for patients with suspected osteomyelitis would be an MRI. Plain radiographs and CT may be useful but are less accurate.

ASSESSMENT OF OSTEOMYELITIS

8. A patient requires imaging for suspected osteomyelitis from a trochanteric pressure sore. What is the sensitivity of MRI in detecting osteomyelitis?

E. 97%

MRI has a high sensitivity and specificity for evaluation of the extent of osteomyelitis. Huang et al[7] conducted a study to assess the accuracy and utility of MRI for diagnosing osteomyelitis in pressure sores, using histologic/microbiologic results as the standard of reference. They compared the extent of infection using MRI and surgical margins. The overall accuracy of MRI was high with only one false-negative MRI study. MRI for the diagnosis of osteomyelitis yielded a sensitivity of 97% and a specificity of 89%.

Twenty-one patients underwent limited surgical resection guided by MRI findings in which only the enhancing area was resected. Osteomyelitis recurred only once, at the surgical margins. The authors concluded that MRI is accurate in the diagnosis of osteomyelitis and associated soft tissue abnormalities in spinal cord–injured patients. It can delineate the extent of infection and help to guide limited surgical resection and preserve viable tissue.

DAKIN'S SOLUTION

9. You are reviewing a patient who has a trochanteric pressure sore, and the nurse suggests cleaning the wound with Dakin's solution. You have not used this before and decide to research the product before you proceed. *Which one of the following statements is correct regarding Dakin's solution?*
   E. It is useful where *Pseudomonas* is suspected.

   Dakin's solution can be useful for cleaning wounds such as pressure sores that have pseudomonas growth, but should be used cautiously and for limited periods because of its toxicity to healthy tissue. It contains sodium hypochlorite and boric acid, not silver sulfadiazine. It should be diluted to quarter strength and used for a few days only (not 14 days). Wounds with *Pseudomonas* typically appear green and have a characteristic malodor. Other popular dressings for pressure sores include hydrogels if there is black eschar, hydrocolloids if there is granulation tissue, and an alginate and absorbent foam in wounds with high exudate. Manuka honey has also become popular for chemical debridement of pressure sores and this works in a number of ways which include antibacterial as well as debriding. Irrespective of dressing used, the propensity for a pressure sore to heal will be dependent on the vascularity of the wound itself and removal of the instigating cause.

PRESSURE SORE SURGERY

10. *When performing surgical debridement and reconstruction of grade IV pressure sores, which one of the following should generally be avoided?*
   C. Excision of unaffected bony prominences

   While any nonviable or infected bone should be fully debrided, healthy bony prominences should not be routinely excised. If healthy bony prominences are excised to relieve pressure at the site of the sore, this can have unintended consequences from pressure transfer to other sites. An example is perineal ulceration following overresection of the ischial tuberosity.

   Coating the bursa with methylene blue dye before excision can help verify that all bursal tissue has been completely excised. Infiltration of the peribursal area with a liposuction solution can help reduce/control bleeding during debridement. During reconstruction, any dead space must be obliterated with the chosen flap. Flaps should always be designed to allow for further revision surgery. For this reason, advancement and rotation flaps are generally preferred.

RECURRENCE RATES AFTER PRESSURE SORE RECONSTRUCTION

11. *Which one of the following statements is correct regarding recurrence rates after pressure sore reconstruction?*
   D. Myocutaneous and fasciocutaneous reconstructions have comparable ulcer recurrence rates in many series.

   Several authors have assessed recurrence rates after reconstruction of pressure sores. The overall rates range from 19% at 3.7 years (Kierney et al[8]) to 69% at 9.3 months (Disa et al[9]). Disa et al indicated that young posttraumatic paraplegics had a particularly high recurrence rate of 79% at 11 months.

   In a meta-analysis of pressure sore recurrence rates from 55 studies, Saneem et al[10] identified similar recurrence rates with myocutaneous (8.9%) and fasciocutaneous (11.2%) flaps. Perforator flaps appeared to fare best overall with a 5.6% recurrence rate, but the differences between the three flap types were not statistically significant.

REFERENCES

1. Waterlow JJ. Pressure sores: a risk assessment card. Nurs Times 81:49-55, 1985.
2. Lindan O, Greenway RM, Piazza JM. Pressure distribution on the surface of the human body. I. Evaluation in lying and sitting positions using a "bed of springs and nails." Arch Phys Med Rehabil 46:378-385, 1965.
3. Kosiak M, Kubicek WG, Olson M, et al. Evaluation of pressure as a factor in production of ischial ulcer. Arch Phys Med Rehabil 39:623-629, 1958.
4. Kosiak M. Etiology and pathology of ischemic ulcer. Arch Phys Med Rehabil 40:62-68, 1959.
5. Kosiak M. Etiology of decubitus ulcers. Arch Phys Med Rehabil 42:19-29, 1961.
6. Dinsdale SM. Decubitus ulcers: role of pressure and friction in causation. Arch Phys Med Rehabil 55:147-152, 1974.
7. Huang AB, Schweitzer ME, Hume E, et al. Osteomyelitis of the pelvis/hips in paralyzed patients: accuracy and clinical utility of MRI. J Comput Assist Tomogr 22:437-443, 1998.
8. Kierney PC, Engrave LH, Isik FF, et al. Results of 268 pressure sores in 158 patients managed jointly by plastic surgery and rehabilitation medicine. Plast Reconstr Surg 102:765-772, 1998.
9. Disa JJ, Carlton JM, Goldberg NH. Efficacy of operative cure in pressure sore patients. Plast Reconstr Surg 89:272-278, 1992.
10. Saneem M, Au M, Wood T, et al. A systematic review of complication and recurrence rates of musculocutaneous, fasciocutaneous, and perforator-based flaps for treatment of pressure sores. Plast Reconstr Surg 130:67e-77e, 2012.

56. Lower Extremity Reconstruction

See *Essentials of Plastic Surgery*, second edition, pp. 651-666.

GUSTILO CLASSIFICATION

1. **For each of the following scenarios, select the option that best describes the patient's injury? (Each answer may be used once, more than once, or not at all.)**
   A. A patient presents with an open tibial fracture after a motor vehicle accident. Surgery reveals extensive soft tissue damage involving skin and muscle with associated periosteal stripping of bone.
   B. A patient presents with an open tibial fracture after a motor vehicle accident. Surgery reveals extensive soft tissue damage involving skin and muscle with associated periosteal stripping of bone and an associated arterial injury that requires repair.
   C. An elderly woman presents with an open ankle fracture after a low-impact fall that occurred while she was using her walking frame. She has a 2.5 cm wound over the medial malleolus, which is clean and without skin flaps. The surrounding skin is bruised but apparently viable.

   Options:
   a. Gustilo I
   b. Gustilo II
   c. Gustilo IIa
   d. Gustilo IIb
   e. Gustilo IIIa
   f. Gustilo IIIb
   g. Gustilo IIIc
   h. Gustilo IV

2. **What is the key difference between a Gustilo type I and type II injury?**
   A. The degree of wound contamination
   B. The presence or absence of a vascular injury
   C. The degree of fracture comminution
   D. The measured wound size
   E. The location of soft tissue injury

BYRD CLASSIFICATION

3. **Which one of the following is considered in the Byrd classification system but not in the Gustilo classification?**
   A. The degree of force involved to sustain the injury
   B. The size of the soft tissue defect
   C. The presence of a vascular injury
   D. The chronicity of the injury
   E. The degree of skin and soft tissue loss

PROGNOSTIC FACTORS

4. Which one of the following has no prognostic significance following an open tibial shaft fracture?
   A. Comminution
   B. Infection
   C. Concomitant fibula fracture
   D. Bone loss
   E. Soft tissue injury

ORDER OF ACUTE TREATMENT

5. After initial resuscitation measures, which one of the following should generally be performed first when managing an open tibial fracture?
   A. Fasciotomies
   B. Soft tissue wound debridement
   C. Arterial repair
   D. Fracture reduction and stabilization
   E. Nerve repair

TIMING OF SOFT TISSUE RECONSTRUCTION

6. Following adequate debridement and external fixator stabilization of a grade IIIb open tibial fracture, when should definitive free flap reconstruction be performed, based on current evidence?
   A. At the same time
   B. Within 24 hours
   C. Within the first week
   D. After two weeks
   E. Once bone healing is complete

BLOOD SUPPLY TO THE TIBIA

7. Which one of the following statements is correct regarding tibial blood supply?
   A. The periosteal circulation derives from the metaphyseal artery.
   B. The inner third of the cortex is supplied by the endosteal circulation.
   C. The outer two thirds of the cortex are supplied by the periosteal vessels.
   D. Endosteal circulation derives from the nutrient artery on the posterior tibia.
   E. When a long bone is fractured, the nutrient artery is disrupted and the entire distal fragment becomes avascular.

BONY RECONSTRUCTION

8. A 60-year-old man sustains an open midshaft tibial fracture with extensive soft tissue loss after being hit by a car. Exploration in the OR shows a segment of nonviable tibia measuring 8 cm, which is removed. Following debridement, a soft tissue defect measuring 16 by 8 cm is planned for reconstruction using an anterolateral thigh flap with vastus lateralis. A spanning external fixation device is used to temporarily stabilize the fracture and a longer term plan is made for bone transport with distraction osteogenesis. **Which one of the following is true of the distraction process?**
   A. After the device is applied, distraction is postponed for 1 month.
   B. Distraction is commonly performed at a rate of 3 mm per day.
   C. Blood transfusions are commonly required intraoperatively.
   D. A corticotomy is performed outside the zone of injury before distraction.
   E. Distraction is usually reserved for bone defects larger than 20 cm.

LOCAL FLAP OPTIONS IN LOWER LIMB RECONSTRUCTION

9. Which one of the following statements is correct regarding reconstruction of lower limb soft tissue defects in physically active patients?
   A. An extensor digitorum longus flap is supplied by the peroneal vessels, and the use of this flap can result in permanent loss of toe extension.
   B. A flexor digitorum longus flap can be used for small to medium sized midshaft defects but leads to a significant functional loss.
   C. A flexor hallucis longus flap should not be used in athletes for middle third defects because of its important role in running.
   D. Sacrifice of the medial head of gastrocnemius to reconstruct anterior knee defects is preferred to the lateral head because the functional deficit is less.
   E. A proximally based soleus flap can be used to cover the tibial tuberosity but leaves a functional deficit.

RECONSTRUCTIVE OPTIONS FOR THE LOWER LIMB

10. Select the most appropriate reconstructive option for each of the following scenarios. (Each answer may be used once, more than once, or not at all.)
    A. A patient has a 10 cm long by 15 cm wide wound to the anterolateral thigh with exposed muscle belly and an underlying femoral fracture. No nerve, bone, or vessel exposure is noted.
    B. A patient has a 5 by 8 cm anterior knee wound with an exposed total knee replacement prosthesis.
    C. A patient has a 3 by 5 cm distal tibial wound with exposed bone over the medial malleolus and posterior tibial vessels.

    Options:
    a. Split-thickness skin graft (STSG)
    b. Direct closure
    c. Medial gastrocnemius and STSG
    d. Lateral gastrocnemius and STSG
    e. Proximally based soleus and STSG
    f. Free gracilis and STSG
    g. Free latissimus dorsi and STSG

RECONSTRUCTION OF TIBIAL AND KNEE SOFT TISSUE DEFECTS

11. You have a patient with a full-thickness soft tissue defect over the proximal tibia with exposure of the tibial tuberosity measuring 7 by 4 cm. The wound is clean and ready for definitive reconstruction. Which one of the following options is best for coverage of this defect?
    A. Distally based on soleus flap
    B. Medial gastrocnemius flap
    C. Lateral gastrocnemius flap
    D. Bipedicled tibialis anterior flap
    E. Reverse sural artery flap

COMPARTMENT SYNDROME

12. Which one of the following is true of compartment syndrome in the lower limb?
    A. It occurs in less than 1% of tibial shaft fractures.
    B. An open tibial fracture usually decompresses the anterior compartment.
    C. Loss of distal pulses is a reliable early sign suggestive of compartment syndrome.
    D. Sensation will be preserved to the medial calf and foot.
    E. Decompression involves release of all three compartments.

OSTEOMYELITIS

13. **Which one of the following statements is correct regarding the prevention and treatment of osteomyelitis in patients with Gustilo type IIIb tibial fracture?**
    A. The most common pathogens leading to osteomyelitis are anaerobic *Streptococcus* spp.
    B. A single dose of prophylactic cephalosporin and aminoglycoside is sufficient in clean wounds.
    C. All small fragments of bone should be removed during surgical debridement.
    D. The expected infection rate is greater than 20% without antibiotic therapy.
    E. Negative-pressure dressings should not be used in cases of osteomyelitis.

CHRONIC WOUNDS OF THE LOWER EXTREMITY

14. You assess a patient with a nonhealing ulcer to the lower limb. Examination shows a 3 by 3 cm ulcer between the malleoli and gastrocnemius myotendinous junction. There is surrounding soft tissue firmness and swelling with pigmentation changes and varicosities. **Which one of the following is the most appropriate management of this ulcer?**
    A. Excision biopsy
    B. Referral for revascularization surgery
    C. Hyperbaric oxygen therapy
    D. Compression bandaging
    E. Negative pressure wound therapy

… Lower Extremity Reconstruction 455

Answers

GUSTILO CLASSIFICATION

1. *For the following scenarios, the best options are as follows:*
   A. *A patient presents with an open tibial fracture after a motor vehicle accident. Surgery reveals extensive soft tissue damage involving skin and muscle with associated periosteal stripping of bone.*
      f. Gustilo IIIb
   B. *A patient presents with an open tibial fracture after a motor vehicle accident. Surgery reveals extensive soft tissue damage involving skin and muscle with associated periosteal stripping of bone and an associated arterial injury that requires repair.*
      g. Gustilo IIIc
   C. *An elderly woman presents with an open ankle fracture after a low-impact fall that occurred while she was using her walking frame. She has a 2.5 cm wound over the medial malleolus, which is clean and without skin flaps. The surrounding skin is bruised but apparently viable.*
      b. Gustilo II

   The Gustilo classification was first published in 1976[1] and was later modified in 1984.[2] It describes three types of open tibial fractures: I, II, and III. The latter is further divided into types a, b, and c, depending on associated soft tissue damage. It is generally accepted that an accurate assessment of the fracture in relation to the Gustilo classification can only be performed intraoperatively. Plastic surgical input is required for most IIIb and IIIc fractures as described in scenarios 1 and 2.

2. *What is the key difference between a Gustilo type I and type II injury?*
   D. The measured wound size

   Measured wound size is the key discriminator between type I and II injuries. The degree of wound contamination and the presence of a vascular injury are considered in type III injuries. The location of soft tissue injury and the degree of comminution are not specifically considered in this classification. The description of types I through IIIc are as follows:

   Type I: An open fracture with a clean laceration less than 1 cm long
   Type II: An open fracture with a clean laceration greater than 1 cm long without extensive soft tissue injury, flaps, or avulsions
   Type IIIa: Open fractures with extensive soft tissue damage, involving muscle, skin, and neurovascular structures, but with adequate soft tissue coverage
   Type IIIb: As above, except a more extensive injury with periosteal stripping, exposed bone, and/or massive contamination
   Type IIIc: Similar to a type IIIb injury with an additional arterial injury that requires repair

   In-depth knowledge of this classification is useful for everyday practice and for clinical exams as it is often tested in both written and viva examinations.

BYRD CLASSIFICATION

3. Which one of the following is considered in the Byrd classification system but not in the Gustilo classification?

A. The degree of force involved to sustain the injury

The Byrd[3] classification is primarily based on the energy level of injury, ranging from low through moderate to high. It also differs from the Gustilo classification in that the fracture pattern and mechanism of injury are considered for some of the gradings. For example, whether the fracture is displaced, comminuted, or a simple oblique or spiral pattern are considered. Similarities between the two systems are that the degree of the soft tissue injury, including defect size and vascular injury, are considered in both classifications. Chronicity is not specifically considered in either classification, as it is assumed that all are acute injuries. See below:

- Type I: Low-energy forces causing a spiral or oblique fracture pattern with a skin laceration less than 2 cm and a relatively clean wound.
- Type II: Moderate energy forces causing a comminuted or displaced fracture pattern with a skin laceration greater than 2 cm and moderate adjacent skin and muscle contusion, but without devitalized muscle.
- Type III: High-energy forces causing a significantly displaced fracture pattern with severe comminution, segmental fracture, or bone defect with extensive associated skin loss and devitalized muscle.
- Type IV: Fracture pattern as in type III but with extreme energy forces as in high-velocity gunshot or shotgun wounds, a history of degloving, or associated vascular injury requiring repair.

PROGNOSTIC FACTORS

4. Which one of the following has no prognostic significance following an open tibial shaft fracture?

C. Concomitant fibular fracture

In 1983 Keller[4] reviewed 10,000 tibial shaft fractures. In this review, neither fracture location or concomitant fibular fracture showed prognostic significance. Complications did increase in the presence of comminution, displacement, bone loss, distraction, soft tissue injury, infection, and polytrauma.

ORDER OF ACUTE TREATMENT

5. After initial resuscitation measures, which one of the following should generally be performed first when managing an open tibial fracture?

D. Fracture reduction and stabilization

Each of the above factors are highly relevant to the acute management of lower limb open tibial fractures. In general, the wound is washed and fully assessed in the OR with joint orthopedic and plastic surgical teams present, then bony stabilization is performed in order to provide a stable base for further management. This often entails application of an external fixation device. The bone ends must, of course, be debrided fully before reduction. Vascular inflow must be established early to ensure distal limb perfusion. Thorough debridement of soft tissues must be performed with removal of any devitalized tissue and fasciotomies undertaken as required.

Recent evidence has shown that the most important factor affecting outcome after an open tibial fracture is a thorough debridement of devitalized tissues. This is because it optimizes healing and minimizes infection risk. Recent advances in both civilian and military experience indicate that an aggressive washout protocol, temporary fracture stabilization, and application of a negative pressure dressing can also buy some time before formal reconstruction is performed.[5,6]

TIMING OF SOFT TISSUE RECONSTRUCTION

6. Following adequate debridement and external fixator stabilization of a grade IIIb open tibial fracture, when should definitive free flap reconstruction be performed, based on current evidence?
C. Within the first week

Based on current evidence, definitive free tissue cover for open tibial fractures should ideally be performed within the first week. Timing will, of course, be affected by factors such as the nature of the injury, the presence of infection, degree of contamination, and bone loss. It will also be affected by other injuries and the general condition of the patient.

Evidence presented by Byrd[3] in the 1980s supported early debridement and soft tissue cover within the first 5 to 6 days. The authors found that this approach resulted in fewest complications and the shortest length of hospital admission. Godina[7] found that patients who had debridement and free flap cover within 3 days had very low flap failure rates (less than 1%) and postoperative infection rates (1.5%). They found that patients who received their flaps between 3 days and 3 months had an increased flap failure rate (12%) and infection rate (17.5%). It should be noted that this is a relatively wide timeframe as it crosses both the acute, subacute, and chronic biologic phases involved in open fracture wounds. Patients who received flaps beyond 3 months had complication rates that fell somewhere between those managed in the early and intermediate phases. Yaremchuk et al[8] had infection rates of 14% in a cohort of patients who received flap coverage at a mean of 17 days. As described in the explanation to question 5, recent military and civilian experiences suggest that soft tissue cover can be safely delayed for a few days providing that adequate debridement has been performed and the wound temporized with a NPWT device.[5,6] Some of the military data relates to injuries sustained with improvised explosive devices that alter the timeframe because of the requirement for multiple debridement procedures.[6]

In the UK, guidelines have been published jointly by the British Orthopaedic and Plastic Surgery associations based on current available evidence.[9] They suggest that most open tibial fractures are initially debrided, stabilized, and scheduled for surgery within 24 hours with both senior plastic surgeons and orthopedic surgeons present. Exceptions are those with vascular compromise or severe contamination, as these need immediate management. The guidelines also suggest that soft tissue free flap cover should ideally be performed within the first week, in part to ensure that the flap recipient vessels are still in a healthy condition.

BLOOD SUPPLY TO THE TIBIA

7. Which one of the following statements is correct regarding tibial blood supply?
D. Endosteal circulation derives from the nutrient artery on the posterior tibia.

The tibia has three types of blood supply: periosteal, metaphyseal, and nutrient artery supply. The periosteal circulation derives from the primary limb vessels (not the metaphyseal artery) to supply the outer third of the cortex. The endosteal circulation derives from the nutrient artery and supplies the inner two thirds (not one third) of the cortex. When a long bone is fractured, the distal blood supply is usually preserved because of the structure of the periosteal circulation in which the vessels are oriented transversely.

BONY RECONSTRUCTION

8. A 60-year-old man sustains an open midshaft tibial fracture with extensive soft tissue loss after being hit by a car. Exploration in the OR shows a segment of nonviable tibia measuring 8 cm, which is removed. Following debridement, a soft tissue defect measuring 16 by 8 cm is planned for reconstruction using an anterolateral thigh flap with vastus lateralis. A spanning external fixation device is used to temporarily stabilize the fracture and a longer term plan is made for bone transport with distraction osteogenesis. *Which one of the following is true of the distraction process?*

D. A corticotomy is performed outside the zone of injury before distraction.

Distraction osteogenesis was pioneered by Ilizarov and this is typically indicated in segmental long bone gaps up to 12 cm. It involves placement of an external distraction device with a corticotomy performed outside the zone of injury. Bone distraction is slow (1 mm per day, not 3 mm), so this method does take an extended time to achieve required bone length but probably represents the benchmark for long segmental defects of the tibia. The amount of bone generated is anatomically correct for the size of the defect and soft tissues can be closed by the docking method during the same process. Intraoperative blood loss is low so transfusion is not generally required. Distraction begins a week after device application. In cases like this scenario where there is segmental bone loss and soft tissue loss, it is appropriate to achieve wound closure with a free tissue transfer such as a latissimus dorsi or anterolateral thigh flap in the subacute setting. Temporary fracture stabilization can be achieved with a simple external frame. Once the soft tissues have healed (2 to 3 weeks), the external frame can be exchanged for a circular frame. The benefit of such fixation is that weight bearing can begin, so general mobility is improved and where bone ends are together, healing is accelerated.

Nonvascularized bone is traditionally used for reconstructing smaller defects but some authors state that they can be used beneath vascularized muscle flaps for defects up to 10 cm.[6] Free osseous flaps such as fibula, scapula, and iliac crest may reliably be used to reconstruct segmental bone gaps. Fibula flaps can be harvested at lengths of up to 20 cm in adult patients, if required. The use of free tissue flaps is generally indicated for segmental gaps larger than 6 cm. Free flaps are still less favorable than bone transport for segmental tibial defect reconstruction because of the difference in bone shape and quality compared with the native tibia. Their role in upper limb segmental defect reconstruction (for example, humerus) is probably more significant.

LOCAL FLAP OPTIONS IN LOWER LIMB RECONSTRUCTION

9. *Which one of the following statements is correct regarding reconstruction of lower limb soft tissue defects in physically active patients?*

C. A flexor hallucis flap should not be used in athletes for middle third defects because of its important role in running.

The flexor hallucis longus flap can be used to reconstruct middle third soft tissue defects. However, this muscle is important in push off for the great toe, therefore it should not be sacrificed in physically active patients.

With the current focus on an availability of surgeons skilled in free tissue transfer, local flap reconstruction in the lower limb is less commonly used, particularly for higher energy injuries. However, there remain some robust flaps that are particularly useful such as the gastrocnemius for mid and upper third defects. The extensor digitorum longus flap is supplied by the anterior tibial vessels (not the peroneal vessels) and can be used to close small wounds of the middle third. It is important to preserve the peroneal nerve during dissection of this flap. If the entire muscle is harvested, then permanent loss of toe extension will occur. A flexor digitorum longus flap can be used for small defects of the lower portion of the middle third, without significant functional loss. The medial head of gastocnemius is preferentially chosen over the lateral head for reconstruction purposes, as it is larger and not because the functional outcome differs between the two. A proximally based soleus flap can be reliably used to cover the middle third anterior leg defects without causing a functional deficit, particularly if it is harvested as a hemisoleus.

RECONSTRUCTIVE OPTIONS FOR THE LOWER LIMB

10. *For the following scenarios, the best options are as follows:*
    A. **A patient has a 10 cm long by 15 cm wide wound to the anterolateral thigh with exposed muscle belly and an underlying femoral fracture. No nerve, bone, or vessel exposure is noted.**
    a. **Split-thickness skin graft (STSG)**
    This wound should be amenable to skin grafting with or without partial closure, because the wound bed is healthy and vascularized. Although it might be tempting to try and close the wound directly if tissue laxity appears to be adequate, this can be risky because of the underlying fracture and anticipated swelling.
    B. **A patient has a 5 by 8 cm anterior knee wound with an exposed total knee replacement prosthesis.**
    c. **Medial gastrocnemius and STSG**
    This wound is best covered with a medial gastrocnemius local flap and SSG. This is preferable to a lateral gastrocnemius because of its greater size. Free tissue transfer is not generally required in such cases unless local flap options have failed or in areas where there has been previous radiotherapy.
    C. **A patient has a 3 by 5 cm distal tibial wound with exposed bone over the medial malleolus and posterior tibial vessels.**
    f. **Free gracilis and STSG**
    This defect can be covered with a range of different free flaps or with a local fasciocutaneous propeller flap. However, because of its small size and the logistics of harvesting a gracilis versus a latissimus dorsi flap, a gracilis free flap is a better option in this case. Other popular alternatives include fasciocutaneous flaps such as the ALT, scapula, groin, or lateral arm flaps. The benefit of such flaps is avoidance of a skin graft. There are no local options that will so reliably reconstruct this defect.

RECONSTRUCTION OF TIBIAL AND KNEE SOFT TISSUE DEFECTS

11. You have a patient with a full-thickness soft tissue defect over the proximal tibia with exposure of the tibial tuberosity measuring 7 by 4 cm. The wound is clean and ready for definitive reconstruction. *Which one of the following options is best for coverage of this defect?*
    B. **Medial gastrocnemius flap**
    A gastrocnemius flap is a very good source for soft tissue coverage in mid to upper anterior tibial defects after trauma or tumor resection. It is particularly useful for reconstruction of anterior knee defects with an exposed knee prosthesis.
    The gastrocnemius muscle has two heads (medial and lateral); the medial is the larger and is most commonly employed for reconstructions as alluded to in question 9. It receives its blood supply from the medial sural artery, which arises from the popliteal artery. When a medial gastrocnemius flap is raised, an incision is typically made on the medial aspect of the leg, 2 cm posterior to the tibia at midcalf level, and is continued proximally to the popliteal fossa. During this part of the dissection, care is required to prevent injury to the large saphenous vein and saphenous nerve. The fascia and overlying skin are then elevated off the medial gastrocnemius to the midline, where the medial and lateral heads meet. During this part of the dissection, the

sural nerve and small saphenous vein are identified and preserved. The medial raphe between the medial and lateral heads should be divided, and the plane is developed down to soleus muscle. Within this plane, the plantaris tendon is identified. Next, the distal tendon is transected so that the flap can be raised from distal to proximal. Visualization of the sural artery pedicle is not usually required for coverage of a lower defect, as in this case. Where the arc of rotation is greater than 100 degrees, it can be useful to continue the dissection proximally and identify the medial sural artery pedicle and medial sural motor nerve supplying the flap. The nerve can also be transected to stop subsequent muscle contractions. The proximal gastrocnemius attachment or hamstring tendons can also be divided to improve flap reach, although this is not usually required in most cases.[10]

The proximally based (not distally based) soleus flap is a reasonable alternative and can be carried to a point 5 cm above its tendinous insertion. The bipedicled tibialis anterior flap is more suitable for middle third coverage. The reverse sural artery flap is used for the distal third.

COMPARTMENT SYNDROME

12. Which one of the following is true of compartment syndrome in the lower limb?
   D. Sensation will be preserved to the medial calf and foot.

Sensation to the medial calf is preserved in compartment syndrome because this area is supplied by the saphenous nerve that is located outside the compartments of the lower leg. Compartment syndrome is a condition where the intracompartmental pressure exceeds perfusion pressure, leading to ischemia and subsequent necrosis of the muscle compartments. It occurs in approximately 1 in 10 tibial fractures and must be recognized and treated early in order to avoid irreversibly tissue damage. It can occur with both open and closed injuries and the fact that a fracture can breach a given compartment does not mean that the compartment is adequately decompressed. The main signs of compartment syndrome are the six p's: **p**ain (out of proportion to the injury and with passive stretch), **p**ressure from swollen compartments, **p**aresthesia of the involved compartment, **p**aralysis or decreased strength of the involved compartment, **p**allor and **p**ulselessness as a result of vascular compromise. Loss of distal pulses is a late sign of compartment syndrome and is more likely because of vascular injury. To supplement clinical examination, intracompartmental pressures can be measured using devices specifically made for this purpose. A difference of 30 mm Hg or less between the measured pressure and diastolic pressure is considered a justification for decompression. When decompression is performed, a number of approaches are available. One example is to use combined medial and lateral approaches where longitudinal incisions are made 1 to 2 cm medial and 1 to 2 cm lateral to the tibial borders overlying the soft tissue compartments. This facilitates decompression of all four (not three) compartments: anterior, lateral, superficial posterior, and deep posterior. This also preserves the medial perforating vessels in case a local fasciocutaneous flap is required.

OSTEOMYELITIS

13. Which one of the following statements is correct regarding the prevention and treatment of osteomyelitis in patients with a Gustilo type IIIb tibial fracture?
   D. The expected infection rate is greater than 20% without antibiotic therapy.

The most common pathogen in osteomyelitis is *S. aureus*. Prophylactic use of antibiotics can significantly reduce the infection rate in lower limb trauma wounds, but a single dose is not sufficient. Thorough debridement and removal of all devitalized tissue are required, but small viable bone fragments can remain in situ. Negative pressure dressings are appropriate for patients with debrided osteomyelitic wounds in conjunction with antibiotic therapy.[11]

CHRONIC WOUNDS OF THE LOWER EXTREMITY

14. You assess a patient with a nonhealing ulcer to the lower limb. Examination shows a 3 by 3 cm ulcer between the malleoli and gastrocnemius myotendinous junction. There is surrounding soft tissue firmness and swelling with pigmentation changes. *Which one of the following is the most appropriate management of this ulcer?*
D. Compression bandaging
   The clinical description above suggests a diagnosis of venous ulcer. These tend to be located in the gaiter region between the malleoli and the gastrocnemius myotendinous junction, sometimes termed "boot strap distribution." The other findings include chronic edema, varicosities, lipodermatosclerosis, and a history of deep vein thrombosis. Either incision or excision biopsy is indicated in suspected skin cancers such as a Marjolin's ulcer arising in a chronic wound. Referral to the vascular team may be warranted in patients with a suspected arterial ulcer. These present as punched-out, painful ulcers with a history of claudication and absent pulses. Hyperbaric oxygen therapy may be indicated in radiation ulcers before surgical resection and soft tissue cover. It is not indicated in venous ulcers and neither is negative pressure wound therapy (see Chapter 57).

REFERENCES

1. Gustilo RB, Anderson JT. Prevention of infection in the treatment of one thousand and twenty-five open fractures of long bones. J Bone Joint Surg Am 58:453-458, 1976.
2. Gustilo RB, Mendoza RM, Williams DN. Problems in the management of type III (severe) open fractures: a new classification of type III open fractures. J Trauma 24:742-746, 1984.
3. Byrd HS, Spicer TE, Cierny G III. Management of open tibial fractures. Plast Reconstr Surg 76:719, 1985.
4. Keller CS. The principles of the treatment of tibial shaft fractures: a review of 10,146 cases from the literature. Orthopedics 6:993, 1983.
5. Hou Z, Irgit K, Strohecker HA, et al. Delayed flap reconstruction with vacuum-assisted closure management of the open IIIB tibial fracture. J Trauma 71:1705, 2011.
6. Kumar AR, Grewal NS, Chung TL, et al. Lessons from operation Iraqi freedom: successful subacute reconstruction of complex lower extremity battle injuries. Plast Reconstr Surg 123:218, 2009.
7. Godina M. Early microsurgical reconstruction of complex trauma of the extremities. Clin Plast Surg 13:619, 1986.
8. Yaremchuk MJ, Brumback RJ, Manson PN, et al. Acute and definitive management of traumatic osteocutaneous defects of the lower extremity. Plast Reconstr Surg 80:1, 1987.
9. British Association of Plastic Reconstructive and Aesthetic Surgeons. Standards for the management of open fractures of the lower limb. London: Royal Society of Medicine Press, 2009. Available at http://www.bapras.org.uk/downloaddoc.asp?id-141.
10. Masquelet AC, Sassu P. Gastrocnemius flap. In Wei FC, Mardini S, eds. Flaps and Reconstructive Surgery. Philadelphia: Saunders Elsevier, 2009.
11. Patzakis MJ, Wilkins J, Moore TM. Use of antibiotics in open tibial fractures. Clin Orthop Relat Res 178:31, 1983.

57. Foot Ulcers

See *Essentials of Plastic Surgery*, second edition, pp. 667-681.

EPIDEMIOLOGY OF FOOT ULCERS

1. You see a 50-year-old patient in your clinic who has a chronic foot ulcer. In Europe and the United States, what is the most likely underlying condition associated with this diagnosis?
   A. Diabetes mellitus
   B. Malignancy
   C. Infection
   D. Venous insufficiency
   E. Arterial insufficiency

RISKS OF FOOT ULCER COMPLICATIONS IN DIABETIC PATIENTS

2. For each of the following statements, select the most likely risk. (Each option may be used once, more than once, or not at all.)
   A. The risk of a diabetic patient developing a foot ulcer in his or her lifetime
   B. The risk of developing infection in an established diabetic foot ulcer
   C. The risk that an infected diabetic foot ulcer will progress to require amputation

   Options:
   a. 1 in 2
   b. 1 in 4
   c. 1 in 5
   d. 1 in 10
   e. 1 in 20
   f. 1 in 50

RISK FACTORS IN DIABETIC FOOT ULCER DEVELOPMENT

3. What is the classic triad of risk factors for diabetic foot ulcer development?
   A. Poor footwear, foot deformity, and peripheral neuropathy
   B. Peripheral neuropathy, foot deformity, and minor trauma
   C. Smoking, minor trauma, and peripheral arterial disease
   D. Elevated blood glucose, foot deformity, and poor hygiene
   E. Peripheral neuropathy, previous amputation, and smoking

Chapter 57 ■ Foot Ulcers   463

CLASSIFICATION OF DIABETIC FOOT ULCERS

4. **Which one of the following statements is correct regarding classification systems for diabetic foot ulcers?**
   A. The Meggitt-Wagner system is most commonly used and consistently considers infection status across all grades.
   B. The University of Texas system assesses wound size, depth, and chronicity, but not tissue perfusion.
   C. When using the PEDIS system as described by the International Working Group on the Diabetic Foot (IWGDF), the *P* stands for paresthesia.
   D. The main strength of the Infectious Disease Society of America (IDSA) classification system is that it incorporates wound size, depth, and sensation.
   E. Wound depth, infection, and vascularity are the key predictive factors and should ideally be featured within a classification system.

THE AMERICAN DIABETES ASSOCIATION ALGORITHM FOR DIABETIC FOOT ULCERATION

5. The American Diabetes Association (ADA) algorithm for managing neuropathic foot ulcers in diabetic patients has six essential components. **Which one of these components represents the most important aspect to facilitate healing?**
   A. Off-loading
   B. Early debridement
   C. Management of infection
   D. Correction of ischemia
   E. Early amputation

MANAGEMENT OF THE DIABETIC FOOT

6. While you are on call, the emergency department refers a 64-year-old diabetic man with a provisional diagnosis of cellulitis of his foot. Erythema has developed over the course of a few days and his entire foot is warm with moderate swelling. Further examination shows bounding pulses, reduced sensation, and absent deep tendon reflexes. The patient is systemically well, pain free, and afebrile. Blood glucose control is chronically poor. Recent blood test findings are unremarkable. **Which one of the following statements is correct regarding the management of this patient?**
   A. He should be given high-dose intravenous floxacillin and metronidazole.
   B. Early mobilization, elevation, and NSAIDs are beneficial to reduce swelling.
   C. Serial radiographs are unlikely to alter management.
   D. Incision and drainage of the swelling within 24 hours is advisable.
   E. Strict immobilization of the affected foot and ankle is critically important.

FOOT DEFORMITY IN DIABETES

7. Which one of the following is the most common site for development of a diabetic foot ulcer?
A. Heel
B. Arch
C. Lateral sole
D. Region of the great toe
E. Tips of the toes

TOTAL CONTACT CASTING

8. You are considering the use of total contact casting for a patient with a problematic diabetic foot ulcer. **Which one of the following statements is correct regarding this technique?**
A. Patient compliance is typically poor.
B. Infection should be aggressively managed simultaneously.
C. Healing rates are only 40% to 50% within the first 6 weeks.
D. The entire plantar aspect of the foot and lower leg should be in contact with the cast.
E. Casts can be easily placed by patients or their caregivers.

ADJUNCTIVE SURGICAL PROCEDURES IN NONRESPONDING DIABETIC FOOT ULCERS

9. For each of the following scenarios, select the most likely surgical intervention required. (Each answer may be used once, more than once, or not at all.)
A. A patient has ankle equinus and recurrent plantar forefoot ulcers.
B. A patient has claw toes and recalcitrant toe ulcers.
C. A patient has recurrent plantar metatarsophalangeal ulceration of the hallux.

Options:
a. Extensor tenotomy
b. Flexor tenotomy
c. Tendon lengthening
d. Amputation
e. Tendon shortening
f. Wedge osteotomy
g. Resection arthroplasty

DEBRIDEMENT OF DIABETIC FOOT ULCERS

10. A patient presents in the diabetic foot clinic with a necrotic, malodorous foot ulcer. **Which one of the following statements is correct regarding selection of a debridement method for such patients?**
A. Wet-to-dry dressings are nonselective in the tissue removed but provide pain-free dressing changes.
B. When used for wound debridement, maggots are effective against methicillin-resistant *Staphylococcus aureus* (MRSA) and vancomycin-resistant *Enterococcus* (VRE).
C. Hydrosurgical debridement will commonly result in excessive removal of healthy granulation tissue.
D. Gangrene should be routinely debrided before revascularization is attempted.
E. *P. sericata* larvae nonselectively debride devitalized and healthy tissue.

DIAGNOSIS AND MANAGEMENT OF LOWER LIMB ULCERS

11. *For each of the following foot ulcer descriptions, select the most likely cause. (Each option may be used once, more than once, or not at all.)*
    A. *A patient has a painful, punched-out ulcer with a yellow, fibrinous base. Further examination reveals shiny, hairless skin and dystrophic toe nails.*
    B. *A patient has a long-standing, shallow ulcer with irregular edges. Further examination reveals chronic edema and lipodermatosclerosis.*
    C. *A patient has a rapidly enlarging ulcer in a previous burn site.*

Options:
a. Radiotherapy
b. Diabetes mellitus
c. Arterial insufficiency
d. Lymphedema
e. Venous insufficiency
f. Squamous cell carcinoma
g. Basal cell carcinoma
h. Melanoma

Answers

EPIDEMIOLOGY OF FOOT ULCERS
1. *You see a 50-year-old patient in your clinic who has a chronic foot ulcer. In Europe and the United States, what is the most likely underlying condition associated with this diagnosis?*
   A. Diabetes mellitus
   Diabetes is now the leading cause of foot ulcers and their complications, with an incidence of 2.0% to 6.8% per year in the Europe and the United States. Other common causes include venous and arterial ulcers. Skin malignancies represent a fair proportion of foot ulcers and suspicious lesions warrant early biopsy. It is clearly important to be able to recognize the different ulcers in clinical practice as their management differs significantly. Diabetic foot ulcer management should focus on prevention as diabetes continues to affect more people worldwide.

RISKS OF FOOT ULCER COMPLICATIONS IN DIABETIC PATIENTS
2. *For the following statements, the best options are as follows:*
   A. *The risk of a diabetic patient developing a foot ulcer in his or her lifetime*
      b. 1 in 4
   B. *The risk of developing infection in an established diabetic foot ulcer*
      a. 1 in 2
   C. *The risk that an infected foot ulcer will progress to require amputation*
      c. 1 in 5
   The risk of developing complications from diabetic foot disease is significant. One quarter of patients with diabetes will develop a foot ulcer during their lifetime. Half of these will become infected at some stage. Of the infected ulcers, a fifth will ultimately require amputation. More than half of all nontraumatic limb amputations are performed because of diabetes. These figures again support the importance of preventing and treating ulcers early in this population group with patient education, tight control of blood glucose, and practical steps to avoid foot trauma.

RISK FACTORS IN DIABETIC FOOT ULCER DEVELOPMENT
3. *What is the classic triad of risk factors for diabetic foot ulcer development?*
   B. Peripheral neuropathy, foot deformity, and minor trauma
   The classic triad of risk factors for development of diabetic foot ulcers is peripheral neuropathy, foot deformity, and minor trauma. Neuropathy is the most significant single factor. Other contributing factors include poor selection of footwear (which can contribute to repeated minor trauma), poor self-care, smoking, peripheral arterial disease, obesity, and hypertension.

CLASSIFICATION OF DIABETIC FOOT ULCERS
4. *Which one of the following statements is correct regarding classification systems for diabetic foot ulcers?*
   E. Wound depth, infection, and vascularity are key predictive factors and should ideally be featured within a classification system.
   Numerous classification systems have been developed for diabetic foot ulcers, suggesting that no uniformly accepted ideal exists. Three factors are particularly relevant to healing and these

are wound depth, infection status, and vascularity as indicated by the presence or absence of peripheral arterial disease. For this reason, the ideal classification should include these three factors as a minimum. The Meggitt-Wagner system is most commonly used and has six grades as follows:

0: Preulcerative/high-risk foot
1: Superficial ulcer
2: Deep to tendon, bone, or joint
3: Deep with abscess/osteomyelitis
4: Forefoot gangrene
5: Whole foot gangrene

Weaknesses of this system are that the presence or absence of wound infection is not considered in grades 0 to 2, and peripheral arterial disease is considered only in grades 4 and 5. The University of Texas Wound Classification System uses a 4-by-4 matrix and considers wound depth, infection, and peripheral arterial disease, so it contains the three key criteria described above. It is therefore a useful system, but does not take into account wound size or chronicity, which are two additional factors that will influence healing. The International Working Group on the Diabetic Foot (IWGDF) developed the PEDIS (perfusion, extent/size, depth/tissue loss, infection, and sensation) system, which does cover the key criteria. The Infectious Disease Society of America (IDSA) system describes the presence of infection in diabetic foot ulcers and has four grades: not infected, mild, moderate, and severe infection. It is essentially the same as the *infection* component of the PEDIS classification. However, it does not assess other key components such as wound size, depth, and sensation.

THE AMERICAN DIABETES ASSOCIATION ALGORITHM FOR DIABETIC FOOT ULCERATION

5. The American Diabetes Association (ADA) algorithm for managing neuropathic foot ulcers in diabetic patients has six essential components. **Which one of these components represents the most important aspect to facilitate healing?**
   A. Off-loading
      According to the ADA, the management of neuropathic diabetic foot ulcers requires six essential factors. Off-loading of pressure is the most important. The goal is to off-load pressure at the ulcer site while the patient is ambulatory. The other essential factors are the following:
      - Debridement early and often
      - Moist wound healing environment
      - Treatment of infection
      - Correction of ischemia (below-the-knee disease)
      - Prevention of amputation

      All factors should be addressed, in conjunction with optimization of medical therapy, to successfully manage diabetic foot ulcers.

MANAGEMENT OF THE DIABETIC FOOT

6. While you are on call, the emergency department refers a 64-year-old diabetic man with a provisional diagnosis of cellulitis of his foot. Erythema has developed over the course of a few days and his entire foot is warm with moderate swelling. Further examination shows bounding pulses, reduced sensation, and absent deep tendon reflexes. The patient is systemically well, pain free, and afebrile. Blood glucose control is chronically poor. Recent blood test findings are unremarkable. *Which one of the following statements is correct regarding the management of this patient?*
   E. Strict immobilization of the affected foot and ankle is critically important.

   This patient demonstrates Charcot foot, which is a condition of unknown cause that occurs in diabetic patients. It presents as a red, hot, swollen foot and ankle and can be confused with either cellulitis or deep venous thrombosis.[1] If it is not diagnosed, the outcome is poor with irreversible destruction of the bony architecture of the foot. Serial radiographs can be useful for monitoring bony changes. If a wound is present, osteomyelitis should be excluded with an MRI. It may be reasonable to begin antibiotic therapy for this patient. However, he is less likely to have infection because he is well and has normal blood results such as white blood cell count.

FOOT DEFORMITY IN DIABETES

7. *Which one of the following is the most common site for development of a diabetic foot ulcer?*
   D. Region of the great toe

   Common sites for diabetic foot ulcers are those where pressure and shear are most likely to occur, in conjunction with the poorest areas of blood supply. Overall, the most common site is under the hallux. Other areas include the heel (because pressure is transmitted when lying or standing), the tips of the toes (especially with clawing and pressure when weight bearing), and those that are exposed to high repetitive trauma during walking.

TOTAL CONTACT CASTING

8. You are considering the use of total contact casting for a patient with a problematic diabetic foot ulcer. *Which one of the following statements is correct regarding this technique?*
   D. The entire plantar aspect of the foot and lower leg should be in contact with the cast.

   The goal of contact casting is to evenly distribute pressure across the foot, rather than to completely relieve the ulcer site of pressure at the expense of other vulnerable areas. Infection and ischemia should be aggressively treated before casting begins. Casts should be applied by a skilled clinician to prevent iatrogenic ulceration. Patient compliance is very good, because it is difficult to remove a full cast. Healing rates are 72% to 100% over 5 to 7 weeks.[2]

Chapter 57 ■ Foot Ulcers   469

ADJUNCTIVE SURGICAL PROCEDURES IN NONRESPONDING DIABETIC FOOT ULCERS

9. For the following scenarios, the best options are as follows:
  A. A patient has ankle equinus and recurrent plantar forefoot ulcers.
   c. Tendon lengthening
  B. A patient has claw toes and recalcitrant toe ulcers.
   b. Flexor tenotomy
  C. A patient has recurrent plantar metatarsophalangeal ulceration of the hallux.
   g. Resection arthroplasty

Corrective surgery for foot deformities may be considered in patients who have failed appropriate off-loading methods or have recurrent ulceration despite proper preventive care. Ankle equinus may be treated with Achilles' tendon lengthening via an open or endoscopic approach. This may risk infection, subsequent rupture and transfer of the ulcer to the heel.

In patients with claw toes and recalcitrant foot ulcers, a long flexor tenotomy may be consider ed if the deformity is not reducible. A Keller arthroplasty can improve the motion and alignment of the first metatarsophalangeal joint by removing the proximal aspect of the proximal phalanx of the great toe. This may benefit patients with recalcitrant MTP joint ulceration.

DEBRIDEMENT OF DIABETIC FOOT ULCERS

10. A patient presents in the diabetic foot clinic with a necrotic, malodorous foot ulcer. **Which one of the following statements is correct regarding selection of a debridement method for such patients?**
  B. When used for wound debridement, maggots are effective against methicillin-resistant *Staphylococcus aureus* (MRSA) and vancomycin-resistant *Enterococcus* (VRE).

Debridement of chronic ulcers is important in order to remove devitalized tissue and reset the acute healing process. Debridement may be achieved mechanically or chemically. Mechanical debridement includes wet-to-dry dressings, surgical debridement, and maggot therapy. Chemical debridement includes enzymatic debridement with collagenases or other active dressings such as honey. Maggots *(Phaenicia sericata)* are the larvae of green blowfly and they selectively consume devitalized tissue in wounds, while preserving healthy tissue. A secondary benefit is that they are resistant to both MRSA and VRE. Not only are wet-to-dry dressings nonselective in the tissue removed, they are also painful for patients, can lead to surface cooling, and are labor intensive. Surgical debridement can be with a traditional blade or with hydrosurgical debridement using systems like the Versajet (Smith & Nephew, Memphis, TN). Such systems are highly effective at debriding wounds accurately using high-velocity streams of saline and a vacuum. This appears to remove necrotic tissue and the biofilm. Wet gangrene should be debrided promptly to minimize systemic illness, but dry gangrene without cellulitis should remain in situ until revascularization is achieved to minimize progressive tissue loss and promote subsequent wound healing.

DIAGNOSIS AND MANAGEMENT OF LOWER LIMB ULCERS

11. *For the following descriptions, the best options are as follows:*

A. *A patient has a painful, punched-out ulcer with a yellow, fibrinous base. Further examination reveals shiny, hairless skin and dystrophic toenails.*
   c. Arterial insufficiency

B. *A patient has a long-standing, shallow ulcer with irregular edges. Further examination reveals chronic edema and lipodermatosclerosis.*
   e. Venous insufficiency

C. *A patient has a rapidly enlarging ulcer in a previous burn site.*
   f. Squamous cell carcinoma

Lower limb ulcers have some distinct features according to the cause. Factors to be considered when assessing an ulcer include location, appearance, symptoms, and risk factors. (see Table 57-3, *Essentials of Plastic Surgery,* second edition).

The hallmark features of an arterial ulcer are a round or punched-out appearance with a well-demarcated border. There may be a fibrinous yellow base or true eschar. Bone and/or tendon may be evident in the wound base. The typical location is over the distal bony prominences. Other features include a shiny appearance to the adjacent skin, loss of hair, dystrophic toenails, and absence of foot pulses.

The hallmark features of a venous lesion are a shallow ulcer with irregular borders located near the medial malleolus. Other features include varicose veins, leg edema, dermatitis, lipodermatosclerosis, and purple pigmentary changes.

The key indicators of a skin malignancy, such as an SCC or melanoma, are rapid growth with bleeding and ulceration. There may well be a keratin scabs itch, an SCC, and the lesion may appear de novo or in the setting of a chronic wound. Wound edges may be poorly defined and such lesions require biopsy to exclude or confirm the suspected diagnosis. Other skin malignancies such as BCC or melanoma can also present with nonhealing ulcerated appearances. Melanomas are often, but not always, pigmented.

Diabetic ulcers as discussed already, arise on pressure points on the feet. There is often callus surrounding the wound with undermined edges, blisters, hemorrhage, or necrosis present. Exposure of deeper structures may be observed. Radiotherapy ulcers arise in previous treatment sites and appear as unstable patches of skin. A high suspicion for malignancy should be maintained until biopsies have been performed.

REFERENCES

1. American Family Physician. The Charcot foot in diabetes: six key points. Available at *http://www.aafp.org/afp/1998/0601/p2705.html.*
2. Sinacore DR, Mueller MJ, Diamond JE. Diabetic plantar ulcers treated by total contact casting. A clinical report. Phys Ther 67:1543-1549, 1987.

58. Lymphedema

See *Essentials of Plastic Surgery*, second edition, pp. 682-690.

DEMOGRAPHICS

1. Which one of the following statements is correct regarding the demographics of lymphedema?
A. It currently affects around one million people worldwide.
B. It is limited to the limbs and genital areas.
C. It affects 1 in 10 patients following mastectomy.
D. Worldwide, 90% of cases affect the lower limb.
E. Globally, the most common cause is iatrogenic.

PHYSIOLOGY OF THE LYMPHATIC SYSTEM

2. Which one of the following statements is correct regarding the lymphatic system?
A. Derived embryologically from the venous system, it serves to move interstitial proteins and lipids from the vascular system.
B. It is comprised of a collection of valveless, superficial interconnecting vessels with no deeper component.
C. Muscle does not contain lymphatic channels but its contraction is vital to lymphatic fluid transport.
D. The basic functional unit of the lymphatic system is the noncontractile lymphangion.
E. Lymphatic channels share very similar basement membrane properties to blood vessels.

STAGING OF LYMPHEDEMA

3. According to the International Society of Lymphology classification system, what disease stage is characterized by resolution of lymphedema with elevation of the limb?
A. Stage 0
B. Stage I
C. Stage II
D. Stage III
E. Stage IV

PRIMARY LYMPHEDEMA

4. Which one of the following statements is correct regarding primary lymphedema?
A. Congenital lymphedema is also known as *Milroy's disease* and usually involves unilateral arm and leg lymphedema.
B. Most cases of primary lymphedema are sporadic but some have autosomal recessive inheritance.
C. Most patients with primary lymphedema, irrespective of cause, present with upper limb swelling.
D. Lymphedema tarda is the least common subtype and occurs in the fourth decade.
E. The most common form of primary lymphedema presents within the first 2 years of life.

CLINICAL PRESENTATION

5. A 14-year-old girl develops new-onset lymphedema involving the left leg and foot. A thorough review suggests a strong family history of this condition on her mother's side. **Which one of the following findings might you expect to see on clinical examination?**
   A. Absence of her eyebrows
   B. Epicanthic folds
   C. Lower lid coloboma
   D. Double row of eyelashes
   E. Blepharoptosis

IMAGING IN CASES OF LYMPHEDEMA

6. **Which one of the following modalities is most commonly used for patients with lymphedema?**
   A. Contrast lymphangiography
   B. Contrast CT scan
   C. Contrast MRI scan
   D. Lymphoscintigraphy
   E. Doppler ultrasound

MANAGEMENT OF LYMPHEDEMA

7. *For each of the following scenarios, select the most appropriate treatment option. (Each option may be used once, more than once, or not at all.)*
   A. A 45-year-old-woman presents with long-standing upper limb lymphedema after treatment for breast cancer, despite compliance with a good compression garment. No axillary tethering is noted, and lymphoscintigraphy reveals evidence of lymphatic vessel activity.
   B. A 50-year-old man presents with lymphedema 6 months after a groin dissection for penile squamous cell carcinoma. No evidence of disease recurrence or infection is present.
   C. A 30-year-old woman presents with persistent, bilateral, nonpitting upper limb lymphedema that has been present since puberty, despite compliance with massage, exercise, and compression therapy.

   Options:
   a. Charles procedure
   b. Lymph node transplantation
   c. Lymphaticovenular bypass anastomoses
   d. Miller procedure
   e. Suction-assisted lipectomy
   f. Complete decongestive therapy
   g. Compression garment

LYMPHEDEMA IN BREAST CANCER PATIENTS

8. **Which one of the following statements is correct when considering lymphedema in patients treated for breast cancer?**
   A. Breast cancer represents the second most common cause of upper limb lymphedema resulting from malignancy.
   B. There is no strong supporting evidence that the affected limb must not be used for venipuncture.
   C. Breast conservation surgery is associated with a similar risk of lymphedema, compared with mastectomy.
   D. The incidence of lymphedema is the same after sentinel lymph node biopsy or axillary clearance.
   E. Obesity and weight gain after breast cancer treatment does not affect development of lymphedema.

GENERAL ASPECTS OF LYMPHEDEMA

9. What does a positive "Stemmer sign" refer to with reference to physical examination of a lymphedematous patient?
A. That there is a significant size discrepancy between the limbs
B. That the skin has a "peau de orange" appearance to it
C. That there is active infection in a lymphedematous limb
D. That there is a doughy swelling of the extremities
E. That the skin cannot be pinched over the dorsum of the second toe

NATURAL COURSE OF LYMPHEDEMA

10. You see a patient years after she had a left mastectomy and axillary dissection for breast cancer. She now presents with evidence of blue-red subcutaneous nodules and ecchymosis in the left upper limb. There has been no history of trauma. **What does this most likely suggest?**
A. The presence of lymphangitis
B. Metastatic spread of breast cancer
C. The presence of pseudosarcoma
D. Development of erysipelas
E. Development of a new malignancy

MANAGEMENT OF SECONDARY LYMPHEDEMA

11. What is the usual drug of choice for management of secondary lymphedema as a result of filiariasis?
A. Suramin
B. Ivermectin
C. Mebendazole
D. Penicillin
E. Erythromycin

Answers

DEMOGRAPHICS

1. **Which one of the following statements is correct regarding the demographics of lymphedema?**
   D. Worldwide, 90% of cases affect the lower limb.
   Lymphedema is the buildup of proteinaceous fluid within the interstitial compartment secondary to abnormalities in the lymphatic transport system. Although estimates vary in the literature, lymphedema probably affects in excess of 200 million people worldwide. The most common cause by far is the parasite *Wuchereria bancrofti,* which is estimated to affect more than 90 million people worldwide. (Again this varies in the literature, as it is difficult to accurately record incidence in many developing countries.) This parasitic disease, transmitted by mosquitoes, results in adult filarial worms physically blocking lymphatic channels. The World Health Organization (WHO) has implemented major programs to target the problem of filariasis.[1] The lower limb is affected far more commonly than any other site. The ratio between lower to upper limb involvement is 9:1 across all causes. Lymphedema is not, however, limited to the limbs and genitalia, as it can occur in the head and neck region in patients treated for head and neck cancer.[2]

   In the developed world, the most common cause of secondary lymphedema is malignancy.[3] This occasionally occurs secondary to a primary tumor but is far more common after surgical excision or radiotherapy of tumor or lymph node basins. Between 25% and 50% of patients develop lymphedema of the ipsilateral upper limb after mastectomy.

PHYSIOLOGY OF THE LYMPHATIC SYSTEM

2. **Which one of the following statements is correct regarding the lymphatic system?**
   C. Muscle does not contain lymphatic channels but its contraction is vital to lymphatic fluid transport.
   Although muscle itself does not have lymphatic channels, it serves an important role in lymphatic function by moving lymph from areas of low to high pressure. This propulsive effect occurs secondary to muscle contraction. Other modalities of propulsion are arterial and respiratory movement.

   The lymphatic system is derived embryologically from the venous system and serves to move fluid, proteins, and lipids from the interstitial space into the venous system (not away from it). The lymphatic system contains both deep and superficial components. Some channels such as those within the dermis contain valves. The superficial components drain into the deep components at three main sites: the cubital fossa, the inguinal fossa, and the popliteal fossa. The cisterna chyli is a sac at the level of L1-2 that receives lymphatic drainage from the lower limbs and trunk. From the cisterna, lymph travels within the thoracic duct from T12 and drains into the confluence of the left internal jugular and left subclavian veins. Knowledge of this anatomy is clinically relevant when undertaking a neck dissection, as damage to the lymphatic system here can result in a chyle leak. The lymphangion is the functional unit of the lymphatic system but is noncontractile. While blood vessels have a defined basement membrane, lymphatics have several intercellular gaps that allow movement of fat and proteins into the lymphatics.

STAGING OF LYMPHEDEMA

3. **According to the International Society of Lymphology classification system, what disease stage is characterized by resolution of lymphedema with elevation of the limb?**
   B. Stage I

   The International Society of Lymphology has developed a four-stage classification for lymphedema.[4] Stage 0 represents a latent or subclinical condition without evidence of edema, even though lymphatic transport is impaired. Stage I involves early accumulation of proteinaceous fluid that can cause pitting or nonpitting edema, which resolves with limb elevation. Stage II involves tissue fibrosis, and limb elevation alone will no longer resolve tissue swelling. Stage III is associated with lymphostatic elephantiasis with absent pitting, acanthosis, and other tropic skin changes.

PRIMARY LYMPHEDEMA

4. **Which one of the following statements is correct regarding primary lymphedema?**
   D. Lymphedema tarda is the least common subtype and occurs in the fourth decade.

   Primary lymphedema most commonly affects the lower limbs and can be unilateral or bilateral. It is classified by age of onset as congenital (younger than 2 years), praecox (puberty), or tarda (35 years of age).[3,5] Of these, lymphedema tarda is the rarest subtype (<10%) and lymphedema praecox is the most common, representing up to 80% of all primary lymphedema. Milroy's disease refers to lymphedema congenita and affects females more commonly than males with a 2:1 ratio. It usually presents with bilateral lower limb lymphedema in children before their second birthday. The inheritance pattern for primary lymphedema varies depending on subtype and is most commonly autosomal dominant, but can be sporadic in Milroy's disease.

   Wolf and Kinmouth[6] have classified primary lymphedema as anaplastic, hypoplastic, or hyperplastic, based on the appearance during lymphangiography. Hypoplastic lymphedema is the most common subtype (67% of cases) and can be obstructive or nonobstructive.

CLINICAL PRESENTATION

5. **A 14-year-old girl develops new-onset lymphedema involving the left leg and foot. A thorough review suggests a strong family history of this condition on her mother's side. Which one of the following findings might you expect to see on clinical examination?**
   D. Double row of eyelashes

   The history suggests this patient has Meige's syndrome, which is a type of primary lymphedema occurring in puberty that usually presents as new-onset unilateral lymphedema affecting the foot and calf. Associated inflammation is often present, and this can be complicated by cellulitis. Associated abnormalities include vertebral and cerebrovascular malformations, sensorineural (as opposed to conductive) hearing loss, and a double row of eyelashes (distichiasis). The latter can result from abnormal development of the meibomian glands.

IMAGING IN CASES OF LYMPHEDEMA

6. Which one of the following modalities is most commonly used for patients with lymphedema?

D. Lymphoscintigraphy

Lymphoscintigraphy is currently considered to be the benchmark for diagnosing lymphedema, although other modalities can be very useful in some circumstances.[3] For example, where deep venous thrombosis or chronic vascular disease is suspected, an ultrasound examination is useful. If malignancy is suspected, then CT or MRI may be helpful. Each of these modalities has a high sensitivity and specificity in confirming the diagnosis of lymphedema while facilitating tumor identification. An MRI is particularly good for providing detail of lymphatic architecture and preventing radiation exposure. Because of the success of these less-invasive imaging modalities, contrast lymphangiography is no longer commonly performed.

MANAGEMENT OF LYMPHEDEMA

7. For the following scenarios, the best options are as follows:

A. A 45-year-old woman presents with long-standing upper limb lymphedema after treatment for breast cancer, despite compliance with a good compression garment. No axillary tethering is noted, and lymphoscintigraphy reveals evidence of lymphatic vessel activity.

c. Lymphaticovenular bypass anastomoses

In the absence of axillary tethering/scarring, an autologous lymph node transplantation is less likely to be beneficial. For lymphaticovenular anastomosis to be effective, some functioning lymphatic vessels need to be present. Three or four bypass anastomoses per patient provide good symptomatic and objective improvements in breast cancer patients.

B. A 50-year-old man presents with lymphedema 6 months after a groin dissection for penile squamous cell carcinoma. No evidence of disease recurrence or infection are present. Recurrent disease or infection is not evident.

f. Complete decongestive therapy

Complete decongestive therapy reduces volume by 40% to 60% in patients with pitting edema. It is administered by a lymphedema therapist and combines an initial reduction phase (manual drainage, exercise, skin care, compression, and education) with a maintenance phase of self-care and compression therapy. A compression garment alone is unlikely to be as effective as these combined measures.

C. A 30-year-old woman presents with persistent, bilateral, nonpitting upper limb lymphedema that has been present since puberty, despite compliance with massage, exercise, and compression therapy.

e. Suction-assisted lipectomy

Liposuction techniques for lymphedema can provide satisfactory results if compression garments are worn after surgery. If this is unsuccessful, the patient can be considered for an excisional procedure such as the Miller procedure. This involves a longitudinal excision of skin and subcutaneous tissue with a layered closure.

A Charles procedure might be of functional benefit, but the cosmesis of extensive skin grafting is far less favorable than the longitudinal scarring associated with a Miller excision. Furthermore, this procedure is historically described for the lower limb.

LYMPHEDEMA IN BREAST CANCER PATIENTS

8. Which one of the following statements is correct considering lymphedema in patients treated for breast cancer?

B. There is no strong supporting evidence that the affected limb should not be used for venipuncture.

It is a myth that venipuncture should not be performed on the affected side after treatment of the axilla (particularly in breast cancer patients), because it will exacerbate lymphedema or result in infection. Green et al[7] reviewed literature from 1966 to 2004 and found no evidence to support this common dictum. They stated that the main theoretical risk for patients with lymphedema having cannulation is the introduction of infection, leading to cellulitis and further lymphatic damage. They found no evidence that aseptic placement of a cannula or needle will regularly cause infection or that such an approach will worsen or exacerbate lymphedema. Injections are required for lymphoscintigraphy, lymphangiography, and liposuction, yet these are not regularly complicated by cellulitis or worsening of lymphedema. In the absence of robust evidence, the alternative limb should probably be used preferentially. However, the affected side can be considered for safe use in venipuncture when required.

van der Veen et al[8] attempted to identify risk factors for the development of lymphedema after breast surgery with axillary clearance. In a cohort of 245 women, they found that risk increased with BMI over 25, axillary radiotherapy, and pathologic lymph node status. In general, the greatest risk of developing lymphedema is after mastectomy but is still high after a lumpectomy or axillary node surgery.

GENERAL ASPECTS OF LYMPHEDEMA

9. What does a positive "Stemmer sign" refer to with reference to physical examination of a lymphedematous patient?

E. That the skin cannot be pinched over the dorsum of the second toe

There are a range of signs that should be noted during examination of a patient with suspected lymphedema. The Stemmer sign is elicited by attempting to pinch skin over the dorsum of the second toe. This will not be possible in a patient with significant lymphedema. Other clinical findings are not specific to the lower limb and include doughy swelling, peau de orange skin changes, and circumferential limb measurements with a side-to-side difference greater than 2 cm. Assessing whether the edema is pitting or nonpitting is also important, as well as looking for evidence of active infection such as cellulitis or lymphangitis.

NATURAL COURSE OF LYMPHEDEMA

10. You see a patient years after she had a left mastectomy and axillary dissection for breast cancer. She now presents with evidence of blue-red subcutaneous nodules and ecchymosis in the left upper limb. There has been no history of trauma. What does this most likely suggest?

E. Development of a new malignancy

The description given is suspicious for development of a new malignancy and this is likely to be Stewart-Treves syndrome. This is a type of lymphangiosarcoma arising within chronic lymphedema, classically described after radical mastectomy. It is difficult to treat and has a very poor prognosis (life expectancy is less than 18 months after diagnosis). Wide local resection of the tumor is the preferred treatment modality.[9]

Erysipelas and lymphangitis both present with a red swollen limb and would not be expected to display the above features. Breast cancer more commonly would metastasize to the lungs, bone, or liver, although it may recur locally in the chest wall. The term *pseudosarcoma* refers to massive local edema in severely obese patients where folds of fat compress the lymphatics leading to edema, thickened epidermis, and dermal fibrosis. It most commonly occurs on the thighs.

MANAGEMENT OF SECONDARY LYMPHEDEMA

11. What is the usual drug of choice for management of secondary lymphedema as a result of filiariasis?

B. Ivermectin

Ivermectin is the drug of choice used for treatment of filariasis and is used in the WHO program.[1] It is a broad spectrum antiparasitic agent that may be combined with albendazole in the case of coendemicity with onchocerciasis (another parasitic disease transmitted by black flies that can lead to skin disease and blindness). The other treatment option is to use diethylcarbamazine citrate with albendazole.

REFERENCES

1. World Health Organization. Global programme to eliminate lymphatic filariasis. Available at *http://www.who.int/lymphatic_filariasis/policy/en/*.
2. Deng J, Ridner SH, Dietrich MS, et al. Prevalence of secondary lymphedema in patients with head and neck cancer. J Pain Symptom Manage 43:244-252, 2012.
3. Warren AG, Brorson H, Borud LJ, et al. Lymphedema: a comprehensive review. Ann Plast Surg 59:464-472, 2007.
4. International Society of Lymphoma. The diagnosis and treatment of peripheral lymphedema. Consensus document of the International Society of Lymphology. Lymphology 36:84-91, 2003.
5. Richards AM. Key Notes on Plastic Surgery. Oxford, UK: Blackwell Press, 2002.
6. Wolfe JH, Kinmonth JB. The prognosis of primary lymphedema of the lower limbs. Arch Surg 116:1157-1160, 1981.
7. Greene AK, Borud L, Slavin SA. Blood pressure monitoring and venipuncture in the lymphedematous extremity. Plast Reconstr Surg 116:2058-2059, 2005.
8. van der Veen P, De Voogdt N, Lievens P, et al. Lymphedema development following breast cancer surgery with full axillary resection. Lymphology 37:206-208, 2004.
9. Sharma A, Schwartz RA. Stewart-Treves syndrome: pathogenesis and management. J Am Acad Dermatol 67:1342-1348, 2012.

Part VI

Hand, Wrist, and Upper Extremity

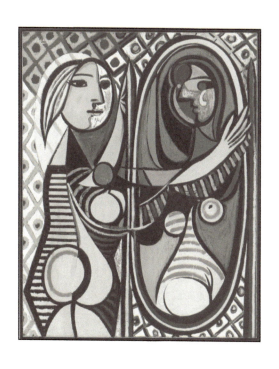

© 2015 Estate of Pablo Picasso / Artists Rights Society (ARS), New York.

59. Hand Anatomy and Biomechanics

See *Essentials of Plastic Surgery*, second edition, pp. 693-707.

ABBREVIATIONS

JOINTS
CMC joint: Carpometacarpal joint
DIP joint: Distal interphalangeal joint
IP joint: Interphalangeal joint
MP joint: Metacarpophalangeal joint
PIP joint: Proximal interphalangeal joint

MUSCLES
AdP: Adductor pollicis
APB: Abductor pollicis brevis
APL: Abductor pollicis longus
BR: Brachioradialis
ECRB: Extensor carpi radialis brevis
ECRL: Extensor carpi radialis longus
ECU: Extensor carpi ulnaris
EDC: Extensor digiti communis
EDM: Extensor digiti minimi
EIP: Extensor indicis proprius
EPL: Extensor pollicis longus
FCR: Flexor carpi radialis
FDM: Flexor digiti minimi
FDP: Flexor digitorum profundus
FDS: Flexor digitorum superficialis
FPB: Flexor pollicis brevis
FPL: Flexor pollicis longus
ODM: Opponens digiti minimi
PL: Palmaris longus
PT: Pronator teres

RETINACULAR SYSTEM

1. *Which one of the following structures can prevent bowstringing of the neurovascular bundle during finger flexion?*
   A. Cleland's ligament
   B. Ligament of Landsmeer
   C. Transverse retinacular ligament
   D. Grayson's ligament
   E. Natatory ligament

DEEP FASCIAL SPACES

2. *For each of the following descriptions, select the space described. (Each option may be used once, more than once, or not at all.)*
   A. *This is the location of a collar button abscess.*
   B. *This space can allow proximal spread of infection from the central palm.*
   C. *This space lies between the pronator quadratus and digital flexor tendons.*

   Options:
   a. Thenar space
   b. Midvolar space
   c. Interdigital space
   d. Parona's space
   e. Hypothenar space

EXTRINSIC EXTENSORS

3. **Which one of the following statements is correct regarding the dorsal wrist compartments?**
   A. There are five dorsal wrist compartments.
   B. EPL is located within the first compartment.
   C. ECRL and ECRB are located within the third compartment.
   D. EDC travels with EIP in the fourth compartment.
   E. EDM and ECU are located within the fifth compartment.

4. You are referred a patient with a zone VI extensor tendon injury who is unable to extend the long finger. **Where will the division have occurred?**
   A. Over the MP joint
   B. At the level of the wrist
   C. Over the proximal phalanx
   D. In the forearm
   E. At the level of the metacarpal

5. *For each of the following descriptions, select the correct answer. (Each option may be used once, more than once, or not at all.)*
   A. *This structure restricts independent action of extensors on a single digit.*
   B. *This structure provides lateral stabilization of the extensor tendon over the MP joint.*
   C. *This structure inserts on the distal phalanx to facilitate DIP joint extension.*

   Options:
   a. Central slip
   b. Juncturae tendinum
   c. Sagittal band
   d. Volar plate
   e. Lateral slip
   f. Lateral band
   g. Transverse retinacular ligament

6. **Which one of the following statements is correct regarding extensor tendon insertions in the hand and wrist?**
   A. EPL passes around Lister's tubercle to insert on the proximal phalanx of the thumb.
   B. The ECRL tendon inserts on the base of the third metacarpal.
   C. The EDC tendons insert directly onto the proximal phalanges.
   D. Both the EIP and EDM insert ulnar to the EDC tendons of the respective digits.
   E. The APL tendon inserts on the base of the proximal phalanx of the thumb.

EXTRINSIC FLEXORS

7. **Which one of the following statements is correct when exploring the contents of the carpal tunnel?**
   A. It usually contains nine structures, including the median nerve and flexor tendons.
   B. The FDS tendons to the middle and ring fingers lie superficial to the FDS tendons to the index and little fingers.
   C. The median nerve lies deep to the FDP tendons.
   D. The FDS tendons to the index and middle fingers lie superficial to the FDS tendons to the ring and little finger.
   E. The FPL lies superficial to the median nerve.

8. Flexor tendon injuries are commonly seen in hand trauma patients. A thorough knowledge of flexor tendon anatomy in the hand is vital to diagnosing and managing these injuries. **Which one of the following statements is correct regarding the anatomy of this area?**
   A. Verdan described six zones of flexor tendon injury that relate to treatment and prognosis.
   B. Even-numbered annular pulleys arise from the volar plates of the MP joint, PIP, and DIP joints.
   C. *No-man's land* describes the flexor sheath from the A1 pulley to the FDP insertion.
   D. The C1 cruciate pulley lies between the A1 and A2 annular pulleys.
   E. The A2 and A4 annular pulleys are considered to be the most important to preserve.

9. You are repairing a complete FPL division from a knife wound over the proximal phalanx. The injury occurred during full flexion of the thumb. **Which one of the following statements is correct regarding the anatomy of this region?**
   A. This represents a zone III injury.
   B. The proximal tendon is unlikely to have retracted proximally.
   C. Preservation of the oblique pulley is most important.
   D. The thumb has both annular and cruciate pulleys.
   E. The neurovascular bundles are more protected than in the fingers.

ARTERIAL SUPPLY TO THE HAND

10. **Which one of the following statements is correct regarding the arterial supply to the hand?**
    A. The princeps pollicis arises consistently from the superficial palmar arch.
    B. The ulnar artery lies ulnar to the ulnar nerve and FCU at the wrist.
    C. In the fingers, the digital vessels lie volar to the digital nerves.
    D. The deep volar arch arises from the larger terminal branch of the ulnar artery
    E. Kaplan's line is a useful marker of the superficial palmar arch.

INNERVATION OF THE HAND AND UPPER LIMB

11. **Which one of the following actions would be lost after an injury to the ulnar nerve at the elbow?**
    A. Flexion of the thumb at the IP joint.
    B. Flexion of the ring finger at the DIP joint.
    C. Flexion of the wrist.
    D. Flexion of the little finger at the PIP joint.
    E. Flexion of the index finger at the DIP joint.

12. **Which one of the following is innervated by a branch of the median nerve?**
    A. FDP to ring finger
    B. Dorsal interossei
    C. APB
    D. Deep portion of FPB
    E. ADM

13. Identify the most accurate sensory nerve supply for each of the following anatomic areas of the hand. (Each option may be used once, more than once, or not at all.)
    A. Dorsum of the hand overlying the index metacarpal
    B. Volar aspect of the wrist overlying the ulnar artery
    C. Nail bed region of the long finger

    Options:
    a. Median nerve
    b. Palmar branch of the ulnar nerve
    c. Lateral antebrachial cutaneous nerve
    d. Posterior antebrachial cutaneous nerve
    e. Medial antebrachial cutaneous nerve
    f. Palmar branch of the median nerve
    g. Superficial branch of the radial nerve

14. Which one of the following is usually spared in a posterior interosseous nerve palsy?
    A. ECRL
    B. ECU
    C. EDM
    D. EDC
    E. EPL

15. Which one of the following is incorrect?
    A. The Martin-Gruber anastomosis is a motor fiber connection between the ulnar and median nerves in the forearm.
    B. The superficial radial nerve passes between the tendons of the brachioradialis and ECRL.
    C. The Riche-Cannieu anastomosis is a sensory fiber connection between the ulnar and median nerves in the hand.
    D. The dorsal sensory branch of the ulnar nerve arises 5 to 7 cm proximal to the ulnar styloid process.
    E. The palmar cutaneous branch of the median nerve arises 5 cm proximal to the wrist crease.

BONES OF THE WRIST

16. Which one of the following bones links the proximal and distal carpal rows?
    A. Trapezoid
    B. Scaphoid
    C. Trapezium
    D. Pisiform
    E. Capitate

Answers

RETINACULAR SYSTEM

1. **Which one of the following structures can prevent bowstringing of the neurovascular bundle during finger flexion?**
   D. Grayson's ligament

   The retinacular system is comprised of palmar (volar) fascia and the retaining ligaments of the fingers. Grayson's and Cleland's ligaments flank the neurovascular bundle and can play a role in anchoring the skin envelope to the digital skeleton without impeding movement. Grayson's ligaments pass transversely from the flexor sheath to the skin and lie volar to the neurovascular bundles. They are thought to prevent bowstringing of the neurovascular bundles. Cleland's ligaments lie dorsally, arising from periosteum and inserting into the skin. The transverse retinacular ligaments anchor the lateral bands to the volar aspect of the proximal phalanx, near the PIP joint. Their function is to prevent excessive dorsal displacement of the lateral bands in PIP joint extension (which occurs in a swan-neck deformity). The ligament of Landsmeer originates on the volar aspect of the middle phalanx and inserts on the dorsal aspect of the distal phalanx. It helps coordinate PIP joint and DIP joint motion. (See Figs. 59-1 and 59-4, *Essentials of Plastic Surgery,* second edition).

DEEP FASCIAL SPACES

2. **For each of the following descriptions, the best options are as follows?**
   A. This is the location of a collar button abscess.
      c. Interdigital space
   B. This space can allow proximal spread of infection from the central palm.
      d. Parona's space
   C. This space lies between the pronator quadratus and digital flexor tendons.
      d. Parona's space

   The fascial spaces of the hand are potential spaces that are clinically relevant with respect to hand infections. The interdigital web space is the site of a collar button abscess. Drainage usually requires both volar and dorsal approaches.

   Parona's space is important with respect to proximal spread of infection from either the midvolar space or from the radial or ulna bursa. It is important to look deep to the digital flexors for pus lying superficial to the pronator quadratus when draining palmar digital infections. The palmar spaces are illustrated in Fig. 59-1.

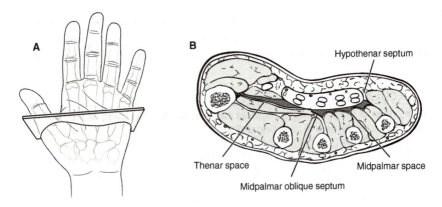

Fig. 59-1 **A** and **B,** Fascial spaces of the hand.

EXTRINSIC EXTENSORS

3. **Which one of the following statements is correct regarding the dorsal wrist compartments?**
   D. **EDC travels with EIP in the fourth compartment.**

   The wrist contains six extensor compartments which are synovial lined fibroosseus tunnels through which extensor tendons pass under the retinaculum (Table 59-1). The EIP and EDC tendons pass through the fourth extensor compartment. The posterior interosseous nerve is also found in this compartment, where it terminates to supply the wrist joint. Knowledge of its anatomic location is useful, because it can be intentionally resected to treat wrist pain or can be a potential donor for digital nerve grafts. EDM and ECU are located in different compartments (fifth and sixth, respectively). ECRL and ECRB are located in the second compartment and EPL within the third compartment.

Table 59-1 *Extensor Compartments of the Wrist*

Compartment	Contents
First	APL, EPB
Second	ECRL, ECRB
Third	EPL
Fourth	EDC, EIP
Fifth	EDM
Sixth	ECU

4. You are referred a patient with a zone VI extensor tendon injury who is unable to extend the long finger. **Where will the division have occurred?**
   E. **At the level of the metacarpal**

   There are nine extensor tendon zones. Odd numbers are over the joints, starting with zone I over the DIP joint, and even numbers are between joints (see Fig. 59-3, *Essentials of Plastic Surgery*, second edition). The injury described is located over the metacarpal. Note that the zones are different in the thumb, with TI at the IP joint, TII at the proximal phalanx, TIII at the MP joint, TIV at the first metacarpal, and TV at the wrist.

5. *For each of the following descriptions, the best options are as follows:*
   A. *This structure restricts independent action of extensors on a single digit.*
      b. **Juncturae tendinum**
   B. *This structure provides lateral stabilization of the extensor tendon over the MCP joint.*
      c. **Sagittal band**
   C. *This structure inserts on the distal phalanx to facilitate DIP joint extension.*
      f. **Lateral band**

      The juncturae tendinum are tendinous interconnections between EDC tendons on the dorsum of the hand. They prevent independent action of EDC on a single digit. They can also transmit MP joint extension to a finger even where the tendon is cut more proximally. The sagittal bands arise from the volar plate and help to stabilize the extensor tendon over the MP joint. The lateral bands are formed by the intrinsics and the lateral slips. They insert onto the distal phalanx as the terminal extensor tendon. The transverse retinacular ligament prevents dorsal subluxation of the lateral bands during PIP joint extension.

6. **Which one of the following statements is correct regarding extensor tendon insertions in the hand and wrist?**
   D. **Both the EIP and EDM insert ulnar to the EDC tendons of the respective digits.**

   All four fingers have an EDC tendon which effects a mass extension action. In addition, the index and little finger each have another tendon (EIP and EDM, respectively), which allow for independent extension. These may be used as tendon transfers and it is important to be able to differentiate them anatomically from EDC (Table 59-2).

Table 59-2 *Extensor Tendon Insertions*

Extensor Tendon	Insertion
APL	Base of the thumb metacarpal
EPB	Base of the proximal phalanx of the thumb (can vary)
ECRL	Base of the index metacarpal
ECRB	Base of the middle metacarpal
EPL	Distal phalanx of the thumb
EDC	Extensor expansion of the index to little fingers
EIP	Extensor expansion of the index finger
EDM	Extensor expansion of the little finger
ECU	Base of the metacarpal of the little finger

EXTRINSIC FLEXORS

7. **Which one of the following statements is correct when exploring the contents of the carpal tunnel?**
   B. The FDS tendons to the middle and ring fingers lie superficial to the FDS tendons to the index and little fingers.
   The carpal tunnel usually contains nine flexor tendons (four FDS, four FDP, and one FPL) and the median nerve (see Fig. 78-1, *Essentials of Plastic Surgery,* second edition). The FDS tendons to the middle and ring fingers lie most superficially alongside the median nerve.

8. Flexor tendon injuries are commonly seen in hand trauma patients. A thorough knowledge of flexor tendon anatomy in the hand is vital to diagnosing and managing these injuries. **Which one of the following statements is correct regarding the anatomy of this area?**
   E. The A2 and A4 annular pulleys are considered to be the most important to preserve.
   In 1959 Verdan[1] described five zones (not six) of flexor tendon injury, which relate to treatment and prognosis (see Fig. 59-5, *Essentials of Plastic Surgery,* second edition). Bunnell[2] had previously described zone II as *no-man's land* because of the poor outcomes of repair in this area. This zone lies between the A1 pulley and the FDS (not the FDP) insertion and represents a tight sheath that contains both flexors. The sheath comprises five annular and three cruciate pulleys (see Fig. 59-6, *Essentials of Plastic Surgery,* second edition). These function to prevent bowstringing and improve the mechanical advantage of tendons. The A2 and A4 pulleys are most important in preventing bowstringing and should be preserved during surgery. The odd-numbered annular pulleys are sited at the joints (MP, PIP, and DIP), whereas the even-numbered pulleys lie over the shafts of the phalanges. All cruciate pulleys lie between the annular pulleys; however, no cruciate pulley exists between A1 and A2.

9. You are repairing a complete FPL division from a knife wound over the proximal phalanx. The injury occurred during full flexion of the thumb. **Which one of the following statements is correct regarding the anatomy of this region?**
   C. Preservation of the oblique pulley is most important.
   The thumb flexor zones differ from those of the other digits (see Fig. 59-5, *Essentials of Plastic Surgery,* second edition) and an injury over the proximal phalanx is located in zone II. The thumb contains only one long flexor and three pulleys (one oblique and two annular) but does not have a cruciate pulley like the fingers. The most important pulley is the oblique pulley and this is at risk of damage in a zone II injury. It is a continuation of the adductor pollicis insertion and lies between the two annular pulleys. These are located at the MP joint and IP joints. When completely divided, the FPL tendon retracts proximally and is usually found just ulnar/deep to the FCR tendon in the wrist. The neurovascular bundles are less well protected in the thumb as they lie more superficially than in the other digits.

ARTERIAL SUPPLY TO THE HAND

10. **Which one of the following statements is correct regarding the arterial supply to the hand?**
    E. Kaplan's line is a useful marker of the superficial palmar arch.
    Kaplan[3] originally described the *cardinal line* in 1953 as a line "drawn from the apex of the interdigital fold between the thumb and index finger toward the ulnar side of the hand, parallel with the middle crease of the hand." It has also been described as a line drawn across the palm

from the first web space to the hook of the hamate (Fig. 59-2). Various authors have identified it as a useful landmark in carpal tunnel release, because the superficial palmar arch is usually distal to this line, ensuring dissection stops here will protect it from damage. The princeps pollicis artery arises from the deep palmar arch or from the radial artery direct (not the superficial arch) and is the dominant blood supply to the thumb. The ulnar artery lies radial (not ulnar) to the nerve and FCU at the wrist. The digital vessels lie dorsal to the nerve within the fingers and when patients describe profuse bleeding after sustaining a knife wound to the volar aspect of the digit, they are likely to have also transected the digital nerve. The deep palmar arch is formed by the largest branch of the radial, not ulnar, artery. (See Fig. 59-7, *Essentials of Plastic Surgery*, second edition.)

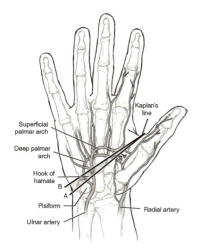

Fig. 59-2 Kaplan's line in relation to vascular anatomy of the hand.

INNERVATION OF THE HAND AND UPPER LIMB

11. Which one of the following actions would be lost after an injury to the ulnar nerve at the elbow?
   B. Flexion of the ring finger at the DIP joint
   Most of the extrinsic flexors are innervated by the median nerve, with the exception of the FDP to the little and ring fingers and the FCU. Loss of ulnar nerve function would affect the ability to flex both the little and ring fingers at the DIP joint. Flexion at the PIP joint would be spared because this is controlled by the median nerve innervated FDS. Flexion at the thumb IP joint and index finger DIP joint would also be spared as they are innervated by the anterior interosseus branch of the median nerve. The main wrist flexor is the FCU; however, wrist flexion is still possible with loss of FCU function because of the action of FCR.

12. Which one of the following is innervated by a branch of the median nerve?
   C. APB
   APB is innervated by the recurrent motor branch of the median nerve. It is a useful guide to median nerve function in the hand in relation to carpal tunnel syndrome. All of the other listed muscles are usually innervated by the ulnar nerve.

13. For each of the following descriptions, the correct nerve supply is as follows:
    A. Dorsum of the hand overlying the index metacarpal
       g. **Superficial branch of radial nerve**
    B. Volar aspect of the wrist overlying the ulnar artery
       e. **Medial antebrachial cutaneous nerve**
    C. Nail bed region of the long finger
       a. **Median nerve**
         The sensory nerve supply to the hand and wrist arises from branches of the radial, ulnar, median, medial antebrachial cutaneous, and musculocutaneous nerves. The lateral antebrachial cutaneous nerve arises from the musculocutaneous nerve, and the posterior antebrachial cutaneous nerve arises from the radial nerve. The sensory distribution differs on the volar surface compared with the dorsal surface (see Fig. 59-8, *Essentials of Plastic Surgery*, second edition.)

14. Which one of the following is usually spared in a posterior interosseous nerve palsy?
    A. **ECRL**
       BR and ECRL are usually supplied by the radial nerve before it branches into the superficial radial nerve and the posterior interosseous nerve (PIN), although sometimes ECRL is also supplied by the PIN. Therefore a patient with a posterior interosseous nerve palsy may still be able to extend their wrist.

15. Which one of the following is incorrect?
    C. **The Riche-Cannieu anastomosis is a sensory fiber connection between the ulnar and median nerves in the hand.**
       A Riche-Cannieu anastomosis is a motor fiber connection from the ulnar to median nerve in the hand and is thought to be present in as many as 70% of individuals. A Martin-Gruber anastomosis is a motor fiber connection from the median to ulnar nerve in the forearm that is present in 10% to 25% of the United States population.[4] A Berretini anastomosis can arise between the common digital nerves derived from the median and ulnar nerves.[5] A Martin-Gruber anastomosis can result in preserved ulnar nerve motor function in the hand after a high ulnar nerve injury. A Riche-Cannieu anastomosis can result in preserved thenar motor function after a more proximal median nerve injury. Therefore its presence can lead to confusion in a clinical examination, particularly in a trauma setting.

BONES OF THE WRIST

16. Which one of the following bones links the proximal and distal carpal rows?
    B. **Scaphoid**
       The distal row includes the trapezium, trapezoid, capitates, and hamate. The proximal carpal row includes the scaphoid, lunate, and triquetrum. The scaphoid links the proximal and distal rows and is the most commonly fractured carpal bone (the pisiform is a sesamoid bone within the FCU tendon and is not a functional part of the carpus) (Fig. 59-3).

Fig. 59-3 The space of Poirier *(white arrows)* is located between the lesser arc *(red dashed line)* and the greater arc *(black line)*. The greater arc represents the zone of fractures and dislocations, the lesser arc represents the zone of dislocations, and the space of Poirier is the vulnerable zone between them. Fibers of the radioscaphocapitate ligament *(left)* and ulnocapitate ligament *(right)* interdigitate and form an arclike ligamentous structure called the *arcuate ligament* in the greater arc region. The lesser arc outlines the lunate. The scapholunate ligament and lunotriquetral ligament are part of the lesser arc, which does not extend to the distal radius and ulna.

REFERENCES

1. Verdan CE. Primary repair of flexor tendons. *J Bone Joint Surg Am* 42:647-657, 1960.
2. Bunnell S. Surgery of the Hand, ed 2. Philadelphia: JB Lippincott, 1948.
3. Kaplan EB. Surface anatomy of the hand and wrist. In Spinner E, ed. Functional and Surgical Anatomy of the Hand. Philadelphia: JB Lippincott, 1953.
4. Rodriguez-Niedenführ M, Vazquez T, Parkin I, et al. Martin-Gruber anastomosis revisited. Clin Anat 15:129-134, 2002.
5. Tagil SM, Bozkurt MC, Ozçakar L, et al. Superficial palmar communications between the ulnar and median nerves in Turkish cadavers. Clin Anat 20:795-798, 2007.

60. Basic Hand Examination

See *Essentials of Plastic Surgery*, second edition, pp. 708-719.

NORMAL RANGE OF MOVEMENT IN THE HAND AND WRIST

1. A 35-year-old mechanic presents with pain and stiffness in his dominant hand and wrist after a fall 6 weeks earlier. **Which one of the following is most likely to represent a normal active joint range for this individual?**
   A. Index finger MP joint: −15 to +80 degrees
   B. Little finger MP joint: 0 to +70 degrees
   C. Middle finger PIP joint: −25 to +55 degrees
   D. Wrist extension/flexion −30 to +75 degrees
   E. Wrist radial/ulnar deviation: −10 to ±10 degrees

EXAMINING MOTOR FUNCTION

2. **When examining a patient following a hand injury, which one of the following is correct?**
   A. The FDP tendon is assessed by testing isolated flexion of the PIP joint.
   B. Isolated active flexion at the MP joint specifically tests integrity of the FPL tendon.
   C. Assessment of FDS requires isolation of the adjacent digits in flexion.
   D. AdP weakness may be masked by thumb IP joint flexion.
   E. APB is assessed with the hand placed flat with the palm down.

3. **When examining a patient following lacerations to the dorsum of the hand and wrist, which one of the following is correct?**
   A. EDC function can be confirmed by extending all four MP joints with IP joints in flexion.
   B. Isolated active extension at the thumb IP joint specifically tests the integrity of the EPL tendon.
   C. ECRL and ECRB cannot normally be independently assessed.
   D. APL and EPB are tested independently with different movements.
   E. ECU is best independently assessed by extending the wrist in neutral.

CLINICAL SIGNS OF PATHOLOGY

4. **When seeing a patient with de Quervain's tenosynovitis, which one of the following movements will most exacerbate their pain?**
   A. Wrist flexion
   B. Finger extension
   C. Thumb extension
   D. Ulnar deviation of the wrist
   E. Radial deviation of the wrist

5. Tinel's test is a technique used to assess nerve pathology in the upper limb. **Which one of the following is correct?**
   A. An advancing Tinel's sign over time is unreliable as a guide to nerve recovery.
   B. A positive Tinel's sign is tingling along the course of the nerve upon percussion.
   C. A positive Tinel's sign at the carpal tunnel is a diagnostic for carpal tunnel syndrome.
   D. The extent of a positive Tinel's sign is proportional to the severity of nerve compression.
   E. Tinel's sign is only applicable to the median nerve and carpal tunnel syndrome.

ASSESSING SPECIFIC NERVES IN THE UPPER LIMB

6. A patient has reduced sensation in the little and ring fingers and hypothenar eminence, with normal sensation on the dorso-ulnar aspect of the hand. **Which one of the following is most likely?**
   A. Diabetic neuropathy
   B. T1 nerve root compression
   C. Brachial plexus tumor
   D. Ulnar nerve compression at the elbow
   E. Ulnar nerve compression at the wrist

7. A patient presents for a medicolegal assessment, claiming a nerve injury 6 weeks ago when he cut his finger at work. He reports reduced sensation in the index finger. The skin feels moist and wrinkles on immersion in water. Static two-point discrimination at the tip is 4 mm. **Which one of the following is most likely?**
   A. Complete division of the digital nerve
   B. 50% division of the digital nerve
   C. No significant digital nerve injury
   D. Neuroma in continuity
   E. Compression of the digital nerve by scar tissue

8. A patient has 6/10 sensation in the dorsal first web space following a night in handcuffs. **Which one of the following is most likely?**
   A. Posterior interosseous nerve neurapraxia
   B. Proximal radial nerve injury from prolonged pronation
   C. Superficial radial nerve neuropraxia
   D. Lateral antebrachial cutaneous nerve neurapraxia
   E. Superficial radial nerve neurotmesis

Answers

NORMAL RANGE OF MOVEMENT IN THE HAND AND WRIST

1. A 35-year-old mechanic presents with pain and stiffness in his dominant hand and wrist after a fall 6 weeks earlier. **Which one of the following is most likely to represent a normal active joint range for this individual?**
   A. **Index finger MP joint −15 to +80 degrees**

   Joint range of motion does vary widely within the general population because of differences in age, joint laxity, and individual anatomy. Furthermore, active and passive ranges frequently differ with range increased on passive movement. The American Society for Surgery of the Hand (ASSH) offers a guide to normal joint ranges, which is worth reviewing[1] (Table 60-1).

   All of the ranges described in the clinical scenario are reduced for a healthy 35-year-old male, with the exception of answer option A. The MP joints have a large range of motion, both passive and active. This also differs between the digits, with most being present in the little finger which can commonly have 40 degrees of extension and 90 degrees of flexion. Range of motion progressively decreases in the MP joints moving radially from the little finger to index. This is in contrast to the PIP joint which normally has a range of 0 to 100 degrees only because of the box ligamentous structure and it is more consistent between the digits. It is vital to have a good understanding of normal and abnormal joint ranges when assessing hand patients in clinic. The best approach is to compare left with right in most cases, as this helps ascertain the "normal" or baseline range for each individual. Joint ranges must be documented in the notes, especially in conditions such as Dupuytren's disease or following a hand injury.

Table 60-1 *Normal Range of Motion Reference Values for the Upper Limb*

Typical Range of Motion (degrees)		
Elbow	Extension/flexion	0/145
Forearm	Pronation/supination	70/85
Wrist	Extension/flexion	70/75
	Radial/ulnar	20/35
Thumb basal joint	Palmar adduction/abduction	Contact or 45
	Radial adduction/abduction	Contact or 60
Thumb IPJ	Hyperextension/flexion	15/80
Thumb MPJ	Hyperextension/flexion	10/55
Finger DIPJ	Extension/flexion	0/80
Finger PIPJ	Extension/flexion	0/100
Finger MPJ	Hyperextension/flexion	(0-45/90)

EXAMINING MOTOR FUNCTION

2. When examining a patient following a hand injury, which one of the following is correct?
   D. AdP weakness may be masked by thumb flexion.

   To assess the AdP, a paper sheet is placed between the thumb and index finger, and the patient is asked to forcibly grasp it against resistance (see Fig. 60-13, *Essentials of Plastic Surgery,* second edition). Flexion at the thumb IP joint can occur to compensate when AdP is weak (positive Froment's test, which is a classic test for ulnar nerve function).

   The FDP is assessed by immobilizing the digit and testing for isolated DIP joint flexion. Assessment of the FDS requires that the adjacent digits are held in extension while flexion of the PIP joint is attempted (see Figs. 60-5 and 60-6, *Essentials of Plastic Surgery,* second edition). Immobilization is required to prevent the FDP from contributing to PIP joint flexion as it also crosses the joint. The FPL is assessed by active flexion of the IP joint, not the MP joint which is flexed by the thenar muscles APB, OP, and FPB (see Figs. 60-4 and 60-12, *Essentials of Plastic Surgery,* second edition).

   The APB is tested with the hand placed on a table and the palm facing upward not downward (see Fig. 60-3, *Essentials of Plastic Surgery,* second edition). The assessment of APB is a classic test for the recurrent motor branch of the median nerve at the wrist.

3. When examining a patient following lacerations to the dorsum of the hand and wrist, which one of the following is correct?
   A. EDC function can be confirmed by extending all four MP joints with IP joints in flexion.

   EDC function is assessed by asking the patient to extend the fingers at the knuckles (MP joint) with IP joints flexed, or asking them to straighten all fingers simultaneously. To independently assess the EIP and EDM/EDQ, the respective digits should be extended independently (see Fig. 60-10, *Essentials of Plastic Surgery,* second edition).

   Isolated active extension at the thumb IP joint does not specifically test for integrity of the EPL tendon, because the EPB can also cross this joint and be responsible for IP joint extension. The EPB insertion is highly variable: it is absent in around 5% of hands, inserts into the MP joint extensor hood in around 25%, into the base of the proximal phalanx in around 25%, and continues right up to the distal phalanx in 25%.[2] Therefore, to accurately assess EPL function, the patient should be asked to put their hand flat on a surface and lift their thumb up off that surface. The full length of the EPL tendon from the extensor retinaculum to IP joint will usually be seen and be palpable (see Fig. 60-9, *Essentials of Plastic Surgery,* second edition).

   ECRL and ECRB share the same action but can be independently assessed by palpation while asking the patient to make a fist and extend the wrist (see Fig. 60-8, *Essentials of Plastic Surgery,* second edition). APL and EPB are tested with the same movement but may also be differentiated by palpation of the tendons. The patient should be instructed to move their thumb out to the side or do a thumbs-up gesture (see Fig. 60-7, *Essentials of Plastic Surgery,* second edition). ECU is best tested by having the patient extend the wrist with ulnar deviation while palpating the tendon at the wrist (see Fig. 60-11, *Essentials of Plastic Surgery,* second edition).

CLINICAL SIGNS OF PATHOLOGY

4. **When seeing a patient with de Quervain's tenosynovitis, which one of the following movements will most exacerbate their plan?**
   D. Ulnar deviation of the wrist
   Patients with de Quervain's tenosynovitis have tenderness and swelling affecting the first extensor compartment. Pain is exacerbated by stretching the tendons passing within this compartment, namely APL and EPB. This can be tested with either Finkelstein's test or Eichoff's test. Both involve stretching of the tendon by pulling the hand into ulnar deviation and applying traction on the thumb. Although the test can be performed with the thumb clasped within the patient's own fingers, it is generally thought to generate more false-positive results than placement of traction on the relaxed thumb (Fig. 60-1, A and B).[3] There may also be discomfort during other movements, such as thumb extension where APL and EPB may be active, but ulnar deviation of the wrist is usually the most painful.

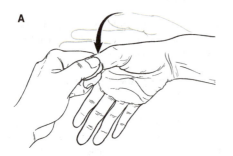
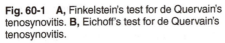
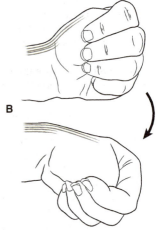

Fig. 60-1 **A,** Finkelstein's test for de Quervain's tenosynovitis. **B,** Eichoff's test for de Quervain's tenosynovitis.

5. **Tinel's test is a technique used to assess nerve pathology in the upper limb. Which one of the following is correct?**
   B. A positive Tinel's sign is tingling along the course of the nerve upon percussion.
   A positive Tinel's sign is indicated by a tingling sensation along the course of a nerve when it is tapped at a site of compression or regeneration. It is a useful method to assess nerve regeneration in cases such as two-stage facial reanimation techniques and following upper limb nerve injury (see Chapters 42 and 80, *Essentials of Plastic Surgery,* second edition). As nerve compression increases, progressive axonal loss can lead to a loss of Tinel's sign in more severe cases, but there is no proportional change relating to greater damage. Although Tinel's sign is used as part of a clinical examination for carpal tunnel syndrome and nerve regeneration, the results are variable and examiner dependent. Therefore this test is not diagnostic or reliable in isolation and should be combined with other information.[4]

ASSESSING SPECIFIC NERVES IN THE UPPER LIMB

6. A patient has reduced sensation in the little and ring fingers and hypothenar eminence, with normal sensation on the dorso-ulnar aspect of the hand. **Which one of the following is most likely?**
   E. Ulnar nerve compression at the wrist
   Sparing of the dorsal sensory branch of the ulnar nerve suggests pathology distal to this branch, which arises 5 to 7 cm proximal to the ulnar styloid. More proximal lesions, or a diffuse neuropathy, would usually affect all the distal functions of the nerve, both motor and sensory.

7. A patient presents for a medicolegal assessment, claiming a nerve injury 6 weeks ago when he cut his finger at work. He reports reduced sensation in the index finger. The skin feels moist and wrinkles on immersion in water. Static two-point discrimination at the tip is 4 mm. **Which one of the following is most likely?**
   C. No significant digital nerve injury
   This patient has objectively normal findings despite his subjective complaints. Although a degree of reduced sensation is reported, a significant digital nerve injury is very unlikely, with the normal two-point discrimination displayed (normal values for two-point discrimination are static, up to 6 mm in the fingertip, and dynamic 2 to 3 mm). Six weeks is too early for normal two-point discrimination to return after a complete or 50% nerve injury. Moist skin suggests preserved sweating, and wrinkling on immersion also suggests a largely intact digital nerve. Sweating is very useful to assess when suspecting digital nerve injury, as where a patient describes altered sensation distal to a laceration and the finger also feels smooth over the same distribution, division of the nerve is likely.

8. *A patient has 6/10 sensation in the dorsal first web space following a night in handcuffs. Which one of the following is most likely?*
   C. Superficial radial nerve neurapraxia
   This patient has most likely had a compression of the superficial radial nerve at the wrist from the handcuffs, resulting in a neurapraxia rather than a complete nerve division. The lateral antebrachial cutaneous nerve territory does not extend onto the hand. The posterior interosseous nerve has mainly motor function with the exception of sensory supply to the dorsal wrist capsule. A proximal radial nerve injury would involve motor weakness with decreased extension and wrist drop.

REFERENCES

1. American Society for Surgery of the Hand. Normal range of motion reference values. Available at http://www.assh.org/Public/HandAnatomy/Anatomy/Pages/Normal-Range-Motion.aspx.
2. Jabir S, Lyall H, Iwuagwu FC. The extensor pollicis brevis: a review of its anatomy and variations. Eplasty 13:e35, 2013.
3. Finkelstein H. Stenosing tenosynovitis at the radial styloid process. J Bone Joint Surg 12:509-540, 1930.
4. Lifchez SD, Means KR Jr, Dunn RE, et al. Intra- and inter-examiner variability in performing Tinel's test. J Hand Surg Am 35:212-216, 2010.

61. Congenital Hand Anomalies

See *Essentials of Plastic Surgery*, second edition, pp. 720-740.

EMBRYOLOGY

1. **Which one of the following is the most likely effect of interference with the zone of polarizing activity in the developing limb?**
   A. A truncated limb
   B. An absent limb
   C. A limb with absent fingernails
   D. A limb with abnormal ulnar development
   E. A limb with a hypoplastic thumb

CLASSIFICATION OF CONGENITAL ANOMALIES

2. **For each of the following clinical conditions, select the correct congenital classification descriptor according to the International Federation of Societies for Surgery of the Hand classification system. (Each option may be used once, more than once, or not at all.)**
   A. Syndactyly
   B. Streeter's syndrome
   C. Trigger thumb

   Options:
   a. Failure of formation
   b. Failure of differentiation
   c. Duplication
   d. Overgrowth
   e. Undergrowth
   f. Constriction band syndrome
   g. Generalized
   h. Does not fit into a classification category

CLASSIFICATION SYSTEMS FOR CONGENITAL LIMB ABNORMALITIES

3. **Which one of the following is predominantly classified according to radiologic features rather than clinical findings?**
   A. Thumb hypoplasia
   B. Constriction ring syndrome
   C. Macrodactyly
   D. Syndactyly
   E. Thumb duplication

SYNDACTYLY

4. A 2-month-old baby with complex syndactyly involving all four fingers is referred to you. **Which one of the following statements is correct regarding this condition?**
   A. The term *complex* implies additional hidden phalanges or joint anomalies.
   B. Radiographs will reliably predict the subtype of syndactyly.
   C. Correctional surgery can be performed in a single stage.
   D. A Buck-Gramko stiletto flap is the only reliable technique for correcting a tip deformity.
   E. This pattern of syndactyly is often associated with a syndrome.

5. You assess a 1-year-old white girl who has syndactyly of both hands. This is her initial presentation. **Which one of the following statements is correct regarding this condition?**
   A. The optimal time for surgery has passed.
   B. It is most likely to affect the middle and index fingers.
   C. Her condition is less common than camptodactyly.
   D. The frequency of this condition is much higher in the black population.
   E. Other family members are unlikely to be affected.

CAMPTODACTYLY

6. A 13-year-old girl presents with lifelong mild flexion contractures to both little finger PIP joints, which have become worse during puberty. Her range of motion in these joints is now 20 to 75 degrees. **Which one of the following statements is correct regarding her condition?**
   A. It more frequently affects the thumb and index finger.
   B. Presentation in girls of this age is fairly unusual.
   C. It is caused by abnormal flexor or extensor tendons.
   D. Her condition is easily correctable with modern surgical techniques.
   E. She should be treated nonoperatively with physiotherapy.

CLINODACTYLY

7. A patient with a diagnosis of clinodactyly is referred to you. **Which one of the following statements is correct regarding this condition?**
   A. Patients often present with painful, stiff digits.
   B. The head of the proximal phalanx is often abnormal.
   C. The ring finger is most commonly affected.
   D. K-wires should be used during surgical correction.
   E. Physiotherapy and splinting are sufficient treatments in many cases.

POLYDACTYLY

8. **Which one of the following statements is correct regarding polydactyly?**
   A. The true incidence is accurately recorded at 1:1000 live births.
   B. Classification systems are the same for preaxial and postaxial subtypes.
   C. Incidence remains fairly consistent across all racial groups.
   D. Treatment is almost always surgery, performed at one year of age.
   E. Other syndromes must be excluded in well-developed ulnar polydactyly.

MACRODACTYLY

9. You are referred a young patient with one digit significantly larger than the others. **Which one of the following is correct?**
   A. This condition only affects the soft tissues.
   B. Amputation is only rarely indicated.
   C. The digit will continue to grow disproportionately unless treated.
   D. The condition is usually bilateral and symmetrical.
   E. The patient may have associated soft tissue nodules and café au lait spots.

CLEFT HAND

10. You receive a referral letter about a child with typical cleft hand. **Which one of the following statements is correct?**
  A. The child is likely to have poor hand function.
  B. Syndactyly is unlikely to be a feature.
  C. Both hands are likely to be involved.
  D. Chest wall deformities are likely to be present.
  E. Metacarpal development is most likely to be normal.

CONSTRICTION BAND SYNDROME

11. You are asked to see a baby in the neonatal unit who has a grossly swollen purple toe distal to a tight band. You notice another constriction band at the ankle in the same limb. **Which one of the following statements is incorrect?**
  A. A hair tourniquet should be promptly excluded before diagnosing constriction ring syndrome in a digit.
  B. The full circumference of the band on the affected toe should be released.
  C. The band at the ankle can cause lymphedema as the child grows.
  D. A distal segment that is blue or purple should receive early surgical intervention.
  E. Plain radiographs can be helpful in planning treatment for the ankle.

PEDIATRIC TRIGGER THUMB

12. You are on call and receive a referral for a toddler whose thumb has spontaneously stuck in flexion at the IP joint. Gentle manipulation resolves the situation in clinic, and the thumb now functions normally. **Which one of the following is correct regarding this condition?**
  A. It is associated with Notta's node on the FPL tendon.
  B. Treatment is usually the same in children as it is in adults.
  C. Imaging should be requested to exclude bony pathology.
  D. The child should be scheduled for definitive correction on an elective basis.
  E. The chance that the contralateral thumb is affected is 50%.

TREATMENT OPTIONS FOR CONGENITAL HAND DEFORMITIES

13. *For each of the following conditions, select the most appropriate treatment option. (Each option may be used once, more than once, or not at all.)*
  A. Wassel type IV thumb duplication
  B. Blauth type 3B hypoplastic thumb
  C. Pouce flottant

  Options:
  a. Deletion of one duplicate, without disturbance of the other
  b. Bilhaut-Cloquet procedure
  c. Reverse (mirror) Z flaps
  d. Deletion of one duplicate and centralization of the other digit
  e. Amputation and pollicization of the index finger
  f. Opponensplasty only
  g. Closing wedge osteotomy
  h. Opponensplasty and first web space deepening

CLINICAL SCENARIOS IN CONGENITAL HAND ANOMALIES

14. Select the option that most appropriately describes each of the following conditions. (Each option may be used once, more than once, or not at all.)
    A. A 3-month-old baby has a radial deviation of the little finger beyond the PIP joint.
    B. A 16-week-old baby has a complete duplication of the left little finger.
    C. A 2-month-old girl has a duplicate thumb. A plain radiograph shows complete duplication of the proximal and distal phalanges.

Options:
a. Wassel type II preaxial polydactyly
b. Wassel type III preaxial polydactyly
c. Wassel type IV preaxial polydactyly
d. Type A postaxial polydactyly
e. Type B postaxial polydactyly
f. Type C postaxial polydactyly
g. Clinodactyly
h. Camptodactyly
i. Kirner's deformity

Answers

EMBRYOLOGY

1. Which one of the following is the most likely effect of interference with the zone of polarizing activity in the developing limb?

D. A limb with abnormal ulnar development

Embryologic development of the limb occurs primarily between weeks 5 and 8. Growth and development occur in three main directions: proximal to distal (axial), radial to ulnar (preaxial and postaxial), and volar to dorsal.

The zone of polarizing activity (ZPA) is a cluster of mesenchymal cells on the postaxial (ulnar) border and plays a role in preaxial/postaxial (radial to ulnar) differentiation. It induces ulnar formation and the four ulnar sided digits in the hand. Consequently, interference with the ZPA results in abnormal ulnar side development such as ulnar longitudinal deficiency. Volar/dorsal development is controlled by the dorsal ectoderm and the wingless-type protein. Altered development in this field can result in absence of the fingernails. The apical ectodermal ridge (AER) is an ectodermal thickening at the leading edge of the limb bud, responsible for axial development. Its removal leads to limb truncation. Progressive loss of FGF function at the AER leads to a loss of radial structures (for example, thumb hypoplasia).

CLASSIFICATION OF CONGENITAL ANOMALIES

2. For the following scenarios, the best options are as follows:

A. Syndactyly
  b. Failure of differentiation
B. Streeter's syndrome
  f. Constriction band syndrome
C. Trigger thumb
  h. Does not fit into a classification category

Swanson[1] described the uniformly accepted classification system for congenital hand anomalies in 1976. This has been adopted by most hand authorities, including the International Federation of Societies for Surgery of the Hand and the American Society for Surgery of the Hand. It has seven categories and is a popular topic for examination questions (Table 61-1). Syndactyly is the congenital fusion of two or more digits and is an example of failure to differentiate. The precise cause is unknown but the theory is that there may be a failure of digital patterning, failure of apoptosis between the digits, or failure of the apical ectodermal ridge regression.[2]

Constriction band syndrome has its own category within the classification system. It is sometimes known as congenital band syndrome or Streeter's syndrome and represents a breadth of abnormalities where limbs or digits become constricted leading to deformity or loss of the distal part. It is also associated with acrosyndactyly and may be confused with symbrachydactyly. It is thought to occur secondary to external amniotic band compression in utero.

Trigger thumb is not a true congenital deformity and so does not fit within the classification scheme. It represents a thickening of the FPL tendon which results in the thumb becoming stuck in flexion at the IP joint.

Chapter 61 ▪ Congenital Hand Anomalies   503

Table 61-1 *Classification for Congenital Hand Anomalies*[1]

Type		Examples
I	Failure of formation	Phocomelia, hypoplastic thumb, radial, central, or ulnar longitudinal deficiency
II	Failure of differentiation	Synostosis, syndactyly, radial head dislocation, symphalangism, camptodactyly, clinodactyly, Kirner's deformity
III	Duplication	Polydactyly, mirror hand, duplicate thumb
IV	Overgrowth	Macrodactyly
V	Undergrowth	Brachydactyly
VI	Constriction band	Constriction band
VII	Generalized	

CLASSIFICATION SYSTEMS FOR CONGENITAL LIMB ABNORMALITIES

3. Which one of the following is predominantly classified according to radiologic features rather than clinical findings?

E. Thumb duplication

Wassel[3] classified thumb duplication according to the underlying bony anatomy (see Fig. 61-4, *Essentials of Plastic Surgery,* second edition).
- Type I: Least common, occurs in 2%[4]
- Type IV: Most common, occurs in 43%[4]
- Type VII: Most complex, requires at least one triphalangeal thumb. Syndactyly is classified into incomplete/complete, simple/complex/complicated, according to both soft tissue and skeletal features.

Classification systems for the other abnormalities have also been described and these are largely based on clinical appearance.

Blauth[5] classified hypoplastic thumb anomalies, and Manske and McCaroll[6] modified them as follows:
- Type 1: Diminution of thenar muscle bulk, smaller thumb elements
- Type 2: Absence of thenar intrinsic muscles, decreased thumb-index web space, MP joint instability from the ulnar collateral ligament
- Type 3A: Type 2 with extrinsic muscle abnormalities, even less bony (metacarpal) element, stable CMCJ
- Type 3B: Type 3A with an unstable CMCJ
- Type 4: Floating thumb (pouce flottant): small pedicle holding a floating thumb
- Type 5: Completely absent thumb

A key point is that the presence or absence of a stable CMCJ will guide surgical management.

Patterson[7] classified constriction ring syndrome as follows:
- Type I: Simple constriction ring
- Type II: Constriction ring with deformity of the distal part
- Type III: Constriction with variable fusion of distal parts (acrosyndactyly)
- Type IV: Complete intrauterine disruption

Upton[8] classified macrodactyly as follows:
- Type I: Macrodactyly with lipofibromatosis of the nerve(s)
- Type II: Associated with neurofibromatosis (von Recklinghausen's disease)
- Type III: Macrodactyly with hyperostosis (very rare)
- Type IV: Macrodactyly with hemihypertrophy

Syndactyly tends to be classified according to both clinical and radiologic findings (see question 4).

SYNDACTYLY

4. A 2-month-old baby with complex syndactyly involving all four fingers is referred to you. *Which one of the following statements is correct regarding this condition?*

E. This pattern of syndactyly is often associated with a syndrome.

This pattern of syndactyly can occur as part of Apert's syndrome. The term *complex syndactyly* refers to bony fusion of the distal phalanges. Additional phalanges (polysyndactyly) and abnormal joints (for example, symphalangism) are classified as *complicated syndactyly*. This term is used inconsistently. It is sometimes used to describe significant neurovascular or tendinous anomalies or syndactyly that occurs as part of a syndrome (Fig. 61-1). (See *Essentials of Plastic Surgery*, second edition.[9])

Upton[10] classified the hand anomalies in Apert's syndrome as follows:
Type I: Complex syndactyly of all four fingers, the first web space is spared
Type II: Complex syndactyly of all four fingers, simple first web syndactyly
Type III: Complex syndactyly of all digits, including the thumb

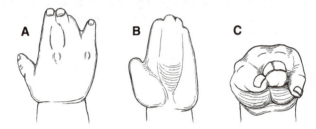

Fig. 61-1 A, Typical type I or spade-shaped hand. **B,** Type II or mitten hand. **C,** Type III or rosebud hand.

Radiographs are critical for evaluating bony involvement but can give false results as a result of incomplete ossification. Tip reconstruction can be performed with a Henty "pulp plasty" (see Fig. 61-2, *Essentials of Plastic Surgery*, second edition) or Buck-Gramko flaps. This case will require multiple surgical stages. A rule of thumb is that surgery should only be performed on one side of a digit at a time to minimize risk to the vascular supply.

5. You assess a 1-year-old white girl who has syndactyly of both hands. This is her initial presentation. *Which one of the following statements is correct regarding this condition?*

C. Her condition is less common than camptodactyly.

In the United States, the incidence of syndactyly is 1:2000 live births. This condition is 10 times more common in white people than in black people. The most common site is the third (not the second) web space. Up to 40% of cases have a family history of syndactyly. Syndactyly is much less common than camptodactyly, the incidence of which is probably closer to 1:100. It is difficult to define the optimal time for surgery, but it is commonly performed between 1 and 2 years of age provided it does not affect the border digits. If border digits are involved, correction is usually carried out earlier so that differential growth of the digits is not affected.

CAMPTODACTYLY

6. A 13-year-old girl presents with lifelong mild flexion contractures to both little finger PIP joints, which have become worse during puberty. Her range of motion in these joints is now 20 to 75 degrees. *Which one of the following statements is correct regarding her condition?*
E. She should be treated nonoperatively with physiotherapy.

Camptodactyly is a common condition typically affecting the little finger. It can be present and first noticed at birth or it can worsen with accelerated growth and only become evident around the time of puberty. Females are more commonly affected than males and presentation is common at this age. The underlying cause is not confirmed, but theories include abnormal flexor tendons (such as additional FDS slips), abnormal extensor tendons, bony deformities, or abnormal lumbrical insertions. Mild contractures should be managed with physiotherapy and extension splinting. More severe contractures may require surgical release. Plain radiographs should be obtained to exclude bony abnormalities.

CLINODACTYLY

7. A patient with a diagnosis of clinodactyly is referred to you. *Which one of the following statements is correct regarding this condition?*
D. K-wires should be used during surgical correction.

Clinodactyly refers to a curvature of the finger in a radial/ulnar direction and often features an abnormal middle phalanx. The physis may be C-shaped (bracketed) around one corner of the phalangeal base. The middle phalanx may be triangular or trapezoidal in shape and the former is termed a "delta" phalanx. These features prevent normal growth on one side resulting in uneven growth of the digit. The presence of a deformed head of the proximal phalanx is more typical of camptodactyly (see Fig. 61-3, *Essentials of Plastic Surgery*, second edition and question 7). Clinodactyly is usually painless and affects the little finger most frequently. Surgical correction nearly always requires a stabilizing K-wire. A Z-plasty may be required to release the soft tissues. Splinting is not an effective treatment for clinodactyly.

POLYDACTYLY

8. *Which one of the following statements is correct regarding polydactyly?*
E. Other syndromes must be excluded in well-developed ulnar polydactyly.

In well-developed ulnar polydactyly, there is a 30% risk of syndromic association, therefore a full workup should be arranged in such cases. Mild ulnar polydactyly is, however, rarely associated with other conditions and represents an isolated finding.

Although conditions such as Holt-Oram syndrome and Fanconi anemia are more common with radial longitudinal deficiency, an association also exists between them and radial polydactyly (specifically, triphalangeal thumb or Wassel type VII). Therefore it is prudent to ensure that the children with radial polydactyly are also fully assessed by a pediatrician.[11,12] Polydactyly is classified as preaxial or postaxial, depending on whether the radial or ulnar digits are duplicated. Postaxial subtypes are classified as A or B, depending on how well the extra digit is formed (A is well formed and B is rudimentary). Preaxial subtypes are classified using the Wassel system[8] as described in question 3. Both classifications are useful to guide management. Incidence is estimated to be between 1:300 and 1:3000 depending on subtype and race. These may be underestimates because of autoamputation of rudimentary digits at an early age. Surgery is not required for the majority of polydactyly cases. Treatment requirements depend on the subtype and extent of the abnormality. For example, mild ulnar polydactyly may autoamputate or be managed with simple ligation.

MACRODACTYLY

9. You are referred a young patient with one digit significantly larger than the others. **Which one of the following is correct?**
   E. **The patient may have associated soft tissue nodules and café au lait spots.**
   Macrodactyly is a condition of overgrowth of a digit and is usually an isolated unilateral finding, but may be associated with other conditions such as neurofibromatosis. For this reason, a full assessment of the other features associated with neurofibromatosis should be explored. The etiology is largely unknown but the most common theory is that the growth is somehow nerve induced. There are different types of macrodactyly (static or progressive) and growth may therefore be proportional or disproportionate to other digits. Both soft tissue and bone are usually affected and amputation may be the best option for some patients, although debulking is generally performed as a first-line treatment. The psychological effects of this condition can be severe, so a multidisciplinary approach including counseling is advised.

CLEFT HAND

10. You receive a referral letter about a child with typical cleft hand. **Which one of the following statements is correct?**
    C. **Both hands are likely to be involved.**
    Typical cleft hand is normally bilateral and familial. Syndactyly is a common finding. Hand function is usually very good but cosmesis is poor. For this reason, Flatt described it as a "functional triumph, but a social disaster." Metacarpal abnormalities are common, as these bones can be absent, bifid, or duplicated. This condition may be associated with cleft lip or cleft palate so the oral cavity should be assessed during examination. Atypical cleft hand differs from typical cleft hand and can occur as part of Poland's syndrome. Therefore it can be associated with any of the other common features of Poland's syndrome such as chest wall deformity, upper limb abnormality, or breast hypoplasia (see *Essentials of Plastic Surgery,* second edition). Atypical cleft hand is unilateral and spontaneous with syndactyly occurring infrequently. The remaining digits can be markedly hypoplastic.

CONSTRICTION BAND SYNDROME

11. You are asked to see a baby in the neonatal unit who has a grossly swollen purple toe distal to a tight band. You notice another constriction band at the ankle in the same limb. **Which one of the following statements is incorrect?**
    B. **The full circumference of the band on the affected toe should be released.**
    Vascular compromise in the toe warrants prompt surgical release. However, it is advisable to release no more than 50% of the circumference at one time to reduce the risk of exacerbating vascular compromise. If the toe were simply lymphedematous, observation and elevation would be sufficient at this early stage. As a child grows, constriction bands can interfere with deeper structures, and plain radiographs can be helpful to monitor the underlying ankle joint. Hair tourniquets around the toes of infants are commonly referred to plastic surgery for review. The hair is usually very difficult to visualize even with loupe magnification and management may require blade division of the hair down to or through the skin to ensure adequate release.

PEDIATRIC TRIGGER THUMB

12. You are on call and receive a referral for a toddler whose thumb has spontaneously stuck in flexion at the IP joint. Gentle manipulation resolves the situation in clinic, and the thumb now functions normally. **Which one of the following statements is correct regarding this condition?**
    A. **It is associated with Notta's node on the FPL tendon.**

    Trigger thumb in a child is treated differently from that in adults. Half of all cases of pediatric trigger thumb will settle without surgery within 6 months. Steroid injections usually provide no benefit. It is bilateral in only a quarter (not half) of cases, and imaging is rarely indicated unless trauma has occurred. Notta's node is a thickening on the FPL tendon that catches on the A1 pulley. This pulley is surgically released in persistent cases. The diagnosis should be explained to the parents and follow-up planned for approximately 6 to 8 weeks.

TREATMENT OPTIONS FOR CONGENITAL HAND DEFORMITIES

13. For the following conditions, the best options are as follows:
    A. Wassel type IV thumb duplication
       d. **Deletion of one duplicate and centralization of the digit**
    B. Blauth type 3B hypoplastic thumb
       e. **Amputation and pollicization of the index finger**
    C. Pouce flottant
       e. **Amputation and pollicization of the index finger**

    Wassel type IV duplications are most commonly treated by removal of the less favorable duplicate. Elements of both duplicates may be combined to produce the best overall function (for example, preservation and reinsertion of tendons onto the remaining digit). The remaining digit should be centralized to a functional axis, which may require a wedge osteotomy to the proximal phalanx or narrowing of the metacarpal head (see Fig. 61-6, *Essentials of Plastic Surgery*, second edition).

    Pollicization is typically preferred for types 3B, 4, and 5 in Blauth's classification of thumb hypoplasia. Pouce flottant is classified as type 4.

CLINICAL SCENARIOS IN CONGENITAL HAND ANOMALIES

14. For the following scenarios, the best options are as follows:
    A. A 3-month-old baby has a radial deviation of the little finger beyond the PIP joint.
       g. **Clinodactyly (Fig. 61-2, *A*)**
    B. A 16-week-old baby has a complete duplication of the left little finger.
       d. **Type A postaxial polydactyly**
    C. A 2-month-old girl has a duplicate thumb. A plain radiograph shows complete duplication of the proximal and distal phalanges.
       c. **Wassel type IV preaxial polydactyly (Fig. 61-2, *B*)**

    As discussed in question 7, clinodactyly presents most commonly as radial deviation of the little finger caused by an underlying bracketed physis. As discussed in question 8, ulnar polydactyly can be grouped as type A (a well-developed supernumerary digit) and type B (a rudimentary, pedunculated digit). The Wassel classification is used to describe thumb duplication and type IV thumb duplication is the most common type. Kirner's deformity is

volar-radial curvature of the distal phalanx caused by an abnormality of the physis of the distal phalanx, with tethering of the distal phalanx by an abnormal FDP insertion. Camptodactyly is a congenital flexion deformity of the little finger PIP joint which may be caused by abnormal lumbricals, flexor tendon slips, or PIP joint capsule.

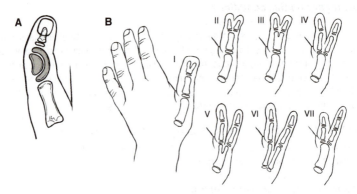

Fig. 61-2 A, Clinodactyly caused by a longitudinally bracketed physis. **B,** Wassel classification of thumb polydactyly.

References

1. Swanson AB. A classification for congenital limb malformations. J Hand Surg Am 1:8-22, 1976.
2. Choi, M, Sharma S, Louie O. Congenital hand abnormalities. In Thorne C, ed. Grabb & Smith's Plastic Surgery, ed 6. Philadelphia: Lippincott Williams & Wilkins, 2006.
3. Wassel HD. The results of surgery for polydactyly of the thumb. A review. Clin Ortho Relat Res 64:175-193, 1969.
4. Flatt AE, ed. The Care of Congenital Hand Anomalies, ed 2. St Louis: Quality Medical Publishing, 1994.
5. Blauth W. [The hypoplastic thumb] Arch Orthop Unfallchir 62:225-246, 1967.
6. Manske PR, McCaroll HR Jr. Index finger pollicization for a congenitally absent or nonfunctioning thumb. J Hand Surg Am 10:606-613, 1985.
7. Patterson TJ. Congenital ring-constrictions. Br J Plast Surg 14:1-31, 1961.
8. Upton J. Congenital anomalies of the hand and forearm. In McCarthy JG, ed. Plastic Surgery, vol 8, ed 2. Philadelphia: WB Saunders, 1990.
9. Janis JE, ed. Essentials of Plastic Surgery, ed 2. St Louis: Quality Medical Publishing, 2014.
10. Upton J. Apert syndrome: classification and pathologic anatomy of limb anomalies. Clin Plast Surg 18:321-355, 1991.
11. Castilla EE, Lugarinho R, da Graça Dutra M, et al. Associated anomalies in individuals with polydactyly. Am J Med Genet 80:459-465, 1998.
12. Wilks DJ, Kay SP, Bourke G. Fanconi's anemia and unilateral thumb polydactyly—don't miss it. J Plast Reconstr Aesthet Surg 65:1083-1086, 2012.

62. Carpal Bone Fractures

See *Essentials of Plastic Surgery*, second edition, pp. 741-749.

THE SCAPHOID BONE

1. **Which one of the following statements is correct regarding the scaphoid bone?**
   A. It is most commonly fractured in children and adolescents.
   B. Its entire surface is covered with articular cartilage.
   C. It is the only bone to bridge the proximal and distal carpal rows.
   D. It is supplied by a single distal vascular pedicle originating from the radial artery.
   E. The volar portion of the scapholunate ligament is stronger than the dorsal component.

DIAGNOSING A SCAPHOID FRACTURE

2. **Which one of the following statements is correct regarding the process of diagnosing a scaphoid fracture?**
   A. Forced hyperextension is the key mechanism causing scaphoid waist fractures.
   B. Tenderness in the anatomical snuffbox is highly specific for a scaphoid fracture.
   C. Comprehensive five-view radiographic imaging can reliably exclude a scaphoid fracture.
   D. An MRI scan of the wrist should normally be obtained in the acute setting.
   E. Bone scans can be a useful aid in fracture diagnosis after a few weeks.

TREATMENT OF SCAPHOID FRACTURES

3. A 20-year-old woman presents with an acute, proximal pole scaphoid fracture. Plain radiographs confirm the fracture is nondisplaced. **Which one of the following statements is correct regarding management of this patient?**
   A. Nonoperative management in a short arm cast should be undertaken.
   B. She will benefit from internal fixation with a differential pitch screw.
   C. Splinting in a thumb spica cast is required for up to 6 weeks.
   D. Her profession will be the main factor in guiding treatment selection.
   E. If internal fixation is selected, a volar approach must be used.

COMPLICATIONS AFTER SCAPHOID FRACTURES

4. A 30-year-old man is referred to you with a persistent nonunion of a scaphoid fracture 8 weeks after immobilization. **Which one of the following statements is correct regarding the sequelae of scaphoid fractures?**
   A. Nonunion of a wrist fracture can result in a volar intercalated segment instability (VISI) deformity.
   B. Scaphoid nonunion can result in a scapholunate advanced collapse (SLAC) wrist deformity.
   C. A humpback deformity following scaphoid malunion requires surgical intervention.
   D. Degenerative arthritis of the wrist is common after proximal scaphoid nonunion.
   E. A delayed union is diagnosed if pain is ongoing and no radiographic evidence of union is seen after 6 to 8 weeks of immobilization.

CARPAL BONE FRACTURES

5. **Which one of the following statements is correct regarding carpal bone fractures?**
   A. Fractures of the hook of the hamate are unlikely to be associated with a nerve injury.
   B. Hamate fractures represent approximately 40% of all carpal bone fractures.
   C. Fractures to the pisiform are easily viewed on AP and lateral radiographs.
   D. Hamate body fractures can occur with fourth and fifth CMC joint dislocations and may require fixation.
   E. The triquetrum tends to fracture with forced thumb hyperextension.

6. **For each of the following descriptions, select the most likely carpal bone involved. (Each option may be used once, more than once, or not at all.)**
   A. *This carpal bone is involved in Kienbock's disease which may develop spontaneously or following carpal bone fracture.*
   B. *This carpal bone may be fractured during a wrist hyperextension injury through the "anvil mechanism."*
   C. *This carpal bone is the least commonly fractured, as a result of the protection of the surrounding bony anatomy and strong carpal ligaments.*

   Options:
   a. Scaphoid
   b. Triquetrum
   c. Hamate
   d. Trapezium
   e. Capitate
   f. Lunate
   g. Trapezoid
   h. Pisiform

DELAYED PRESENTATION OF CARPAL BONE FRACTURES

7. A young male patient presents with a spontaneous inability to flex the little finger at the PIP and DIP joints. There has been no recent trauma to the little finger itself, but about 3 months ago he sustained a fall onto his outstretched hand while mountain biking. He sought no medical intervention but has continued to have a tender wrist. Plain radiographs confirm evidence of a carpal bone fracture. **Which one of the following is most likely to be involved?**
   A. Hook of hamate
   B. Body of hamate
   C. Body of triquetrum
   D. Volar pole of lunate
   E. Body of capitate

Answers

THE SCAPHOID BONE

1. Which one of the following statements is correct regarding the scaphoid bone?
C. It is the only bone to bridge the proximal and distal carpal rows.

The scaphoid is a component of the proximal carpal row and is the only bone to bridge both proximal and distal rows. It is an important component in normal wrist function. While it is the most commonly fractured bone of the carpus, fractures are uncommon in children while it remains cartilaginous. Approximately 80% of the surface is covered with articular cartilage, leaving a thin strip around the dorsal waist where most blood supply enters. The scaphoid has two (not one) vascular pedicles, both of which originate from the radial artery; one at the distal tubercle, supplying 20%, and one along the dorsal ridge which supplies the remaining 80%. There are no vessels entering proximal to the wrist, hence the higher rate of nonunion and avascular necrosis with proximal fractures. During surgery, care should be taken to preserve the dorsal ridge region of vascular supply.[1] The dorsal scapholunate ligament is much stronger and this helps to prevent excessive flexion of the scaphoid relative to the lunate.

DIAGNOSING A SCAPHOID FRACTURE

2. Which one of the following statements is correct regarding the process of diagnosing a scaphoid fracture?
E. Bone scans can be a useful aid in fracture diagnosis after a few weeks.

The standard approach to imaging for suspected scaphoid fractures is five-view radiographs. There are variations between institutions regarding the series of images acquired. A typical series includes PA, lateral, oblique, clenched fist, and scaphoid views. Despite this, normal radiographs cannot always exclude a scaphoid fracture, so they may need to be repeated after 2 or 3 weeks or augmented by additional investigations. CT imaging can provide a more detailed examination of the scaphoid. After a few weeks, bone scans can also be useful because they show increased isotope activity along the fracture line. While CT is helpful in identifying the scaphoid and its alignment,[2] MRI is preferred by many in the acute phase, as other causes of pain (such as bone contusions) may also be demonstrated. However, the cost of this modality and the difficulties in getting timely access to scans precludes its routine use in most patients. There are two main mechanisms of injury for scaphoid fracture: axial loading from a punch injury and hyperextension injuries, such as occur during a fall onto the outstretched hand. Axial loading frequently results in fractures of the wrist (see Fig. 62-2, *Essentials of Plastic Surgery,* second edition). Although tenderness in the anatomic snuffbox is common in scaphoid fractures, it is nonspecific and is seen in some normal people and with many other conditions. When there is an acute scaphoid fracture present, there is normally additional volar or dorsal tenderness identified.

TREATMENT OF SCAPHOID FRACTURES

3. A 20-year-old woman presents with an acute, proximal pole scaphoid fracture. Plain radiographs confirm the fracture is nondisplaced. **Which one of the following statements is correct regarding management of this patient?**
B. She will benefit from internal fixation with a differential pitch screw.

Most nondisplaced scaphoid fractures heal well with immobilization. However, internal fixation is recommended for proximal pole fractures because of high rates of nonunion. Otherwise, internal fixation is usually reserved for displaced fractures and those with delayed union. Internal fixation uses a solid or cannulated screw placed across the fracture site. Screws with a differential pitch are preferred to provide compression across the fracture site. Nonoperative management requires an extended duration of immobilization for a total of 12 weeks. The first 6 weeks should be in a long arm thumb spica cast and the second 6 weeks in a short arm thumb spica cast. Consequently, a patient's profession should be taken into account when selecting treatment as internal fixation may be preferable to reduce the immobilization period. It is not the main factor, however, in guiding treatment for a proximal pole fracture. Either a dorsal or volar approach can be used for internal fixation, but the dorsal approach provides a better exposure of the proximal pole.

COMPLICATIONS AFTER SCAPHOID FRACTURES

4. A 30-year-old man is referred to you with a persistent nonunion of a scaphoid fracture 8 weeks after immobilization. **Which one of the following statements is correct regarding the sequelae of scaphoid fractures?**
   D. **Degenerative arthritis of the wrist is common after proximal scaphoid nonunion.**
   One of the main problems with inadequately treated scaphoid fractures is chronic wrist pain and development of degenerative osteoarthritis. Scaphoid nonunion can result in instability of the intercalated segment of the wrist (the lunate and associated components of the proximal carpal row). This usually results in extension of or a dorsal angulation of the lunate (that is, dorsal intercalated segment instability [DISI, not VISI]). Over time, the resulting degenerative change in the wrist can lead to a scaphoid nonunion-advanced collapse (SNAC) wrist deformity.[3] A humpback deformity can be associated with DISI deformity and reduced function but it is not always symptomatic and does not therefore always require surgical correction.[4] Delayed union is diagnosed if symptoms persist with no radiographic evidence of healing after 4 months of immobilization, although some would diagnose this earlier than four months. If the fracture lines appear sclerotic, this is nonunion.

CARPAL BONE FRACTURES

5. **Which one of the following statements is correct regarding carpal bone fractures?**
   D. **Hamate body fractures can occur with fourth and fifth CMC joint dislocations and may require fixation.**
   Hamate fractures either involve the body or the hook (hamulus). Fractures of the body most commonly occur because of the axial load through the wrist, such as occurs during a punch injury. In patients who present with fourth and fifth metacarpal base fractures following an axial loading, careful examination of the CMC joints and hamate is required during assessment. These injuries may cause a hamate body fracture in the coronal plane with dorsal translation of the fractured segment. A CT scan is warranted in this situation and the hamate fracture may require K-wire or screw fixation. Hamulus fractures may directly injure the ulnar nerve and artery, or cause compression due to hematoma in Guyon's canal. Therefore careful examination of the ulnar nerve must be performed.

   While hamate fractures are relatively common, they represent fewer than 40% of all carpal bone fractures. The scaphoid is most commonly fractured (70%) followed by the triquetrum. The pisiform is a sesamoid bone in the FCU that can be fractured due to direct trauma. Plain radiographs frequently do not demonstrate these injuries and specific carpal tunnel views or CT scans are required. Trapezium (not triquetrum) fractures are thought to occur with combined hyperextension and abduction forces to the thumb.

Chapter 62 • Carpal Bone Fractures

6. *For each of the following descriptions, the best options are as follows:*
   A. *This carpal bone is involved in Kienbock's disease which may develop spontaneously or following carpal bone fracture.*
      f. Lunate
   B. *This carpal bone may be fractured during a wrist hyperextension injury through the "anvil mechanism."*
      e. Capitate
   C. *This carpal bone is the least commonly fractured, as a result of the protection of the surrounding bony anatomy and strong carpal ligaments.*
      g. Trapezoid

   Kienbock's disease is a condition of avascular necrosis of the lunate. It may occur spontaneously or following a nonunion of a lunate fracture. Alternatively, Kienbock's may first present with a pathologic fracture of the lunate. Prompt management of displaced lunate body fractures is advocated to minimize the risk of nonunion or Kienbock's. The capitate is at risk of transverse body fracture during forced hyperextension when the capitate is forced against the distal radius through the anvil mechanism (see Fig. 62-4, *Essentials of Plastic Surgery*, second edition). This can result in 180-degree rotation of the proximal fragment which cannot heal without formal reduction and stabilization. Patients remain at risk of avascular necrosis of the proximal fragment. The trapezoid is the least commonly fractured carpal bone, as it is well protected by surrounding tissues. However, chronic injuries may require second CMC joint arthrodesis.

DELAYED PRESENTATION OF CARPAL BONE FRACTURES

7. A young male patient presents with a spontaneous inability to flex the little finger at the PIP and DIP joints. There has been no recent trauma to the little finger itself, but about 3 months ago he sustained a fall onto his outstretched hand while mountain biking. He sought no medical intervention but has continued to have a tender wrist. Plain radiographs confirm evidence of a carpal bone fracture. **Which one of the following is most likely to be involved?**
   A. Hook of hamate

   Untreated hook of hamate fractures can present with delayed spontaneous rupture of the little finger flexor tendons. Attrition ruptures of the tendon occur secondary to degenerative bony changes at the fracture site where nonunion has occurred. In this case, the hamulus fragment should be excised in addition to addressing the flexor tendon ruptures.

REFERENCES

1. Nakamura R, Imaeda T, Horii E, et al. Analysis of scaphoid fracture displacement by three-dimensional computed tomography. J Hand Surg Am 16:485-492, 1991.
2. Gelberman RH, Menon J. The vascularity of the scaphoid bone. J Hand Surg Am 5:508-513, 1980.
3. Taleisnik J, Watson HK. Midcarpal instability caused by malunited fractures of the distal radius. J Hand Surg Am 20:57-62, 1995.
4. Jiranek WA, Ruby LK, Millender LB, et al. Long-term results after Russe bone-grafting: the effect of malunion of the scaphoid. J Bone Joint Surg Am 74:1217-1228, 1992.

63. Carpal Instability and Dislocations

See *Essentials of Plastic Surgery*, second edition, pp. 750-772.

CARPAL INSTABILITY

1. **Which one of the following statements is correct when describing carpal instability?**
   A. Carpal instability dissociative (CID) is instability between the distal radius and the carpus.
   B. Carpal instability nondissociative (CIND) is instability that does not show on a plain radiograph.
   C. Carpal instability adaptive (CIA) is usually due to a deformity of the distal radius.
   D. A dorsal intercalated segment instability (DISI) deformity is characterized by extension of the lunate and scaphoid.
   E. A volar intercalated segment instability (VISI) deformity is characterized by an increased scapholunate angle.

RECOGNITION OF A CARPAL INJURY

2. **Which one of the following statements is correct regarding assessment of a plain radiograph of an injured wrist?**
   A. Lesser arc injuries involve ligamentous disruption with a scaphoid fracture.
   B. The cortical ring sign represents hyperflexion of the scaphoid.
   C. A scapholunate angle of less than 30 degrees implies a scapholunate ligament disruption.
   D. Dorsal angulation of the lunate implies disruption of the lunotriquetral ligament.
   E. A proximal pole capitate fracture may be an isolated injury.

EXAMINATION FINDINGS IN CARPAL INSTABILITY

3. A patient with chronic wrist pain has a positive Watson test on examination. **Which one of the following structures is most likely to be injured?**
   A. Scaphoid bone
   B. Radial styloid
   C. Radioscapholunate ligament
   D. Lunotriquetral ligament
   E. Scapholunate ligament

4. A patient is referred with a stage III perilunate injury. **Which one of the following findings is least likely to be present?**
   A. Median nerve paresthesias
   B. A fracture of the radial styloid
   C. A tear in the space of Poirier
   D. Lunate dislocation into the carpal tunnel
   E. Lunotriquetral ligament rupture

LIGAMENTS OF THE WRIST

5. You are opening a wrist to reduce and repair a perilunate dislocation. ***Which one of the following statements is correct?***
   A. A dorsal capsular flap must be used to preserve the ligaments.
   B. A triangular capsular flap is required to preserve the volar ligaments.
   C. The dorsal scapholunate ligament usually requires repair.
   D. The lunate is commonly dislocated into the carpal tunnel.
   E. A volar incision should be avoided to protect the median nerve.

MANAGEMENT OF CARPAL INSTABILITY

6. A young patient presents with persistent pain and instability 6 months after a closed wrist injury. A scapholunate ligament disruption is confirmed. ***Which one of the following is the most likely treatment?***
   A. Bone anchor repair of the ligament
   B. Radiolunate fusion
   C. FCR ligament reconstruction
   D. Radioscapholunate fusion
   E. Percutaneous K-wiring

WRIST ARTHROSCOPY

7. You are performing arthroscopy to investigate chronic wrist pain in a 40-year-old woman. ***Which one of the following is correct?***
   A. Your first portal is likely to be the 1-2 interval portal.
   B. The EPL tendon is at risk of injury at the 4-5 interval portal.
   C. The 4-5 interval portal is the most common viewing portal.
   D. Ligamentous injuries should be graded according to the Geissler system.
   E. A 4 mm wide, 30-degree viewing scope is most appropriate.

Answers

CARPAL INSTABILITY

1. Which one of the following statements is correct when describing carpal instability?

C. Carpal instability adaptive (CIA) is usually due to a deformity of the distal radius.

CIA refers to compensatory changes in the carpus to accommodate an extrinsic problem, the most common of which is an uneven platform following a distal radius fracture. CID refers to instability between bones of the same carpal row (for example, scaphoid and lunate or lunate and triquetrum). CIND refers to instability of the entire proximal row (for example, scaphoid, lunate, and triquetrum), relative to either the distal carpal row or the radius and TFCC.

A dorsal intercalated segment instability (DISI) deformity is characterized by extension of the lunate in the lateral view with flexion of the scaphoid, giving a scapholunate angle greater than 60 degrees (Fig. 63-1). A volar intercalated segment instability (VISI) deformity is characterized by a reduced scapholunate angle less than 30 degrees (see Table 63-1, *Essentials of Plastic Surgery*, second edition).

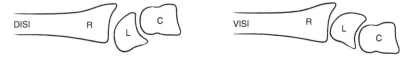

Fig. 63-1 In dorsal intercalated segment instability *(DISI)* the lunate *(L)* tilts dorsally. In volar intercalated segment instability *(VISI)* the lunate tilts volarly. (*C*, Capitate; *R*, radius.)

RECOGNITION OF A CARPAL INJURY

2. Which one of the following statements is correct regarding assessment of a plain radiograph of an injured wrist?

B. The cortical ring sign represents hyperflexion of the scaphoid.

A flexed scaphoid gives a cortical ring appearance in the AP view (see Fig. 63-12, *Essentials of Plastic Surgery*, second edition). The proximal carpal row includes the scaphoid, lunate, and triquetrum (see Fig. 63-7, *Essentials of Plastic Surgery*, second edition). The lunate is referred to as the *intercalated segment*, because its movements are heavily influenced by the ligamentous complexes between these three bones. When the lunotriquetral ligament complex is disrupted, the lunate becomes volarly angulated giving a scapholunate angle of less than 30 degrees. When the scapholunate ligament complex is disrupted, the lunate becomes more dorsally angulated under the influence of the lunotriquetral ligament complex. This increases the scapholunate angle to more than 60 degrees in the lateral view. Progressive perilunate injuries may be purely ligamentous, passing along the lesser arc. When fractures of either the radial styloid, scaphoid, capitate, or triquetrum occur, this is considered a greater arc injury (see Fig. 63-7, *Essentials of Plastic Surgery*, second edition). A proximal pole capitates fracture is usually part of a greater arc injury and therefore not an isolated injury.

Chapter 63 ▪ Carpal Instability and Dislocations   517

EXAMINATION FINDINGS IN CARPAL INSTABILITY

3. A patient with chronic wrist pain has a positive Watson test on examination. **Which one of the following structures is most likely to be injured?**
   E. Scapholunate ligament
   A positive Watson test corresponds to a "clunk" felt during dynamic wrist loading. The Watson (scaphoid shift) test assesses scaphoid instability (see Fig. 63-10, *Essentials of Plastic Surgery, second edition*). It particularly stresses the scapholunate ligament but may be positive in other problems affecting carpal stability. The test is performed as follows:
   The examiner holds the scaphoid in full extension by placing pressure over the tubercle on the volar side while the wrist is in full extension and ulnar deviation. The examiner's thumb prevents normal flexion of the scaphoid as the wrist is moved from ulnar to radial deviation and pressure is maintained over the tubercle on the volar aspect. The movement is then reversed. As the rest of the carpus moves, the restrained scaphoid has to "catch up" with the lunate and other bones. This occurs gradually if ligament integrity is normal. If the scapholunate ligament is damaged, or another disruption to carpal integration is present, the scaphoid can be restrained in the abnormal position for a prolonged period and palpated as a bulge on the dorsum of the wrist. As the other carpal bones move, the scaphoid has to jump back into position in the scaphoid fossa of the radius. This usually reproduces pain or a clunk. However, a slight clunk or discomfort can occur even in individuals with normal ligament integrity.

4. A patient is referred with stage III perilunate injury. **Which one of the following findings is least likely to be present?**
   D. Lunate dislocation into the carpal tunnel
   Mayfield et al[1] described four stages of progressive perilunate injury:
   Stage I: Scapholunate diastasis
   Stage II: Dorsal dislocation of capitate
   Stage III: Lunotriquetral dissociation
   Stage IV: Dislocation of the lunate volarly
   Any of the features described in options A through E may be seen in a stage III injury with the exception of dislocation of the lunate into the carpal tunnel, which would render this a stage IV injury. Median nerve paresthesias are common following perilunate injury, and extended carpal tunnel decompression is frequently required as a result. Purely ligamentous injuries occur along the lesser arc, while fracture dislocations such as with a styloid or scaphoid fracture occur along the greater arc. As such, a radial styloid fracture or lunotriquetrial ligament rupture could be seen in a stage III injury. The space of Poirier represents a weak zone in the volar wrist capsule and is usually torn in perilunate injuries.

LIGAMENTS OF THE WRIST

5. You are opening a wrist to reduce and repair a perilunate dislocation. **Which one of the following statements is correct?**
   C. The dorsal scapholunate ligament usually requires repair.
   Unless there is a transscaphoid fracture dislocation, there is always some scapholunate ligament damage in perilunate injuries. A dorsal ligament-sparing capsular flap has been described by Berger[2] which comprises a chevron with the apex ulnar ward over the triquetrum to preserve integrity of the dorsal radiocarpal (DRC) and dorsal intercarpal (DIC) ligament fibers (Fig. 63-2). While this approach is popular with many surgeons, there is insufficient outcome data to prove superiority over a simple dorsal capsular incision and some would argue that the wrist will be immobilized any way for a sufficient period to avoid subsequent instability due to dorsal ligament insufficiency.

As discussed in question 4, the lunate is only found in the carpal tunnel in stage IV injuries. A volar incision is often employed to decompress the median nerve, to repair the volar capsule, and to aid in relocation of a completely dislocated lunate.

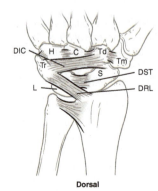

Fig. 63-2 Dorsal ligaments of the wrist. (*C*, Capitate; *DIC*, dorsal intercarpal ligament; *DRL*, dorsal radiocarpal ligament; *DST*, dorsal scaphotriquetral ligament; *H*, hamate; *L*, lunate; *S*, scaphoid; *Td*, trapezoid; *Tm*, trapezium; *Tr*, triquetrum.)

MANAGEMENT OF CARPAL INSTABILITY

6. A young patient presents with persistent pain and instability six months after a closed wrist injury. A scapholunate ligament disruption is confirmed. **Which one of the following is the most likely treatment?**
   C. FCR ligament reconstruction
   Brunelli and Brunelli[3] described using a distally based strip of half of the FCR tendon passed volar to dorsal through the scaphoid and anchored onto the distal radius. This has since been modified by several authors. Six months after the injury is too late to undertake successful K-wire stabilization or direct ligament repair. A ligament reconstruction with FCR or ECRL should only be considered if the joint surfaces are healthy. If degenerative changes are seen, denervation of the wrist or various methods of intercarpal fusion may be considered instead.

WRIST ARTHROSCOPY

7. You are performing arthroscopy to investigate chronic wrist pain in a 40-year-old woman. **Which one of the following is correct?**
   D. Ligamentous injuries should be graded according to the Geissler system.
   The Geissler grading system is based on the appearance of the scapholunate ligament, the alignment of the carpus, and the ability to pass a probe between the scaphoid and lunate (see Table 63-2, *Essentials of Plastic Surgery*, second edition).
   The usual equipment for a wrist arthroscopy is a 2.7 mm, 30-degree viewing scope with traction apparatus and a wet technique to aid inspection of the tightly packed carpus. The numbered portals are described according to the extensor compartments. Therefore the 3-4 portal lies between the third and fourth compartments. The 3-4 portal is the most common first portal, and this is where the EPL tendon is at most risk. It is also the most common viewing portal.

REFERENCES

1. Mayfield J, Johnson RP, Kilcoyne RK, et al. Carpal dislocation: pathomechanics and progressive perilunar instability. J Hand Surg Am 5:226-241, 1980.
2. Berger RA. A method of defining palpable landmarks for the ligament-splitting dorsal wrist capsulotomy. J Hand Surg Am 32:1291-1295, 2007.
3. Brunelli GA, Brunelli GR. A new technique to correct carpal instability with scaphoid rotary subluxation: a preliminary report. J Hand Surg Am 20(3 Pt 2): S82-S85, 1995.

64. Distal Radius Fractures

See *Essentials of Plastic Surgery*, second edition, pp. 773-784.

DISTAL RADIUS FRACTURE NOMENCLATURE
1. **When describing the radiographic appearance of a distal radius fracture, which one of the following is correct?**
   A. A die punch fracture is characterized by depression of the scaphoid fossa.
   B. A Barton's fracture is characterized by a volarly displaced distal radius fracture with shortening.
   C. A Colles' fracture is dorsally angulated distal radius fracture with shortening and dorsal comminution.
   D. A Smith's fracture is a displaced intraarticular oblique fracture of the radial styloid.
   E. A chauffeur's fracture is characterized by depression of the lunate fossa.

IMAGING OF THE DISTAL RADIUS
2. **When reviewing radiographs for signs of injury to the distal radius, which one of the following is correct?**
   A. A true lateral view of the wrist shows a 50% overlap of the pisiform and distal pole of the scaphoid.
   B. The normal distal radius has an average dorsal tilt of 10 degrees.
   C. The distal ulnar articular surface is in negative variance when sitting distal to the radial articular surface.
   D. The average radial inclination is 10 degrees on a PA radiograph of the wrist.
   E. The minimum clinically significant articular step-off for intervention is 2 mm.

NONOPERATIVE MANAGEMENT OF DISTAL RADIAL FRACTURES
3. You are discussing the merits of nonoperative management of a Colles' fracture with a fit 52-year-old patient. The radiograph confirms 20-degree dorsal angulation of the articular surface. ***Which one of the following is incorrect?***
   A. An initial closed reduction and splint application should be attempted.
   B. If the postreduction views are satisfactory, a review with repeat imaging at 1 week is important.
   C. The patient needs to know the warning signs of acute carpal tunnel syndrome.
   D. If the fracture has moved again at 1 week, remanipulation and splinting should be attempted.
   E. There is a risk of EPL tendon rupture with both operative and nonoperative management.

EXTERNAL FIXATION

4. You are planning percutaneous fixation to stabilize a Colles' fracture in a frail, osteoporotic 70-year-old woman. **Which one of the following statements is true?**
  A. K-wire fixation will allow earlier mobilization than nonoperative care.
  B. Percutaneous wiring alone should be adequate.
  C. If the dorsal angulation is 10 to 20 degrees, further intervention is not required.
  D. External fixation is contraindicated in this scenario.
  E. Splinting beyond 4 weeks should be avoided to minimize stiffness.

INTERNAL FIXATION OF DISTAL RADIUS FRACTURES

5. *When planning fixation of a comminuted distal radius fracture, which one of the following is correct?*
  A. Conventional spanning plates rely on purchase on the near cortex.
  B. Locking plates rely on purchase on the far cortex.
  C. Buttress plates have an antiglide effect to support intraarticular fracture fragments.
  D. Dorsal plating is more popular than volar plating because it involves a simpler anatomic approach.
  E. Bone grafting and substitutes should not be used in osteoporotic distal radius fractures.

COMPLICATIONS FOLLOWING DISTAL RADIUS FRACTURES

6. *When discussing open fixation of a distal radius fracture with a patient, which one of the following is correct?*
  A. The risk of chronic regional pain syndrome is approximately 40%.
  B. Open fixation avoids the risk of superficial radial nerve injury.
  C. Wrist strength will reach its maximum at 6 months with physiotherapy.
  D. The postoperative splint may include the elbow, leading to stiffness.
  E. The risk of malunion is avoided by operative intervention.

DISTAL RADIUS FRACTURE OUTCOMES

7. *Which one of the following is proven to give the best outcome for a Colles' type fracture in a patient with good bone stock?*
  A. Volar locking plate internal fixation.
  B. Closed manipulation and percutaneous pinning.
  C. Closed manipulation and splinting.
  D. Volar nonlocking plate internal fixation.
  E. No single modality has proven to be superior.

Answers

DISTAL RADIUS FRACTURE NOMENCLATURE

1. **When describing the radiographic appearance of a distal radius fracture, which one of the following is correct?**
   C. A Colles' fracture is a dorsally angulated distal radius fracture with shortening and dorsal comminution.
   Colles' original 1814 description is reported to be a low-energy extraarticular fracture of the distal radius, as described above, occurring in elderly individuals. It may be associated with an ulnar styloid or TFCC injury. A die punch fracture is a depression of the lunate fossa from impaction of the lunate into the distal radius. A Barton's fracture is an unstable volar or dorsally displaced intraarticular fracture-subluxation of the distal radius with displacement of the carpus along with the fracture fragment. A Smith's fracture is referred to as a reverse Colles' fracture (that is, with volar angulation). A chauffeur's fracture features an intraarticular distal radius fracture where the fragment includes the radial styloid, which displaces with the carpus (Fig. 64-1).

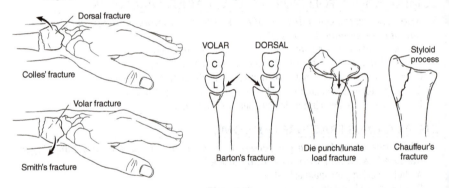

Fig. 64-1 Types of fractures.

IMAGING OF THE DISTAL RADIUS

2. **When reviewing radiographs for signs of injury to the distal radius, which one of the following is correct?**
   A. A true lateral view of the wrist shows a 50% overlap of the pisiform and distal pole of the scaphoid.
   The quality of a lateral radiograph can be assessed in part by referencing the relative position of the pisiform to the distal pole of the scaphoid. In a true lateral view, they will overlap by 50%. A rough guide to interpretation of distal radius fracture radiographs is given by the "Rule of 11's":
   Average volar tilt 11 degrees (not dorsal)
   Average radial height 11 mm
   Average radial inclination 22 degrees (for example, double 11)
   Radial height refers to the distance that the radial styloid projects beyond the sigmoid notch (at the distal tip of ulnar articulation) and is usually 11 to 12 mm. Ulnar variance describes the

position of the transverse distal ulnar joint surface relative to the distal radius joint surface at the wrist. Positive variance is present if the ulnar sits greater than 2 mm more distally than the radius, and in negative variance if the ulnar surface sits greater than 2 mm more proximally (Fig. 64-2). Most surgeons consider a 1 mm intraarticular step-off to be sufficient to indicate intervention.

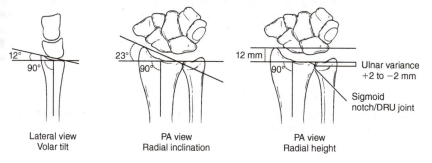

Fig. 64-2 Normal anatomic parameters of the distal radius.

NONOPERATIVE MANAGEMENT OF DISTAL RADIAL FRACTURES

3. You are discussing the merits of nonoperative management of a Colles' fracture with a fit 52-year-old patient. The radiograph confirms 20-degree dorsal angulation of the articular surface. *Which one of the following is incorrect?*
   D. If the fracture has moved again at 1 week, remanipulation and splinting should be attempted.
   A Colles' fracture is an extraarticular injury. All displaced extraarticular fractures would normally be manipulated and placed in a splint in the first instance. If the position is satisfactory following this, a trial of nonoperative management is warranted. If the fracture is behaving in an unstable fashion at 1 week, particularly in a fairly young, active patient, it should be formally stabilized rather than making further attempts at nonoperative management (see Fig. 64-6, *Essentials of Plastic Surgery,* second edition).

   Patients should be advised to seek help if they develop tingling or numbness in their digits, and signs of carpal tunnel syndrome should be sought before and after manipulation of a fracture. Attrition rupture of the EPL tendon can occur with either operative or nonoperative management of distal radius fractures.

EXTERNAL FIXATION

4. You are planning percutaneous fixation to stabilize a Colles' fracture in a frail, osteoporotic 70-year-old woman. *Which one of the following statements is true?*
   C. If the dorsal angulation is 10 to 20 degrees, further intervention is not required.
   While dorsal angulation greater than 10 degrees and radial shortening greater than 3 mm after reduction is usually an indication for intervention, up to 20 degrees dorsal angulation and 5 mm shortening can be tolerated in elderly inactive patients.

   K-wire fixation in osteoporotic bone is not sufficiently stable to allow early mobilization. Furthermore, it would usually be supplemented with an external fixator. Four weeks of splintage, either in the form of a plaster splint or external fixator, would be insufficient for healing. A minimum of 6 weeks is required.

INTERNAL FIXATION OF DISTAL RADIUS FRACTURES

5. When planning fixation of a comminuted distal radius fracture, which one of the following is correct?

C. Buttress plates have an antiglide effect to support intraarticular fracture fragments.

Conventional spanning plates rely on purchase into the far cortex, whereas locking plates may be adequate with only the near cortex. Volar plating is preferred to dorsal plating because there are fewer associated complications, and there is a more favorable surface contour to the radius. Bone grafting with autologous or substitute materials is important where there are metaphyseal defects following disimpaction. This can be useful in osteoporotic bone where additional strength may be conferred by use of a substitute.

COMPLICATIONS FOLLOWING DISTAL RADIUS FRACTURES

6. When discussing open fixation of a distal radius fracture with a patient, which one of the following is correct?

D. The postoperative splint may include the elbow, leading to stiffness.

A sugar-tong splint is sometimes required following surgery to prevent forearm rotation when the DRU joint needs to be immobilized, for example, if there has been an associated TFCC injury. This interferes with elbow movements and can lead to stiffness, which usually settles with physiotherapy. Although chronic regional pain syndrome has been reported to be as high as 40% with distal radius fractures in the past, it is currently thought to be less common at a rate of less than 3% after surgery.[1] The superficial radial nerve is at risk during both open and percutaneous fixation techniques. Wrist strength may continue to improve over the first year with physiotherapy. Patients should always be aware that malunion and nonunion can both still occur despite surgical intervention.

DISTAL RADIUS FRACTURE OUTCOMES

7. Which one of the following is proven to give the best outcome for a Colles' type fracture in a patient with good bone stock?

E. No single modality has proven to be superior.

Extraarticular fractures in patients with good bone stock will often do well with manipulation and splinting, or a variety of fixations, and there is no conclusive evidence to mandate one option over another. The treatment is tailored to the patient's requirements, their health status, and the skill set of the treating surgeon. For a treatment algorithm for distal radius fractures, see Fig. 64-6, *Essentials of Plastic Surgery,* second edition.

REFERENCE

1. Johnson NA, Cultler L, Dias JJ, et al. Complications after volar locking plate fixation of distal radius fractures. Injury 45:528-533, 2014.

65. Metacarpal and Phalangeal Fractures

See *Essentials of Plastic Surgery*, second edition, pp. 785-800.

FRACTURE TERMINOLOGY

1. For each of the following descriptions, select the correct fracture terminology. (Each option may be used once, more than once, or not at all).
   A. A fracture that occurs in elderly females after minimal trauma.
   B. A unicortical fracture commonly seen in children.
   C. A fracture type that results in more than two bone fragments.

   Options:
   a. Comminuted
   b. Stress
   c. Pathologic
   d. Greenstick
   e. Spiral
   f. Impaction
   g. Open

SALTER-HARRIS CLASSIFICATION SYSTEM

2. You are referred a child with a phalangeal fracture passing through both the epiphysis and physis. *According to the Salter-Harris classification system, what type of fracture does this represent?*
   A. Type I
   B. Type II
   C. Type III
   D. Type IV
   E. Type V

FRACTURE HEALING

3. *Which one of the following medications should be avoided in the early phases of fracture healing?*
   A. Acetaminophen
   B. Ibuprofen
   C. Codeine
   D. Tramadol
   E. Gabapentin

SAFE SPLINTING FOR HAND INJURIES

4. *When applying a splint after closed reduction of a hand fracture, which one of the following is correct?*
   A. The wrist should be placed in neutral.
   B. The IP joints should be flexed.
   C. The MP joints should be extended.
   D. The thumb should be abducted from the palm.
   E. The wrist should be placed in ulnar deviation.

HAND INJURIES DUE TO PUNCHING

5. **Which one of the following hand injuries is most commonly observed in professional boxers?**
   A. Metacarpal neck fracture
   B. Metacarpal shaft fracture
   C. Damage to the extensor mechanism
   D. Damage to the collateral ligaments
   E. Phalangeal shaft fracture

CLOSED REDUCTION OF HAND FRACTURES

6. **For which one of the following displaced fracture types is the Jahss maneuver useful?**
   A. Metacarpal neck
   B. Metacarpal base
   C. Proximal phalanx condyles
   D. Proximal phalanx shaft
   E. Proximal phalanx base

DEFORMING FORCES IN HAND FRACTURES

7. Most metacarpal fractures result in apex dorsal angulation. **Which one of the following anatomic features is usually responsible?**
   A. The fracture pattern
   B. The extensor tendons
   C. The flexor tendons
   D. The shape of the bone
   E. The intrinsic muscles

METACARPAL FRACTURES

8. You are seeing a patient one week after a punch injury leading to a closed, 40-degree apex dorsally angulated fifth metacarpal neck fracture. **Which one of the following statements is correct?**
   A. This degree of angulation mandates surgical intervention.
   B. This fracture is likely to be unstable and require careful splinting.
   C. There is unlikely to be any associated extensor lag.
   D. Functional outcomes following this injury are usually poor.
   E. This can be treated with buddy taping to the ring finger and mobilization.

9. A 30-year-old woman presents with an acute spiral fracture of the fifth metacarpal shaft with 4 mm shortening and scissoring of the digits. **Which one of the following statements is correct?**
   A. Closed reduction with transverse K-wires is unsuitable for treating this fracture.
   B. The digital overlap on flexion suggests rotation at the fracture site.
   C. Manipulation and splinting in a resting volar cast are adequate to maintain correction.
   D. Fixation with a lag screw and compression plate should be used for this fracture.
   E. Intramedullary K-wires should be used to treat this fracture.

10. **Which one of the following statements is correct regarding fractures of the metacarpal base?**
    A. When stabilizing a closed Bennett fracture with percutaneous wires, the proximal fragment needs to be captured by at least one wire.
    B. A reverse Bennett fracture involves the distal shaft of the first metacarpal and usually requires fixation.
    C. Rolando fractures of the first metacarpal are extraarticular basal fractures best treated with K-wires.
    D. Intraarticular fracture dislocations of the fourth and fifth metacarpal bases are inherently unstable and require stabilization into the carpus following reduction.
    E. Fracture dislocations of the second and third metacarpal bases are common following axial loading and require external fixation devices.

PHALANGEAL FRACTURES

11. **Which one of the following is correct regarding intraarticular fractures of the PIP joint?**
    A. Pilon fractures result in two main fragments with dorsal subluxation of the middle phalanx shaft.
    B. A hemi-hamate bone graft may be used to resurface the middle phalanx base after a pilon fracture.
    C. Dynamic external fixators require a minimum of three wires in order to adequately stabilize the middle phalanx shaft.
    D. A volar plate avulsion fracture with 10% of the articular surface and no subluxation should initially be splinted in extension.
    E. Open reduction and internal fixation is generally preferable to closed methods to ensure accurate reduction.

FRACTURES OF THE PHALANGES

12. **When considering whether a phalangeal fracture is stable, which one of the following is correct?**
    A. Fractures of the base of the proximal phalanx base tend to angulate apex dorsal because of the pull of the interossei on the proximal fragment.
    B. Oblique fractures are unlikely to lead to sufficient shortening to interfere with tendon balance.
    C. Volar avulsion fractures of the base of the middle phalanx remain stable even where more than 40% of the articular surface is avulsed.
    D. Fractures of the middle phalanx shaft angulate apex volar if the fracture is distal to the FDS tendon insertion.
    E. Oblique unicondylar fractures tend to be very stable, so rarely lead to lateral deviation or rotational deformities.

13. A 30-year-old man has sustained a displaced transverse extraarticular fracture of the ring finger middle phalanx base. There is angulation with the apex dorsal and there are no visible wounds. **Which one of the following statements is correct?**
    A. Internal fixation with lag screws is the best option for this fracture.
    B. This fracture is stable and should be manipulated and buddy taped to the ring finger.
    C. The basal (proximal) fragment is being displaced by the FDS tendon.
    D. A dynamic external fixator is required to enable ligamentotaxis to reduce the deformity.
    E. Crossed K-wires should provide a satisfactory method for stabilizing this fracture.

14. *In which one of the following scenarios can a Seymour fracture be present?*
   A. A 30-year-old man with a distal phalanx crush injury
   B. A 10-year-old girl with a nail bed injury
   C. A 45-year-old woman with a rotational deformity
   D. A 7-year-old boy with a PIP joint extensor lag
   E. A 14-year-old boy with loss of DIP joint flexion

COMPLICATIONS FOLLOWING HAND FRACTURE FIXATION

15. You are discussing treatment options with a patient who has a 40-degree angulated (apex volar) extraarticular transverse basal fracture of the ring finger proximal phalanx. The patient is reluctant to have any manipulation or surgery. **Which one of the following is correct?**
   A. Nonoperative management in this position will give completely normal function.
   B. Closed reduction followed by a dorsal MP joint extension blocking splint may be sufficient.
   C. There is no risk of tendon adhesions with nonoperative management.
   D. Failed nonoperative management can only be salvaged in the first week.
   E. The risks of infection and nerve injury are less with percutaneous pins than with internal fixation.

Answers

FRACTURE TERMINOLOGY

1. For each of the following descriptions, the best options are as follows:
   A. A fracture that occurs in elderly females after minimal trauma.
      c. Pathologic
   B. A unicortical fracture commonly seen in children.
      d. Greenstick
   C. A fracture type that results in more than two bone fragments.
      a. Comminuted

   Fracture terminology is useful when describing either the cause or appearance of a fracture and may help guide treatment. Fractures are open or closed according to whether the skin overlying the fracture site is intact or not. They are further described according to the number of bony fragments as either simple or comminuted. Simple fractures contain two bone fragments, while comminuted fractures have multiple fragments. The radiologic appearance of a fracture can be described as transverse, oblique, spiral, or longitudinal. Causal terminology includes pathologic fractures that occur in bones that are weakened such as by tumor or osteoporosis, stress fractures that occur in normal bone in response to cyclical loading, or greenstick fractures that occur in children where the cortices are more pliable and the periosteum thicker, tending to lead to buckling rather than complete fractures.

SALTER-HARRIS CLASSIFICATION SYSTEM

2. You are referred a child with a phalangeal fracture passing through both the epiphysis and physis. *According to the Salter-Harris classification system, what type of fracture does this represent?*
   C. Type III

   This fracture represents a Salter-Harris type III injury.[1] The Salter-Harris classification applies to fractures that occur at the growth plate (physis) in developing limbs. The classification system is well known and is often tested in examination settings. The most common fracture pattern is a type II injury which involves the metaphysis and physis. These fractures can result in abnormal growth if the epiphyseal plates are permanently damaged (Fig. 65-1).

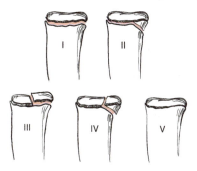

Fig. 65-1 Salter-Harris classification system of pediatric fractures.

FRACTURE HEALING

3. Which one of the following medications should be avoided in the early phases of fracture healing?

B. Ibuprofen

There is mixed evidence on the effects of NSAIDs on fracture healing but a number of animal studies suggest that healing is adversely affected by the administration of NSAIDs. In addition, clinical studies in humans also support this finding. NSAIDs interfere with the inflammatory stage of bone healing. Based on current evidence, they are probably best avoided in patients with acute fractures.[2]

SAFE SPLINTING FOR HAND INJURIES

4. When applying a splint after closed reduction of a hand fracture, which one of the following is correct?

D. The thumb should be abducted from the palm.

The safe position for hand splinting involves IP joints fully extended, MP joints flexed to 70 to 90 degrees, and the wrist in slight extension. This places the MP joint collateral ligaments and IP joint volar plates under maximal stretch and decreases subsequent joint stiffness. It also maximizes function if stiffness persists. The thumb should be abducted from the palm as if holding a beer glass; otherwise it will be difficult to subsequently regain full range of motion (Fig. 65-2).

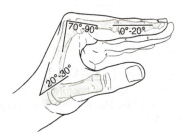

Fig. 65-2 Safe position for splinting of the hand (also known as intrinsic plus position).

HAND INJURIES DUE TO PUNCHING

5. Which one of the following hand injuries is most commonly observed in professional boxers?

C. Damage to the extensor mechanism

The term "boxer's" fracture is used to describe a fifth metacarpal neck fracture occurring during a punch injury. This is a misnomer because professional boxers rarely sustain such an injury. True boxers are more likely to sustain sagittal band ruptures at the MP joint, resulting in extensor tendon subluxation known as "boxer's knuckle," or fractures affecting the index and middle rays.

CLOSED REDUCTION OF HAND FRACTURES

6. For which one of the following displaced fracture types is the Jahss maneuver useful?

A. Metacarpal neck

The Jahss maneuver is used to reduce a metacarpal neck fracture, for example if malrotation or pseudoclawing is present. It is performed under local anesthetic block by flexing the MP joints to

90 degrees and applying force to the metacarpal head in a dorsal direction through the proximal phalanx, while stabilizing the metacarpal shaft. Holding the MP joint in flexion relaxes the intrinsic muscles while tightening the collateral ligaments and locates the proximal phalanx base under the metacarpal head such that reduction may be achieved (Fig. 65-3).

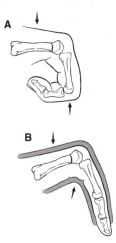

Fig. 65-3 **A** and **B,** Jahss maneuver.

DEFORMING FORCES IN HAND FRACTURES

7. Most metacarpal fractures result in apex dorsal angulation. *Which one of the following anatomic features is usually responsible?*
   E. The intrinsic muscles
   Most metacarpal fractures display apex dorsal angulation because of the intrinsic muscles. For example, metacarpal neck fractures angulate apex dorsally because the intrinsic muscles lie volar to the axis of rotation of the MP joint, maintaining flexion of the head. The mechanics of phalangeal fractures are more complex with basal fractures of the proximal phalanx tending to angulate apex volar due to the pull of the interossei, whereas middle phalanx fracture angulation depends on the position of the fracture relative to the FDS insertion.

METACARPAL FRACTURES

8. You are seeing a patient one week after a punch injury leading to a closed, 40-degree apex dorsally angulated fifth metacarpal neck fracture. *Which one of the following statements is correct?*
   E. This can be treated with buddy taping to the ring finger and mobilization.
   Fifth metacarpal neck fractures are usually very stable after a punch injury as the distal fragment is highly impacted. A significant degree of apex dorsal angulation can be tolerated without functional deficit and 40-degree angulation is unlikely to cause a functional problem in the little finger.[3] Due to the blunt impact over a flexed MP joint, there may be an associated injury to the extensor apparatus. Extensor lag is often present initially and is usually due to altered joint mechanics and relative shortening of the bony skeleton versus the tendon. On occasion, the extensor apparatus is also injured, or may be tethered by a bony spicule. Although functional

outcomes are good, patients will be left with the appearance of a depressed knuckle. There is no clear consensus on the best nonoperative management of fifth metacarpal fractures and patients tend to do well with either early mobilization with buddy strapping or short-term casting.[4]

9. A 30-year-old woman presents with an acute spiral fracture of the fifth metacarpal shaft with a 4 mm shortening and scissoring of the digits. **Which one of the following statements is correct?**
   B. The digital overlap on flexion suggests rotation at the fracture site.
   While there can sometimes be a mild degree of pseudorotation with fifth metacarpal neck fractures as a result of swelling of the interosseous muscles, malrotation seen in the context of a spiral fracture is much more likely to be of clinical significance. The shortening seen makes true malrotation likely, as shortening along a spiral fracture line will generate rotation. Frank scissoring of the digits is always abnormal.
   Closed reduction and transverse percutaneous wires may provide relative stability for this fracture, provided that accurate reduction is produced during manipulation and adequate stabilization against the fourth metacarpal is provided. This will require 2 to 3 transverse wires through the fifth into the fourth metacarpal. A protective splint is still required for the initial 1 to 2 weeks. Many surgeons find this method unacceptable and prefer not to pass K-wires through the interossei.
   Internal fixation with multiple lag screws or a lag screw and neutralization plate (not a compression plate) provides a more rigid fixation than K-wires, but at the expense of visible scarring and potentially extensive soft tissue dissection. Early mobilization is preferred following internal fixation to minimize adhesion of gliding surfaces. The choice between multiple lag screws or a screw and plate is determined by the length of the fracture relative to the width and length of the bone. A shorter fracture is unlikely to be stable with screws alone. A noncompressing neutralization plate is applied to support lag screw fixation of a short spiral fracture rather than a compression plate which would place strain on the lag screw fixation and potentially cause rotation. While intramedullary K-wires can be useful for transverse fifth metacarpal shaft and neck fractures, they cannot control rotation.

10. **Which one of the following statements is correct regarding fractures of the metacarpal base?**
    D. Intraarticular fracture dislocations of the fourth and fifth metacarpal bases are inherently unstable and require stabilization into the carpus following reduction.
    Fracture dislocations of the fourth and fifth metacarpals may be termed "reverse Bennett fractures" and can occur following axial loading such as during a punch injury. They are relatively common injuries and may be associated with a fracture of the hamate, which can be missed on plain radiographs. The metacarpal bases can dislocate dorsally and should be reduced and stabilized with percutaneous K-wires into the carpus and adjacent metacarpal.
    A Bennett fracture is a two-part fracture of the first metacarpal base that leaves a small fragment attached to the carpus due to the strong volar beak ligament. The remainder of the metacarpal shaft is displaced and requires reduction and stabilization with K-wires, usually passing into the trapezium and often into the index metacarpal base. The proximal fragment is usually small and stable. It is used as a guide to ensure adequate reduction of the metacarpal base, but does not have to be included in the K-wire passes (Fig. 65-4).

Chapter 65 ■ Metacarpal and Phalangeal Fractures

Rolando fractures are comminuted intraarticular fractures of the first metacarpal. They are treated with either open reduction and plate fixation of larger fragments or closed K-wiring. The second and third CMC joints are very stable and are rarely fractured or dislocated.

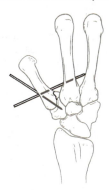

Fig. 65-4 Reduction and stabilization of Bennett's fracture using Kirschner wires into the trapezium and index metacarpal base.

PHALANGEAL FRACTURES

11. Which one of the following is correct regarding intraarticular fractures of the PIP joint?

B. A hemi-hamate bone graft may be used to resurface the middle phalanx base after a pilon fracture.

Not all intraarticular PIP joint fractures are pilon fractures. A pilon fracture occurs following an axial load, causing impaction and comminution of the base of the middle phalanx, often with splaying of the fragments. Treatment options for intraarticular fractures range from simple buddy taping to dynamic external fixators (e.g., Suzuki pins and rubber band system), which use ligamentotaxis to hold the joint space open while allowing movement to encourage a better final joint surface and minimize stiffness.[5] While a third transverse pin/wire is sometimes needed to control dorsal subluxation of the middle phalanx shaft in flexion, it is often possible to achieve adequate control with two pins/wires. When there is a significant impaction of joint surface fragments, open reduction and fixation may be achieved through either a volar or dorsal approach.

In select circumstances, a bone/cartilage graft may be harvested from the dorsal aspect of the hamate articulation with the fourth/fifth metacarpal bases and used to replace the damaged volar PIP joint surface of the middle phalanx.

Stiffness is minimized by avoiding additional soft tissue injury and encouraging early movement, therefore closed techniques are generally preferred where possible for fractures involving the PIP joint.

Minor, stable volar plate avulsion fractures may be managed with either buddy strapping and mobilization, or with a short period using a dorsal extension blocking splint and active flexion exercises. Splinting in extension will tend to distract the bony fragment and lead to delayed healing and stiffness (see Figs. 65-12 and 66-3, *Essentials of Plastic Surgery*, second edition).

FRACTURES OF THE PHALANGES

12. When considering whether a phalangeal fracture is stable, which one of the following is correct?
D. Fractures of the middle phalanx shaft angulate apex volar if the fracture is distal to the FDS tendon insertion.

Proximal phalangeal shaft fractures usually angulate apex volar because of flexion of the proximal fragment by the interossei. However, middle phalanx shaft fractures can angulate either apex volar or apex dorsal, depending on the location of the fracture in relation to the insertion of the FDS tendon. Oblique phalangeal shaft fractures have a tendency to shorten as the bone fragments slide relative to one another because of the surrounding soft tissue forces. This can lead to shortening which may interfere with tendon balance.

Volar avulsion fractures at the base of the middle phalanx are commonly stabilized by the intact collateral ligaments (Fig. 65-5). While the accessory collateral ligaments attach to the volar plate and therefore cannot exert any stabilizing force on the middle phalanx once the volar plate attachment is avulsed, the true collateral ligaments insert broadly onto the volar 40% of the proximal phalanx. Therefore if some of the true collateral ligament insertion is preserved, the joint may remain fairly stable, but if more than 40% of the middle phalanx is avulsed, there is no longer any stabilizing force from these ligaments acting on the distal fragment, which then usually subluxes dorsally.

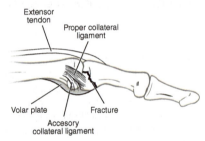

Fig. 65-5 Volar avulsion fracture at the base of the middle phalanx.

Oblique unicondylar fractures tend to be very unstable, so they can commonly lead to lateral deviation or rotational deformities.

13. A 30-year-old man has sustained a displaced transverse extraarticular fracture of the ring finger middle phalanx base. There is angulation with the apex dorsal and there are no visible wounds. Which one of the following statements is correct?
E. Crossed K-wires should provide a satisfactory method for stabilizing this fracture.

The apex dorsal angulation suggests that the proximal (basal) fragment is being pulled by the insertion of the central slip while the distal (shaft) fragment is being pulled by the strong FDS insertion. This is likely to be unstable after reduction and therefore liable to fall into the same position when the patient flexes the fingers. Closed reduction and percutaneous K-wires should stabilize the fracture adequately. Crossed wires from each midlateral line could be used, either antegrade or retrograde (Fig. 65-6). Opening the digit to use plate fixation increases the soft tissue injury and the likelihood of postoperative adhesions, but could be considered for this fracture if the basal fragment is of sufficient size. Lag screws are not suited to transverse fractures and are used for oblique or spiral fracture patterns. Dynamic external fixators are generally reserved for intraarticular fractures of the phalanges.

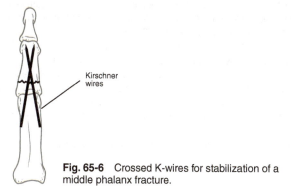

Fig. 65-6 Crossed K-wires for stabilization of a middle phalanx fracture.

14. In which one of the following scenarios can a Seymour fracture be present?
B. A 10-year-old girl with a nail bed injury

A Seymour fracture is an open epiphyseal injury of the distal phalanx. When assessing a child in clinic with a nail bed injury, it is important to look for the presence of a Seymour fracture, which can be mistaken for a simple mallet deformity or soft tissue swelling after a crush injury. This is an open Salter-Harris type fracture where a nail bed injury and distal phalanx fracture coexist. The clue is that the nail plate usually lies superficial to the nail fold, rather than tucked underneath it. If the fracture is not reduced, there may be subsequent growth disturbance. Furthermore, part of the proximal nail bed may flip into the fracture site, preventing healing or closed reduction. These injuries are more likely to be treated surgically to ensure that the fracture is properly reduced and stabilized, in addition to cleaning and repairing the nail bed.[6]

COMPLICATIONS FOLLOWING HAND FRACTURE FIXATION

15. You are discussing treatment options with a patient who has a 40-degree angulated (apex volar) extraarticular transverse basal fracture of the ring finger proximal phalanx. The patient is reluctant to have any manipulation or surgery. **Which one of the following is correct?**
B. Closed reduction followed by a dorsal MP joint extension blocking splint may be sufficient.

The pull of the flexor tendons will tend to help maintain the correction, provided an extension block is in place to prevent redisplacement in the early stages. Pseudoclawing occurs when a basal proximal phalanx fracture unites in apex-volar angulation. This may result in reduced composite flexion of the digit, and also lead to an extensor lag. Tendon adhesions can occur with nonoperative and operative management, but they are most common following open internal fixation. Failed nonoperative management can be salvaged at most stages but remanipulation and fixation of the original fracture is easiest in the first 10 to 14 days. There may be a greater risk of nerve injury if care is not taken during closed cutaneous pinning, because the tip of the wire can easily slide off the small, curved phalanx (particularly at the narrow phalangeal neck), whereas the digital nerves can be readily seen and protected during open fixation. There is also a higher risk of infection at pin track sites with external wires than with internal fixation.

REFERENCES

1. Salter RB, Harris WR. Injuries involving the Epiphyseal plate. J Bone Joint Surg Am 45:587-622, 1963.
2. Pountos I, Georgouli T, Calori GM, et al. Do nonsteroidal anti-inflammatory drugs affect bone healing? A critical analysis. ScientificWorldJournal 2012:606404, 2012.
3. Hunter JM, Cowen JN. Fifth metacarpal fractures in a compensation clinic population. A report on one hundred and thirty-three cases. J Bone Joint Surg Am 52:1159-1165, 1970.
4. Statius Muller MG, Poolman RW, van Hoogstraten MJ, et al. Immediate immobilization gives good results in boxer's fractures with volar angulation up to 70 degrees: a prospective randomized trial comparing immediate mobilization with cast immobilization. Arch Orthop Trauma Surg 123:534-537, 2003.
5. Suzuki Y, Matsuhaga T, Sato S, et al. The pins and rubbers traction system for treatment of comminuted intraarticular fractures and fracture-dislocations in the hand. J Hand Surg Br 19:98-107, 1994.
6. Seymour N. Juxta-epiphysial fracture of the terminal phalanx of the finger. J Bone Joint Surg Br 48:347-349, 1966.

66. Phalangeal Dislocations

See *Essentials of Plastic Surgery*, second edition, pp. 801-809.

CLINICAL EVALUATION OF THE JOINT

1. **When assessing the small joints of the hand for evidence of a ligamentous injury, which one of the following is correct?**
   A. A grade I collateral ligament tear will be grossly unstable during lateral stress testing.
   B. Lateral stability in extension does not exclude the presence of a collateral ligament tear.
   C. Stener lesions are nonspecific to a particular small joint and can occur with all injury grades I through III.
   D. Dislocations are described according to the position of the proximal bone to normal joint alignment.
   E. Two radiographic views are required involving joints proximal and distal to the injury.

FINGER MP JOINT ANATOMY

2. **Which one of the following is responsible for the cam effect in MP joint flexion?**
   A. The volar plate
   B. The flexor tendons
   C. The collateral ligaments
   D. The joint contour
   E. The deep transverse metacarpal ligament

DORSAL DISLOCATION OF THE FINGER MP JOINT

3. You assess a young man with a dorsal index finger MP joint dislocation after a fall. The MP joint is in 70 degrees of extension and the IP joint is flexed. There are no fractures seen on three plain radiograph views. **Which one of the following is correct?**
   A. Wrist and MP joint extension will aid closed reduction.
   B. The metacarpal head may be trapped between the long flexor tendons and the lumbrical.
   C. It can be reliably assumed that the collateral ligaments are intact.
   D. If an open reduction is required, a dorsal approach is best.
   E. If an open reduction is required, the A1 pulley must be preserved.

THUMB MP JOINT INJURY

4. A patient has sustained a closed injury to the thumb during a fall onto an outstretched hand. Ligamentous damage is suspected. **Which one of the following is correct regarding thumb MP joint collateral ligament injuries?**
   A. UCL injuries are twice as common as RCL or volar plate injuries.
   B. UCL tears are most likely to occur at the proximal origin from the metacarpal.
   C. Complete RCL injuries always need operative intervention because of the risk of a Stener lesion.
   D. Grade II UCL and RCL injuries are treated similarly, with 4 weeks of immobilization in a cast.
   E. UCL injuries involving avulsion fractures are most commonly intraarticular and require surgical intervention.

CHRONIC MP JOINT INJURY OF THE THUMB

5. A 59-year-old man complains of pain and weakness affecting his dominant thumb, which has been getting worse over 5 years. On examination the IP joint and CMC joint are unremarkable. The MP joint sits in radial deviation, but there is an endpoint on radial stressing at 45 degrees. The RCL is intact. There is sclerosis and a small radial osteophyte on radiographs. *Which one of the following is correct?*
   A. Fusion of the MP joint may be the most appropriate long-term solution.
   B. Repeated steroid injections may be all that is required for symptomatic management.
   C. A palmaris longus tendon graft should be used to reconstruct the UCL.
   D. If the patient cannot recall a specific injury, it is unlikely that the UCL is the problem.
   E. A period of 8 to 12 weeks in a thumb spica cast may allow this injury to stabilize.

ANATOMY OF THE PIP JOINT

6. *Which one of the following is correct regarding PIP joint?*
   A. The ligament box complex comprises the volar plate and true collateral ligaments only.
   B. The PIP joint is less commonly dislocated than the DIP joint.
   C. A normal PIP joint range of motion involves a 70-degree arc of rotation.
   D. Dorsal dislocation of the PIP joint is most common, given the joint anatomy.
   E. Volar plate avulsion usually occurs at the proximal phalanx.

CLASSIFICATION OF DORSAL PIP JOINT DISLOCATIONS

7. A patient presents with a type II dorsal dislocation of the PIP joint. *What does this description suggest?*
   A. That there is an associated bony injury.
   B. That some joint congruity is maintained.
   C. That the volar plate is still intact.
   D. That the collateral ligaments are still intact.
   E. That both volar plate and collateral ligaments are injured.

TREATMENT OF ACUTE PIP JOINT DISLOCATIONS

8. You see a patient in the hand trauma clinic following reduction of a dorsal dislocation of the ring finger PIP joint. Postreduction radiographs reveal a 30% volar articular fragment at the base of the middle phalanx that is well aligned. *Which one of the following is the most appropriate management plan?*
   A. Mobilize with buddy strapping to the middle finger and see again in 2 to 3 weeks.
   B. Immobilize for 2 to 3 weeks in extension to prevent joint contracture, then progressively mobilize with buddy strapping.
   C. Protect and mobilize within a dorsal blocking splint at 20 to 30 degrees for 3 weeks, reducing the splint angle weekly.
   D. Perform open reduction and mini-lag screw fixation of the bony fragment and begin early mobilization.
   E. Apply a dynamic skeletal traction frame across the PIP joint and begin early mobilization.

9. A patient presents after a fall during which he injured his little finger PIP joint. He states that immediately after the fall his finger was pointing away from the ring finger at about 60 degrees, but he was able to manipulate the finger back into place. Examination shows a residual 30 degrees of lateral instability on stress testing. Radiographs are all normal. **Which one of the following is correct?**
A. Although the RCL will have been injured, the volar plate will be spared.
B. This injury will require surgical intervention with a bone anchor device.
C. Buddy taping to the ring finger and mobilization may be all that is required.
D. The outcome following this injury is likely to be excellent with normal function by six weeks.
E. This mechanism of injury is less common than a volar dislocation of the PIP joint.

Answers

CLINICAL EVALUATION OF THE JOINT

1. When assessing the small joints of the hand for evidence of a ligamentous injury, which one of the following is correct?

B. Lateral stability in extension does not exclude the presence of a collateral ligament tear.

When assessing the stability of the small joints of the hand, stress testing should be performed in both flexion and extension to ensure that the collateral ligaments and volar plate are independently and accurately tested. For example, the PIP joint can remain stable in extension despite a collateral ligament tear because of volar plate stability. Flexion of the joint relaxes the volar plate and facilitates assessment of the collateral ligaments. Local anesthetic blocks are often required to perform this assessment.

Collateral ligament injuries are graded I through III, according to increasing instability. A grade I injury is grossly stable with only a microscopic tear. A grade II injury results in relative instability in lateral stress testing (around 20 degrees), but with a definite endpoint. A grade III injury results in gross instability with no firm endpoint. Only grade III injuries (complete) lead to a Stener lesion which is specific to the thumb MP joint.[1,2]

Dislocations are described according to the position of the distal bone (not proximal) relative to normal joint alignment. While the joints proximal and distal to the injury must be imaged, this must be in three (not two) views.

FINGER MP JOINT ANATOMY

2. Which one of the following is responsible for the cam effect in MP joint flexion?

D. The joint contour

All of the listed options contribute to the stability of the MP joint, but during flexion it is particularly stable from the *cam effect* of the joint. A cam effect converts a rotational motion into a linear one (Fig. 66-1). The metacarpal head is nonspherical, and when flexion occurs the collateral ligaments are placed on stretch. This explains why splints are designed to maintain the joint in flexion, and why Dupuytren's contractures can be left longer before treatment when involving this joint. There is also more stable bony contact when the MP joint is placed in 70 degrees or more of flexion, which also contributes to overall stability.

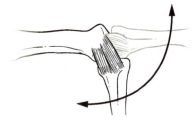

Fig. 66-1 The *cam effect* is created by eccentric movement of the proximal phalanx on the metacarpal head, causing a dynamic change in collateral ligament length.

Chapter 66 ▪ Phalangeal Dislocations   541

DORSAL DISLOCATION OF THE FINGER MP JOINT

3. You assess a young man with a dorsal index finger MP joint dislocation after a fall. The MP joint is in 70 degrees of extension and the IP joint is flexed. There are no fractures seen on three plain radiograph views. *Which one of the following is correct?*

B. The metacarpal head may be trapped between the long flexor tendons and the lumbrical.
The head of the metacarpal is commonly found to be trapped between the lumbrical radially and the flexor tendons ulnarly and this is often the reason why reduction is challenging. Closed reduction is most likely to be successful if the wrist is flexed, because this will slacken off the long flexors. This is a fairly high-energy injury and the radial collateral ligament may have been avulsed. A volar approach provides the best access to the key structures during open reduction. Either the radial digital nerve to the index finger or the lumbrical may lie very superficially over the metacarpal head, so care must be taken when elevating the skin flaps and exploring the joint to avoid damage.

Dividing the A1 pulley is sometimes used to slacken off the flexor pull and give more flexibility to the volar joint structures during reduction. Loss of this pulley would not have any negative functional consequences.

THUMB MP JOINT INJURY

4. A patient has sustained a closed injury to the thumb during a fall onto an outstretched hand. Ligamentous damage is suspected. *Which one of the following is correct regarding thumb MP joint collateral ligament injuries?*

D. Grade II UCL and RCL injuries are treated similarly with 4 weeks of immobilization in a cast.
UCL injuries of the thumb are ten times more common than RCL injuries. UCL tears are five times more likely to occur distally at the insertion into the proximal phalanx than at the proximal site. Stener lesions only occur at the UCL, since on the radial side the abductor insertion is too wide to become interposed between the RCL fragments. Failure to recognize and treat a Stener lesion of the UCL may result in chronic instability and degenerative change at the MP joint. All grade III UCL injuries require surgical intervention, and grade III injuries to the RCL will also do so if there is volar subluxation. Grade II RCL/UCL injuries are treated similarly, with cast immobilization for 4 weeks then protected mobilization for a further 2 weeks.

Avulsion fractures of the proximal phalanx can occur with UCL tears. Typically they are small fracture fragments that do not involve the articular surface and are managed with cast immobilization. Large fracture fragments with more than 2 mm of displacement require intervention.

CHRONIC MP JOINT INJURY OF THE THUMB

5. A 59-year-old man complains of pain and weakness affecting his dominant thumb, which has been getting worse over 5 years. On examination the IP joint and CMC joint are unremarkable. The MP joint sits in radial deviation, but there is an endpoint on radial stressing at 45 degrees. The RCL is intact. There is sclerosis and a small radial osteophyte on radiographs. *Which one of the following is correct?*

A. Fusion of the MP joint may be the most appropriate long-term solution.
Gamekeeper's thumb is a term for chronic thumb MP joint UCL injuries. It may be the result of a missed grade III UCL rupture with a Stener lesion, or it may be caused by repeated minor injuries that culminate in gradual attrition of the ligament. Either way, direct delayed repair of the UCL

is not usually possible. The joint should always be assessed for signs of osteoarthritis before considering UCL reconstruction. If arthritis is present, it is usually more appropriate to fuse the MP joint instead of reconstructing the UCL. Fusion of this joint is well tolerated if there is good IP joint and CMC joint function.

ANATOMY OF THE PIP JOINT

6. Which one of the following is correct regarding PIP joint?
   D. Dorsal dislocation of the PIP joint is most common, given the joint anatomy.
   The PIP joint is the most commonly dislocated small joint in the hand, and dorsal dislocation because of hyperextension is the most common mechanism. The joint is normally very stable because of the anatomy of the ligament box complex which comprises the volar plate as well as the proper and accessory collateral ligaments (see Fig. 66-2, *Essentials of Plastic Surgery*, second edition). This ligament complex must be disrupted in at least two planes for dislocation to occur. The volar plate most commonly (80%) avulses distally from the middle phalanx, and when it avulses proximally it can become trapped within the joint necessitating open reduction. The collateral ligaments usually avulse proximally (85%). The normal range of PIP joint motion varies between digits, but is typically more than 100 degrees. The arc of rotation of the DIP joint is usually 90 degrees.

CLASSIFICATION OF DORSAL PIP JOINT DISLOCATIONS

7. A patient presents with a type II dorsal dislocation of the PIP joint. *What does this description suggest?*
   E. That both volar plate and collateral ligaments are injured.
   The classification system for dorsal dislocations of the PIP joint has three categories. The system is useful as it guides treatment. Injury types I and II are soft tissue injuries only. Type III injuries have associated fractures. Types I and II differ in the degree of soft tissue damage and joint congruity. Type I is a hyperextension injury with either partial or complete volar plate avulsion and partial articulation of the joint remains intact. Type II is also a hyperextension injury but results in complete dorsal dislocation of the middle phalanx. The volar plate must be completely divided for this to occur and the collateral ligaments must also be damaged.

TREATMENT OF ACUTE PIP JOINT DISLOCATIONS

8. You see a patient in the hand trauma clinic following reduction of a dorsal dislocation of the ring finger PIP joint. Postreduction radiographs reveal a 30% volar articular fragment at the base of the middle phalanx that is well aligned. *Which one of the following is the most appropriate management plan?*
   C. Protect and mobilize within a dorsal blocking splint at 20 to 30 degrees for 3 weeks, reducing the splint angle weekly.
   Following adequate reduction of a dorsal PIP joint dislocation, the size of any volar fragment at the middle phalanx base tends to indicate the degree of stability and subsequent treatment. Fragments less than 40% of the articular surface, as in this case, are often stable. This is because a portion of the true collateral ligament insertion to the base of the middle phalanx is preserved on each side. If the injury is stable with good alignment of the fragment, operative intervention is not required. A splint regimen should protect against recurrent dorsal dislocation, while mobilizing the joint early to reduce subsequent fibrosis and stiffness.[3,4]

9. A patient presents after a fall during which he injured his little finger PIP joint. He states that immediately after the fall his finger was pointing away from the ring finger at about 60 degrees, but he was able to manipulate the finger back into place. Examination shows a residual 30 degrees of lateral instability on stress testing. Radiographs are normal. **Which one of the following is correct?**
   C. **Buddy taping to the ring finger and mobilization may be all that is required.**
      Lateral dislocations of the PIP joint are relatively common and can usually be treated nonoperatively with buddy taping to the adjacent finger and early mobilization. Surgical intervention is not usually required. The main injury involves the RCL but there will also be a degree of damage to the volar plate. Outcomes following PIP joint dislocation are generally poor, even with good compliance and physiotherapy. The range of movement may take several months to recover and may not return to normal. There is often some long-term residual thickening around the PIP joint because of fibrosis after an injury, which some patients find distressing. Lateral dislocations of the little finger PIP joint are more common than volar dislocations, which are rare.

REFERENCES

1. Glickel SZ, Barron OA, Catalano LW. Dislocations and ligament injuries in the digits. In Green DP, Hotchkiss RN, Pederson WC, et al, eds. Green's Operative Hand Surgery, ed 5, Philadelphia: Churchill Livingstone 2005.
2. Stener B. Skeletal injuries associated with rupture of the ulnar collateral ligament of the metacarpophalangeal joint of the thumb: a clinical and anatomic study. Acta Chir Scand 125:583-586, 1963
3. Deitch MA, Kiefhaber TR, Comisar BR, et al. Dorsal fracture dislocations of the proximal interphalangeal joint: surgical complications and long-term results. J Hand Surg Am 24:914-923, 1999.
4. Eaton RG, Malerich MM. Volar plate arthroplasty of the proximal interphalangeal joint: a review of ten years' experience. J Hand Surg Am 5:260-268, 1980.

67. Fingertip Injuries

See *Essentials of Plastic Surgery*, second edition, pp. 810-823.

ANATOMY

1. **Which one of the following statements is true regarding the vascular anatomy of the fingertip?**
   A. The volar venous supply is dominant.
   B. The digital artery bifurcates at the DIP joint.
   C. Valves are absent in the vasculature of the digits.
   D. The arterial supply is interconnected by two anastomotic arches.
   E. Common digital nerves are located deep to the digital arteries distally.

HOMODIGITAL FLAPS

2. **Which one of the following is a bilateral V-Y flap technique based on the lateral aspects of the injured digit that is used for reconstruction of transverse and lateral oblique injuries?**
   A. Atasoy V-Y advancement
   B. Furlow V-Y advancement
   C. Kutler V-Y advancement
   D. Venkataswami V-Y advancement
   E. Souquet advancement

3. **Why are Moberg-type advancement flaps usually avoided in the fingers?**
   A. Subsequent IP joint stiffness
   B. Cold intolerance to the fingertip
   C. Abnormal sensation to the fingertip
   D. Dorsal skin necrosis
   E. Partial flap failure

4. **What is the main benefit of using "Dellon's modification" when using a Moberg flap to reconstruct a thumb defect?**
   A. Flap viability is increased
   B. Flap reach is increased
   C. Both digital blood vessels are preserved
   D. Both digital nerves are preserved
   E. The surgical time is reduced

HETERODIGITAL FLAPS

5. **What is the main drawback of using the cross-finger flap to reconstruct an index fingertip defect?**
   A. The limited availability of donor tissue
   B. The technical difficulty of elevating the flap
   C. The lack of postoperative protective sensation
   D. The lack of postoperative tactile sensation
   E. The high risk of long-term postoperative stiffness

6. **Which one of the following flaps cannot be used to reconstruct finger or thumb tip defects?**
   A. First dorsal metacarpal artery perforator flap (Quaba)
   B. First dorsal metacarpal artery flap (Foucher)
   C. Heterodigital neurovascular pedicled island flap (Littler)
   D. Cross-finger flap
   E. Volar advancement flap (Moberg)

7. **Which one of the following statements is true of the pedicled island flap described by Littler?**
   A. It is most commonly used for radial thumb tip defects.
   B. It is always harvested from the middle finger.
   C. It involves extended dissection into the palm.
   D. The donor defect can normally be closed directly.
   E. It preserves the normal vascular supply to the donor digit.

REGIONAL FLAPS

8. **What is the main problem with using a thenar flap to reconstruct a volar oblique injury to the index or middle finger?**
   A. The limited availability of donor tissue
   B. The high flap failure rate
   C. The need for a second stage
   D. The risk of postoperative stiffness
   E. The need for a donor site skin graft

RECONSTRUCTIVE PRINCIPLES

9. **Why is it particularly important to maintain joint mobility in the ring and little fingers?**
   A. To maintain the aesthetic balance of the hand
   B. To maintain pinch grip strength
   C. To maintain power grip strength
   D. To maintain key pinch strength
   E. To maintain support grip

COMPOSITE GRAFTING

10. **Which one of the following statements is true of composite fingertip grafts?**
    A. They are only successful in children.
    B. They act only as biologic dressings.
    C. Graft take is improved by postoperative warming.
    D. Graft take is improved by bone removal and defatting.
    E. They are generally useful after crush injuries.

REVISION AMPUTATION

11. Three months after a revision amputation through the DIP joint of the middle finger, a patient is unable to actively flex his PIP joint. Each time he tries to do so the PIP joint extends instead. **What is the correct term used to describe this problem?**
    A. Interosseous plus
    B. Intrinsic minus
    C. Quadrigia effect
    D. Lumbrical plus
    E. Lumbrical minus

RECONSTRUCTIVE OPTIONS FOR THE FINGERTIP

12. Match each of the following defects to the best available reconstructive option. Assume in each case that the patient is a healthy, nonsmoking young woman with no time pressure to achieve healing and that maximum length is to be preserved. (Each option may be used once, more than once, or not at all.)
    A. Transverse index tip amputation through the mid-nail bed with exposed bone
    B. Volar oblique middle fingertip amputation, 1 cm^2, no exposed bone
    C. Lateral oblique index fingertip amputation from the DIP joint crease distally on the radial side with exposed bone

Options:
  a. Healing by secondary intention
  b. Split-thickness skin graft
  c. Full-thickness skin graft
  d. Volar advancement flap (Moberg)
  e. Volar V-Y advancement flap (Atasoy)
  f. Neurovascular pedicled island flap (Littler)
  g. Homodigital neurovascular island flap (Venkataswami)
  h. Cross-finger flap

MANAGEMENT OF THUMB TIP INJURIES

13. For each of the following clinical scenarios, select the most appropriate reconstructive technique for a healthy patient. (Each option may be used once, more than once, or not at all.)
    A. A defect of the thumb affecting the entire nail bed from the extensor insertion to the tip. The defect measures 1.5 by 2 cm, leaving only exposed distal phalanx in this area.
    B. A pulp defect of the thumb, 1.7 by 3 cm in diameter. The FPL tendon is exposed but intact, and the distal phalanx is exposed to the tip. The dorsal aspect is completely intact, with the nail complex unaffected.
    C. Circumferential degloving of the distal phalanx of the thumb. The bone length is preserved and the FPL and EPL are intact. There is complete loss of pulp and the nail bed complex.

Options:
  a. Dorsal metacarpal artery flap (Foucher)
  b. V-Y advancement flap (Atasoy)
  c. Groin flap
  d. Reverse cross-finger flap
  e. Thenar flap
  f. Terminalization at IP joint
  g. Advancement flap (Moberg)

Answers

ANATOMY

1. Which one of the following statements is true regarding the vascular anatomy of the fingertip?
D. The arterial supply is interconnected by two anastomotic arches.
The arterial supply to the fingertip arises from the proper digital arteries which divide into three branches at the level of the DIP joint. The three branches are connected by two anastomotic arches. The dorsal venous supply is dominant and veins around the lateral nail wall and distal pulp form an arch over the distal phalanx. A second arch is formed more proximally over the middle phalanx. The presence of these arches is relevant to distal tip replantation surgery (see Chapter 73).

HOMODIGITAL FLAPS

2. Which one of the following is a bilateral V-Y flap technique based on the lateral aspects of the injured digit that is used for reconstruction of transverse and lateral oblique injuries.
C. Kutler V-Y advancement
The Kutler V-Y advancement flap is a bilateral technique that was described for transverse amputations, but may be more suited to lateral oblique injuries of the digits. Two triangular flaps are designed and centrally placed to cover the defect (Fig. 67-1).[1-4]

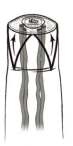 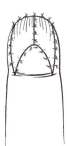

Fig. 67-1 Kutler flap dissection.

The Atasoy and Furlow flaps are both types of volar advancement flaps that are indicated for reconstructing dorsal oblique and some transverse injuries. The Venkataswami flap is an oblique triangular flap used for volar oblique injuries. The Souquet flap is a rectangular flap not a V-Y flap, rotated so that the free edge advances to cover a defect in the fingertip. It is based on the neurovascular bundle but does not advance especially well. It has been modified by Lloyd and Sammut to maintain sensation and yet improve reach.[5]

3. Why are Moberg-type advancement flaps usually avoided in the fingers?
D. Dorsal skin necrosis
Although a Moberg advancement flap is feasible for reconstruction of the index fingertip it is not recommended, as it requires division of the dorsal branches of the digital vessels and this can lead to subsequent dorsal skin necrosis. While it is possible to preserve many of these

branches using a tissue spreading technique, the Moberg flap is generally best reserved for thumb reconstruction. There is a small risk of subsequent IP joint stiffness, partial flap failure, and cold intolerance to the tip with most reconstructions, but these risks are not specific to the Moberg flap.[6]

4. **What is the main benefit of using "Dellon's modification" when using a Moberg flap to reconstruct a thpumb defect?**
   B. Flap reach is increased
   The Moberg flap is a volar advancement flap described for reconstruction of thumb tip defects. It has a robust vascularity because it is elevated on both neurovascular pedicles simultaneously. It is useful for closing volar soft tissue defects of the thumb 1 to 1.5 cm in diameter. Dellon's modification involves extension of the flap base into the first web space and this can increase advancement to around 3 cm. The surgical time is most likely to be increased (not decreased) in Dellon's modification, as a result of the extended dissection involved.

HETERODIGITAL FLAPS

5. **What is the main drawback of using the cross-finger flap to reconstruct an index fingertip defect?**
   D. The lack of postoperative tactile sensation
   The main drawback to using the cross-finger flap to reconstruct an index fingertip defect is the postoperative lack of tactile gnosis, which is reported to occur in all patients.[7] Normal tactile gnosis is very important to maintain in the index finger given its key role in pinch grip, key grip, and precision activity. Protective sensation is generally well maintained with this flap, although it requires cortical relearning. There is plenty of donor soft tissue available from the cross-finger flap in most cases, as this is harvested from the dorsum of the middle finger. It is a technically straightforward procedure that can be accomplished under local anesthetic in a few minutes. The risk of long-term postoperative stiffness is low because splinting can be achieved in the safe position (or close to it) with the IP joints in full extension.

6. **Which one of the following flaps cannot be used to reconstruct finger or thumb tip defects?**
   A. First dorsal metacarpal artery perforator flap (Quaba)
   The Quaba flap is not useful for fingertip reconstruction because it does not have sufficient reach to move much beyond the PIP joint. Flow can be antegrade through perforators from the dorsal metacarpal artery (DMA) or retrograde from the volar system or the dorsal digital arteries. Perforators are primarily distal to the junctura tendinea in the distal third of the dorsum of the hand. All of the other flaps are useful for thumb or fingertip reconstruction.

7. **Which one of the following statements is true of the pedicled island flap described by Littler?**
   C. It involves extended dissection into the palm.
   The pedicled island flap described by Littler[8] is used to reconstruct large defects of the thumb tip and is most commonly used for ulnar (not radial) defects. It can be harvested from either the ring or middle fingers and involves sacrifice of one of the digital arteries and nerves to the donor

digit. It involves significant dissection into the palm in order to obtain sufficient reach and to tunnel the pedicle. The donor defect requires a skin graft (Fig. 67-2).

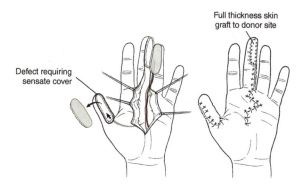

Fig. 67-2   Neurovascular pedicled flap.

REGIONAL FLAPS

8. **What is the main problem with using a thenar flap to reconstruct a volar oblique injury to the index or middle finger?**
   D. **The risk of postoperative stiffness**

   The thenar flap involves a two-stage process. In the first stage, an area of skin and subcutaneous fat is raised from the thenar eminence and inset into a volar defect of the index (or middle) fingertip. In the second stage, at 10 to 14 days, the flap is divided and inset is completed. The donor site is closed, grafted, or left to heal by secondary intention. The main problem with this flap is that the index finger is flexed at the PIP joint between the first and second stages. This can result in stiffness and loss of motion to the PIP joint secondary to collateral ligament and volar plate tightening that may not fully recover. For this reason, it should be avoided in older patients and those with comorbidities such as arthritis and Dupuytren's disease. The flap has a low failure rate and availability of suitable (glabrous) tissue is good for fingertip reconstruction. The need for a second stage and the potential for a donor site graft represent limitations, but these are less of a problem (Fig. 67-3).

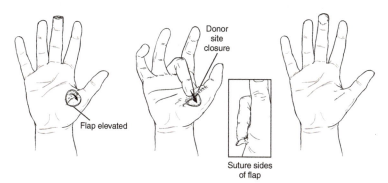

Fig. 67-3   Thenar flap.

RECONSTRUCTIVE PRINCIPLES

9. Why is it particularly important to maintain joint mobility in the ring and little fingers?

C. To maintain power grip strength

The ring and little fingers have an important functional role in the power grip of the hand. For this reason, it is important to maintain joint mobility (flexion, in particular combines with wrist extension) while minimizing pain. Sensibility and aesthetics are generally less important features.

COMPOSITE GRAFTING

10. Which one of the following statements is true of composite fingertip grafts?

D. Graft take is improved by bone removal and defatting.

Nonmicrosurgical replantation of the amputated fingertip is known as composite grafting and is not usually recommended in adults. The main indication is in children younger than six years of age. Some authorities think that composite grafts act only as biologic dressings that allow granulation and healing from underneath, while others believe they are able to successfully act as true grafts. Attempts have been made to improve take by cooling (not warming) the grafts postoperatively. In spite of recommendations to reserve the technique for use in children, there have been successful reports of their use in adults. Graft survival has been improved by excision of bone, defatting, tie oversuturing, and finger splinting.[9,10] Composite fraying is best suited to clean sharp lacerations rather than crush injuries.

REVISION AMPUTATION

11. Three months after a revision amputation through the DIP joint of the middle finger, a patient is unable to actively flex his PIP joint. Each time he tries to do so the PIP joint extends instead. **What is the correct term used to describe this problem?**

D. Lumbrical plus

The lumbrical plus deformity may occur following a partial amputation of the finger. The PIP joint extends during attempts to actively flex the joint because the retracted FDP tendon remains attached to the lumbrical muscles in the palm. FDP contraction, therefore, pulls on the lumbrical muscle, causing flexion of the MP joint and extension of the IP joint. The lumbrical plus deformity can be prevented by securing the FDP to the A4 pulley during revision amputation, however care must be taken when performing such a procedure as there is a risk of causing a quadrigia effect instead. For this reason it is not commonly performed. If the FDP tendon is overly advanced or tensioned in the injured digit, the action of FDP in the remaining digits is compromised. This is because the FDP tendons share a common muscle belly and if one is significantly tighter than the others, normal flexion in the remaining digits is restricted. Intrinsic minus deformity is a condition where the finger MP joints are hyperextended and the PIP joints are flexed. This is because the normal function of the intrinsics is restricted, causing an imbalance between the strong extrinsics and the deficient intrinsics. It is typically observed in association with an ulnar motor nerve injury.

Chapter 67 ■ Fingertip Injuries   551

RECONSTRUCTIVE OPTIONS FOR THE FINGERTIP

12. *For the following defects, the best reconstructive options are as follows. Assume in each case that the patient is a healthy, nonsmoking young woman with no time pressure to achieve healing and that maximum length is to be preserved.*
   A. *Transverse index tip amputation through mid-nail bed with exposed bone*
      e. **Volar V-Y advancement flap (Atasoy)**
   B. *Volar oblique middle fingertip amputation, 1 cm^2, no exposed bone*
      a. **Healing by secondary intention**
   C. *Lateral oblique index fingertip amputation from the DIP joint crease distally on the radial side with exposed bone*
      g. **Homodigital neurovascular island flap (Venkataswamy)**

      In scenarios A and C there are available local flaps that should provide sensate, durable cover for the defect. Since scenario B has no critical structures exposed and is no more than 1 cm^2 in size, healing by secondary intention should be fairly quick and give good cover, color, contour, and sensation to the finger over time.

MANAGEMENT OF THUMB TIP INJURIES

13. *For the following scenarios, the best options for a healthy patient are as follows:*
   A. *A defect of the thumb affecting the entire nail bed from the extensor insertion to the tip. The defect measures 1.5 by 2 cm, leaving only exposed distal phalanx in this area.*
      d. **Reverse cross-finger flap**

      The options for the patient in scenario A are a reverse cross-finger flap from the index proximal phalanx or a Foucher flap from the same area. Because sensation is not a major requirement for the dorsum of the thumb, the reverse cross-finger flap is an appropriate and simpler option with a smaller donor site scar than the Foucher flap.
   B. *A pulp defect of the thumb 1.7 by 3 cm in diameter. The FPL tendon is exposed but intact, and the distal phalanx is exposed to the tip. The dorsal aspect is completely intact, with the nail complex unaffected.*
      a. **Dorsal metacarpal artery flap (Foucher)**

      The options for the patient in scenario B include a cross-finger flap from the index finger or a Foucher flap. A Moberg flap would not be large enough. A Littler flap would leave a large defect on the donor finger and is perhaps better suited to smaller defects. A cross-finger flap would fail to provide sensation, which is a key requirement for the thumb pulp.
   C. *Circumferential degloving of the distal phalanx of the thumb. The bone length is preserved and the FPL and EPL are intact. There is complete loss of pulp and the nail bed complex.*
      c. **Groin flap**

      The options for the patient in scenario C include a free wraparound toe transfer or a free (or pedicled) groin flap. As there is an intact skeleton with joint function, cover with a groin flap is preferred from the options given. Amputation would not normally be undertaken in a young healthy patient without ruling out all other reconstructive options.

      The common principle in thumb reconstruction is maintenance of length, so with bone length preserved in these scenarios, the aim should be to find soft tissue cover.

REFERENCES

1. Atasoy E, Ioakimidis E, Kasdan ML, et al. Reconstruction of the amputated finger tip with a triangular volar flap. A new surgical procedure. J Bone Joint Surg Am 52:921-926, 1970.
2. Furlow LT Jr. V-Y "cup" flap for volar oblique amputation of fingers. J Hand Surg Br 9:253-256, 1984.
3. Kutler W. A new method for fingertip amputation. JAMA 133:29-30, 1947.
4. Venkataswami R, Subramanian N. Oblique triangular flap: a new method of repair for oblique amputations of the fingertip and thumb. Plast Reconstr Surg 66:296-300, 1980.
5. Lloyd N, Sammut D. A modification of the Souquet advancement flap in fingertip reconstruction. J Hand Surg Eur 38:395-398, 2013.
6. Moberg E. Aspects of sensation in reconstructive surgery of the upper extremity. J Bone Joint Surg Am 46:817-825, 1964.
7. Nishikawa H, Smith PJ. The recovery of sensation and function after cross-finger flaps for fingertip injury. J Hand Surg Br 17:102-107, 1992.
8. Littler JW. The neurovascular pedicle method of digital transposition for reconstruction of the thumb. Plast Reconstr Surg 12:303-319, 1953.
9. Elsahy NI. When to replant a fingertip after its complete amputation. Plast Reconstr Surg 60:14-21, 1977.
10. Moiemen NS, Elliot D. Composite graft replacement of digital tips. A study in children. J Hand Surg Br 22:346-352, 1997.

68. Nail Bed Injuries

See *Essentials of Plastic Surgery*, second edition, pp. 824-833.

DEMOGRAPHICS OF NAIL BED INJURIES
1. Which one of the following is correct regarding nail bed injuries?
   A. They most commonly occur in children under two years of age.
   B. The border digits are most commonly affected.
   C. More than 90% have a concomitant distal phalanx fracture.
   D. Most injuries spare the soft tissues of the fingertip.
   E. They account for two thirds of hand injuries in children.

NAIL BED ANATOMY
2. Label the five marked regions of the nail bed complex using the options listed (Fig. 68-1). (Each option may be used once only or not at all.)

   Options:
   a. Paronychia
   b. Paronychium
   c. Perionychium
   d. Hyponychium
   e. Eponychium
   f. Sterile matrix
   g. Germinal matrix
   h. Extensor origin

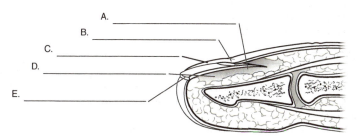

Fig. 68-1 Anatomy of the fingertip and nail bed.

NORMAL NAIL GROWTH

3. *For each of the following descriptions of nail growth, select the anatomic area of the nail apparatus responsible. (Each option may be used once, more than once, or not at all.)*
A. This area is responsible for creating a shine to the nail plate.
B. This is the key site for nail growth through gradient parakeratosis.
C. This area is responsible for increasing nail strength.

Options:
a. Lunula
b. Hyponychium
c. Sterile matrix
d. Nail fold
e. Eponychium
f. Germinal matrix

NAIL GROWTH RATES

4. You see a patient following avulsion of the nail plate. She asks how long it will take for the nail to regrow and what factors may affect this. ***Which one of the following is not associated with increased nail growth?***
A. Summer season
B. Younger age
C. Female sex
D. Digital length
E. Onychophagia

CLASSIFICATION OF NAIL BED INJURIES

5. ***When considering the Van Beek classification, what is the clinical relevance of a type I or II nail bed injury?***
A. That no intervention is required.
B. That splinting is required.
C. That nail trephination is required.
D. That nail bed repair is required.
E. That nail bed grafting is required.

NAIL BED REPAIR

6. You are planning to undertake a nail bed repair on a 5-year-old child following a "door shut injury" which has resulted in a comminuted tuft fracture and nail bed laceration distal to the lunula. ***Which one of the following is correct regarding the procedure?***
A. Neither postoperative antibiotics nor a finger tourniquet are warranted.
B. Reliable bony stabilization will require a kirschner wire.
C. Wound extension is required proximal to the nail fold for access.
D. Repair outcomes using tissue glue are poor and should be avoided.
E. The nail bed should be minimally debrided and repaired with a 6-0 or 7-0 suture.

PERFORMING A STANDARD NAIL BED REPAIR

7. When performing a nail bed repair, use of the nail plate as a postoperative splint is often advocated. *What is the other key benefit to replacing the nail plate?*
   A. To prevent subsequent nail ridging
   B. To increase nail regrowth
   C. For improved cosmesis until a new nail has formed
   D. To decrease postoperative pain
   E. To reduce rates of infection

HOOK-NAIL DEFORMITY

8. *Which one of the following is true of the hook-nail deformity?*
   A. It is primarily because of damage to the germinal matrix.
   B. It is best prevented by using a postoperative splint.
   C. Surgical correction of an established deformity may require a local flap.
   D. It is a consequence of injury to the sterile matrix.
   E. It can be corrected with placement of a skin graft under the distal nail bed.

DEMOGRAPHICS OF NAIL BED INJURIES
1. **Which one of the following is correct regarding nail bed injuries?**
   E. They account for two thirds of hand injuries in children.
   Nail bed injuries are extremely common in children and young adults, with most occurring in males between the ages of 4 and 30. The middle finger is most commonly affected because of its increased length compared with the other digits. Most injuries involve the nail bed and soft tissue of the fingertip. Many (50%) also involve fractures of the distal phalanx.

NAIL BED ANATOMY
2. **For Fig. 68-2, the anatomic components of the nail bed complex are as follows:**
   The fingertip includes the volar pulp and dorsal nail complex. The perionychium is a collective description of the nail bed, nail plate, hyponychium, and eponychium. The paronychial regions are the lateral borders adjacent to the nail plate; i.e., they run parallel to the nail edge. The hyponychium is the area between the distal nail and pulp and has a keratin plug that acts as a mechanical barrier. The eponychium is the distal portion of the nail fold where it is attached to the nail plate. Paronychia refers to an infection of the soft tissues surrounding the nail complex. The germinal and sterile matrices are both important in nail growth.

   A. g. Germinal matrix
   B. e. Eponychium
   C. b. Paronychium
   D. f. Sterile matrix
   E. d. Hyponychium

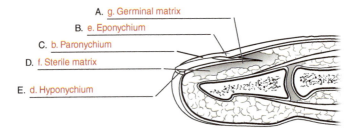

Fig. 68-2 Anatomy of the fingertip and nail bed.

NORMAL NAIL GROWTH
3. **For each of the following descriptions of nail growth, select the anatomic area of the nail apparatus responsible.**
   A. This area is responsible for creating a shine to the nail plate.
   d. Nail fold
   B. This is the key site for nail growth through gradient parakeratosis.
   f. Germinal matrix
   C. This area is responsible for increasing nail strength.
   c. Sterile matrix
   Nail growth occurs at three key sites: the germinal matrix, the dorsal roof of the nail fold, and the sterile matrix. Of these, the germinal matrix is the most important area, as it is responsible for 90% of nail production. It lies immediately distal to the extensor tendon insertion. Production occurs through gradient parakeratosis with cells initially moving in a volar-dorsal direction before

growing in a proximal-distal direction. The lunula represents the distal part of the germinal matrix. The nail fold has a ventral floor and dorsal roof, both of which are involved in nail growth. The ventral floor is the site of the distal germinal matrix and the dorsal roof hosts cells that impart nail shine. The sterile matrix is important for contributing to nail strength and thickness by adding squamous cells to the nail plate.

NAIL GROWTH RATES

4. You see a patient following avulsion of the nail plate. She asks how long it will take for the nail to regrow and what factors may affect this. *Which one of the following is not associated with increased nail growth?*
   C. Female sex
   Normal nail growth is variable but is typically 3 to 4 mm per month.[1,2] It therefore takes about 4 months to regrow a nail fully. Factors that seem to increase growth include greater digital length (the nail of the middle finger grows faster than that of the little finger), time of year (growth is increased in the summer), younger age, and a nail-biting habit (onychophagia). There may be a slight sex difference, with growth in males being greater than in females, although this is not confirmed and may simply be a factor of differences in digit length.

CLASSIFICATION OF NAIL BED INJURIES

5. *When considering the Van Beek classification, what is the clinical relevance of a type I or II nail bed injury?*
   C. That nail trephination is required.
   The classification system described by Van Beek has five categories.[3] Types I and II are both subungual hematomas and are differentiated by their size. Type I is less than 25% and type II is greater than 50%. The difference is arbitrary, since both are usually treated the same using a trephination technique under local anesthetic to drain the hematoma. Type III injuries involve a nail bed laceration and a distal phalangeal fracture. These are treated with repair of the laceration and splinting of the fracture. Types IV and V involve more significant damage to the nail bed that precludes simple repair. They do not necessarily involve a distal phalangeal fracture, although they may well do so. These are best managed using nail bed grafts from the same digit or the great toe, because leaving them to heal by secondary intention will lead to misshapen and nonadherent nail plates.

NAIL BED REPAIR

6. You are planning to undertake a nail bed repair on a 5-year-old child following a "door shut injury" which has resulted in a comminuted tuft fracture and nail bed laceration distal to the lunula. *Which one of the following is correct regarding the procedure?*
   E. The nail bed should be minimally debrided and repaired with a 6-0 or 7-0 suture.
   Nail bed tissue is highly specialized and debridement must be minimal to optimize preserved tissue. Furthermore, crushed and bruised nail bed tissue often survives. Following debridement, careful repair of the nail bed should be performed with a fine suture (e.g., 6-0 or 7-0) under loupe magnification. A finger tourniquet should be used to provide a blood-free field and the application and removal times must be noted by the surgeon and documented by the OR staff. Strict adherence to this will reduce the chances of inadvertently leaving a tourniquet in situ. A general rule of thumb is to prescribe antibiotics for nail bed injuries that have a distal phalanx fracture, but not for those without. Tuft fractures do not require K-wire stabilization as the nail plate and soft tissues provide adequate support. Unstable shaft fractures close to the DIP joint will frequently require K-wiring. Wound extension proximal to the nail fold is only required when

access to the germinal matrix is required. Use of glue instead of sutures has shown comparable results for nail bed repair and may be considered.[4]

PERFORMING A STANDARD NAIL BED REPAIR

7. When performing a nail bed repair, use of the nail plate as a postoperative splint is often advocated. *What is the other key benefit to replacing the nail plate?*
   A. To prevent subsequent nail ridging
   The main theoretical benefit of replacing the nail plate within the nail fold is to keep the fold open in the early stages of regrowth and prevent nail fold adhesions (synechiae). Nail fold adhesions are thought to lead to ridging of the nail. There is no effect on nail regrowth, postoperative pain, or rates of infection. Although cosmesis may be improved in the short term, the nail plate only remains in situ for a short period of time and will not remain in place until a new nail has completely regrown.

HOOK-NAIL DEFORMITY

8. *Which one of the following is true of the hook-nail deformity?*
   C. Surgical correction of an established deformity may require a local flap.
   The hook-nail deformity is caused by a lack of distal phalanx bone support beneath the nail bed which continues to grow distally over the top of the short bone end. It is best prevented by matching bone length and nail bed length so that underlying support is achieved for the full length of the nail bed. Therefore, preservation of distal phalanx length and primary shortening of the nail bed during a revision amputation may avoid subsequent development of this deformity. Neither germinal or sterile matrix damage is the cause of a hook-nail deformity as evidenced by continued growth of the nail, and splinting alone will not prevent it. Once established, the deformity may be corrected using the antennae procedure, which was described by Atasoy.[5] This is a two-stage procedure that addresses the lack of support for the nail bed and the relative lack of volar soft tissue. In the first stage, the pulp and nail bed are elevated off the distal phalanx and the nail bed is then splinted in a straight position with two or three small K-wires (hence the term "antennae"). The residual soft tissue pulp deficit is then reconstructed using a cross-finger flap from the adjacent index finger.

REFERENCES

1. Yaemsiri S, Hou N, Slining MM, et al. Growth rate of human fingernails and toenails in healthy American young adults. J Eur Acad Dermatol Venereol 24:420-423, 2010.
2. Wu Z, Xu J, Jiao Y, et al. Fingernail growth rate and macroelement levels determined by ICP-OES in healthy Chinese college students. Pol J Environ Stud 21:1067-1070, 2012.
3. Van Beek AL, Kassan MA, Adson MH, et al. Management of acute fingernail injuries. Hand Clin 6:23-35; discussion 37-38, 1990.
4. Strauss EJ, Weil WM, Jordan C, et al. A prospective, randomized, controlled trial of 2-octylcyanoacrylate versus suture repair of nail bed injuries. J Hand Surg Am 33:250-253, 2008.
5. Atasoy E, Godfrey A, Kalisman M. The "antenna" procedure for the "hook-nail" deformity. J Hand Surg Am 8:55-58, 1983.

69. Flexor Tendon Injuries

See *Essentials of Plastic Surgery*, second edition, pp. 834-844.

FLEXOR ANATOMY

1. **Which one of the following is true regarding the anatomy of the flexor tendons?**
   A. The FDS tendons insert into the distal phalanges.
   B. The FDP tendons are attached to the lumbricals in the palm.
   C. Camper's chiasm lies at the level of the PIP joint.
   D. At the wrist, the index and middle FDS tendons lie most superficial.
   E. FPL originates from the lateral epicondyle of the humerus.

2. **Which one of the following flexor muscles is entirely supplied by the anterior interosseous nerve?**
   A. The FDS
   B. The FDP
   C. The FPL
   D. Both FDS and FDP
   E. Both FDP and FPL

PULLEY SYSTEM

3. **When repairing a digital flexor tendon injury, which combination of pulleys is it most important to preserve?**
   A. A1 and A3
   B. A2 and A4
   C. A3 and A5
   D. A1 and A4
   E. A2 and A5

TENDON NUTRITION

4. **Which one of the following represents the major nutritional supply to the flexor tendons within the digits?**
   A. Sharpey's fibers at the bony tendon insertion
   B. Blood vessels at the myotendinous junction
   C. Vinculum longus and vinculum brevis to each tendon
   D. Synovial diffusion from the flexor sheath
   E. Axial nutrient vessels in the palmar surface of the tendon

PRINCIPLES OF REPAIR

5. **What represents the recommended threshold for performing formal repair using a core suture in partially divided flexor tendon injuries?**
   A. Any degree of division
   B. 15% division
   C. 25% division
   D. 50% division
   E. 75% division

6. **When repairing a zone II digital flexor tendon injury, which one of the following is correct?**
   A. The core suture should lie as dorsal as possible within the tendon to preserve vascularity.
   B. A continuous two-strand repair is recommended to facilitate early rehabilitation.
   C. The core suture should pass 5 mm proximal and distal to the repair.
   D. A Pulvertaft weave should be used, as it is stronger than other suture techniques.
   E. An epitendinous suture will add approximately 15% to 20% strength to the core suture repair.

ZONE I FLEXOR TENDON INJURIES

7. A 20-year-old rugby player is seen 1 day after sustaining a closed injury while grabbing the shirt of an opponent during a game. He is unable to flex the DIP joint of his right ring finger but is able to flex the PIP joint. A radiograph confirms the presence of a bony fragment at the level of the PIP joint. **Which one of the following best describes this injury?**
   A. Leddy type I
   B. Leddy type II
   C. Leddy type III
   D. Leddy type IV
   E. Leddy type V

8. **Which one of the following is correct regarding zone I digital flexor tendon injuries?**
   A. Bone anchor devices are useful for primary repair.
   B. A braided suture is best for a pull-out suture repair.
   C. 10 mm of distal stump is the minimum required to perform a primary repair.
   D. Repair must always be performed within one week of injury.
   E. In sharp injuries the tendon usually retracts into the palm.

REPAIR WITHIN DIFFERENT FLEXOR ZONES

9. Different zones of flexor tendon injury require different principles of management. **Which one of the following statements is correct?**
   A. The use of epitendinous sutures is necessary for all injury zones.
   B. FDS and FDP should always be individually repaired.
   C. Zone III injuries are traditionally associated with the poorest functional outcomes.
   D. The carpal ligament should not be repaired following zone IV repair.
   E. The oblique pulley is most important to preserve during FPL repairs.

CLINICAL SCENARIOS

10. You are assessing a 23-year-old patient who is no longer able to flex the DIP joint of his dominant ring finger 5 weeks after a game of rugby. A lateral radiograph is unremarkable. **When discussing treatment options with him, which one of the following is correct?**
    A. The proximal tendon end may have to be retrieved at the level of the wrist crease.
    B. Direct repair should not present a problem in this case.
    C. An immediate palmaris longus tendon graft may be required.
    D. Consent should be obtained for both primary and staged repair.
    E. A single-stage direct repair under tension is preferable to a staged reconstruction.

Chapter 69 ▪ Flexor Tendon Injuries

11. *In which one of the following intraoperative scenarios should delayed primary tendon repair at a second operation be considered?*
A. Zone I middle FDP division from a glass injury 3 days earlier
B. Zone III index FDS division from a knife wound 12 days earlier
C. Zone II ring FDS and FDP division from a circular saw injury that day
D. Zone I index FDP division from a human bite wound the previous night
E. Zone II middle FDP division from a knife wound 2 days earlier with clear, pale fluid in the sheath

12. *For each of the following clinical scenarios, select the most likely diagnosis from the options listed. (Each option may be used once, more than once, or not at all.)*
A. A 53-year-old man sustains a stab injury to the volar aspect of his palm in line with the ring finger. On examination he is able to flex the ring finger at both the PIP and DIP joints, but this is painful on resisted flexion.
B. An 18-year-old girl falls onto glass while on a night out. She sustains a 1 cm laceration over the radial aspect of the wrist. Clinical examination reveals no significant deficit, except she is unable to flex the little finger PIP joint independently.
C. A 25-year-old patient is seen in clinic after physiotherapy following repair of a partial FPL zone II tendon division. Her thumb flexion is good, but she is unable to flex the thumb without the index finger DIP joint flexing.

Options:
a. Partial division of a zone V flexor tendon
b. Complete division of zone III flexor tendon
c. Linburg's anomaly
d. Wartenburg sign
e. Complete division of a zone II flexor tendon
f. Hematoma only
g. Absent flexor tendon
h. Adhesions secondary to repair
i. Partial division of a zone III flexor tendon

POSTOPERATIVE CARE

13. *When applying a splint after flexor tendon repair, which one of the following is correct?*
A. The MP joints should all be flexed to 90 degrees.
B. The splint should be placed on the volar aspect.
C. The wrist should be extended or in neutral.
D. The IP joints should be almost fully extended.
E. Elastic band traction should routinely be used.

COMPLICATIONS FOLLOWING FLEXOR TENDON REPAIR

14. *Which one of the following is correct regarding outcomes after flexor tendon repair?*
A. Rupture after primary repair occurs in 15% of cases.
B. Contractures after primary repair occur in 60% of cases.
C. FPL is the most frequently ruptured flexor tendon after primary repair.
D. Most contractures that occur after flexor repair require tenolysis.
E. Poor surgical technique is usually to blame for rupture.

Answers

FLEXOR ANATOMY

1. **Which one of the following is true regarding the anatomy of the flexor tendons?**
   B. The FDP tendons are attached to the lumbricals in the palm.

   Flexion of the digits is controlled by the FDS, FDP, and FPL muscles. The FDP originates from the proximal ulna and interosseous membrane and inserts into the distal phalanges to provide flexion at the DIP joints and contributes to PIP joint flexion. It is also attached to the lumbricals in the palm and this is important after flexor tendon division, as the proximal end of the FDP tendon will therefore not retract further proximal than the midpalm. The FDS originates from the medial epicondyle of the humerus and coronoid process of the ulna and inserts into the middle phalanges to provide flexion at the PIP joints. The FPL originates at the proximal radius, interosseous membrane, coronoid process, and sometimes from the medial epicondyle of the humerus. It inserts into the distal phalanx of the thumb to provide flexion of the IP joint. Camper's chiasm represents the division of FDS into two slips on either side of the FDP tendon distal to the level of the MP joint. The two slips insert separately to the middle phalanx. Knowledge of the anatomic position of the FDS tendons at the wrist is useful during spaghetti wrist repair, as this can help to identify the tendons accurately. The index and little finger FDS tendons lie deep, not superficial to the ring and middle FDS tendons.

2. **Which one of the following flexor muscles is entirely supplied by the anterior interosseous nerve?**
   C. The FPL

   The anterior interosseous nerve is a branch of the median nerve in the forearm. It supplies the FPL, the pronation quadratus, and the radial two FDP tendons. The ulna two FDP tendons are supplied by the ulnar nerve and the FDS are supplied by the median nerve directly (see Chapters 59 and 78, *Essentials of Plastic Surgery*, second edition). When not due to neuritis, anterior interosseous nerve palsy can occur secondary to compression of the nerve by the tendinous edge of the deep head of the pronator teres or tendinous origin of FDS. Patients with this condition cannot flex the index DIP joint or thumb IP joint normally, resulting in an abnormal tip pinch grip. Patients cannot make the "ok" sign in this scenario. There is no sensory deficit present because the anterior interosseous has no cutaneous sensory branches.

PULLEY SYSTEM

3. **When repairing a digital flexor tendon injury, which combination of pulleys is it most important to preserve?**
   B. A2 and A4

   The pulley system in the digits involves five annular pulleys and three cruciate pulleys. The annular pulleys are located along the flexor sheath starting at the MP joint with A1. The even numbered annular pulleys are located over the phalangeal shafts (A2-proximal phalanx and the A4-middle phalanx), while the odd numbered pulleys are located over the small joints (A1-MP, A3-PIP, A5-DIP). Their collective function is to prevent bowstringing of the tendon during flexion and provide a mechanical advantage. Ideally they should be preserved during flexor tendon repair. However, the A2 and A4 pulleys are thought to be the most important (see Fig. 69-2, *Essentials of Plastic Surgery*, second edition).

Chapter 69 ▪ Flexor Tendon Injuries 563

TENDON NUTRITION

4. Which one of the following represents the major nutritional supply to the flexor tendons within the digits?

D. Synovial diffusion from the flexor sheath

Tendon nutrition in the digits depends significantly on diffusion from the synovial sheath. The other sources of nutrition listed each make a variable contribution to tendon nutrition, but the vascular network within the digital flexor tendons is sparse. The bony insertion and musculotendinous junction blood supply is limited to around 1 cm of tendon length at each site, with the remaining blood supply arising from the vinculae. In the forearm and proximal digit there is also a vascular supply from segmental vessels in the paratenon.

Axial blood supply within the flexors tends to be located in the dorsal portion of the tendon, so many surgeons prefer to place sutures in the volar portion during repair in the hope of maximizing blood supply. In contrast, there is some evidence that placing the core sutures dorsally within the tendon may be biomechanically advantageous.[1]

PRINCIPLES OF REPAIR

5. What represents the recommended threshold for performing formal repair using a core suture in partially divided flexor tendon injuries?

D. 50% division

The management of partial flexor tendon repairs will depend on a number of factors such as the location, the flexor tendon involved, and the type of injury sustained. It will also be affected by surgeon preference. However, most agree that tendon lacerations involving more than 50% of the tendon diameter should be formally repaired with core and epitendinous sutures. Lesser divisions should be smoothed off or repaired with simple sutures to avoid the edges catching and to ensure the tendon ends are neatly apposed.

6. When repairing a zone II digital flexor tendon injury, which one of the following is correct?

E. An epitendinous suture will add approximately 15% to 20% strength to the core suture repair.

The main benefit of using an epitendinous suture is that it adds up to 20% additional strength to the repair. In addition, it helps to smooth the repair and improve gliding within the flexor sheath. A meta-analysis of complications after flexor tendon repair also suggested that the rate of reoperation is reduced by 84% if an epitendinous suture is used.[2]

There is debate surrounding the optimal positioning of core sutures as discussed in the explanation to question 4, with volar positioning considered to be best for tendon vascularity and dorsal positioning considered more biomechanically favorable during active flexion. In reality, many tendons are sufficiently thin that reliably placing the suture anywhere other than centrally is challenging.

A minimum four-strand (not two) core suture repair is required in order to commence early active mobilization. This may be undertaken as a two-strand core suture combined with a two-strand mattress, as two separate two-strand core sutures, or as a single four-strand core suture repair. There is no definitive evidence that a four-strand single-knot technique is superior to two adjacent two-strand core sutures. Some surgeons prefer to use a six-strand technique when the tendon diameter is sufficient to allow this. The core suture should ideally have 10 mm (not 5 mm) proximal and distal to the repair. A Pulvertaft weave cannot be used in primary tendon repair in the digit, as it would entail significant tendon shortening and would create too much bulk to fit within the tendon sheath.

ZONE I FLEXOR TENDON INJURIES

7. A 20-year-old rugby player is seen 1 day after sustaining a closed injury while grabbing the shirt of an opponent during a game. He is unable to flex the DIP joint of his right ring finger but is able to flex the PIP joint. A radiograph confirms the presence of a bony fragment at the level of the PIP joint. **Which one of the following best describes this injury?**
   B. Leddy type II
   Zone I closed avulsion injuries of the FDP were classified by Leddy and Packer in 1977 into three categories based on the presence of a bony fragment on radiograph, the blood supply, and the position of the retracted proximal tendon end.[3] Additional fourth and fifth categories were subsequently added.[4] The classification is useful to guide management. The patient described has a type II injury based on the bony fragment position and should undergo an open repair using a pull-out suture or bone anchor device.

   The modified Leddy-Packer classification includes the following:
   Type I: The FDP tendon retracts into the palm with rupture of both vincula.
   Type II: The FDP tendon avulses with a small fragment of distal phalanx, the long vinculum remains intact, and the tendon retracts to the level of the PIP joint (A3 pulley).
   Type III: A large bony fragment is avulsed with the tendon and is prevented from retraction beyond the middle phalanx by the A4 pulley.
   Type IV: An avulsion fracture of the distal phalanx combines with tendon avulsion from the fragment, along with tendon retraction.
   Type V: A bony avulsion of the FDP is coupled with a distal phalanx fracture (either intraarticular or extraarticular).

8. **Which one of the following is correct regarding zone I digital flexor tendon injuries?**
   A. Bone anchor devices are useful for primary repair.
   Bone anchor devices may be used successfully in primary tendon repairs. The outcomes using bone anchors are comparable to pull-out suture techniques. The recommended technique is to insert either a mini-Mitek or two micro-Mitek anchors at a 45-degree angle from distal/volar to proximal/dorsal, while taking care not to violate the DIP joint surface or nail bed.[5,6]
   When using a pull-out suture technique where the core suture is passed externally over the nail, a monofilament such as nylon or polypropylene is preferred. Braided sutures glide less well, are difficult to remove, and are also more prone to infection. FDP avulsion may also be repaired by drilling a small hole transversely through the distal phalanx for the core suture to pass through, enabling a fully internal repair. Although the normal recommendation for core suture repair is that there is 10 mm of tendon proximal and distal to the repair, a distal stump of 5 mm is considered sufficient for standard core suture repair of zone I flexor tendon injuries. For most flexor tendon injuries, repair within a week of injury is recommended. However, some injuries that involve avulsion of the tendon insertion from the distal phalanx, with minimal proximal retraction (due to either intact vinculae or a bony fragment anchored against a pulley), may still be repaired after several weeks. A delay repairing a retracted tendon can lead to a shortening, a quadriga effect, and collapse of the flexor sheath.

REPAIR WITHIN DIFFERENT FLEXOR ZONES

9. Different zones of flexor tendon injury require different principles of management. **Which one of the following statements is correct?**
   E. The oblique pulley is most important to preserve during FPL repairs.
   The most important pulley to preserve in the thumb, is the oblique pulley. Although the use of an epitendinous suture can add a further 15% to 20% strength to a flexor tendon repair, it is not necessary for zone V repairs. A four- or six-strand core repair is advocated for most injuries (see Fig. 69-6, *Essentials of Plastic Surgery*, second edition). Zone II injuries have the poorest functional outcomes. This zone was previously termed "no man's land" because of the difficulties with achieving satisfactory repair and outcomes. The carpal ligament should be repaired in zone IV injuries to prevent bowstringing during rehabilitation.

   In most cases it is best to repair both FDS and FDP. However, many people do not have an FDS in the little finger and the FDS may not always be repaired in zone II if it is very small and likely to interfere with satisfactory movement of the FDP repair. Where there is a problem with bulk, some surgeons opt to repair only one slip of FDS and trim the other in zone II.

CLINICAL SCENARIOS

10. You see a 23-year-old patient who is no longer able to flex the DIP joint of his dominant ring finger 5 weeks after a game of rugby. A lateral radiograph is unremarkable. **When discussing treatment options with him, which one of the following is correct?**
    D. Consent should be obtained for both primary and staged repair.
    This is likely to be a Leddy-Packer type I FDP tendon avulsion injury, with the tendon end lying in the palm. The FDP tendon does not usually retract to the wrist because of the lumbrical attachments and the tendinous interconnections between the FDP tendons to the four fingers.

    In this scenario, the window for successful direct repair is reduced to 7 to 10 days compared to type II and III injuries, because the tendon has lost both the vincular and synovial nutrient supplies, and the flexor sheath is largely empty and able to shrink down. There is a chance that this will actually be a type II injury, with an intact vinculum longum and the tendon end at the A3 pulley, in which case a direct repair might still be possible. However, this is much less likely, and beyond 4 weeks there may have been sufficient musculotendinous contraction to lead to an excessively tight repair, causing a troublesome quadriga effect. A quadriga effect occurs when shortening or tethering of one FDP tendon reduces power and excursion in the remaining three healthy tendons, as described by Verdan.[7]

    If a primary repair is not possible in a delayed presentation, it is not advisable to perform an immediate palmaris graft, because the sheath is usually scarred and contracted. Even if there is adequate space for a primary graft, the risk of adhesions is much higher than if a staged approach is used. A silicone (Hunter) rod spacer is usually placed to generate a pseudosheath for subsequent tendon grafting within 8 weeks.

11. *In which one of the following intraoperative scenarios should delayed primary tendon repair at a second operation be considered?*
    D. Zone I index FDP division from a human bite wound the previous night
    Immediate repair is not recommended in bite wounds because of contamination and an element of crush injury. A thorough debridement and washout in addition to antibiotic therapy is preferable, followed by a delayed primary tendon repair if the wound is clean at 48 to 72 hours. When exploring an open tendon injury, serous fluid in the sheath is not uncommon; however, turbid or frankly purulent fluid is a contraindication to immediate repair.

12. *For each of the following clinical scenarios, select the most likely diagnosis from the options listed.*
   A. *A 53-year-old man sustains a stab injury to the volar aspect of his palm in line with the ring finger. On examination he is able to flex the ring finger at both the PIP and DIP joints, but this is painful on resisted flexion.*
      i. **Partial division of zone III flexor tendon**
         The patient in this scenario has sustained an injury in zone III. There are two possible explanations for his pain on flexion. Either there is a partial flexion tendon injury or a hematoma from the injury causing discomfort. The safest management is to proceed with formal exploration to confirm the nature of the injury. Although many partial flexor tendon injuries do not require repair, exploration is warranted, because the tendon may subsequently rupture or cause triggering without repair.
   B. *An 18-year-old girl falls onto glass while on a night out. She sustains a 1 cm laceration over the radial aspect of the wrist. Clinical examination reveals no significant deficit, except she is unable to flex the little finger PIP joint independently.*
      g. **Absent flexor tendon**
         The patient in this scenario is at risk of FCR and radial artery injury. Clinically these structures do not appear to be injured, although exploration may still be warranted, because glass injuries usually penetrate to the bone. The chances of her sustaining an isolated FDS little finger injury are slim given the site of injury. It is far more likely that she has a congenital absence of the FDS; this occurs in approximately 15% of the population. It is important to assess the contralateral limb, since the condition may well be bilateral.
   C. *A 25-year-old patient is seen in clinic after physiotherapy following repair of a partial FPL zone II tendon division. Her thumb flexion is good, but she is unable to flex the thumb without the index finger DIP joint flexing.*
      c. **Linburg's anomaly**
         The patient in this scenario displays the Linburg anomaly (Linburg-Comstock anomaly), in which there are attachments between the FPL and index FDP tendons in the carpal tunnel. This occurs in approximately a third of the population and will have been present before the tendon repair, but was not recognized and documented.

POSTOPERATIVE CARE

13. *When applying a splint after flexor tendon repair, which one of the following is correct?*
   D. **The IP joints should be almost fully extended.**
      Precise postoperative care after flexor tendon repair is critical to achieving a good outcome. The patient must be placed in a dorsal blocking splint to prevent excessive extension of the repair. The wrist should be placed in slight flexion, as this weakens the flexor tendons and can reduce the risk of postoperative rupture.
      The dorsal blocking splint should usually maintain the MP joints in approximately 60 to 70 degrees of flexion. There is a wide range of preferred MP joint splint angles reported (20 to 90 degrees); however, most authors agree that the IP joints should be able to straighten fully, otherwise flexion contractures will develop. Trying to force all four MP joints into 90 degrees of flexion often results in an MP joint angle of around 70 degrees and unintended flexion at the IP joints. Not all techniques require elastic band use in conjunction with the splint. The Kleinert protocol uses elastic band traction to facilitate active extension and passive flexion after repair. Other techniques rely on early, active mobilization and splinting alone.

COMPLICATIONS FOLLOWING FLEXOR TENDON REPAIR

14. Which one of the following is correct regarding outcomes after flexor tendon repair?

C. FPL is the most frequently ruptured flexor tendon after primary repair.

The most commonly reruptured flexor tendon is the FPL, but ring and little finger FDP tendons also have higher rates of rerupture. The overall rate of rerupture after primary repair is around 5% (not 15%). Although rerupture can be due to poor surgical technique during the repair, the main factors tend to be related to the postoperative care, such as patients removing the splint or not complying with rehabilitation advice. Contractures occur in around 20% of cases, and again this is affected by the rehabilitation and aftercare provided and patient compliance. Few patients require joint release (capsulotomy) for managing this complication. Tenolysis may be required in patients with adhesions that are unresponsive to focused hand therapy. These patients typically display an intact tendon repair with good passive ROM but poor active ROM.

REFERENCES

1. Komanduri M, Phillips CS, Mass DP. Tensile strength of flexor tendon repairs in a dynamic cadaver model. J Hand Surg Am 21:605-611, 1996.
2. Dy CJ, Hernandez-Soria A, Ma Y, et al. Complications after flexor tendon repair: a systematic review and meta-analysis. J Hand Surg Am 37:543-551, 2012.
3. Leddy JP, Packer JW. Avulsion of the profundus tendon insertion in athletes. J Hand Surg Am 2:66-69, 1977.
4. Al-Qattan MM. Type 5 avulsion of the insertion of the flexor digitorum profundus tendon. J Hand Surg Br 26:427-431, 2001.
5. Brustein M, Pellegrini J, Choueka J, et al. Bone suture anchors versus the pullout button for repair of distal profundus tendon injuries: a comparison of strength in human cadaveric hands. J Hand Surg 26A:489-496, 2001.
6. McCallister W, Ambrose H, Katolik L, et al. Comparison of pullout button versus suture anchor for zone 1 flexor tendon repair. J Hand Surg Am 31:246-251, 2006.
7. Verdan C. Syndrome of the quadriga. Surg Clin North Am 40:425-426, 1960.

70. Extensor Tendon Injuries

See *Essentials of Plastic Surgery*, second edition, pp. 845-854.

EXTENSOR TENDON ANATOMY

1. **Which one of the following is correct regarding extensor tendon anatomy?**
   A. The EDC to little finger is absent in 10% of patients.
   B. The ECU is the only extensor with a true sheath.
   C. The EDC is the only structure within the fourth compartment.
   D. The EPL travels in the same compartment as the EPB.
   E. The ECRL and ECRB insert into the same metacarpal.

EXTENSOR COMPARTMENTS OF THE WRIST

2. **For each of the following structures, select the correct extensor compartment through which they pass at the wrist. (Each option may be used once, more than once, or not at all.)**
   A. Extensor carpi ulnaris
   B. Abductor pollicis longus
   C. Extensor indicis

   Options:
   a. First compartment
   b. Second compartment
   c. Third compartment
   d. Fourth compartment
   e. Fifth compartment
   f. Sixth compartment

INTRINSIC MUSCLES OF THE HAND

3. **Which one of the following is correct regarding the intrinsic muscles of the hand?**
   A. There are eight interossei, all innervated by the ulnar nerve.
   B. The sole function of the interossei is adduction and abduction of the digits.
   C. The lumbricals originate from the FDP tendons and are all innervated by the ulnar nerve.
   D. The lumbricals facilitate extension at the IP joints and are weak MP joint flexors.
   E. The intrinsic muscles all share a similar bipennate structure.

DIGITAL EXTENSOR TENDON ANATOMY

4. **Correctly identify the anatomic components of the extensor mechanism on the diagram below (Fig. 70-1). Five of the nine options will be used.**

   Options:
   a. Extrinsic extensor
   b. Central slip
   c. Oblique retinacular ligament
   d. Triangular ligament
   e. Interosseous muscle/tendon
   f. Lumbrical
   g. Sagittal band
   h. Bare triangle
   i. Lateral band

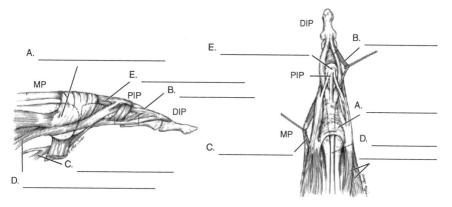

Fig. 70-1 Anatomy of the extensor mechanism of the finger.

VASCULAR ANATOMY

5. **Which one of the following provides a source of blood supply in flexor but not extensor tendons?**
   A. Myotendinous junction
   B. Bony insertion
   C. Paratenon
   D. Synovial fluid
   E. Vinculae

ZONES OF INJURY

6. For each of the following clinical scenarios, select the most likely extensor injury zone from the options listed. (Each option may be used once, more than once, or not at all.)
   A. A patient sustains a transverse laceration to the distal forearm when falling through a glass door.
   B. A patient has an open mallet deformity of the thumb from glass.
   C. A patient has a punch/bite injury to the ring finger MP joint with purulent discharge.

   Options:
   a. Zone I
   b. Zone II
   c. Zone III
   d. Zone IV
   e. Zone V
   f. Zone VI
   g. Zone VII
   h. Zone VIII
   i. Zone IX

7. Which extensor zone of injury is a Seymour fracture sometimes mistaken for?
   A. Zone I
   B. Zone II
   C. Zone III
   D. Zone IV
   E. Zone V

8. Which zone of injury does the term "fight bite" refer to?
   A. Zone II
   B. Zone III
   C. Zone IV
   D. Zone V
   E. Zone VI

MALLET DEFORMITIES

9. Which one of the following does not affect the grading of a mallet deformity according to the Doyle classification?
   A. The presence of an open wound
   B. The presence of soft tissue loss
   C. The presence of an intraarticular fracture
   D. The presence of a transepiphyseal plate injury
   E. The presence of infection

10. **What is the typical management of a closed mallet deformity with a small bony fragment (type I) in a compliant patient?**
   A. Splint immobilization of the DIP joint in full extension for a total of four weeks.
   B. Splint immobilization of the DIP and PIP joints in full extension for a total of four weeks.
   C. K-wire immobilization of the DIP joint in extension for a total of six weeks.
   D. K-wire immobilization of the DIP joint in hyperextension for a total of six weeks.
   E. Splint immobilization of the DIP joint in full extension for a total of six weeks.

11. You see a patient in clinic with a closed soft tissue mallet deformity that has been splinted for three weeks. The patient informs you that they removed the splint at home two days before this visit and left the digit unsupported. There is an extensor lag. **What duration of further continuous splinting is most likely to be required?**
   A. 2 weeks
   B. 3 weeks
   C. 6 weeks
   D. 10 weeks
   E. No set time

CENTRAL SLIP INJURIES

12. A young diabetic patient has sustained a closed soft tissue injury to the index finger PIP joint which has resulted in a new boutonniere deformity. There is no fracture present. **What is the best initial management of the PIP joint in this scenario?**
   A. Active mobilization
   B. External splinting in extension
   C. K-wire stabilization in extension
   D. Direct suture repair
   E. Reconstruction with a flap of proximal tendon

13. A patient presents with a healing 3-day-old incised wound from glass over the dorsum of the PIP joint. Active extension against resistance is preserved, and radiographs reveal that there is no foreign body. **Which one of the following is correct?**
   A. The wound should be left to heal without further intervention.
   B. Full, active extension against resistance implies that the central slip is intact.
   C. The PIP joint capsule is unlikely to be injured.
   D. A turnover tendon flap will be needed if the tendon is divided.
   E. A bone anchor may be required to repair the central slip.

14. A 65-year-old woman presents complaining of recurrent problems extending her middle finger. On examination she is able to fully flex the MP joint with some discomfort beyond 45 degrees but is unable to then actively extend the joint. She can passively straighten the finger and hold it straight against resistance. The joint appears swollen, but there is no subluxation or dislocation. **What is the most likely cause of her problem?**
   A. Intrinsic muscle tightness interfering with the extensor mechanism balance
   B. An osteophyte at the metacarpal head tethering the MP joint collateral ligament in flexion
   C. Radial sagittal band rupture of the middle finger EDC tendon
   D. A dorsal MP joint capsular tear
   E. A loose osteochondral body in the MP joint caused by osteoarthritis

CLOSED EXTENSOR TENDON RUPTURES

15. **Which one of the following closed extensor tendon injuries is most likely to require operative intervention?**
    A. A mallet deformity of the ring finger with a 2 by 2 mm bony avulsion fragment from the distal phalanx
    B. An acute soft tissue central slip injury following a blow from a cricket ball
    C. An acute ECU injury with a small bony avulsion fragment after digging frozen ground with a spade
    D. An acute central slip injury with a 2 by 1 mm bony avulsion fragment from the base of the middle phalanx
    E. A soft tissue mallet deformity of the thumb after a distal radius fracture

CLINICAL CONCEPTS IN EXTENSOR TENDON MANAGEMENT

16. **How should the hand be placed in a splint following repair of multiple zone VIII extensor tendon injuries that involve the myotendinous junction?**
    A. Wrist neutral, MP joints extended
    B. Wrist neutral, MP joints flexed 20 degrees
    C. Wrist extended 70 degrees, MP joints flexed 70 degrees
    D. Wrist extended 20 degrees, MP joints flexed 40 degrees
    E. Wrist extended 40 degrees, MP joint flexed 20 degrees

MANAGEMENT OF EXTENSOR TENDON INJURIES

17. **When managing extensor tendon injuries, which one of the following is correct?**
    A. Acute sagittal band ruptures should be managed nonoperatively.
    B. A swan neck deformity may develop secondary to a zone I extensor rupture.
    C. EPL ruptures are more common at the IP joint than at the wrist.
    D. Tendon ruptures in rheumatoid arthritis can generally be repaired directly.
    E. Extensor tendon repairs are less vulnerable than flexor tendon repairs and require less strict splinting regimens.

EXTRINSIC AND INTRINSIC EXTENSOR PROBLEMS

18. You are asked by the senior hand therapist to give a second opinion on a patient who has difficulty flexing his little and ring fingers 6 months after repair of divided EDC tendons in zone V. When you passively flex the MP joints, he is unable to flex the IP joints. When you extend the MP joints, he is able to flex the IP joints. **What is the recommendation that most likely will address this issue?**
    A. Release of the tight intrinsic muscle insertions from the extensor mechanism
    B. An intensive period of active and passive physiotherapy without splints
    C. Extensor tenolysis around the site of repair only
    D. Extensor tenolysis around the site of repair and into the finger as required
    E. An intensive period of active and passive physiotherapy with an MP joint blocking splint

Answers

EXTENSOR TENDON ANATOMY

1. Which one of the following is correct regarding extensor tendon anatomy?
  B. The ECU is the only extensor with a true sheath.
   The fact that the ECU has a true sheath has clinical relevance, since a tear to the sheath can lead to ulnar-sided wrist pain and subluxation of the ECU. The EDC to the little finger is absent in approximately half of the population (not 10%). Extension of the little finger is achieved by the EDM alone in these patients. The fourth compartment contains the EDC and EIP. In addition, the posterior interosseous nerve lies in the floor of the fourth compartment. It is a useful potential donor site for nerve grafts for digital nerve defects, because harvest incurs minimal donor-site morbidity and the nerve diameter is similar to that of the digital nerves. The EPL and EPB are located in different extensor compartments. The EPL is within the third compartment and has a path that passes around Lister's tubercle. This useful bony landmark is found between the second and third compartments. The EPL is angled around the tubercle as it passes through the compartment and this is a potential site of friction and subsequent attrition rupture (as seen in rheumatoid arthritis or distal radius fractures). The EPB is within the first compartment with the APL. This compartment is positioned on the radial aspect of the wrist and may be spared in dorsal lacerations. The ECRL and ECRB both insert into different metacarpal bones. The ECRL inserts into the base of the index finger, and the ECRB inserts into the base of the middle finger.[1,2]

EXTENSOR COMPARTMENTS OF THE WRIST

2. For the following structures, the best options are as follows:
  A. Extensor carpi ulnaris
   f. Sixth compartment
  B. Abductor pollicis longus
   a. First compartment
  C. Extensor indicis
   d. Fourth compartment
     There are six extensor compartments at the wrist. The ECU is the only tendon to run within the sixth compartment. The APL runs with the EPB within the first compartment. The EIP runs with the EDC in the fourth compartment. Fig. 70-2 shows the various compartments and the structures which they contain. Knowledge of the extensor compartments of the wrist is often tested in clinical exams and is highly relevant to trauma and tendon transfer.

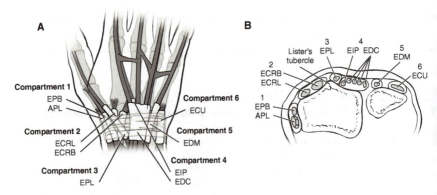

Fig. 70-2 Extensor compartments. (*APL*, Abductor pollicis longus; *ECRB*, extensor carpi radialis brevis; *ECRL*, extensor carpi radialis longus; *EDC*, extensor digitorum communis; *ECU*, extensor carpi ulnaris; *EDM*, extensor digiti minimi; *EIP*, extensor indicis proprius; *EPB*, extensor pollicis brevis; *EPL*, extensor pollicis longus.)

INTRINSIC MUSCLES OF THE HAND

3. **Which one of the following is correct regarding the intrinsic muscles of the hand?**

   D. The lumbricals facilitate extension at the IP joints and are weak MP joint flexors.

   The intrinsic muscles of the hand include the lumbricals and interossei. There are seven interossei (four dorsal and three palmar), all of which are innervated by the ulnar nerve (see Fig. 70-2, *Essentials of Plastic Surgery*, second edition). Their main purpose is abduction (dorsal) and adduction (palmar) of the digits but they also contribute to MP and IP joint extension. The lumbricals do originate from the FDP tendons and insert on the extensor hood. They have dual innervation with the ulnar two receiving innervation from the ulnar nerve and the radial two receiving innervation from the median nerve. The palmar interossei are unipennate muscles.

DIGITAL EXTENSOR TENDON ANATOMY

4. **For Fig. 70-3, the anatomic components of the extensor mechanism are as follows:**

   The extensor mechanism is complex and receives both intrinsic and extrinsic muscle contribution. The extensor digitorum communis trifurcates into the central slip and two lateral slips. The central slip inserts into the base of the middle phalanx along with fibers from the lumbricals and interossei. The lateral bands are formed from the lateral slips and the lateral bands of the intrinsics, and these reunite over the distal portion of the middle phalanx to form the terminal extensor tendon inserting at the distal phalanx. The sagittal bands originate from the intermetacarpal plate on either side of the metacarpal head to form a dorsal hood. They maintain the central slip of the extensors over the MP joint preventing lateral subluxation.

Chapter 70 ■ Extensor Tendon Injuries

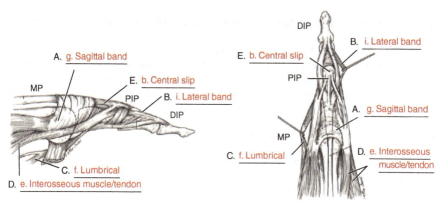

Fig. 70-3 Anatomy of the extensor mechanism of the finger.

VASCULAR ANATOMY

5. **Which one of the following provides a source of blood supply in flexor but not extensor tendons?**
   E. Vinculae
   The extensor tendons receive blood supply from a number of sources as do the flexor tendons. These include the myotendinous junction, the bony insertion, the paratenon along the length of the tendon, and synovial lined tissue (such as under the reinaculum). Unlike the flexor tendons, however, there are no vinculae vessels supplying the extensor tendons.

ZONES OF INJURY

6. **For the following scenarios, the best options are as follows:**
   A. **A patient sustains a transverse laceration to the distal forearm when falling through a glass door.**
      h. Zone VIII
   B. **A patient has an open mallet deformity of the thumb from glass.**
      a. Zone I
   C. **A patient has a punch/bite injury to the ring finger MP joint with purulent discharge.**
      e. Zone V

   The established nomenclature for extensor tendons contains nine different zones for the fingers and five zones for the thumb starting with zone I most distal over the DIP joint or IP joint, respectively. The finger zones can then be counted as odd numbers over the joints (DIP, PIP, MP, and carpus I, III, V, and VII). The even numbers refer to the middle phalanx, proximal phalanx, metacarpal, and distal forearm (II, IV, VI, and VIII, respectively). Zone IX refers to the proximal to midforearm where muscle bellies are present (see Fig. 70-5, *Essentials of Plastic Surgery,* second edition).

7. **Which extensor zone of injury is a Seymour fracture sometimes mistaken for?**
   A. **Zone I**
   Zone I injuries involve the extensor tendon near the DIP joint. A Seymour fracture is a type of open fracture with the nail bed trapped in the physis. It often presents with the nail plate sitting on top of the nail fold and is mistaken for a simple nail bed or mallet zone I extensor injury. It requires careful management, because without treatment the nail bed will remain in the physis and affect healing and growth. The extensor tendon inserts on the epiphysis, therefore is intact in this injury.

8. **Which zone of injury does the term "fight bite" refer to?**
   D. **Zone V**
   Open zone V extensor tendon injuries commonly occur following a punch injury to the face where the attacker's fist contacts the tooth of the other person during the punch. It is effectively a self-inflicted human bite injury, hence the term "fight bite." This injury mechanism often results in partial division of the extensor over the MP joint and also involves the joint itself. Presentation is typically delayed until infection begins with swelling, inflammation, and pain in the joint. Management involves admission for intravenous antibiotics, formal exploration, and wash out of the wound including the joint. The extensor should be repaired, if necessary, only once infection is controlled. The wound may be left to heal by secondary intention or closed as a delayed secondary procedure.

MALLET DEFORMITIES

9. **Which one of the following does not affect the grading of a mallet deformity according to the Doyle classification?**
   E. **The presence of infection**
   A mallet injury is a zone I extensor injury with loss of continuity of the extensor close to the DIP joint. A clear classification system is clinically relevant to a mallet injury, as it guides treatment and enables comparison of clinical outcomes between patients. Mallet injuries are open or closed, can involve a fracture or soft tissue injury, and in some circumstances both are present. The Doyle classification has four grades. Type I is a closed injury with or without a small bony avulsion. Type II is an open injury with a laceration close to the DIP joint that results in a loss of tendon continuity. Type III is an open injury with soft tissue loss. Type IV is an injury with a fracture of the distal phalanx that may involve the articular surface or the epiphyseal region.[3]

10. **What is the typical management of a closed mallet deformity with a small bony fragment (type I) in a compliant patient?**
    E. **Splint immobilization of the DIP joint in full extension for a total of six weeks.**
    Most closed mallet injuries can be satisfactorily managed nonoperatively with external splinting. The splint may be placed volar or dorsal and should hold the DIP joint in extension for at least six weeks, then a night splint should be used for another two weeks. The PIP and MP joints should be free to mobilize. K-wire immobilization may be considered in cases where compliance is not possible, in patients with occupations that may find continuous external splinting unacceptable, or in cases where reduction with splinting alone is inadequate.

Chapter 70 ■ Extensor Tendon Injuries   577

11. You see a patient in clinic with a closed soft tissue mallet deformity that has been splinted for three weeks. The patient informs you that they removed the splint at home two days before this visit and left the digit unsupported. There is an extensor lag. *What duration of further continuous splinting is most likely to be required?*
C. 6 weeks
   The normal duration of splinting following a mallet deformity is six weeks of continuous splinting followed by two weeks of night-time splinting. The patient must understand that the splint is to be worn continuously for the entire six weeks and that removal resulting in DIP joint flexion, at any stage before this, will restart the clock and a minimum of an additional six weeks splinting will be required. In general, soft tissue mallet injuries take longer to heal than bony mallet injuries and this must be kept in mind when selecting a suitable management plan. Patients should be shown how to safely remove and reapply the splint for skin care without flexing the DIP joint.

CENTRAL SLIP INJURIES

12. A young diabetic patient has sustained a closed soft tissue injury to the index finger PIP joint which has resulted in a new boutonniere deformity. There is no fracture present. *What is the best initial management of the PIP joint in this scenario?*
B. External splinting in extension
   The boutonniere deformity occurs secondary to injury to the digital extensor in zone III. A closed avulsion can occur following trauma and is often misdiagnosed as a sprained finger. The deformity develops as the lateral bands migrate volarly, changing their vector of pull, to cause PIP joint flexion and DIP joint hyperextension. Closed zone III avulsion injuries are best treated nonoperatively with external splinting of the PIP joint in extension. Regimens vary, but a typical example is six weeks continuous splinting and another two weeks splinting at night only. It is important to keep the remaining finger joints free to actively mobilize throughout, in order to avoid stiffness. K-wires are not normally required to hold the PIP joint in extension and are best avoided, as they can cause damage to the articular surface and also carry a risk of infection. Extra care should be taken to avoid their use in higher risk patients such as diabetics. Active mobilization is not required until the period of splinting is complete. It is, however, very important at this stage in order to minimize subsequent joint stiffness. Some regimens include early graduated flexion with flexion blocking splints, or active flexion and passive extension in a Capener splint which is a type of dynamic spring-loaded splint that holds the PIP joint in extension but allows flexion against resistance. The name is generated from the individual who first described the splint; however, this has now become a generic term used by many manufacturers and hand therapists.[4] Specialized surgical repair is usually only required in open injuries. A proximal extensor tendon turnover flap may be used where there is substance loss.

13. A patient presents with a healing 3-day-old incised wound from glass over the dorsum of the PIP joint. Active extension against resistance is preserved, and radiographs reveal that there is no foreign body. *Which one of the following is correct?*
E. A bone anchor may be required to repair the central slip.
   Glass injuries often penetrate easily until resistance is met, usually against bone. At PIP joint level, the dorsal soft tissues and tendon are thin, therefore the joint capsule may well have been injured. At 3 days, the wound has barely started healing and the benefits of identifying and repairing a central slip injury early (avoiding a boutonniere deformity) outweigh the downsides of exploring the wound under a local anesthetic block.

If the central slip is divided, the patient may well be able to fully extend against resistance. Two intact lateral bands will still give strong extension, and a single intact lateral band is enough to fully extend in the early stages. If a central slip injury is missed, the finger will gradually collapse into a boutonniere deformity as the lateral bands sublux volar to the pivot point of the PIP joint. Contracture of the volar plate and joint capsule can develop quickly, and the central slip remnants become retracted and scarred, making delayed repair more challenging.

With an acute, sharp division of the central slip, direct repair will normally be possible, but a bone anchor or drill hole through the middle phalanx may be required if the distal stump is insufficient to hold a suture. Turnover flaps, such as described by Snow,[5] are reserved for occasions where a gap prevents direct repair, such as circular saw or abrasive central slip injuries.

14. A 65-year-old woman attends clinic complaining of recurrent problems extending her middle finger. On examination she is able to fully flex the MP joint with some discomfort beyond 45 degrees, but is unable to then actively extend the joint. She can passively straighten the finger and hold it straight against resistance. The joint appears swollen, but there is no subluxation or dislocation. **What is the most likely cause of her problem?**
   C. Radial sagittal band rupture of the middle finger EDC tendon
   This woman's symptoms are in keeping with a sagittal band rupture, which can present acutely or as a chronic problem. This injury allows the EDC tendon to sublux into the gutters on either side of the prominent metacarpal head when the MP joint is flexed. When the patient tries to extend the MP joint from full flexion, this can be difficult because the EDC has lost its tension and therefore its mechanical advantage by slipping off the metacarpal head.

   Another typical scenario for this injury is a young male boxer or fighter with an acutely painful and swollen dorsal aspect of the MP joint after a punch injury. There will be pain with increasing flexion and a point beyond which the tendon slips into the gutter.

CLOSED EXTENSOR TENDON RUPTURES

15. **Which one of the following closed extensor tendon injuries is most likely to require operative intervention?**
   E. A soft tissue mallet deformity of the thumb after a distal radius fracture
   A distal radius fracture is a risk factor for an EPL attrition rupture, which usually occurs around Lister's tubercle. It is important not to miss this diagnosis by mistaking a proximal injury for a simple zone I mallet injury, as the patient may end up with weeks of unnecessary splinting to no avail and will be better served by an EIP to EPL tendon transfer. Closed zone I EPL ruptures can, of course, occur, but these are rare. A combination of the clinical findings (such as swelling and tenderness around either the IP joint or Lister's tubercle) and ultrasound may be helpful in distinguishing the different levels of injury. Many authors advocate a similar management plan for zone I EPL ruptures to finger mallet injuries, i.e., splinting of closed soft tissue injuries.[6] However, there are also concerns that the EPL tendon tends to retract more than the lateral bands of the fingers, and many patients normally have significant hyperextension possible at the thumb IP joint, so some authors would advocate surgical repair regardless of zone in the thumb. There is no strong evidence either way in zone I EPL injuries, and imaging may be helpful to identify those whose tendon has retracted more and who may therefore fail nonoperative management.

CLINICAL CONCEPTS IN EXTENSOR TENDON MANAGEMENT

16. *How should the hand be placed in a splint following repair of multiple zone VIII extensor tendon injuries that involve the myotendinous junction?*

E. Wrist extended 40 degrees, MP joint flexed 20 degrees

The correct position of postoperative splinting following repair of the extensor tendons is dependent on the zone of injury involved. The normal "safe" position for splinting, is the wrist in slight extension, MP joints flexed between 70 and 90 degrees, and IP joints in extension. This position is modified following extensor repair in order to minimize tension across the repair sites. For example, the recommended position following a zone VIII repair is to have the wrist extended 40 degrees, the MP joints flexed 20 degrees, and the fingers free to mobilize into active extension within the splint.

MANAGEMENT OF EXTENSOR TENDON INJURIES

17. *When managing extensor tendon injuries, which one of the following is correct?*

B. A swan neck deformity may develop secondary to a zone I extensor rupture.

Swan neck deformities may result from a chronic zone I extensor tendon rupture or from pathology around the PIP joint, such as volar plate laxity or an FDS tendon rupture.

Acute closed sagittal band ruptures may be managed with an MP joint flexion blocking splint if they are identified within the first 2 weeks; however, there is still a risk of subsequent extensor tendon subluxation. Furthermore, delayed presentations and open injuries should ideally be repaired. Surgical treatment involves either directly repairing the sagittal band or reanchoring the EDC tendon to a firm structure, such as the volar plate or volar transverse metacarpal ligament. This may be achieved with either a suturing technique or a strip of EDC tendon used as a lasso (Watson technique).[7] Operative treatment requires a similar method of splinting to nonoperative care, but should give a greater chance of subsequent tendon stability. Extensor tendon repairs in the flat tendon zones within the fingers are more vulnerable to stretching and rupture in the early stages than flexor tendon repairs. Careful protection with splints is required.

EXTRINSIC AND INTRINSIC EXTENSOR PROBLEMS

18. You are asked by the senior hand therapist to give a second opinion on a patient who has difficulty flexing his little and ring fingers 6 months after repair of divided EDC tendons in zone V. When you passively flex the MP joints, he is unable to flex the IP joints. When you extend the MP joints, he is able to flex the IP joints. *What is the recommendation that most likely will address this issue?*

D. Extensor tenolysis around the site of repair and into the finger as required

The scenario given is typical of extrinsic extensor tethering. When the MP joints are in extension, the extrinsic mechanism is slackened and the patient is able to flex the IP joints. If the problem was of intrinsic tightness, extending the MP joints would make the problem worse and prevent IP joint flexion. Accepting this diagnosis and the fact that the patient is already seeing a senior therapist, it is unlikely that further physiotherapy and splinting is going to correct this 6 months after repair. An extensor tenolysis will require release of the expected adhesions around the site of repair, but also usually requires a more extensive release into the surrounding extensor zones due to additional adhesion formation.

References

1. Reissis N, Stirrat A, Manek S, et al. The terminal branch of posterior interosseous nerve: a useful donor for digital nerve grafting. J Hand Surg Br 17:638-640, 1992.
2. Waters PM, Schwartz JT. Posterior interosseous nerve: an anatomic study of potential nerve grafts. J Hand Surg Am 18:743-745, 1993.
3. Doyle JR. Extensor tendons-acute injuries. In Green DP, ed. Green's Operative Hand Surgery, ed 3. New York: Churchill Livingstone, 1993
4. Capener N. Lively splints. Physiotherapy 53:371, 1967.
5. Snow JW. Use of a retrograde tendon flap in repairing a severed extensor in the PIP joint area. Plast Reconstr Surg 51:555-558, 1973.
6. Tabbal GN, Bastidas N, Sharma S. Closed mallet thumb injury: a review of the literature and case study of the use of magnetic resonance imaging in deciding treatment. Plast Reconstr Surg 124:222-226, 2009.
7. Watson HK, Weinzweig J, Guidera PM. Sagittal band reconstruction. J Hand Surg Am 22:452-456, 1997.

71. Tendon Transfers

See *Essentials of Plastic Surgery*, second edition, pp. 855-863.

Box 71-1 FOREARM AND HAND MUSCLE ABBREVIATIONS

ADM: Abductor digiti minimi
APB: Abductor pollicis brevis
APL: Abductor pollicis longus
BR: Brachioradialis
ECRB: Extensor carpi radialis brevis
ECRL: Extensor carpi radialis longus
ECU: Extensor carpi ulnaris
EDC: Extensor digitorum communis
EDM: Extensor digiti minimi
EIP: Extensor indicis proprius
EPB: Extensor pollicis brevis
EPL: Extensor pollicis longus
FCR: Flexor carpi radialis
FCU: Flexor carpi ulnaris
FDM: Flexor digiti minimi
FDP: Flexor digitorum profundus
FDS: Flexor digitorum superficialis
FPB: Flexor pollicis brevis
FPL: Flexor pollicis longus
ODM: Opponens digiti minimi
OP: Opponens pollicis
PL: Palmaris longus
PQ: Pronator quadratus
PT: Pronator teres
SORL: Spiral oblique retinacular ligament

PRINCIPLES OF TENDON TRANSFER

1. **Which one of the following is a usual feature of a donor muscle selected for tendon transfer?**
   A. A power grading greater than the muscle it is replacing
   B. A synergistic action to the muscle it is replacing
   C. The potential to perform multiple new functions
   D. A greater excursion than the muscle it is replacing
   E. A different vector to the muscle it is replacing

2. **What is the most common indication for tendon transfer?**
   A. Nerve injury alone
   B. Tendon injury alone
   C. Combined nerve and tendon injuries
   D. Spasticity
   E. Muscle injury

3. **Which one of the following conditions is the most significant contraindication to tendon transfer?**
   A. Diabetes mellitus
   B. Fluctuating spasticity
   C. Stabilized function following poliomyelitis
   D. Rheumatoid arthritis
   E. Failure of prior tendon grafting

4. **In which one of the following scenarios might an immediate tendon transfer be indicated in a young, otherwise healthy patient?**
   A. Active leprosy with clawing of the hand
   B. Untreated carpal tunnel syndrome with thenar wasting
   C. Radial nerve repair at midhumeral level
   D. Resurfacing of scarred forearm after trauma
   E. Recent ulnar nerve repair at wrist level

TRANSFERS IN MEDIAN NERVE PALSY

5. You see a 20-year-old patient with poor recovery following a median nerve division at the wrist 2 years earlier. She asks about potential reconstructive options. **Which one of the following tendon transfers could be used to address thenar muscle denervation?**
   A. An EIP transfer around the radial border of the wrist
   B. A ring finger FDP transfer through a flexor retinaculum window
   C. An abductor digiti minimi transfer across the palm
   D. A palmaris longus plus fascial strip transfer around an FCU pulley
   E. An FDS ring transfer around an FCR pulley

TRANSFERS IN ULNAR NERVE PALSY

6. A patient presents with full FCU (MRC grade V) and incomplete FDP (MRC grade IV) recovery but persistent clawing 18 months after an ulnar nerve repair at the elbow. **Which one of the following is contraindicated in this case?**
   A. An MP joint hyperextension-blocking splint for the long term
   B. A ring finger FDS tendon transfer to the lateral bands to correct the clawing
   C. An FCR transfer with PL grafts to the A1/A2 pulleys to correct the clawing
   D. Postponement of tendon transfers until passive joint range improves, if clawing is not passively correctable
   E. An ECRB transfer with PL graft aid thumb adduction

TENDON TRANSFERS IN RADIAL NERVE PALSY

7. You are considering tendon transfers for a young, healthy man 4 months after repair of a radial nerve injury at the elbow. **Which one of the following statements is correct?**
   A. Recovery of some wrist extension would be expected by this stage.
   B. If there is no sign of EPL recovery by now, a tendon transfer will be needed.
   C. An EMG is unlikely to be helpful this long after injury.
   D. Recovery of strong digital extension would be expected by this stage.
   E. If motor recovery is seen, but is slower than expected, rerepair of the nerve may be required.

8. **When treating a radial nerve palsy, which one of the following is most likely to cause a functional problem when planning a combined transfer with PT to ECRB?**
   A. PT to ECRB, FDS ring to EDC, FDS middle to EPL/EIP
   B. PT to ECRB, FCR to APL, FDS ring to EDC, FDS middle to EPL
   C. PT to ECRL, FCR to EDC, PL to EPL
   D. PT to ECRB, FCR to APL, FCU to EDC, PL to EPL
   E. PT to ECRL, FCR to EDC, PL to EPL

TRANSFERS IN COMBINED NERVE PALSIES

9. You have a patient with persistent wasting of the thenar eminence muscle group and mild clawing of the digits after a midforearm laceration that required repair of both the median and ulnar nerves 4 years earlier. *Which one of the following is correct when considering tendon transfers for this patient?*
   A. Previous compliance with physiotherapy is no longer relevant to this scenario.
   B. One single tendon transfer can be used to address the deficits described.
   C. An EIP tendon transfer is more likely to be successful than a PL (Camitz) or FDS tendon transfer for thumb opposition.
   D. An ADM (Huber) transfer is more likely to be successful than a PL (Camitz) or FDS tendon transfer for thumb opposition.
   E. Previously denervated MRC grade II muscles may be used as donors for transfer.

COMPLICATIONS AFTER TENDON TRANSFERS

10. *Which one of the following scenarios is most likely to lead to a failed tendon transfer?*
    A. A PT to ECRB transfer at the same time as radial nerve exploration in the arm
    B. An EIP to EPL transfer three months after a distal radius fracture
    C. A tibialis posterior to tibialis anterior transfer at the same time as a tumor excision from the common peroneal nerve
    D. A tendon transfer in the forearm under a mature, pliable ALT flap
    E. A lateral band transfer to correct a stiff swan neck deformity

TENDON TRANSFERS IN RHEUMATOID ARTHRITIS

11. A patient with rheumatoid arthritis presents with spontaneous inability to extend the IP joint of the thumb. The remaining digits are unaffected. *Which one of the following tendons is commonly transferred to reinstate function in this situation?*
    A. FCR
    B. EDC
    C. APL
    D. EIP
    E. FDP

Answers

PRINCIPLES OF TENDON TRANSFER

1. Which one of the following is a usual feature of a donor muscle selected for tendon transfer?
   B. A synergistic action to the muscle it is replacing
   When considering tendon transfers it is vital that passive motion of any joints involved is optimized and the soft tissue envelope is supple. Beyond this, there are six key principles that underpin tendon transfer in relation to the donor and recipient muscles. These can be remembered with the mnemonic SPEEPS: **S**ingle function, **P**ower (adequate), **E**xpendable, **E**xcursion, **P**ull, **S**ynergistic.
   When considering a transfer, each transferred tendon should ideally restore a single function. The donor must be adequately powered, so ideally the transferred muscle/tendon will have similar power to the unit being replaced. Medical Research Council (MRC) grade for the donor muscle should ideally be grade V, although grade IV can also be adequate. The donor muscle must be expendable (e.g., one wrist flexor or extensor should be preserved.) The excursion or amplitude of the transferred tendon should be similar to the excursion being replaced, but it does not have to be greater. The line of pull or vector should be similar between donor and recipient action and avoid pulleys wherever possible. The transferred donor and recipient muscles should ideally be synergistic. For example, finger flexion is optimal with wrist extension, so using a wrist extensor for finger flexion is advantageous when it comes to rehabilitation.[1]

2. What is the most common indication for tendon transfer?
   A. Nerve injury alone
   The most common indication for tendon transfer is nerve injury. This may be required because repair or grafting of the nerve is not possible (e.g., some brachial plexus injuries) or if previous attempts at repair have failed. Tendon transfer may be indicated when reinnervation will take so long that permanent damage to the motor endplates will have occurred. The other options listed each represent potential reasons for tendon transfer. Medical diseases where limb function is impaired, such as poliomyelitis or leprosy, represent potential indications for tendon transfer but the disease must be well controlled before surgery.

3. Which one of the following conditions is the most significant contraindication to tendon transfer?
   B. Fluctuating spasticity
   Although sometimes very useful, tendon transfers can also be unpredictable in spasticity, such as in cerebral palsy. This is particularly true where spasticity is variable, such as in athetoid movements. Where a deficit or ability is variable, tendon transfer should be avoided.
   Diabetes mellitus is not a significant contraindication to tendon transfer, but glycemic control should be optimized as for any surgery. A stable deficit postpoliomyelitis can respond well to a tendon transfer where a suitable donor is available; however, sufficient recovery time should have elapsed before surgery is considered.
   Rheumatoid arthritis can provide many opportunities for a tendon transfer, such as EIP to EPL or crossed intrinsic transfer during MP joint realignment. It is important to address the

Chapter 71 ▪ Tendon Transfers 585

underlying cause first by controlling the disease medically, debriding active synovitis and excising osteophytes, or addressing other bony prominences (such as a prominent ulnar head).

A tendon transfer can be helpful if grafting of a tendon defect has failed; however, any causes for the first failure should be addressed (e.g., prominent metalwork, abnormal bony prominences, poor patient compliance with therapy, or infection).

4. **In which one of the following scenarios might an immediate tendon transfer be indicated in a young, otherwise healthy patient?**
   C. **Radial nerve repair at midhumeral level**

   Tendon transfers are more commonly performed as delayed procedures, as there are many factors to optimize before surgery, such as allowing any recovery to develop, allowing scar tissue to improve, or infection to settle. One good indication for an immediate tendon transfer is to augment function while waiting for prolonged nerve recovery, or where the prognosis for nerve or muscle recovery is poor. A good example of this is using a PT to ECRB transfer to act as an internal wrist splint for a patient with a high radial nerve injury while recovery is awaited. This potentially frees the patient from an external splint and puts the hand in a better position for using the remaining median and ulnar innervated muscles.

   Tendon transfers can be helpful in leprosy, but the disease must be controlled first. While an immediate PL transfer for thumb abduction/opposition (Camitz procedure) is sometimes used in carpal tunnel syndrome with thenar wasting, which is more common in elderly patients or others expected to make a poor recovery. In a young, healthy patient with only partial thenar wasting, it would be more common to simply decompress the carpal tunnel and allow a period of recovery before considering a tendon transfer.

   When resurfacing a scarred limb, it is usual to allow the soft tissue envelope to mature and soften before undertaking tendon transfers, as there is a high risk of adhesions and poor excursion if an immediate transfer is done. Following an immediate distal nerve repair, such as the ulnar nerve at the wrist, recovery is expected to occur much sooner than with a proximal injury, so tendon transfer in this setting is unlikely to be required.

TRANSFERS IN MEDIAN NERVE PALSY

5. You see a 20-year-old patient with poor recovery following a median nerve division at the wrist 2 years earlier. She asks about potential reconstructive options. **Which one of the following tendon transfer could be used to address thenar muscle denervation?**
   C. **An abductor digiti minimi transfer across the palm**

   The Huber[2] transfer uses abductor digiti minimi as a transfer across the palm to restore thumb abduction/opposition.[3,4] It is more commonly performed in children, where it can be helpful in addressing thumb hypoplasia. It is less common in adults, as there are other options which may be simpler and the cosmetic appearance can be disappointing because of the bridge of muscle crossing the palm.

   Common options include a radial innervated EIP transfer around the ulnar border of the hand,[4] or a proximal median nerve innervated ring finger FDS transfer. The FDP should not be sacrificed because of the unacceptable digital flexion deficit that would result. The PL can also be transferred with a strip of palmar fascia to augment length (Camitz transfer). However, the vector would be poor and the length insufficient if passed around the FCU, and in this scenario the PL may well have been injured. The FCR is not a good pulley to route an FDS transfer for thumb opposition/abduction around as the vector is incorrect.

TRANSFERS IN ULNAR NERVE PALSY

6. A patient presents with full FCU (MRC grade V) and incomplete FDP (MRC grade IV) recovery but persistent clawing 18 months after an ulnar nerve repair at the elbow. *Which one of the following is contraindicated in this case?*
   B. A ring finger FDS tendon transfer to the lateral bands to correct the clawing
   Although a transfer of the ring finger FDS tendon to the lateral bands could provide good correction of clawing, it would leave the ring finger unacceptably weak, since the FDP to this digit has been denervated and is not fully recovered. Many patients manage perfectly well with a long-term ulnar claw splint, so it is important to check whether they are content with a splint before embarking on complex reconstruction. Options C and E can also be used in ulnar clawing.

TENDON TRANSFERS IN RADIAL NERVE PALSY

7. You are considering tendon transfers for a young, healthy man 4 months after repair of a radial nerve injury at the elbow. *Which one of the following statements is correct?*
   A. Recovery of some wrist extension would be expected by this stage.
   When considering tendon transfers, it is important to understand the expected timescale for nerve regeneration after repair/graft and the likely extent of nerve and muscle recovery, otherwise an unnecessary transfer might be undertaken. The ERCL and the ECRB are supplied very proximally, hence there should be some wrist extension by four months. Although there may be signs of EDC reinnervation, it is unlikely to be strong at this stage. EPL recovery occurs late and may still remain sufficient up to 1 year after injury, as the PIN motor branch enters the muscle more distally in the forearm. Nerve recovery is typically 1 mm/day. EMG studies are helpful to demonstrate early signs of reinnervation before significant clinical signs of recovery. If EPL displayed early recovery on EMG, a transfer would usually be postponed. Rerepair of a recovering nerve will sacrifice the recovered function and prolong the time to reinnervation of distal muscles. It is therefore unlikely to produce a superior outcome.

8. When treating a radial nerve palsy, which one of the following is most likely to cause a functional problem when planning a combined transfer with PT to ECRB?
   D. PT to ECRB, FCR to APL, FCU to EDC, PL to EPL
   Tendon transfers are tailored to each individual patient and according to surgeon experience and preference. One of the core principles is to avoid creating an unacceptable donor deficit. Scenario D would give good wrist and digital extension but at the unacceptable cost of preventing adequate wrist flexion, because both wrist flexors have been used (FCU and FCR). All of the other combinations address the deficits following radial nerve palsy without severe donor morbidity. PT is usually transferred to ECRB in radial nerve injuries to provide wrist extension, but ECRL and ECU are not usually reconstructed. FCR may be transferred to EPB and APL together to provide thumb extension and abduction. FCU or FCR may be used to provide digital extension by transfer to EDC. PL or FDS ring may be used to provide thumb extension by transfer to EPL.

TRANSFERS IN COMBINED NERVE PALSY

9. You have a patient with persistent wasting of the thenar eminence muscle group and mild clawing of the digits after a midforearm laceration that required repair of both the median and ulnar nerves 4 years earlier. *Which one of the following is correct when considering tendon transfers for this patient?*
C. An EIP tendon transfer is more likely to be more successful than a PL (Camitz) or FDS tendon transfer for thumb opposition.

A radial nerve innervated EIP transfer[4] will be preferable to either a PL or FDS transfer for thumb opposition/abduction, as these muscles are innervated by the median nerve and may also have had direct damage to the muscle belly at the time of injury. A Huber transfer[2,3] which uses the abductor digiti minimi muscle, is innervated by the ulnar nerve and is unlikely to have recovered well, given that the patient still has other signs of intrinsic muscle denervation. "One tendon transfer, one function" is one of the core principles when planning a series of transfers, and it is always sensible to review compliance with physiotherapy before undertaking complex upper limb reconstruction. While previously denervated muscles may be used if adequately recovered, it is preferable to use an uninjured donor where possible and MRC grade II power is insufficient for use as a transfer.

COMPLICATIONS AFTER TENDON TRANSFERS

10. *Which one of the following scenarios is most likely to lead to a failed tendon transfer?*
E. A lateral band transfer to correct a stiff swan neck deformity

Scenario E demonstrates a violation of one of the core principles of tendon transfer, which is that joints must already be supple enough for functional range of motion before tendon transfer is undertaken. There will likely be an early recurrence of the original deformity, or adhesions leading to stiffness if a transfer is performed in this scenario. Therefore the PIP joint should be released as a first stage, with a delayed lateral band transfer once a stable range of joint movement is obtained and the soft tissue envelope has settled again.

Scenarios A through D demonstrate tendon transfers that may be appropriate. It is often sensible to perform an early tendon transfer, despite anticipated nerve recovery to improve quality of life, if this spares the patient from requiring an external splint and the recovery time is likely to be prolonged. As such, PT to ECRB transfer can allow a patient with radial nerve palsy to manage without a bulky wrist splint; likewise, a tibialis posterior to anterior transfer can obviate the need for a foot drop splint in patients with common peroneal nerve injury. EPL rupture can occur with distal radius fractures due to direct injury or ischemia in the third extensor compartment. The EIP passes through a different compartment and is therefore unlikely to rupture following transfer to the EPL. Transfers can be routed beneath a flap reconstruction, but the soft tissue envelope must be soft and pliable.

TENDON TRANSFERS IN RHEUMATOID ARTHRITIS

11. A patient with rheumatoid arthritis presents with spontaneous inability to extend the IP joint of the thumb. The remaining digits are unaffected. *Which one of the following tendons is commonly transferred to reinstate function in this situation?*

D. EIP

This patient demonstrates spontaneous rupture of the EPL tendon with inability to extend the IP joint. This can occur in advanced rheumatoid arthritis where attrition rupture develops from synovitis or abrasion on bony spurs along the course of the EPL, particularly under the extensor retinaculum and over the carpus. The advantage of using the EIP tendon is that index finger extension can be maintained by the EDC and the path of the tendon transfer avoids some of the areas of previous damage. It is a straightforward procedure to undertake with minimal exposure required. The distal EPL is identified by making a longitudinal incision over the first metacarpal. The EIP is identified as the index MP joint and is differentiated from the EDC tendon by its more ulnar position and insertion. A small incision allows this tendon to be divided at the extensor expansion. A second, proximal incision over the base of the second metacarpal allows the tendon to be retrieved before being rerouted subcutaneously to the distal stump of the EPL. A Pulvertaft weave is performed with the thumb and wrist in full extension. It is, of course, important to ensure that the EDC to the index finger is intact before transferring the EIP, as there may be multiple tendon ruptures in rheumatoid arthritis (see Chapter 84, *Essentials of Plastic Surgery*, second edition).

Other tendon transfers for EPL rupture include ring finger FDS and palmaris longus. The FCR is sometimes used for APL and EPB but not EPL. The EDC is usually avoided, as this would give a mass extension action to the digits and thumb. The FDP tendon harvest would sacrifice the DIP joint flexion, which is not generally acceptable.

REFERENCES

1. Beasley RW. Principles of tendon transfer. Orthop Clin North Am 1:433-438, 1970.
2. Huber E. Hilfsoperation bei Medianuslähmung. Deutsche Zeitschrift für Chirurgie 162:271-275, 1921.
3. Littler JW, Cooley SG. Opposition of the thumb and its restoration by abductor digiti quinti transfer. J Bone Joint Surg Am 45:1389-1396, 1963.
4. Burkhalter WE. Early tendon transfer in upper extremity peripheral nerve injury. Clin Orthop Relat Res 104:68-79, 1974.

72. Hand and Finger Amputations

See *Essentials of Plastic Surgery*, second edition, pp. 864-868.

DIGITAL AMPUTATIONS

1. You have evaluated a 28-year-old manual worker for acute revision of a traumatic amputation of the ring finger after a circular saw injury. The amputation is at the level of the middle phalanx just proximal to the FDS insertion. **Which one of the following is correct regarding the surgical procedure?**
   A. The digital nerve stumps should be buried subperiosteally.
   B. The proximal FDP tendon should be secured to the bone.
   C. The amputation level should remain at the base of the middle phalanx.
   D. The dorsal and volar skin flaps should be equal length.
   E. Articular cartilage at the PIP joint will need to be removed.

RAY AMPUTATIONS

2. **Which one of the following is a benefit of performing a ray amputation of the ring finger after traumatic amputation through the proximal phalanx?**
   A. Improved power grip
   B. Improved key pinch
   C. Improved pronation
   D. Improved interdigital gap
   E. Improved supination

3. *At what level should the index finger metacarpal normally be resected during a ray amputation?*
   A. The neck
   B. The distal shaft
   C. The midshaft
   D. The metacarpal base
   E. The entire metacarpal should be removed

4. *In which ray amputations might you consider metacarpal transposition?*
   A. Index or middle finger
   B. Index or ring finger
   C. Index or little finger
   D. Middle or ring finger
   E. Ring or little finger

WRIST AND FOREARM AMPUTATIONS

5. When treating patients with traumatic amputations at the wrist or forearm, **which one of the following is correct?**
   A. Transection of the radius and ulnar in the forearm should be performed at different levels.
   B. Preservation of the radiocarpal joint at the wrist may allow a functional prosthesis to be used.
   C. Fusion of the distal radioulnar joint should be performed during a radiocarpal amputation for improved stability.
   D. Tendon length in the forearm can be minimized if hand transplantation is felt to be a viable future option.
   E. The minimum recommended forearm length for a useful forearm prosthesis is 15 cm.

COMPLICATIONS FOLLOWING AMPUTATION

6. A 28-year-old man complains of an unpleasant tingling and burning sensation with light touch over the stump of his amputated index finger stump 6 weeks after surgery. *Which one of the following is the most likely cause?*
   A. A neuroma of the digital nerve
   B. A mild postoperative infection
   C. Complex regional pain syndrome
   D. Allodynia caused by nerve injury and reinnervation
   E. Cold intolerance caused by sympathetic denervation

… Chapter 72 ■ Hand and Finger Amputations   591

Answers

DIGITAL AMPUTATIONS

1. You have evaluated a 28-year-old manual worker for acute revision of a traumatic amputation of the ring finger after a circular saw injury. The amputation is at the level of the middle phalanx just proximal to the FDS insertion. *Which one of the following is correct regarding the surgical procedure?*
   E. Articular cartilage at the PIP joint will need to be removed.
   With no flexor tendon attachment, there is little point in keeping the residual middle phalanx. The proximal phalanx must be shortened to at least remove all articular cartilage in order to avoid a pseudobursa, and more commonly to the neck of the proximal phalanx to avoid the stump being too long when the patient makes a fist. During initial amputation, the digital nerves should simply be divided proximal to the skin flaps and allowed to retract back into the soft tissues. If a subsequent neuroma develops, that can be dealt with by a number of techniques. The tendon ends should be allowed to retract in order to avoid a quadriga effect (see Chapter 69). If the FDS insertion is intact, there may be useful PIP joint flexion, in which case it may be worth using a local flap to preserve digital length. FDP retraction may result in paradoxical extension of the injured digit when trying to flex the fingers caused by tension through the lumbrical. This is uncommon and is dealt with on an elective basis with division of the lumbrical. The fishmouth incision should be designed to provide a longer volar skin flap as this is sensate and provides better soft tissue padding for the new fingertip.[1,2]

RAY AMPUTATIONS

2. *Which one of the following is a benefit of performing a ray amputation of the ring finger after traumatic amputation through the proximal phalanx?*
   D. Improved interdigital gap
   Ray amputation is usually an elective procedure following initial care of a proximal digital amputation. The main purpose is to close the interdigital gap to stop objects falling through. A secondary potential benefit is an improvement in cosmesis. Power grip, key grip, pronation, and supination power are usually reduced after ray amputation, so must be considered when pursuing a ray amputation for cosmetic reasons.[3,4,5]

3. *At what level should the index finger metacarpal normally be resected during a ray amputation?*
   D. The metacarpal base
   When performing a ray amputation of the index or little fingers, the osteotomy is usually made at the metacarpal base (metaphyseal flare), preserving tendon attachments to the base and maintaining CMC joint integrity. The tendon insertions for the index finger are FCR and ECRL, while those for the little finger are FCU and ECU. Preservation of these is important. The bony amputation level for a middle or ring finger may also be through the base, but some surgeons prefer a total base resection.

4. *In which ray amputations might you consider metacarpal transposition?*
   D. Middle or ring finger
   The border digits can be transposed to close the gap from the third or fourth ray amputations.[6] The base of the fifth metacarpal should still be preserved in order to protect the insertions of the ECU and FCU tendons as discussed in question 3. Likewise, the index metacarpal base should be preserved to protect the ECRL and FCR tendon insertions. The osteotomy is performed at the metaphyseal flare. Ray amputations usually result in 15% to 20% reduction in grip strength and narrowing of the palm.[3,4,5]

WRIST AND FOREARM AMPUTATIONS

5. When treating patients with traumatic amputations at the wrist or forearm, *which one of the following is correct?*
   B. Preservation of the radiocarpal joint at the wrist may allow a functional prosthesis to be used.
   Transection of the radius and ulna should be at the same level. The DRU joint should be preserved rather than fused where possible to allow pronation and supination. While the tendons are often divided under traction to allow proximal retraction, this is not appropriate if future hand transplantation is a possibility. The minimum length considered useful for a forearm prosthesis is 8 to 10 cm of residual radius and ulna length.

COMPLICATIONS FOLLOWING AMPUTATION

6. A 28-year-old man complains of an unpleasant tingling and burning sensation with light touch over the stump of his amputated index finger 6 weeks after surgery. *Which one of the following is the most likely cause?*
   D. Allodynia caused by nerve injury and reinnervation
   Allodynia is the perception of a painful sensation following what is normally a nonnoxious stimulus, such as a burning sensation in response to a light touch. Mild symptoms can be quite common after digital amputation during the early stages of scar maturation and reinnervation; however, this usually settles with desensitization exercises. If allodynia persists, becomes severe, or is associated with trophic changes to the soft tissues, it may be part of complex regional pain syndrome.

   Six weeks is too early for formation of a neuroma, and this would usually present as a pinpoint site of tenderness over the digital nerve stump or external scar, leading to an "electric shock" sensation or "shooting pain." It is rather late for development of a postoperative infection and if infection was present the digit would be painful, swollen, tender, and warm. Cold intolerance is a recognized complication of digital amputation but would not present in this way.

REFERENCES

1. Adamson GJ, Palmer RE. Amputations. In Achauer BM, Erikson E, Guyuron B, et al, eds. Plastic Surgery: Indications, Operations, and Outcomes. St Louis: Mosby–Year Book, 2000.
2. Louis DS, Jebson PJ, Graham T. Amputations. In Green DP, Hotchkiss RN, Pederson WC, eds. Green's Operative Hand Surgery, ed 4. Philadelphia: Churchill Livingstone, 1999.
3. Murray JF, Carman W, Mackenzie JK. Transmetacarpal amputation of the index finger: a clinical assessment of hand strength and complications. J Hand Surg Am 2:471-481, 1977.
4. Garcia-Moral CA, Putman-Mullins J, Taylor PA, et al. Ray resection of the index finger. Orthop Trans 15:71, 1991.
5. Melikyan EY, Beg MS, Woodbridge S, et al. The functional results of ray amputation. Hand Surg 8:47-51, 2003.
6. Carroll RE. Transposition of the index finger to replace the middle finger. Clin Orthop 15:27-34, 1959.

73. Replantation

See *Essentials of Plastic Surgery*, second edition, pp. 869-880.

INDICATIONS FOR REPLANTATION
1. **Which one of the following represents a relative contraindication to digital replantation in an adult because of likely poor long-term function?**
   A. Middle finger amputation through neck of middle phalanx
   B. Ring finger amputation through neck of proximal phalanx
   C. Little finger amputation through the DIP joint
   D. Thumb amputation through midshaft proximal phalanx
   E. Thumb amputation through the IP joint

CLASSIFICATION OF DIGITAL AMPUTATIONS
2. A neighboring hospital refers a patient with multiple fingertip amputations. The injury is described according to the Tamai classification system. **On which one of the following is this classification based?**
   A. The mechanism of injury
   B. The level of injury
   C. The time since injury
   D. The predicted outcome after replantation
   E. The number of digits involved

PRESERVATION OF AMPUTATED DIGITS
3. **When arranging transport of an amputated digit, which one of the following is correct?**
   A. The digit should be placed in saline-soaked gauze in a bag or specimen container.
   B. The bag containing the digit should be transported on dry ice.
   C. The optimal temperature for storage of the amputated digit is approximately 4° C.
   D. The maximum cold ischemia time for a digit is 12 hours.
   E. The maximum warm ischemia time for a digit is 3 hours.

PREOPERATIVE WORKUP
4. **Which one of the following is correct when preparing a patient for replantation of a digit?**
   A. A local anesthetic ring block is advisable to ensure patient comfort.
   B. Plain radiographs of the hand and the amputated digit are required.
   C. Tetanus prophylaxis is only required if surgery will be delayed.
   D. Aspirin 150 mg should be given in the ER to improve distal circulation.
   E. Oral antibiotics are only indicated in contaminated injuries.

MANAGEMENT OF PROXIMAL LIMB AMPUTATIONS

5. A patient sustains a midhumeral guillotine amputation. **Which one of the following is correct when undertaking replantation in this case?**
A. Fasciotomy are not required and risk further unnecessary tissue injury.
B. Skeletal stabilization should be achieved before creating a vascular shunt.
C. Carpal and cubital tunnel decompression is generally recommended.
D. The maximum warm ischemia time is 2 hours.
E. The maximum cold ischemia time is 12 hours.

SURGICAL PRINCIPLES

6. Which one of the following is correct when performing an upper limb replantation?
A. Regional anesthesia should be avoided as it may compromise blood flow.
B. Use of a tourniquet should be avoided to reduce ischemia time.
C. The full arm and a leg should be prepared for nerve or vein graft harvest.
D. The maximum tourniquet time allowed is 90 minutes at 250 mm Hg.
E. A two-team approach is rarely justified for proximal amputations.

OPERATIVE SEQUENCE

7. In what order should structures usually be repaired when replanting a digit?
A. Bone, tendon, nerve, vessel
B. Bone, vessel, nerve, tendon
C. Vessel, bone, tendon, nerve
D. Vessel, nerve, bone, tendon
E. Bone, vessel, tendon, nerve

VESSEL INJURY

8. When assessing the vessels for replantation of a digit, which one of the following is correct?
A. A pearly gray translucent appearance indicates a friable vessel wall.
B. A tortuous "corkscrew" appearance indicates an intraluminal thrombus.
C. The presence of a terminal thrombus means that the vessel is unsalvageable.
D. A "red-line" appearance along the distal vessel makes salvage less likely.
E. The *sausage sign* requires further vessel resection and a vein graft will be required.

PHARMACOLOGIC ADJUNCTS

9. There are a number of useful pharmacologic agents to improve the success rate in replantation. **Which one of the following is correct?**
A. Topical papaverine may be used to aid vascular anastomosis.
B. If leech therapy is required, amoxicillin prophylaxis is indicated.
C. Systemic heparinization is recommended for distal amputations.
D. Systemic prostaglandin therapy is commonly used after replantation.
E. Oral aspirin is not useful in the early phase, as it has a 48-hour lag time.

OUTCOMES OF REPLANTATION

10. Before replantation of a digit, you are discussing likely outcomes with a patient. *Which one of the following is correct?*
    A. Fewer than 50% of replanted digits survive the first 24 hours after surgery, irrespective of injury mechanism or replantation technique.
    B. Arterial insufficiency is the main reason for early failure and requires an urgent return to the OR.
    C. Most patients will regain normal fingertip two-point discrimination by 6 months.
    D. Cold intolerance is common in many patients and is usually a permanent feature.
    E. Few patients will require subsequent secondary surgery providing an adequate rehabilitation protocol is followed.

11. *Following digital replantation, which one of the following is the most likely secondary procedure a patient will subsequently require?*
    A. Joint fusion
    B. Neurolysis
    C. Tenolysis
    D. Web space release
    E. Correction of nonunion

Answers

INDICATIONS FOR REPLANTATION

1. **Which one of the following represents a relative contraindication to digital replantation in an adult because of likely poor long-term function?**
   B. Ring finger amputation through neck of proximal phalanx
   A single digit amputation in flexor tendon zone II is a relative contraindication to replantation, since there is a high likelihood of poor functional outcome because of stiffness and immobility. Almost all patients are likely to require secondary surgery to release tendon adhesions or joint contractures. A detailed discussion with the patient regarding the likely outcome following replantation should be undertaken before proceeding with surgery. In many cases, a single digit amputation proximal to the FDS insertion is best managed with a revision amputation rather than replantation (see Chapter 72, *Essentials of Plastic Surgery*, second edition).

   However, there may still be reasons to pursue replantation in this scenario: for example, the patient may prefer a stiff, potentially painful digit to an absent digit for social, aesthetic, or psychological reasons. In Japan, for example, a missing digit has criminal connotations. In female patients, preservation of length in the left ring finger may be preferred for wearing or receiving a wedding or engagement band. In children, zone II single-digit injuries should still be replanted where possible, as children tend to have significantly better outcomes after surgery with regard to mobility and sensation.

   In contrast to zone II flexor level replants, zone I flexor level replants tend to have far better outcomes even when DIP joint motion is not preserved.[1] Therefore replantation of these is often indicated. All thumb amputations should be replanted where possible, given the importance of thumb function in opposition. The thumb remains functionally very useful even when it is stiff and relatively immobile.

CLASSIFICATION OF DIGITAL AMPUTATIONS

2. **A neighboring hospital refers a patient with multiple fingertip amputations. The injury is described according to the Tamai classification system. On which one of the following is this classification based?**
   B. The level of injury
   The two main classification systems for fingertip amputation are the Tamai[2] and Sebastin and Chung[3] classifications. They are each based on the level of injury and the clinical relevance of this is in relation to the anticipated difficulty of vascular repair, in particular the venous outflow. For example, in injuries distal to the lunula (Tamai zone I and Chung zone IA), direct anastomosis of venous outflow is not possible. Instead, anastomosis to the volar venous plexus may sometimes be performed; otherwise, leech therapy, nail bed bleed, or heparin therapy is required to provide adequate venous drainage. In more proximal injuries it may be possible to repair both arteries and veins but this is still very difficult beyond the FDP insertion. The zones of these two classification systems are shown in Figs. 73-1 and 73-2. The mechanism of injury and degree of soft tissue damage is more relevant to the Urbaniak[4] classification. This is a classification of ring avulsion injuries and does not relate to level of injury. The time since injury and the number of digits involved does not form part of any of these classification systems.

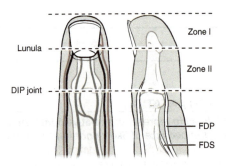

Fig. 73-1 Tamai's classification of fingertip amputation. (*DIP joint,* Distal interphalangeal joint; *FDP,* flexor digitorum profundus; *FDS,* flexor digitorum superficialis.)

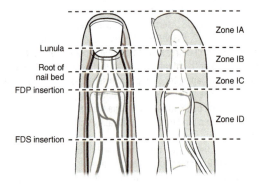

Fig. 73-2 Chung's classification of digital amputations.

PRESERVATION OF AMPUTATED DIGITS

3. When arranging transport of an amputated digit, which one of the following is correct?

C. The optimal temperature for storage of the amputated digit is approximately 4° C.

The optimal storage temperature for an amputated digit is 4° C, which can be achieved by refrigeration of the transport container. The digit is preferably wrapped in damp gauze and placed in a bag, which may then be kept on iced water. Heavily soaked gauze may result in waterlogging of the tissues and should be avoided. It is essential to avoid the error of allowing contact between the tissues and ice, which may result in freezing and subsequent cell necrosis.

In general, revascularization of amputated parts should be achieved as soon as possible. Digits are more tolerant of warm ischemia than the hand or forearm, as they contain no muscle. Warm ischemia times for digits should ideally be less than 6 hours. Cold ischemia times should be less than 24 hours.

In spite of these guidance figures, successful digital replantation has been reported in several cases after up to 30 hours of cold ischemia, with one procedure after 94 hours.[5] Such prolonged ischemia times are not generally recommended.

PREOPERATIVE WORKUP

4. Which one of the following is correct when preparing a patient for replantation of a digit?
B. Plain radiographs of the hand and the amputated digit are required.

Preoperative imaging of both the patient's injured hand and the amputated part is important to anticipate the functional outcome, plan skeletal stabilization, and assess any bone loss. A local anesthetic ring block may seem a good idea for patient comfort, but is contraindicated because it can decrease vascular flow or risk damage to proximal vessels. Also, repeated manipulation of the digit may result in vasospasm so it should be avoided. This is particularly relevant to partial amputations. The patient should be kept warm and well perfused with adequate intravenous fluids before, during, and after surgery. All patients should receive both tetanus and intravenous antibiotic prophylaxis in the ER. (Tetanus management is discussed further in Chapter 29, Table 29-1, *Essentials of Plastic Surgery*, second edition.) Aspirin is not required before surgery, but is commonly given during or after at a dose of 325 mg pr/po, as it inhibits platelet aggregation at the anastomosis at this dose level.

MANAGEMENT OF PROXIMAL LIMB AMPUTATIONS

5. A patient sustains a midhumeral guillotine amputation. Which one of the following is correct when undertaking replantation in this case?
C. Carpal and cubital tunnel decompression is generally recommended.

There is always a degree of edema and relative ischemia following a major replantation, in part because only the major inflow and outflow are restored and also because of the ischemia-vascular response. As such, it is prudent to decompress major nerves at their common sites of compression to minimize further insults.

Fasciotomy is recommended for the same reason to decompress the forearm and intrinsic hand muscle compartments following a major replantation. It is perfectly reasonable to proceed with a temporary vascular shunt before bony stabilization to minimize ischemia time, while careful debridement is undertaken or a difficult bony fixation planned.[6] Although the most common shunt is a specifically designed PVC vascular shunt, other materials such as chest drains or pediatric feeding tubes may be used as a substitute if required.

Tolerable ischemia times vary according to the proportion of muscle in the amputated part and whether appropriate cooling has occurred. For an arm or forearm amputation, a maximum of 4 to 6 hours warm ischemia and a maximum of 10 to 12 hours cold ischemia are generally quoted.

SURGICAL PRINCIPLES

6. Which one of the following is correct when performing an upper limb replantation?
C. The full arm and a leg should be prepared for nerve or vein graft harvest.

When planning an upper limb replantation, the possibility of vessel and nerve gaps should be anticipated, therefore the full arm and at least one leg should be adequately prepared for donor tissue harvest. In digital replantation, the posterior interosseous nerve (PIN) can be a useful donor graft for the digital nerves with minimal donor site disturbance. It is found in the fourth extensor compartment at the wrist. Suitable donor vessel grafts include both volar and dorsal wrist veins for digital vessels. Suitable leg grafts for larger structures in proximal replantations include the sural nerve and dorsal foot or saphenous veins. Graft harvest can proceed while other repairs are performed at the replantation site.

Regional anesthesia is a useful adjunct to general anesthesia, as it improves postoperative comfort and reduces vasospasm. It can also reduce the anesthetic agent requirement, and therefore nausea and vomiting, during the procedure. Use of a tourniquet is standard practice for exploration and debridement of any upper limb wound, as it provides a clear blood-free field, making surgery more efficient. Inflation of the tourniquet should be avoided once revascularization has been performed, as stopping flow may increase thrombosis at the anastomotic site. The standard pressure used for an adult upper limb is 250 mm Hg and a safe maximum continuous time is 120 minutes. After this time, the tourniquet must be deflated and the arm allowed to perfuse for at least 20 minutes. Where possible, a two-team approach is recommended for replantation, so one team can prepare the amputated part while the other prepares the injured digit and harvests grafts. This approach should minimize further ischemia time.

OPERATIVE SEQUENCE

7. In what order should structures usually be repaired when replanting a digit?

A. Bone, tendon, nerve, vessel

The usual order for digital replant is bone first in order to set length and provide a stable functional base for further reconstruction. The tendons should be repaired second as these will take tension off of nerve and vessel repairs. Furthermore, leaving tendon repairs until after the microsurgery risks inadvertent damage to the more delicate nerve and vessel repairs. Repairing the nerves before the vessels is often recommended, as it keeps the operating field clear of blood from bleeding adjacent tissues and means that following revascularization no other structure repair is required.[2,3,7] It would still be reasonable to repair the vessels before the nerves, especially when ischemia time is already extended, and some surgeons would do so routinely.

VESSEL INJURY

8. When assessing the vessels for replantation of a digit, which one of the following is correct?

D. A "red-line" appearance along the distal vessel makes salvage less likely.

A normal, clean digital vessel appears somewhat translucent and gray. The "corkscrew" appearance usually indicates a traction injury. A terminal thrombus may be evacuated, leaving a potentially healthy vessel end. The red-line sign along the distal neurovascular bundle may indicate damage to the vessel and is associated with a poorer prognosis. A sausage appearance occurs when the vessel is blocked with a thrombus, which may be evacuated.

PHARMACOLOGIC ADJUNCTS

9. There are a number of useful pharmacologic agents to improve the success rate in replantation. *Which one of the following is correct?*

A. Topical papaverine may be used to aid vascular anastomosis.

Papaverine is a potent smooth muscle relaxant that appears to work through inhibition of phosphodiesterases and by influencing calcium channels. It may be used topically during microsurgery to dilate both arteries and veins before and after anastomosis. Other agents used for this purpose include the calcium channel blocker verapamil and the local anesthetic sodium channel blocker lidocaine. Leech therapy is useful for venous congested digits, but carries a small risk of infection with *Aeromonas hydrophila*. The usual prophylaxis for this is ciprofloxacin or a third-generation cephalosporin. Although systemic heparinization might occasionally be used where there is higher concern than usual regarding thrombosis, this has to be balanced against the risk of hemorrhage and is not routine. Systemic prostaglandin therapy has been used by some microsurgeons, but this is not commonplace, whereas oral aspirin therapy is regularly administered after replantation.[8]

OUTCOMES OF REPLANTATION

10. Before replantation of a digit, you are discussing likely outcomes with a patient. **Which one of the following is correct?**
B. Arterial insufficiency is the main reason for early failure and requires an urgent return to the OR.
The main reason for early replantation failure is arterial insufficiency (up to 60% of cases). This presents with a pale, cold finger with no bleeding on pinprick testing. Patients must be warned about the risk of both an extended initial procedure time and a potential return to the OR following replantation. Unfortunately, digits that struggle to survive tend to have poor long-term function with atrophy, reduced sensation, and stiffness.

Survival rates following digital replantation are generally above 50% and will depend on factors such as injury mechanism, digit involved, level of injury, timing of replantation, and surgical skill. The overall survival for distal digital amputation was 86%, according to a systematic review published in 2011.[3] Other published success rates range from 54% to 84%, and, as expected, the success for guillotine-type injuries is much better than for crush injuries (77% versus 49%).[9]

Most patients do regain useful sensation but this does not reach normal two-point discrimination. A normal two-point discrimination is 3 mm for dynamic and 6 mm for static (see Chapter 59, *Essentials of Plastic Surgery,* second edition). A review of 293 distal replants showed two-point discrimination at less than 15 mm. In the systematic review, mean two-point discrimination was 7 mm. While cold intolerance is common and should be explained to the patient preoperatively, it will usually improve over time (2 years). A large number of patients will require secondary surgery even when the vascularity of the digit remains satisfactory (see question 11).

11. *Following digital replantation, which one of the following is the most likely secondary procedure a patient will subsequently require?*
C. Tenolysis
More than half of patients undergoing digital replantation are likely to require secondary surgery. This will be affected by the nature of the original injury and rehabilitation protocol. For example, as discussed in question 1, secondary surgery is more likely in zone II flexor level replantations. The most common procedures are flexor or extensor tenolysis and/or release of joint contractures. This is probably because newly revascularized digits are often immobilized longer than in the early postoperative phase, and subsequent stiffness soon develops as the requirements of the extensor and flexor tendon repairs and the fracture union compete in the rehabilitation regimen. Other common secondary procedures are revision fixation of a nonunion, neurolysis and/or nerve grafting, web-space release, and amputation where function remains poor.

REFERENCES

1. O'Brien BM. Replantation surgery. Clin Plast Surg 1:405-426, 1974.
2. Tamai S. Twenty years' experience of limb replantation: review of 293 upper extremity replants. J Hand Surg 7:549-556, 1982.
3. Sebastin SJ, Chung KC. A systematic review of the outcomes of replantation of distal digital amputation. Plast Reconstr Surg 128:723-737, 2011.
4. Urbaniak JR, Evans JP, Bright DS. Microvascular management of ring avulsion injuries. J Hand Surg Am 6:25-30, 1981.
5. Wei FC, Chen HC, Chuang CC. Three successful digital replantations in a patient after 84, 86, and 94 hours cold ischemia time. Plast Reconstr Surg 82:346-350, 1988.
6. Subramanian A, Vercruysse G, Dente C, et al. A decade's experience with temporary intravascular shunts at a civilian level I trauma center. J Trauma 65:316-324, 2008.
7. Chao JJ, Castello JR, English JM, et al. Microsurgery: free tissue transfer and replantation. Sel Read Plast Surg 9:1, 2000.
8. Rodríguez Vegas JM, Ruiz Alonso ME, Terán Saavedra PP. PGE-1 in replantation and free tissue transfer: early preliminary experience. Microsurgery 27:395-397, 2007.
9. Wilhelmi BJ, Lee WP, Pagensteert GI, et al. Replantation in the mutilated hand. Hand Clin 19:89-120, 2003.

74. Hand Transplantation

See *Essentials of Plastic Surgery*, second edition, pp. 881-889.

LEVEL OF AMPUTATION

1. A patient is referred for consideration of hand transplantation and currently uses a prosthesis. **Which once of the following amputation levels is optimal for an upper limb prosthesis?**
   A. Transmetacarpal
   B. Radiocarpal
   C. Midforearm
   D. Proximal forearm
   E. Transhumeral

INDICATIONS AND CONTRAINDICATIONS

2. A 21-year-old right-hand-dominant patient had a left transmetacarpal amputation following meningococcal septicemia 12 months ago. He would like a hand transplant. **What is the main contraindication to hand transplant in this case?**
   A. His age
   B. The level of injury
   C. His hand dominance
   D. The mechanism of injury
   E. The time interval since injury

3. There are a number of medical contraindications to hand transplant. **In which one of the following scenarios may transplant still be indicated?**
   A. During early pregnancy
   B. Following medical treatment for hepatitis A infection
   C. A year after mastectomy and radiotherapy
   D. In a healthy patient with symbrachydactyly
   E. In a patient with well-controlled HIV

TRANSPLANTATION CRITERIA

4. **Why is it particularly important for one of the hand transplant team to physically meet a potential donor before embarking on a hand transplant?**
   A. To confirm ABO blood type
   B. To confirm a positive crossmatch
   C. To meet the donor family members
   D. To assess donor limb integrity, size, and appearance
   E. To take written informed consent for limb donation

OPERATIVE STEPS

5. When performing a distal forearm hand transplant, which one of the following is correct?
A. The donor limb is removed with a humeral fishmouth incision and a transelbow amputation.
B. A single-team approach to the second stage is preferable for optimal matching of nerve, vessel, and tendon length.
C. The sequence of reconstruction is bone, extensor tendons, flexor tendons, arteries, veins, and nerves.
D. Tension should be set for the extensors so that the fingers are extended when the wrist is extended.
E. Epineurial repair is the preferred technique for the ulnar and median nerves at this level.

IMMUNOSUPPRESSION

6. Which one of the following is correct regarding immunosuppressive therapy in hand transplantation?
A. Tacrolimus is normally used as a depletion agent before a transplant.
B. The most common maintenance regimen is rapamycin with corticosteroids.
C. Mycophenalate mofetil is restricted to cases with late rejection due to hepatotoxicity.
D. Antihypertensive and hypoglycemic agents are commonly required.
E. Metabolic complications of immunosuppressive therapy are permanent.

7. Which one of the following is the most antigenic tissue?
A. Fat
B. Muscle
C. Endothelium
D. Bone
E. Skin

OUTCOMES

8. Which one of the following is true regarding hand transplantation performed at forearm level?
A. Proximal forearm transplants tend to provide the best extrinsic motor function.
B. Distal forearm transplants consistently provide near normal intrinsic motor function.
C. Tactile and discriminative sensation are regained in most transplant cases.
D. Peak functional recovery can be expected at 1 year after surgery.
E. Functional outcome is best measured using the DASH score which specifically relates to hand transplant.

9. Which one of the following is expected at 6 months after hand transplantation?
A. A 5% risk of medication-induced diabetes
B. A 10% chance of acute rejection
C. A 25% chance of opportunistic infection
D. A 50% chance of graft loss
E. A 75% chance of patient satisfaction

MANAGEMENT OF COMPLICATIONS

10. You are asked to assess a patient following hand transplantation as there are concerns regarding acute rejection. *In order to assess rejection according to the Banff classification, what test will be required?*
    A. MRI
    B. Blood sample
    C. Doppler ultrasound
    D. Cytology sample
    E. Skin biopsy

11. You have confirmed the presence of acute rejection clinically by using the Banff scoring system. *Which one of the following represents the first-line agent you should use to manage this rejection?*
    A. Tacrolimus
    B. Sulfasalazine
    C. Mycophenalate mofetil
    D. Corticosteroid
    E. Monoclonal antibodies

Answers

LEVEL OF AMPUTATION

1. A patient is referred for consideration of hand transplantation and currently uses a prosthesis. *Which once of the following amputation levels is optimal for an upper limb prosthesis?*
   C. Midforearm
   When considering the merits of hand transplantation, the ability to successfully use a prosthesis must first be considered. There are many options for a prosthesis in patients with a midforearm amputation. Patients with a transmetacarpal stump are usually able to use their wrists well to perform many activities and the additional values of a prosthesis can be limited. Amputations at the radiocarpal level preserve length well but have very little function without a prosthetic; yet fitting a useful prosthesis at this level can be difficult. A transhumeral amputation can work well with a prosthesis but the success of this is dependent on shoulder mobility, and overall function is likely to be poorer than a midforearm prosthesis.

INDICATIONS AND CONTRAINDICATIONS

2. A 21-year-old right-hand-dominant patient had a left transmetacarpal amputation following meningococcal septicemia 12 months ago. He would like a hand transplant. *What is the main contraindication to hand transplant in this case?*
   C. His hand dominance
   Transplantation is considered for traumatic amputations (as opposed to congenital absences) with strict inclusion criteria. The main indication for hand transplantation is a bilateral upper or quadrimembral amputee, or an amputee who has lost their dominant upper limb. This patient has retained his dominant upper limb so is very unlikely to warrant the risks associated with the procedure and lifelong immunosuppression. Other criteria include age over 18 years, a good state of general health, and an adequate period of using a prosthesis (which can be arranged after the initial assessment if not already undertaken). He would therefore not be excluded on these grounds. Each case must be judged on its own merits and due thought given to the quality of the remaining tissues at the stump, which is influenced by the mechanism of injury. Level of injury is also important, as removal of a failed transplanted limb should ideally not leave the patient in a worse functional position than when they started; this is difficult to avoid in a transmetacarpal amputation. In general, a transmetacarpal amputation in the dominant hand of a young patient following meningococcal sepsis could be considered for transplant.

3. There are a number of medical contraindications to hand transplant. *In which one of the following scenarios may transplant still be indicated?*
   B. Following medical treatment for hepatitis A infection
   Hepatitis A is an acute, self-limiting viral infection that does not lead to chronic infection. Although there may be liver damage if the initial infection is severe, this can be screened for during assessment for transplant. Active hepatitis infection or HIV represent contraindications to transplant as do a current diagnosis of cancer, high risk of cancer recurrence (such as shortly

after mastectomy and radiotherapy), pregnancy, immunologic dysfunction, and hypercoagulable states.

Hand transplantation is generally contraindicated in the management of congenital limb anomalies. In congenital limb absence, the patient will have no prior experience of a functioning limb at the defect site and will have lifelong learned behavior patterns and cortical representation that are based on the limb deficit being their normal state. Also, in the trauma setting there are predictable recipient structures to unite, which is often not the case in congenital anomalies.

TRANSPLANTATION CRITERIA

4. Why is it particularly important for one of the hand transplant team to physically meet a potential donor before embarking on a hand transplant?

D. To assess donor limb integrity, size, and appearance

Assessment of the physical characteristics of the limb is critical in achieving a good outcome following hand transplant. This affects the functional, cosmetic and psychological outcome, and also affects practical steps such as completing osteosynthesis of the radius and ulna in the forearm. It is the responsibility of the transplant team to optimize this match and therefore they will be closely involved in selection. Skin tone, hair density, and overall physical match with the recipient are important, so even when there may be a suitable donor match in terms of blood grouping, etc., transplant may be stopped based on physical criteria.

While correct ABO typing and crossmatching are key to a successful transplant, the surgical team do not need to meet the donor to gather this information. During immunological screening, a positive crossmatch is a major problem as it means that the recipient has preformed antibodies to the donor tissue and will likely undergo a hyperacute rejection.

In many transplant programs, contact with the donor family is through the specialist in organ donation who is seeking consent for donation of all (or selected) organs. The upper limb transplant team will usually have made arrangements for the additional consent elements (such as pointing out that the donated limbs will be visible and that media attention is not always avoidable) to be included in this process.

OPERATIVE STEPS

5. When performing a distal forearm hand transplant, which one of the following is correct?

A. The donor limb is removed with a humeral fishmouth incision and a transelbow amputation.

This method of removing the donor limb is swift, minimizing the impact on solid organ retrieval. It also preserves all the required distal tissues with excess length to allow accurate preparation in the recipient OR.

A two-team approach is preferred within the recipient OR area so the ischemic time is kept to a minimum. The teams must coordinate closely to ensure matched osteotomies and clear tagging of important structures at an appropriate length. The sequence of reconstruction varies according to amputation level and tissue type. The urgency to revascularize depends on composite tissue types included, with greater urgency in grafts having a significant muscle component (in more proximal transplants). For a distal forearm transplantation, a typical sequence would be bony fixation, extensor tendons (set to full extension with the wrist flexed), dorsal veins, nerves, arteries, and flexor tendons. At this level, a grouped fascicular repair technique is recommended over an epineurial repair where possible.

IMMUNOSUPPRESSION

6. Which one of the following is correct regarding immunosuppressive therapy in hand transplantation?

D. Antihypertensive and hypoglycemic agents are commonly required.

Patients taking immunosuppressive drugs for transplant surgery may develop hypertension or hyperglycemia as a consequence, often requiring medications to address this. Gastroprotective medication may also be required as a result of prolonged corticosteroid use. Metabolic complications reported following hand transplant in a 28-patient review included hyperglycemia in 13 patients (46.42%), hypertension in 7 patients (25%), and hyperlipidemia in 4 patients (14.28%). Preparation for this is an important component of the preoperative counseling and consent process. While metabolic complications are a common side effect of immunosuppressive regimens, these changes are usually reversed as immunosuppressive medication doses are reduced or stopped.

Induction immunotherapy is performed before surgery to prevent acute rejection. Lymphocyte depleting agents are used and include antithymocyte globulin and alemtuzumab. Tacrolimus (Prograf) is also used in the induction phase; however, it is a calcineurin inhibitor that reduces lymphocyte activation and not a depleting agent. Tacrolimus also appears to have an additional secondary beneficial effect on nerve recovery/regeneration.

The most common maintenance regimen is triple therapy with tacrolimus, mycophenolate mofetil (MMF), and corticosteroids. Many protocols attempt to reduce tacrolimus and it may be replaced by rapamycin. MMF is a common component of both induction and maintenance regimens, having a role in B- and T-lymphocyte suppression. It is considered to be much less hepatotoxic than its predecessors: cyclophosphamide and azathioprine.[1]

7. Which one of the following is the most antigenic tissue?

E. Skin

Vascularized composite allografts (VCAs) will contain a number of different tissue types such as skin, bone, muscle, and nerve within a single graft. Of these tissue components, skin is the most antigenic and, as a result, direct inspection is important to identify acute rejection. This will manifest as erythematous macules, diffuse redness, or asymptomatic papules (see Chapter 7). For this reason, patients should be seen in clinic on a regular basis after transplant and must be educated in reporting potential signs of rejection.

OUTCOMES

8. Which one of the following is true regarding hand transplantation performed at forearm level?

C. Tactile and discriminative sensation are regained in most transplant cases.

It is reasonable to expect a good sensory recovery after hand transplant, with more than 90% reported rates of return for tactile, pain, and temperature sensation. While extrinsic motor function is expected in all cases, the rate of intrinsic recovery is less predictable. A midforearm transplant is more likely to produce a good result than a more proximal transplant; there is a shorter distance for nerve recovery to reinnervate distal muscles, there is a functioning elbow, and there is the possibility of strong Pulvertaft tendon weaves for uniting the extrinsic motor units (rather than muscle belly repairs). Peak recovery is not at 1 year, as recovery is expected to continue for several years.

The DASH score (disability of arm and shoulder) is a well-regarded scoring system used for upper limb function. However, it is not specific to hand transplantation. A hand transplantation score has been developed (HTSS) and this has six key areas including appearance, sensibility, movement, psychological and social acceptance, activities of daily living, and patient satisfaction.[2]

9. **Which one of the following is expected at 6 months after hand transplantation?**
   E. A 75% chance of patient satisfaction
   In spite of the rigorous medical regimen, the side effects from medications, and the intrusive therapy and monitoring schedule, more than 75% of patients have a subjective improvement in quality of life after a hand transplant. Most patients perform ADLs independently and some have returned to full employment. The risk of metabolic complications was discussed in question 6 and the overall rate is approximately 70%. The risk of hyperglycemia-induced problems secondary to immunotherapy is around 45%.

   Acute rejection has been a consistent problem after limb transplant, with 85% incidence within the first year. These episodes are, however, treatable with immunotherapy modification. The risk of opportunistic infection is high because of immunosuppression. This is estimated to be approximately 60% to 65%. Infections include CMV, herpes, and bacterial subtypes, and appropriate prophylaxis is required, particularly in the first 6 to 12 months. The risk of graft loss is low across all series of vascularized transplant, although the Chinese series on limb transplant reported losses over 40% because of poor patient compliance with medical therapy.[3]

MANAGEMENT OF COMPLICATIONS

10. You are asked to assess a patient following hand transplantation as there are concerns regarding acute rejection. *In order to assess rejection according to the Banff classification, what test will be required?*
    E. Skin biopsy
    Vascularized composite allograft rejection is graded according to the Banff classification,[4] which is based upon the histological appearances of a 4 mm punch biopsy specimen. The grades of rejection range from 0 to 4 based upon evidence of the extent and severity of inflammatory change and the presence or absence of cell necrosis.

11. You have confirmed the presence of acute rejection clinically by using the Banff scoring system. *Which one of the following represents the first-line agent you should use to manage this rejection?*
    D. Corticosteroid
    The first-line agent in an acute rejection episode is a high-dose corticosteroid (prednisolone/hydrocortisone), while ensuring that tacrolimus or MMF doses are optimized. Second-line agents include high-dose tacrolimus, monoclonal antibodies, and sirolimus (see Chapter 7).

REFERENCES

1. Landin L, Bonastre J, Casado-Sanchez C, et al. Outcomes with respect to disabilities of the upper limb after hand allograft transplantation: a systematic review. Transpl Int 25:424-432, 2012.
2. Petruzzo P, Lanzetta M, Dubernard JM, et al. The international registry on hand and composite tissue transplantation. Transplantation 86:487-492, 2008.
3. Pei G, Xiang D, Gu L, et al. A report of 15 hand allotransplantations in 12 patients and their outcomes in China. Transplantation 94:1052-1059, 2012
4. Cendales LC, Kanitakis J, Schneeberger S, et al. The Banff 2007 working classification of skin-containing composite tissue allograft pathology. Am J Transplant 8:1396-1400, 2008.

75. Thumb Reconstruction

See *Essentials of Plastic Surgery*, second edition, pp. 890-900.

GENERAL CONSIDERATIONS

1. **When planning thumb reconstruction, which one of the following is correct?**
   A. Even distal third amputations require reconstruction to preserve function.
   B. A stiff replanted thumb usually achieves better function than an alternative reconstruction.
   C. In extensive mutilating injuries, reconstruction should occur in less than 72 hours for optimal cortical plasticity.
   D. Additional bone length is only required for proximal third amputations.
   E. Amputation through the IP joint is a good indication for a toe transfer.

RECONSTRUCTIVE OPTIONS IN THE THUMB

2. **Which one of the following statements is correct when considering thumb reconstruction?**
   A. An index finger cross-finger flap is ideal for a 2 by 2 cm volar defect over the MP joint and proximal phalanx.
   B. A full-thickness skin graft will ultimately achieve similar sensation to a homodigital flap on the thumb pulp.
   C. The wraparound procedure is ideal for children, because it expands well with growth.
   D. A great toe transfer is the preferred option for CMC joint amputations to achieve ideal length and aesthetics.
   E. Free toe transfer can be carried out as a single stage immediately after the initial debridement.

VOLAR ADVANCEMENT FLAPS

3. You have a patient with a 1.5 by 1.5 cm defect of the thumb pulp with exposed bone. **Which one of the following is correct when using a Moberg flap for this patient?**
   A. The IP and MP joints will be fully straight following physiotherapy.
   B. The midlateral incisions should form a "zigzag" to improve flap advancement.
   C. Release of skin proximally may be required to achieve closure.
   D. A full-thickness skin graft will also be required.
   E. The standard flap can easily be advanced to cover this size of defect.

MANAGEMENT OF THE FIRST WEB SPACE

4. You are planning to release a contracted first web space 18 months after a crush injury to the thumb that resulted in amputation through the proximal phalanx and has left the patient with a stiff CMC joint and a short thumb. *Which one of the following is correct?*
   A. Adductor pollicis should never be released.
   B. The optimal Z-plasty design involves multiple 30-degree flaps.
   C. If the skin is released properly, deeper structures need not be disturbed.
   D. The first dorsal interosseous muscle may need to be released.
   E. A dorsal rotation/transposition skin flap avoids the need for a skin graft.

PROCEDURES THAT ADD BONE LENGTH

5. When considering distraction osteogenesis to lengthen the metacarpal of a partially amputated thumb, *which one of the following is correct?*
   A. A minimum of 50% of the metacarpal is required.
   B. Up to 5 cm of lengthening can be reliably produced.
   C. Approximately 2 mm of advancement per week is optimal for lengthening.
   D. Bone grafting may be required in patients over 25 years of age.
   E. The soft tissue envelope will always stretch to accommodate lengthening.

POLLICIZATION

6. When pollicizing the index finger, *which one of the following is correct?*
   A. The index CMC joint becomes the new thumb CMC joint.
   B. The first dorsal interosseous muscle becomes the new APL.
   C. The FDS tendon becomes the new FPL tendon.
   D. The proximal phalanx becomes the middle phalanx.
   E. The EIP tendon becomes the new EPL tendon.

FREE TOE TRANSFER

7. When planning a free toe transfer for thumb reconstruction, *which one of the following is correct?*
   A. Second toe transfers are equal in strength to great toe transfers.
   B. An oblique osteotomy through the toe metatarsal can improve function in the new thumb.
   C. The arterial supply to the great toe is consistently from the first metatarsal artery arising from dorsalis pedis.
   D. The contralateral great toe is preferred to favorably align the arterial anastomosis in the first web space.
   E. The second toe donor site often requires skin grafting for closure.

Answers

GENERAL CONSIDERATIONS

1. **When planning thumb reconstruction, which one of the following is correct?**
   B. A stiff replanted thumb usually achieves better function than an alternative reconstruction.

   Thumb injuries are classified as proximal, middle, and distal third injuries and their management is typically guided by this classification (see Fig. 75-1, *Essentials of Plastic Surgery*, second edition).

   In general, as much tissue as possible should be salvaged and attempts made to preserve length, sensibility, and function. A stiff replanted thumb is normally superior in aesthetics and function to an alternative reconstruction. However, there are always exceptions to any rule, and each case should be assessed individually (e.g., some patients may opt for terminalization to facilitate a more speedy return to work).

   Although attempts are usually made to salvage all viable tissue and length in the thumb, distal third (IP joint and distal) amputations are usually well compensated for, since there is sufficient length for reasonable function; again, this depends on the individual patient's requirements and anatomy.

   Middle third (metacarpal neck to IP joint) amputations may be sufficiently short to require bone lengthening in addition to first web deepening, particularly when proximal to the MP joint. IP joint amputations are not typical cases for a free toe transfer. This is more commonly reserved for amputations through the distal half of the metacarpal or proximal part of the proximal phalanx. However, a distal third injury might benefit from partial toe tissue transfer, such as for pulp or nail replacement.

   Extensive mutilating injuries often need a delayed reconstruction to preserve and stabilize the remaining skeleton and soft tissue envelope before any additional surgical insult. For example, the first web and thumb base might be covered with a groin flap, followed by an elective free toe transfer or pollicization at a later date.

RECONSTRUCTIVE OPTIONS IN THE THUMB

2. **Which one of the following statements is correct when considering thumb reconstruction?**
   E. Free toe transfer can be carried out as a single stage immediately after the initial debridement.

   Free toe transfer is more commonly used for delayed reconstructions, but it may be carried out acutely if there are suitable recipient bony and soft tissues, the wound is clean and healthy, and appropriate informed consent has been obtained. Wraparound flaps are more likely to be performed urgently, such as when there is exposed bone and immediate soft tissue cover is required, but are not usually recommended for young children because of subsequent growth restriction.

   A cross-finger flap from the index finger would not reach the proximal or radial extent of a defect overlying the proximal phalanx and MP joint. This flap is better suited to defects over the distal phalanx (see Fig. 75-3, *Essentials of Plastic Surgery*, second edition.)

   Full-thickness skin grafts are sometimes used for pulp defects, but sensory return is better with split-thickness grafts or homodigital flaps. An amputation through the CMC joint might be better reconstructed with pollicization. The great toe would not provide sufficient length and, because it is usually around 20% wider than the thumb, the aesthetic outcome is not ideal. The donor site is also not aesthetically pleasing and may require skin grafting.

VOLAR ADVANCEMENT FLAPS

3. You have a patient with a 1.5 by 1.5 cm defect of the thumb pulp with exposed bone. ***Which one of the following is correct when using a Moberg flap for this patient?***
   C. Release of skin proximally may be required to achieve closure.
   The standard Moberg advancement flap may be used for thumb tip defects of up to 50% of the volar pulp surface. The standard Moberg flap can be advanced about 1 cm but requires further release to move the 1.5 cm required in this case (Fig. 75-1). Straight midlateral incisions are made and the volar skin is advanced with the neurovascular bundles superficial to the flexor tendon sheath. This generally requires flexion of both the MP and IP joints during inset, which is not always fully corrected with physiotherapy. A number of modifications have been described, such as advancing the flap in a V-Y fashion proximally, or transversely releasing the proximal skin and applying a full-thickness skin graft to the donor site. Dellon's modification is reported to allow up to 3 cm of advancement (see Fig. 67-6, *Essentials of Plastic Surgery*, second edition).

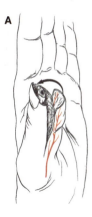
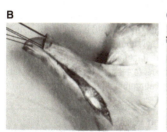
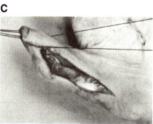

Fig. 75-1 Volar advancement flap (Moberg flap). **A,** Arc to the distal phalanx of the thumb. **B,** Elevation of the flap. **C,** Coverage of the distal phalanx of the thumb.

MANAGEMENT OF THE FIRST WEB SPACE

4. You are planning to release a contracted first web space 18 months after a crush injury to the thumb that resulted in amputation through the proximal phalanx and has left the patient with a stiff CMC joint and a short thumb. ***Which one of the following is correct?***
   D. The first dorsal interosseous muscle may need to be released.
   If the CMC joint is stiff and the web space contracted, it is unlikely that skin release alone will be sufficient. It may be necessary to release both the first dorsal interosseous and adductor pollicis muscles, often reinserting the adductor muscle more proximally. The dorsal rotation flap for first web deepening requires a skin graft to the donor site (see Fig. 75-5, *Essentials of Plastic Surgery*, second edition). When using a Z-plasty technique for first web release, a 60-degree Z-plasty is preferred (see Fig. 75-4, *Essentials of Plastic Surgery*, second edition). Alternatively, the four-flap "jumping man" flaps may be used (see Fig. 61-7, *Essentials of Plastic Surgery*, second edition).

"CADBury" refers to the order of the transposed skin flaps ABCD following inset. It is a caption term in the United Kingdom because of the popular confectionary company Cadburys.

PROCEDURES THAT ADD BONE LENGTH

5. When considering distraction osteogenesis to lengthen the metacarpal of a partially amputated thumb, which one of the following is correct?
D. Bone grafting may be required in patients over 25 years of age.

According to many surgeons, patients over 25 years of age may benefit from additional bone grafting at the site of distraction osteogenesis to improve the rate of union.[1] A minimum of two thirds of the metacarpal is preferred prior to distraction, and a maximum 3.5 cm gain is most common. After the initial rest period, 1 mm per day is the usual rate of distraction. The soft tissue envelope may not tolerate distraction, particularly if there is scarring or previous skin grafts, therefore this may require revision prior to distraction. (See Chapter 23 for further information on distraction osteogenesis.)

POLLICIZATION

6. When pollicizing the index finger, which one of the following is correct?
E. The EIP tendon becomes the new EPL tendon.

Pollicization is a useful and reliable procedure for complete thumb reconstruction. It results in minimal sacrifice of hand function and can provide excellent cosmetic and functional results when performed well. The index finger is classically used and the EIP becomes the new EPL. The MP joint (not CMC joint) becomes the new thumb CMC joint as the digit is shortened. The first dorsal interosseous muscle becomes the new abductor pollicis brevis (not the APL), the FDP (not FDS) becomes the new FPL, and the proximal phalanx becomes the metacarpal. The key structures involved in converting the index finger to a thumb are shown below (Table 75-1). Kozin[2] described the concept, technical details, and outcome of pollicization.

Table 75-1 *Structural Changes During Pollicization*

Initial Index Finger Structure	Reconstructed Thumb Structure
Metacarpal head	Trapezium
Proximal phalanx	Metacarpal
Middle phalanx	Proximal phalanx
Distal phalanx	Distal phalanx
Extensor digitorum communis	Abductor pollicis longus
Extensor indices proprius	Extensor pollicis longus
First dorsal interosseous	Abductor pollicis brevis
First palmar interosseous	Adductor pollicis

FREE TOE TRANSFER

7. When planning a free toe transfer for thumb reconstruction, which one of the following is correct?
B. An oblique osteotomy through the toe metatarsal can improve function in the new thumb.

There is often sufficient length in a transferred great toe without using the metatarsal. When it is required, an oblique osteotomy through the metatarsal helps to improve alignment and range of motion in the new thumb, as the toe MTP joints naturally tend to hyperextend, a great deal of which can be undesirable in the reconstructed thumb.

Great toe transfers are generally stronger than second toe transfers. Although there is debate about which is more aesthetically pleasing, the great toe is usually about 20% broader than the thumb which it is replacing, whereas the second toe is usually noticeably thinner with a short nail. This is variable between individuals. The arterial supply to both is most commonly via the first dorsal metatarsal artery; however, there is considerable variation. An ipsilateral great toe orients the first dorsal metatarsal artery more favorably in the first dorsal web space for anastomosis. The second toe donor site usually closes directly, but the great toe may require skin grafting.

REFERENCES

1. Matev I. Thumb metacarpal lengthening. Tech Hand Up Extrem Surg 7:157-163, 2003.
2. Kozin SH. Pollicization: the concept, technical details, and outcome. Clin Orthop Surg 4:18-35, 2012.

76. Soft Tissue Coverage of the Hand and Upper Extremity

See *Essentials of Plastic Surgery*, second edition, pp. 901-911.

SKIN GRAFTS ON THE HAND

1. **Which one of the following is correct when using a skin graft in the hand?**
   A. Full-thickness grafts are best harvested from the contralateral upper limb.
   B. The heel is a good donor site for glabrous skin graft harvest.
   C. Split-thickness skin grafts should be meshed to improve graft take.
   D. It is normal for glabrous skin grafts to appear sloughy at 1 to 2 weeks.
   E. Split-thickness skin grafts will contract more immediately after harvest than full-thickness grafts.

LOCAL FLAPS FOR FINGER RECONSTRUCTION

2. **Which one of the following is correct regarding local flaps used to reconstruct the digit?**
   A. The Kutler bilateral V-Y flaps are best applied to large dorsal oblique fingertip amputations.
   B. The Atasoy V-Y flap is ideal for reconstructing volar oblique fingertip injuries.
   C. The reverse cross-finger flap is mainly indicated for volar defects over the phalanges.
   D. Homodigital island flaps are contraindicated for fingertip reconstruction following digital vessel injury.
   E. The Moberg flap is ideal for reconstruction of volar defects of the middle finger pulp.

LOCAL FLAPS FOR THUMB TIP RECONSTRUCTION

3. A 21-year-old man presents with a transverse soft-tissue tip amputation to his dominant thumb at the level of the lunula. There is exposed distal phalanx and the soft tissue defect measures 2 by 1 cm. He is generally fit and well and a nonsmoker.
   Which one of the following would be the best reconstructive option in this case?
   A. Healing by secondary intention
   B. Revision amputation
   C. Distally based dorsal hand flap (Quaba)
   D. Thenar flap
   E. Neurovascular island flap (Littler)

Chapter 76 ■ Soft Tissue Coverage of the Hand and Upper Extremity 617

FLAP RECONSTRUCTION OF THE HAND

4. A 40-year-old woman sustains an 8 by 7 cm degloving injury to the dorsum of her right hand, leaving exposed extensor tendons without paratenon. She is generally fit and well and of slim build. **Which one of the following is correct regarding reconstruction in her case?**
   A. A pedicled posterior interosseous artery flap could cover this defect, but will leave a numb patch on the dorsal forearm as the posterior interosseous nerve is sacrificed.
   B. A reverse radial forearm flap could comfortably cover this defect but will give a poor cosmetic outcome.
   C. Free tissue transfer for reconstruction of this defect with an anterolateral thigh flap would be unnecessary and is best avoided in this patient.
   D. An Allen's test should be performed before using a radial forearm flap to reconstruct the defect to ensure flap flow is adequate.
   E. Centering the skin paddle for a reverse radial forearm flap in the middle third of the forearm would provide the most reliable skin perfusion for reconstruction.

5. **When reconstructing a soft tissue defect of the hand using the reverse radial forearm flap, which one of the following is true?**
   A. The flap design should be checked for adequate reach, assuming the pivot point is the radial styloid.
   B. The radial artery is found within an intramuscular septum between the FDS and the FCR.
   C. The cephalic vein is usually incorporated within the flap to aid venous drainage.
   D. The donor site is best closed with meshed split-thickness graft.
   E. The radial artery is routinely reconstructed with a vein graft after flap harvest.

6. **When reconstructing a soft tissue defect of the hand using the posterior interosseous flap, which one of the following is true?**
   A. The flap is centered on a line between the wrist and medial epicondyle.
   B. Flap markings should be performed with the elbow in extension.
   C. The PIA is located distally between the ECU and EDM tendons.
   D. The flap pivot point is 1 cm distal to the ulnar styloid.
   E. The PIA arises proximally from the radial artery at the level of the antecubital fossa.

FLAPS USED FOR ELBOW SOFT TISSUE COVERAGE

7. For each of the following descriptions, select the most likely reconstructive option from the list. (Each option may be used once, more than once, or not at all.)
   A. This reconstruction can be used to reconstruct small soft tissue elbow defects, but is contraindicated in a young laborer.
   B. This flap is based on the posterior radial collateral artery and can only provide coverage of a distal elbow defect if used as a free tissue transfer.
   C. This flap is based on the radial recurrent artery and is a workhorse flap for elbow reconstruction.

   Options:
   a. Reverse lateral arm flap
   b. Flexor carpi ulnaris flap
   c. Posterior interosseous artery flap
   d. Lateral arm flap
   e. Latissimus dorsi flap
   f. Reverse radial forearm flap

VASCULAR SUPPLY TO FREE FLAPS USED IN THE UPPER LIMB

8. *Free tissue transfer may be required for reconstruction of soft tissue defects of the upper limb. For each of the following flaps, select the correct vascular supply from the options listed. (Each option may be used once, more than once, or not at all.)*
   A. *The scapula and parascapular flaps*
   B. *The gracilis flap*
   C. *The serratus anterior flap*
   D. *The groin flap*

   Options:
   a. Lateral femoral circumflex
   b. Thoracodorsal
   c. Circumflex scapular
   d. Medial femoral circumflex
   e. Thoracoacromial
   f. Superficial circumflex iliac
   g. Deep circumflex iliac
   h. Deep inferior epigastric

Answers

SKIN GRAFTS ON THE HAND

1. Which one of the following is correct when using a skin graft in the hand?
D. It is normal for glabrous skin grafts to appear sloughy at 1 to 2 weeks.

The appearance of a glabrous graft can be concerning at 1 to 2 weeks as the thick stratum corneum sloughs. This can give the impression the graft has failed to take. It does, however, regrow in most cases, so it may be helpful to warn the patient and the nursing staff about this before surgery. Glabrous skin grafts can be useful for defects on the palm. They should be harvested from the hypothenar eminence or from a non-weight-bearing part of the foot such as the instep (rather than the heel).

Split-thickness skin grafts are best used as sheet grafts to minimize contraction and improve cosmesis when reconstructing the hand. This is especially true for larger areas, such as burns where early grafting is also prioritized over many other body areas. There are benefits to using split versus full-thickness grafts in general. Split-thickness grafts show less primary contraction than full-thickness grafts, but are more prone to later secondary contraction. Full-thickness grafts are the reverse, so they provide less secondary contraction over time. Split-thickness graft donor sites have to heal by the process of reepithelialization, where full-thickness graft donor sites are closed directly. Split-thickness grafts can provide cover for much larger defects and graft take can be more predictable. Smaller defects are best reconstructed with full-thickness grafts where possible, as a better color and texture match is achieved. Furthermore, the skin cover is likely to be more robust which is highly relevant to the hand and upper limb. Most potential full-thickness graft donor sites are suitable, providing hair-bearing skin is avoided. Common sites include the upper arm, forearm, groin, and supraclavicular fossa. The contralateral upper limb should generally be avoided as then both limbs will have temporary limited function which makes activities of daily living difficult for the patient. It is often possible to use the same limb as a donor for smaller grafts by harvesting skin from the forearm.

LOCAL FLAPS FOR FINGER RECONSTRUCTION

2. Which one of the following is correct regarding local flaps used to reconstruct the digit?
D. Homodigital island flaps are contraindicated for fingertip reconstruction following digital vessel injury.

Homodigital island flaps require sacrifice of one digital vessel, therefore they are contraindicated in single-vessel digits. They are useful for reconstructing fingertip defects unsuitable for skin grafts or healing by secondary intention. The neurovascular bundle is dissected proximally into the palm and the flap is advanced in a V-Y or step-cut fashion. As discussed in Chapter 67, Kutler[1] flaps are two small lateral V-Y flaps than are usually indicated in selected cases for primary repair of transverse or lateral oblique injuries. The main indication is for secondary revision of fingertip amputations. The Atasoy[2] flap is a small volar V-Y advancement flap indicated for dorsal oblique injuries and some transverse amputations (see Fig. 67-5, *Essentials of Plastic Surgery*, second edition). It is contraindicated in volar oblique injuries, as the flap should not extend proximal to the DIP joint crease. It should be elevated in the plane just above the periosteum in order to preserve vascularity.

The reverse cross-finger flap involves raising a thin (subdermal) skin flap away from the defect site and then a subcutaneous flap in the opposite direction at the level of paratenon. It is indicated for coverage of exposed tendon or bone on the dorsum of the adjacent digit. A standard cross-finger flap is used for volar defects. The Moberg flap is contraindicated in finger reconstruction because of the location of the neurovascular bundles. It is generally indicated for volar defects of the thumb tip/pulp.[3]

LOCAL FLAPS FOR THUMB TIP RECONSTRUCTION

3. A 21-year-old man presents with a transverse soft tissue tip amputation to his dominant thumb at the level of the lunula. There is exposed distal phalanx and the soft tissue defect measures 2 by 1 cm. He is generally fit and well and a nonsmoker.
   Which one of the following would be the best reconstructive option in this case?
   E. Neurovascular island flap (Littler)

   The Littler[4] neurovascular island flap is useful for reconstruction of thumb soft tissue defects. It involves elevation of a flap from the middle or ring finger based on one of the neurovascular bundles. Dissection of the bundle is performed proximally into the palm and tunneled radially across to the thumb. The donor site is skin grafted.

   The key principles in thumb reconstruction are to preserve length and achieve sensate, durable soft tissue cover. Reconstruction is therefore often (but not always) best achieved with a local flap. Other options depend on the level of injury and the amount of bone exposed, but range from trimming of the exposed bone and leaving to heal by secondary intention to burying the thumb temporarily in the groin or performing free toe or soft tissue transfer. Given that this is a young patient and the dominant thumb is involved, preservation of length with sensation is important, so neither revision amputation or healing by secondary intention are appropriate given the defect size and location in this case.

   A first dorsal metacarpal artery perforator flap (Quaba flap)[5] would not reach this area and is used for reconstructing the dorsum of the hand and proximal digits (see Fig. 67-11, *Essentials of Plastic Surgery,* second edition). However, a first dorsal metacarpal artery flap (Foucher) with a skin flap harvested from the dorsum of the index finger could be used (see Fig 67-10, Essentials of Plastic Surgery, second edition)

   The thenar flap is occasionally used to reconstruct volar defects of the digits as a two-stage procedure. However, it results in significant stiffness at the IP joints given that the finger is held in flexion for 2 weeks before flap division. It would not be possible to cover the defect described in this scenario using a thenar flap, as the thumb would not flex sufficiently to enable flap reach.[6]

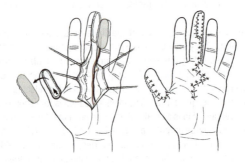

Fig. 76-1 Littler neurovascular island flap, for thumb reconstruction.

Chapter 76 ▪ Soft Tissue Coverage of the Hand and Upper Extremity   621

Even if it could, the stiffness incurred would be counterproductive. The Moberg[3] flap might also be able to cover this defect but may struggle to reach even with Dellon's modification[7] as discussed in Chapter 67 (see Fig. 67-6, *Essentials of Plastic Surgery,* second edition).

FLAP RECONSTRUCTION OF THE HAND

4. A 40-year-old woman sustains an 8 by 7 cm degloving injury to the dorsum of her right hand, leaving exposed extensor tendons without paratenon. She is generally fit and well and of slim build. *Which one of the following is correct regarding reconstruction in her case?*
   B. A reverse radial forearm flap could comfortably cover this defect but will give a poor cosmetic outcome.
   This defect may be adequately reconstructed using a reverse radial forearm flap, but the donor site scarring is a real disadvantage in a young female patient. Other locoregional reconstructive options for this defect include the posterior interosseous and ulnar artery–based flaps, such as the Becker[8] flap, but each of these are also likely to require a skin graft to the donor site. For this reason, free tissue transfer with a thin pliable fasciocutaneous flap such as an anterolateral thigh flap or scapula flap may be better for this patient.
   The posterior interosseous flap may leave a numb patch on the forearm if the posterior, medial, or lateral antebrachial cutaneous nerves are divided during flap harvest. However, division of the posterior interosseous nerve would not cause paresthesia of the skin, since its sensory supply is to the dorsal wrist capsule. Furthermore, this nerve should not be divided when using this flap.
   An Allen's test is performed to confirm that the hand is perfused independently by the radial and ulnar arteries. It involves the application of external pressure over the radial and then ulnar arteries in turn while assessing distal limb perfusion. It is not intended to be used as a test of flap viability.
   When designing the reverse radial forearm flap, it is important to remember that skin perforators are predominantly found in the proximal and distal forearm with a relative paucity in the middle, so ideally the skin paddle should be located in one of these two areas.

5. *When reconstructing a soft tissue defect of the hand using the reverse radial forearm flap, which one of the following is true?*
   A. The flap design should be checked for adequate reach, assuming the pivot point is the radial styloid.
   The radial forearm flap is a fasciocutaneous flap based on the radial artery and associated venae comitantes. It may be used as a free flap or a pedicled flap. When pedicled it may be used based on a reversed flow such that a proximal skin paddle is used to reconstruct a more distal defect.
   The reverse pedicled radial forearm has its pivot point at the radial styloid, and it is important to confirm adequate reach before elevating the flap using a template. As discussed in question 4, good perforating vessels are found proximally and this will provide a long flap reach. Venous outflow is generally adequate using the venae comitantes alone. However, when raising the radial forearm flap as a free flap, it is common practice to include the cephalic vein as this can provide a reliable venous outflow with a good size vein for subsequent anastomosis. The radial artery lies within an intramuscular septum between the FCR and brachioradialis. These two muscles need to be retracted in order to visualize the flap vessels during harvest. Closure of radial forearm donor sites larger than a few centimeters wide will usually require a graft. A full-thickness graft from the groin will provide a reasonable scar, and meshed split grafts should be avoided. It is unusual to reconstruct the radial artery after flap harvest and this should not be necessary, providing the distal perfusion was checked first with an Allen's test. However, in cases where the hand is compromised after tourniquet release, a vein graft would be indicated.

6. **When reconstructing a soft tissue defect of the hand using the posterior interosseous flap, which one of the following is true?**
   C. The PIA is located distally between the ECU and EDM tendons.
   The PIA courses between the ECU and EDM in the distal forearm where it gives off perforating vessels to supply the flap skin paddle. The skin paddle is made approximately 6 cm wide over the distal aspect of the dorsal forearm along a line made between the DRU joint and the lateral, not medial epicondyle. The markings should be performed with the elbow *flexed*, not extended. The pivot point for this flap is 2 cm *proximal* to the ulnar styloid, so adequate reach must be confirmed before the flap elevation. The PIA arises from the interosseous membrane 5 to 6 cm *distal* to the lateral epicondyle. It arises from the ulnar and not the radial artery.

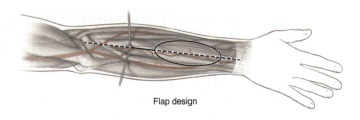

Flap design

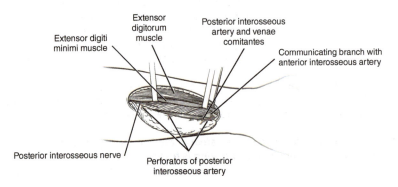

Approach to PIA

Fig. 76-2 Bony landmarks and locations of skin paddle for the posterior interosseous artery flap.

FLAPS USED FOR ELBOW SOFT TISSUE COVERAGE

7. **For the following descriptions, the best options are as follows:**
   A. This reconstruction can be used to reconstruct small soft tissue elbow defects, but is contraindicated in a young laborer.
      b. Flexor carpi ulnaris flap
      A flexor carpi ulnaris muscle flap can be useful in elderly patients who require 3 to 4 cm of muscle cover at the elbow. However, this flap should be avoided in young, active patients because of the important contribution this muscle makes to power grip and the "dart-throwing" motion that the wrist makes during many manual activities.

Chapter 76 ▪ Soft Tissue Coverage of the Hand and Upper Extremity

B. This flap is based on the posterior radial collateral artery and can only provide coverage of a distal elbow defect if used as a free tissue transfer.
   d. Lateral arm flap

   The lateral arm flap is based on the posterior radial collateral artery (see Fig. 76-2, *Essentials of Plastic Surgery,* second edition). It can be pedicled to cover defects of the shoulder and proximal arm. It is also a popular choice for free tissue transfer to the hand because it restricts surgery to a single limb and the donor site can be closed directly.

C. This flap is based on the radial recurrent artery and is a workhorse flap for elbow reconstruction.
   a. Reverse lateral arm flap

   The reverse lateral arm flap is based on the radial recurrent artery and is useful for elbow reconstruction as a pedicled flap (see Fig. 76-2, Essentials of Plastic Surgery, second edition). A key advantage is that the donor site is within the same operative field as the defect and the scarring can be kept to a single limb. A disadvantage is that the arc of rotation may not always allow complete defect coverage.

   As discussed in question 6, the posterior interosseous flap is based on the posterior interosseous artery (a branch of the ulnar artery). It is indicated for reconstruction of the dorsum of the hand. The main advantage is that no major vessels are sacrificed. However, there is a risk that the source vessel may have thrombosis in trauma cases. In addition, flap harvest risks damage to the posterior interosseous nerve which supplies motor innervation to the extensor muscles. The latissimus dorsi flap is based on the thoracodorsal artery and has a broad range of reconstructive uses throughout the body as either a pedicled or free flap. It can be used to fill soft tissue defects or used as functional transfer to provide flexion at the elbow joint.

VASCULAR SUPPLY TO FREE FLAPS USED IN THE UPPER LIMB

8. For each of the following flaps, the correct vascular supply is as follows:

A. The scapular and parascapular flaps
   c. Circumflex scapular

   The scapular and parascapular flaps are reliable thin, pliable fasciocutaneous flaps useful for upper limb reconstruction. They are both supplied by the cutaneous branch of the circumflex scapular vessels and differ slightly in their skin paddle location and precise blood supply. The scapular flap is supplied by the transverse branch of the circumflex scapular, while the parascapular flap is supplied by the descending branch. The skin paddle for the scapular flap is therefore positioned transversely over the middle part of the scapula, while the parascapular flap skin paddle is positioned over the lower lateral border of the scapula. The donor site is generally closed directly and is well hidden in clothing.

B. The gracilis flap
   d. Medial femoral circumflex

   The gracilis flap is a real workhorse flap for both defect and functional reconstruction in the upper limb. It is an excellent flap for achieving dynamic elbow flexion following brachial plexus injury. It is generally raised as a muscle-only flap and is an ideal donor because morbidity is low, with no discernible functional loss and a well-hidden scar passing along the medial thigh. The blood supply to the gracilis is the medial femoral circumflex (which is a branch of the profunda femoris). The muscle differs in size according to age and sex but typically provides 6 by 20 cm of muscle in adult males. It is possible to take a skin paddle with the gracilis, although a longitudinal paddle is generally considered to be unreliable. A transverse skin paddle may be taken as a transverse upper gracilis flap (TUG) when skin is required. This is more often used for breast or perineal reconstruction.

C. The serratus anterior flap
b. Thoracodorsal
The serratus muscle flap is more commonly harvested in conjunction with a latissimus dorsi or bony scapular flap, but can be harvested individually where a small muscle flap is required. This muscle is important in stabilization of the scapula so must not be sacrificed in its entirety. However, the last three digitations can safely be raised without functional impairment. The serratus receives its blood supply from a number of different sources, but the component harvested for free tissue transfer is based on the serratus branch of the thoracodorsal artery. This is why it can be raised along with a latissimus dorsi flap.

D. The groin flap
f. Superficial circumflex iliac
The groin flap has perhaps fallen out of favor with the advent of the anterolateral thigh and other perforator flaps; however, many surgeons continue to use this flap, particularly in reconstruction of upper limb defects in children. This fasciocutaneous flap is generally thin and reliable and allows for the donor defect to be closed directly with well-hidden scars. A perforator flap based on this vascular pedicle has also been described.

The other vascular pedicles listed within the options each supply a flap that may be used for upper limb, chest wall, or head and neck reconstruction. The lateral circumflex femoral supplies the anterolateral thigh flap, the thoracoacromial supplies the pectoralis major and pectoralis minor muscle flaps, the deep circumflex iliac supplies the iliac crest flap, while the deep inferior epigastric supplies the rectus abdominis muscle flap.[9]

REFERENCES
1. Kutler W. A new method for fingertip amputation. JAMA 133:29-30, 1947.
2. Atasoy E, Ioakimidis E, Kasdan ML, et al. Reconstruction of the amputated finger tip with a triangular volar flap. A new surgical procedure. J Bone Joint Surg Am 52:921-926, 1970.
3. Moberg E. Aspects of sensation in reconstructive surgery of the upper extremity. J Bone Joint Surg Am 46:817-825, 1964.
4. Littler JW. The neurovascular pedicle method of digital transposition for reconstruction of the thumb. Plast Reconstr Surg 12:303-319, 1953.
5. Quaba AA, Davison PM. The distally based dorsal hand flap. Br J Plast Surg 43:28-39, 1990.
6. Foucher G, Braun JB. A new island flap transfer from the dorsum of the index to thumb. Plast Reconstr Surg 63:344-349, 1979.
7. Dellon AL. The extended palmar advancement flap. J Hand Surg Am 8:190-194, 1983.
8. Becker C, Gilbert A. The ulnar flap—description and applications. Eur J Plast Surg 11:79-82, 1988.
9. Masquelet AC, Gilbert A. An Atlas of Flaps of the Musculoskeletal System. Boca Raton, FL: CRC Press, 2001.

77. Compartment Syndrome

See *Essentials of Plastic Surgery*, second edition, pp. 912-921.

INTRACOMPARTMENTAL PRESSURES

1. **What is the threshold intracompartmental pressure that would require intervention when a potential compartment syndrome is being assessed?**
   A. An absolute pressure of 10 mm Hg
   B. An absolute pressure of 20 mm Hg
   C. An absolute pressure of 30 mm Hg
   D. Within 40 mm Hg of systolic pressure
   E. Within 80 mm Hg of diastolic pressure

LOWER LIMB COMPARTMENTS

2. You are asked to review a patient following a tibial fracture because there is concern regarding compartment syndrome. **Which one of the following lower leg compartments is most likely to develop compartment syndrome in a patient with a tibial fracture?**
   A. Deep posterior
   B. Superficial posterior
   C. Lateral
   D. Anterior
   E. Medial

FOREARM COMPARTMENTS

3. **Which one of the following muscles is most likely to be damaged by a forearm compartment syndrome?**
   A. Flexor digitorum superficialis (FDS)
   B. Flexor pollicis longus (FPL)
   C. Flexor carpi radialis (FCR)
   D. Flexor carpi ulnaris (FCU)
   E. Pronator teres (PT)

CLINICAL ASSESSMENT

4. The six Ps are often described for the assessment of an awake patient with suspected compartment syndrome. **Which one of these is the best early indicator of this condition?**
   A. Pallor
   B. Pulselessness
   C. Paresthesia
   D. Pain
   E. Poikilothermia

INDICATIONS FOR FASCIOTOMY

5. A patient sustains a high voltage electrical injury stealing copper wire from a substation. He complains of pain in his right forearm. *Which one of the following is the strongest indicator for prompt fasciotomies?*
  A. Three consecutive intracompartmental pressure readings of 20 mm Hg
  B. Paresthesia in the median nerve distribution
  C. Severe pain on passive finger extension
  D. A circumferential superficial burn to the forearm
  E. Radius and ulna fractures on plain radiographs

DELAYED PRESENTATION OF COMPARTMENT SYNDROME

6. A 40-year-old man crushed his arm at work 3 days ago and has been referred from a peripheral hospital because his hand has markedly reduced sensation and power, despite his pain improving. The working diagnosis had been neurapraxia; however, a blood creatinine phosphokinase (CPK) level was checked and is 21,000. His hand is well perfused and his forearm is a little firm and tender. *Which one of the following is correct?*
  A. He should have prompt fasciotomies to the forearm.
  B. His renal function should be checked, then he should have prompt fasciotomies to the forearm.
  C. Serial observation and measurement of intracompartmental pressures should be initiated.
  D. He should be closely observed, with the hand elevated and maintenance of good urine output.
  E. He should undergo urgent ultrasonography of the forearm.

PERFORMING A LEG FASCIOTOMY

7. There are a number of accepted approaches to fasciotomies in the lower leg. *When undertaking a combined lateral and medial two-incision approach, which one of the following is correct?*
  A. The superficial and deep peroneal nerves are at high risk of damage during the lateral release.
  B. Flexor hallucis longus is the first muscle encountered after the lateral incision.
  C. The interosseous membrane must be divided after locating the tibialis anterior.
  D. The medial approach risks inadvertent damage to the posterior tibial vessels and tibial nerve.
  E. The medial incision should be placed 10 cm behind the tibial border.

COMPARTMENTS OF THE LEG

8. *Which one of the following nerves is found in the anterior compartment of the leg?*
  A. Superficial peroneal nerve
  B. Common peroneal nerve
  C. Deep peroneal nerve
  D. Anterior tibial nerve
  E. Saphenous nerve

FASCIOTOMIES IN DIFFERENT ANATOMIC SITES
9. *Which one of the following is correct regarding fasciotomies?*
   A. The arm is decompressed using volar and dorsal incisions.
   B. The 10 hand compartments are decompressed using two dorsal and one midpalmar incision.
   C. All four of the major foot compartments can be decompressed through a single medial approach.
   D. The thigh has three compartments traditionally decompressed through a single medial approach.
   E. A single medial approach remains popular for decompression of the four leg compartments.

Answers

INTRACOMPARTMENTAL PRESSURES

1. What is the threshold intracompartmental pressure that would require intervention when a potential compartment syndrome is being assessed?

C. An absolute pressure of 30 mm Hg

The normal intracompartmental pressure (ICP) is less than 10 mm Hg. Elevated compartment pressure occurs when either the contents of an osseofascial compartment increase in volume, or when the compartment itself reduces in volume (e.g., after a circumferential deep burn, secondary to external constriction). In compartment syndrome, elevated interstitial pressure overwhelms perfusion pressure. As the ICP rises venous pressure rises, and when venous pressure is higher than capillary perfusion pressure the capillaries collapse. The accepted threshold above which there is occlusion of capillary flow is 30 mm Hg or a relative difference between the ICP and the diastolic blood pressure of less than 30 mm Hg, which is a very important point.

LOWER LIMB COMPARTMENTS

2. You are asked to review a patient following a tibial fracture because there is concern regarding compartment syndrome. Which one of the following lower leg compartments is most likely to develop compartment syndrome in a patient with a tibial fracture?

D. Anterior

The anterior compartment is most likely to be involved in a lower limb compartment syndrome. McQueen et al[1] reviewed 59 cases of leg compartment syndrome that included both open and closed tibial injuries. They found that all cases involved the anterior compartment but only 18 involved all four compartments. For intracompartmental pressure monitoring, the anterior compartment is easy to access. The deep posterior is probably the most difficult to reliably decompress but is the second most at-risk compartment. In six of the 59 cases the lateral compartment was also involved, and in five cases the deep posterior compartment was also involved. The deep posterior is probably the most difficult to reliably assess and is the second most at-risk compartment. A more recent study by McQueen et al, retrospectively reviewed 1407 patients who had sustained an open tibial shaft fracture, in order to identify predictors of compartment syndrome. Their analysis showed that the main predictor was age, with males between the ages of 12 and 29 to be at most risk. They did not comment on the compartment involved in this study; however, they postulated that the increased risk in younger patients is due to the increased physical size of muscles in this patient group. The anterior compartment may be most at risk of developing compartment syndrome because it is a particularly tight compartment with well-developed musculature. The close proximity to the tibia is also likely to be a factor.[2]

FOREARM COMPARTMENTS

3. Which one of the following muscles is most likely to be damaged by a forearm compartment syndrome?

B. Flexor pollicis longus (FPL)

Compartment syndrome affects the deep muscles of the volar compartment (FDP and FPL) most significantly. They are more susceptible to damage, since they are compressed against the forearm bones and interosseous membrane (Fig. 77-1). A retrospective study on acute compartment syndrome of the forearm in 93 patients by Duckworth et al,[3] showed that the volar compartment was most commonly decompressed (99% of cases), and this included the carpal tunnel in around half of these cases. The decision on which compartment to decompress was based on clinical examination and intracompartmental measurement. The most common complication was a neurological deficit (18%) followed by contracture (4%). Muscle necrosis with associated weakness was observed in around 3% of cases in this series.

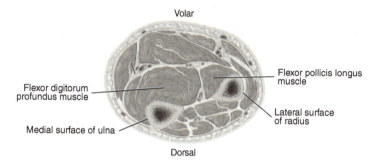

Fig. 77-1 Cross-sectional view of the right proximal forearm.

CLINICAL ASSESSMENT

4. The six Ps are often described for the assessment of an awake patient with suspected compartment syndrome. **Which one of these is the best early indicator of this condition?**

   D. Pain

   The six Ps (**p**ain, **p**allor, **p**oikilothermia, **p**ressure, **p**aralysis/parasthesias, **p**ulselessness) are useful to consider in suspected compartment syndrome. They must be placed in the context of the injury and patient history. Pain is the single most important early aspect and should be disproportionate to the expected pain and exacerbated by passive extension of the compartmental muscles. Progressive loss of nerve function begins with sensory nerves and progresses to motor nerves and is usually a later sign. Pulselessness is another late sign of compartment syndrome, and if present early in the episode, a vascular injury or occlusion is more likely to be the cause. The presence of one of the six Ps alone remains a poor indicator of compartment syndrome. When more than two features coexist in the lower leg, the likelihood increases to above 90%.[4]

INDICATIONS FOR FASCIOTOMY

5. A patient sustains a high voltage electrical injury stealing copper wire from a substation. He complains of pain in his right forearm. **Which one of the following is the strongest indicator for prompt fasciotomies?**

   C. Severe pain on passive finger extension

   As discussed in question 4, pain on passive stretch of the muscles in a compartment is one of the cardinal signs of compartment syndrome. Patients who suffer a high voltage electrical injury are at risk of developing acute compartment syndrome. The bone has a high resistance and becomes disproportionately hot during electrical current conduction. The surrounding muscle is damaged by both the electrical current itself and the heat from the underlying bone. This leads to a massive amount of swelling, which may result in compartment syndrome.

As discussed in question 1, an ICP reading of 30 mm Hg (not 20 mm Hg) or above would be in keeping with compartment syndrome, as would a series of rising pressure readings in association with clinical signs.

Tingling in the median nerve distribution can be an early indicator of rising pressure in the volar compartment of the forearm, but the strongest indication in this scenario is the pain on muscle stretch. The presence of radius and ulna fractures indicates that significant force has been applied to the arm, increasing the risk of elevated compartment pressures, but this is not necessarily an indication for decompression in isolation.

DELAYED PRESENTATION OF COMPARTMENT SYNDROME

6. A 40-year-old man crushed his arm at work 3 days ago and has been referred from a peripheral hospital because his hand has markedly reduced sensation and power, despite his pain improving. The working diagnosis had been neurapraxia; however, a blood creatinine phosphokinase (CPK) level was checked and is 21,000. His hand is well perfused and his forearm is a little firm and tender. **Which one of the following is correct?**

   D. He should be closely observed, with the hand elevated and maintenance of good urine output.

   This man has several features of missed compartment syndrome, with a high-risk mechanism of injury. The elevated CPK levels are concerning, and it is important to maintain good diuresis and monitor renal function while he clears myoglobinuria to avoid renal injury. Unfortunately, the window of opportunity to decompress his forearm has passed. Late decompression converts a closed injury with nonviable muscle into an open injury with little additional benefit, running the risk of secondary infection, compartmentectomy, and in some case series, death.[4] If he still had worsening pain this might indicate viable muscle that could still be salvaged, but as his pain has largely subsided, this does not apply. Ultrasonography is not helpful in diagnosis of compartment syndrome, although it can add information in elimination of other diagnoses. In this case an ultrasound is not likely to add any clinical value so is not indicated. In the absence of raised CPK, but with a swollen limb, a scan may be indicated to exclude DVT or other soft tissue swelling.

PERFORMING A LEG FASCIOTOMY

7. There are a number of accepted approaches to fasciotomies in the lower leg. **When undertaking a combined lateral and medial two-incision approach, which one of the following is correct?**

   D. The medial approach risks inadvertent damage to the posterior tibial vessels and tibial nerve.

   The two-incision approach to leg fasciotomy involves a posteromedial incision combined with either a lateral or anterolateal incision (Fig. 77-2). This access facilitates decompression of the two posterior and anterior/lateral compartments respectively.[5] The medial incision is generally placed 1 to 2 cm posterior to the tibial border to preserve perforating skin vessels from the posterior tibial artery that may be required for local transposition flaps. The incision passes into the superficial posterior compartment and dissection continues around the soleus to access the deep compartment. During this dissection care must be taken to avoid damage to the posterior tibial neurovascular bundle.

The lateral incision is placed anterior to the fibula border and the first compartment entered would be either the lateral or anterior; therefore the peroneal or anterior compartment muscles (not FHL) would be seen first. The anterolateral incision is placed 2 cm posterior to the lateral tibial border, and the first muscle encountered in this approach is the tibialis anterior as the anterior compartment is entered. Dissection then continues subfascially in a lateral direction toward the peroneal septum, which is then divided to release the lateral compartment. The superficial and deep peroneal nerves lie within these two compartments but are unlikely to be damaged using these approaches. The interosseous membrane does not need to be divided, as this separates the anterior and deep posterior compartments.

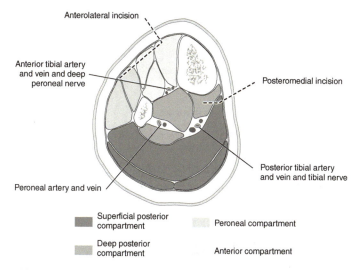

Fig. 77-2 Incisions and anatomic structures for leg fasciotomies.

COMPARTMENTS OF THE LEG

8. Which one of the following nerves is found in the anterior compartment of the leg?
   C. Deep peroneal nerve
   The anterior compartment of the leg contains the anterior tibial vessels and deep peroneal nerve. There is no anterior tibial nerve. It also contains the following four muscles: the tibialis anterior; the extensor hallucis longus; the extensor digitorum longus; and the peroneus tertius, which runs with the digitorum longus (Fig. 77-3). The saphenous nerve is located on the medial aspect of the leg and lies superficial to the leg compartments. The superficial peroneal nerve is located in the lateral compartment along with peroneus longus and brevis. The tibial nerve is located in

the posterior compartment with the posterior tibial vessels, the gastrocnemius, soleus, tibialis posterior, and the long flexors.[5]

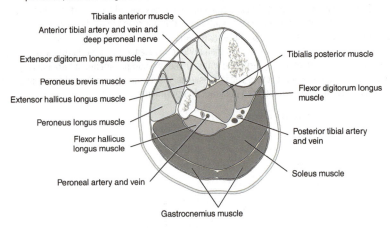

Fig. 77-3 Cross-section of the lower leg.

FASCIOTOMIES IN DIFFERENT ANATOMIC SITES

9. Which one of the following is correct regarding fasciotomies?
   C. All four of the major foot compartments can be decompressed through a single medial approach.
   The foot is considered to have either four or nine compartments (depending on how they are classified), all of which can be decompressed using a single medial incision along the plantar border of the first metatarsal (Fig. 77-4).
   The arm has two compartments (anterior and posterior) that are usually decompressed through medial and lateral incisions (see Fig. 77-6, *Essentials of Plastic Surgery*, second edition). The hand is normally considered to have 10 compartments and is commonly decompressed using two dorsal and two volar incisions. The dorsal incisions are placed over the index and ring metacarpals, while the volar incisions are placed on the ulnar and radial borders of the glabrous palmar skin (see Fig. 77-8, *Essentials of Plastic Surgery*, second edition).
   The anterior and posterior thigh compartments are decompressed using a lateral incision. A separate medial incision is required for decompression of the medial compartment (see Fig. 77-5, *Essentials of Plastic Surgery*, second edition).

The common options for decompression of the four leg compartments include combined medial and lateral incisions or a single lateral approach (see question 7, *Question and Answer* and Fig. 77-4, *Essentials of Plastic Surgery*, second edition).

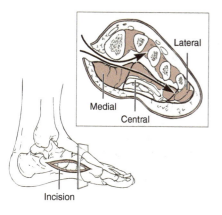

Fig. 77-4 Foot fasciotomy by medial incision. To decompress the four compartments of the foot using a medial approach, an incision is made along the plantar border of the first metatarsal, allowing access to all four compartments. The incision can be extended proximally if the posterior tibial neurovascular bundle requires decompression as well.

REFERENCES

1. McQueen MM, Gaston P, Court-Brown CM. Acute compartment syndrome. Who is at risk? J Bone Joint Surg Br 82:200-203, 2000.
2. McQueen MM, Duckworth AD, Aitken SA, et al. Predictors of compartment syndrome after tibial fracture. J Orthop Trauma. 2015 Apr 9. [Epub ahead of print]
3. Duckworth AD, Mitchell SE, Molyneux SG et al. Acute compartment syndrome of the forearm. J Bone Joint Surg Am 94:e63, 2012.
4. Ulmer T. The clinical diagnosis of compartment syndrome of the lower leg: are clinical findings predictive of the disorder? J Orthop Trauma 16:572-577, 2002.
5. Standards for the management of open fractures of the lower limb. British Orthopaedic Association and British Association of Plastic Reconstructive and Aesthetic Surgeons. London, 2009.

78. Upper Extremity Compression Syndromes

See *Essentials of Plastic Surgery*, second edition, pp. 922-933.

MEDIAN NERVE PATHOLOGY

1. A patient presents with isolated abnormal sensation to the thenar eminence. The forearm and digits are spared. Motor function of the digits and wrist is normal. **Where is the median nerve most likely to be compressed in this case?**
   A. Proximal forearm
   B. Midforearm
   C. Distal forearm
   D. Wrist
   E. Distal end of carpal tunnel

RADIAL NERVE PATHOLOGY

2. *What is the most common site for compression of the radial nerve?*
   A. Proximal to the radial tunnel
   B. The vascular leash of Henry
   C. Proximal margin of ECRB
   D. Arcade of Frohse
   E. Biceps tendon

ULNAR NERVE PATHOLOGY

3. *Which one of the following represents a simple test for ulnar nerve motor function?*
   A. Making a thumb's-up sign
   B. Making an "OK" ring sign
   C. Crossing the middle and ring fingers
   D. Abducting the thumb
   E. Extending the index finger

NERVE COMPRESSION PHYSIOLOGY

4. *Which one of the following is correct regarding nerve compression?*
   A. Axonal damage is always the first sign of a nerve compression injury.
   B. Compressive forces of more than 10 mm Hg are sufficient to impair nerve function.
   C. Symptoms of nerve compression can be caused by adhesions rather than pressure.
   D. Demyelination is an isolated and late sign following chronic nerve compression.
   E. Decreased saltatory conduction is reflected by reduced sensory latency in nerve conduction studies (NCS).

CARPAL TUNNEL SYNDROME

5. **Which one of the following is true regarding carpal tunnel syndrome?**
   A. The prevalence of carpal tunnel syndrome is 1% of the adult population.
   B. Only adults are affected by this compression neuropathy.
   C. Sensory disturbance is limited to the thumb, index, and middle fingers.
   D. When appropriately selected, more than 90% of patients improve after carpal tunnel release.
   E. The main advantage of endoscopic carpal tunnel release is reduced nerve injury risk.

6. An obese 30-year-old office worker presents with symptoms of carpal tunnel syndrome. The NCS shows moderate median nerve compression in the carpal tunnel. His symptoms include discomfort radiating up the forearm. **Which one of the following is correct?**
   A. Use of a wrist splint at night may be effective at reducing his symptoms.
   B. If he frequently uses a computer keyboard, this is likely to be causing his symptoms.
   C. His weight is not a relevant factor in carpal tunnel syndrome.
   D. His forearm discomfort is unlikely to be improved by carpal tunnel release.
   E. If he also had cervical nerve root compression, carpal tunnel release would be contraindicated.

PRONATOR SYNDROME

7. **Which one of the following is true of a patient with pronator syndrome?**
   A. Sensation to the thenar eminence will usually be normal.
   B. Nerve compression is likely due to pronator quadratus at the wrist.
   C. Motor weakness of the digits and wrist will generally be evident.
   D. Paresthesia on resisted FDS contraction is a characteristic finding.
   E. Resolution of symptoms is unlikely after surgical decompression.

ANTERIOR INTEROSSEOUS SYNDROME

8. **What is a typical clinical finding in anterior interosseous syndrome?**
   A. Abnormal sensation to the thenar eminence
   B. Abnormal sensation to the radial digits
   C. Weakness of little finger flexion
   D. Weakness of thumb IPJ flexion
   E. Weakness of thumb abduction

RADIAL NERVE PATHOLOGY

9. A patient has paralysis of the digital and thumb extensors, but some preservation of wrist extension. **What is the most likely cause of his radial nerve palsy?**
   A. Plating of a humeral shaft fracture
   B. Posterior dislocation of the shoulder
   C. Dislocation of the radial head
   D. Plating of a distal radius fracture
   E. An antecubital fossa lipoma

RADIAL TUNNEL SYNDROME

10. A patient is referred with a diagnosis of radial tunnel syndrome. *What is the most likely differential diagnosis or coexisting condition?*
  A. Lateral epicondylitis (tennis elbow)
  B. Medial epicondylitis (golfer's elbow)
  C. Anterior interosseous nerve syndrome
  D. Posterior interosseous nerve syndrome
  E. Wartenberg's syndrome

WARTENBERG'S SYNDROME

11. *What is a typical finding in Wartenberg's syndrome?*
  A. Inability to extend the thumb
  B. Inability to extend the index finger
  C. Abnormal sensation over the dorsum of the fifth metacarpal
  D. Pain over the dorsoradial aspect of the hand
  E. Inability to adduct the little finger

ULNAR NERVE COMPRESSION AT THE ELBOW

12. *When exploring a compressed ulnar nerve at the elbow, which one of the following is least likely to be a site of compression?*
  A. The origin of flexor carpi ulnaris
  B. The roof of the cubital tunnel/Osborne's ligament
  C. The medial intermuscular septum of the arm
  D. Lesions in the floor of the cubital tunnel (e.g., osteophytes)
  E. The vascular leash of Henry

MANAGEMENT OF CUBITAL TUNNEL SYNDROME

13. *Which one of the following is correct regarding the management of cubital tunnel syndrome?*
  A. There is good evidence that a medial epicondylectomy is superior to in situ decompression.
  B. Submuscular nerve transposition produces better outcomes than subcutaneous transposition.
  C. Medial epicondylectomy requires complete resection of the epicondyle to be effective.
  D. Splint therapy is well tolerated and should always be tried before surgery.
  E. Results of surgical decompression are quite unpredictable.

ULNAR NERVE COMPRESSION IN GUYON'S CANAL

14. *Which one of the following is correct regarding ulnar nerve compression in Guyon's canal?*
  A. Ulnar nerve compression here will only produce motor symptoms and signs.
  B. Guyon's canal is divided into two zones according to the branching of the ulnar nerve.
  C. The underlying cause may be an aneurysm of the ulnar artery.
  D. Surgical release requires a different incision to that of a carpal tunnel release.
  E. There is no advantage to imaging if nerve conduction studies clearly show ulnar nerve compression in Guyon's canal.

UPPER LIMB COMPRESSION SYNDROMES

15. For each of the following clinical scenarios, select the most likely diagnosis. (Each option may be used once, more than once, or not at all.)
   A. A patient presents with pain and paresthesia over the dorsoradial aspect of the distal forearm and hand but has no motor symptoms or signs.
   B. A patient presents with weakness and pain during finger and wrist extension but has no discernible sensory deficit.
   C. An elderly patient complains that his little finger sticks out all the time and his grip on his walking stick is weak.

Options:
a. Radial tunnel syndrome
b. Cubital tunnel syndrome
c. Pronator syndrome
d. Ulnar tunnel syndrome
e. Wartenberg's syndrome
f. Posterior interosseous syndrome
g. Anterior interosseous syndrome
h. Carpal tunnel syndrome

Answers

MEDIAN NERVE PATHOLOGY

1. A patient presents with isolated abnormal sensation to the thenar eminence. The forearm and digits are spared. Motor function of the digits and wrist is normal. **Where is the median nerve most likely to be compressed in this case?**

   C. Distal forearm

   This patient has dysfunction of the thenar sensory branch (palmar cutaneous branch) of the median nerve. This arises from the main nerve approximately 5 cm proximal to the wrist and initially runs parallel to the main nerve before passing volarly to the skin. It may be compressed by localized swellings such as hematoma, lipoma, or ganglion cysts. It may also be injured following penetrating trauma to the distal forearm. Further investigation or exploration is warranted in either scenario.

RADIAL NERVE PATHOLOGY

2. *What is the most common site for compression of the radial nerve?*

   D. Arcade of Frohse

   The Arcade of Frohse refers to the proximal edge of the superficial supinator muscle and is the most common site of radial nerve compression. Radial nerve compression is much less common than ulnar or median nerve compression. The radial nerve passes through the radial tunnel which is formed by the radiocapitellar joint bursa, the brachioradialis tendon, the ECRL and the ECRB tendons, and the biceps tendon. There are three other key sites of compression and these are fibrous bands anterior to the radiocapitellar joint (just proximal to the radial tunnel), the vascular leash of Henry (which represents the radial recurrent artery), and the proximal tendon of the ECRB.

ULNAR NERVE PATHOLOGY

3. *Which one of the following represents a simple test for ulnar nerve motor function?*

   C. Crossing the middle and ring fingers

   Ulnar nerve motor palsy is demonstrated by the inability to cross the index and middle fingers or to deviate the extended middle finger ulnarly or radially when the hand is placed on a flat surface. Both of these tests are quick and simple to perform in clinic.

   These clinical findings are because the intrinsic muscles (dorsal and palmar interossei) are paralyzed. In addition, the FDP to the little and ring fingers may be affected, depending on compression/injury level. Making a thumb's-up sign relies on radial nerve innervation of the EPL, EPB, and APL. The "OK" ring sign requires anterior interosseous nerve innervation of the FPL and FDP index finger. Thumb abduction requires innervations of the abductor pollicis by the median nerve. (See Chapter 60, *Essentials of Plastic Surgery*, second edition, for further key examination tests.)

NERVE COMPRESSION PHYSIOLOGY

4. Which one of the following is correct regarding nerve compression?
  C. Symptoms of nerve compression can be caused by adhesions rather than pressure.
  Although external compression is readily considered as a cause of nerve pathology, common symptoms (such as those of carpal or cubital tunnel syndrome) may arise from repeated traction on a nerve. Adhesions may limit nerve excursion, such as around the medial epicondyle during elbow flexion. One study demonstrated that while isolated elbow flexion from 10 to 90 degrees requires only 5 mm of ulnar nerve excursion, combined movements of the shoulder, elbow, and wrist can require up to 22 mm excursion at the cubital tunnel.[1]

  Where this movement is prevented by adhesions, repeated traction insults may lead to the same changes of vascular injury, inflammation and fibrosis with demyelination or axonal degeneration that may occur with recurrent compression. If adhesions are the cause of nerve pathology, it can be difficult to prevent a recurrence.

  Demyelination occurs early in repeatedly compressed nerve segments, whereas axonal damage is a later finding. Compressive forces above 20 mm Hg are considered to be sufficient to impair many aspects of nerve function. Reduced nerve conduction would be reflected by reduced conduction speeds and prolonged latencies on nerve conduction studies.

CARPAL TUNNEL SYNDROME

5. Which one of the following is true regarding carpal tunnel syndrome?
  D. When appropriately selected, more than 90% of patients improve after carpal tunnel release.
  Carpal tunnel syndrome is a compression neuropathy of the median nerve at the wrist within the carpal tunnel. Treatment is commonly with surgical decompression by release of the carpal ligament using an open approach. More than 90% of patients with confirmed carpal tunnel syndrome will have an improvement in their symptoms after adequate median nerve decompression.

  Carpal tunnel syndrome represents the most common upper extremity compression neuropathy and prevalence is estimated to be between 3% and 4%.[2] The condition is not restricted to adults, as children may also develop carpal tunnel syndrome, although much less frequently. The main concern with carpal tunnel syndrome in children is that it presents late, often with bilateral disease and established thenar wasting. It is, however, still treated in the same way as adult carpal tunnel syndrome.

  In addition to altered sensation in the first three digits, the radial border of the ring finger is also commonly affected by sensory changes. As discussed in question 1, the thenar eminence is spared because the palmar cutaneous branch that supplies this area does not pass through the carpal tunnel. The main reported advantages of endoscopic carpal tunnel release are an earlier return to work and reduced scar sensitivity; however, there are higher rates of neurapraxia and recurrent symptoms as a result of incomplete release.

6. An obese 30-year-old office worker presents with symptoms of carpal tunnel syndrome. The NCS shows moderate median nerve compression in the carpal tunnel. His symptoms include discomfort radiating up the forearm. *Which one of the following is correct?*
  A. Use of a wrist splint at night may be effective at reducing his symptoms.
  Neutrally positioned wrist splints can be very effective for relieving symptoms and are usually tolerated best at night. In mild to moderate carpal tunnel syndrome, many patients may choose to avoid surgery after a trial of splint therapy. Splints may also help with symptom management while a patient is waiting for surgery. If splints are helpful but are difficult to tolerate, steroid

injection into the tunnel may be an effective alternative to surgery. Around one-fifth of patients will have a sustained improvement in symptoms after a steroid injection.

The frequency of carpal tunnel syndrome in keyboard workers with variable intensity of use has been reviewed and found to be most common in workers with a low keyboard activity.[3] Obesity is recognized as a common association with carpal tunnel syndrome, along with pregnancy, diabetes, and thyroid disorders.[4]

Although forearm discomfort is not a classic feature of carpal tunnel syndrome, many patients may also experience this. Following carpal tunnel release, many such patients report improvement in their pain symptoms. This is thought to be a result of the "multiple crush phenomenon" in which there are multiple additive insults influencing axonal transport along the length of a nerve.[5] Relieving one factor may sufficiently improve overall nerve function that symptoms relating to other segments of the nerve are also improved. This is not a predictable outcome and patients should not be led to expect an improvement in symptoms which are not directly attributable to compression of the median nerve at the wrist following carpal tunnel release. However, in a patient with coexisting nerve root or thoracic outlet nerve compression and peripheral nerve compression, it is prudent to relieve the peripheral compression in the first instance, since this may give sufficient relief to obviate the need for more complex proximal surgery.

PRONATOR SYNDROME

7. Which one of the following is true of a patient with pronator syndrome?
   D. Paresthesia on resisted FDS contraction is a characteristic finding.

Pronator syndrome is a nerve compression affecting the median nerve in the forearm. It presents with forearm and hand pain, paresthesia, and hypoesthesia including the thenar eminence. It is often worse during resisted FDS contraction. This is because the compression commonly occurs proximally within the forearm at the fibrous arch of FDS. Other key sites of compression include pronator teres (not pronator quadratus, which is deep at the wrist), the ligament of Struthers (ligament between the distal humerus and pronator teres fascia) just proximal to the elbow, and the bicipital aponeurosis (lacertus fibrosus) at the elbow. Compression may also be due to abnormal vasculature in the distal forearm.

Pronator syndrome is predominantly a sensory pathology with no motor weakness usually evident. Occasionally, however, there may be additional signs of weak flexion of the thumb and index finger. Diagnosis is confirmed by history and examination which shows increased tingling on elbow flexion, forearm pronation, resisted FDS contraction, and tapping over the pronator teres. Surgical decompression is usually successful with resolution of symptoms.

ANTERIOR INTEROSSEOUS SYNDROME

8. What is a typical clinical finding in anterior interosseous syndrome?
   D. Weakness of thumb IPJ flexion

The anterior interosseous nerve is a branch of the median nerve that supplies the radial slips of the FDP, FPL, and pronator quadratus. Compression of the nerve is therefore characterized by loss of thumb flexion and index/middle finger DIP joint flexion. Sensation is unaffected. Compression can occur at the tendinous edge of the pronator teres (deep head) or the tendinous origin of the FDS. However, there is also the possibility of other noncompressive causes such as an inflammatory cause (amyotrophy). Diagnosis involves assessment of pinch strength and nerve compression studies are often useful. Surgical decompression with neurolysis is considered by some to be highly effective, but may not always be so. For example, a study reviewing a case series of 16 patients found that resolution of symptoms following decompression was similar to patients who were managed nonoperatively, and the authors suggested that surgery should be restricted to those patients with isolated and complete anterior interosseous motor loss that is persistent at 6 months.[6]

RADIAL NERVE PATHOLOGY

9. A patient has paralysis of the digital and thumb extensors but some preservation of wrist extension. *What is the most likely cause of his radial nerve palsy?*
C. Dislocation of the radial head

The motor branches to the ECRL usually arise before the radial nerve splits around the supinator muscle into the PIN and the superficial radial nerve. Therefore, following an injury or compression at or around the region of the supinator muscle (such as a dislocation of the radial head), there is likely to be preservation of some wrist extension as a result of ECRL function. More proximal injuries to the radial nerve, such as secondary to a humeral shaft fracture or posterior dislocation of the shoulder, would be likely to affect all radial nerve function. Plating of a distal radius fracture should not cause a loss of digital or wrist extension as a result of nerve injury, as the muscles will have been innervated by this level.

RADIAL TUNNEL SYNDROME

10. *A patient is referred with a diagnosis of radial tunnel syndrome. What is the most likely differential diagnosis or coexisting condition?*
A. Lateral epicondylitis (tennis elbow)

Patients with radial tunnel syndrome experience pain in the proximal forearm on movement at the elbow, wrist, or digits similar to tennis elbow, with radiation distally to the dorsum of the hand. There is often tingling of the hand and a secondary weakness of grip due to pain. The pain is typically more distal to that of lateral epicondylitis and is described as being induced by resisted middle finger extension.

Medial epicondylitis or golfer's elbow is similar but affects the ulnar aspect of the forearm. Anterior interosseous syndrome, which was discussed in question 8, is a motor condition with weakness of the FPL and FDP index. Posterior interosseous syndrome is predominantly a motor weakness with difficulty extending the wrist and digits because of nerve compression or traction neuropraxia along the path of the nerve in the forearm. Pain can be a feature but normal sensation is preserved. Wartenberg's syndrome involves pain over the radial aspect of the hand and wrist due to compression of the superficial radial nerve. There is no motor weakness (see question 11).

WARTENBERG'S SYNDROME

11. *What is a typical finding in Wartenberg's syndrome?*
D. Pain over the dorsoradial aspect of the hand

Wartenberg's syndrome is compression of the superficial radial nerve as it emerges from beneath brachioradialis, resulting in pain and paresthesia to the dorsoradial aspect of the hand and wrist. On examination there will usually be a positive Tinel's sign over the superficial radial nerve proximal to the radial styloid. Differential diagnoses include intersection syndrome, which is tenosynovitis caused by friction between the tendons of the first and second extensor compartments (APL and EPB over ECRL and ECRB). Initial treatment includes splinting, activity modification ± steroid injections, and these modalities may be sufficient for most patients. Some patients may go on to benefit from surgical release of the surrounding fascia. Motor function of the index and thumb will be preserved in Wartenberg's syndrome. In contrast, this function will be reduced in posterior interosseous nerve (PIN) compression. The PIN is primarily a motor nerve to the extensor compartment of the forearm with no cutaneous sensory supply. However, patients may complain of unpleasant sensations or pain in the forearm or wrist due to the nociceptive and proprioceptive roles of the PIN. Sensation will be preserved over the fifth MP joint dorsally in either condition, as this is ulnar nerve territory. The inability to adduct the little finger is called Wartenberg's sign and is due to ulnar nerve palsy.

ULNAR NERVE COMPRESSION AT THE ELBOW

12. When exploring a compressed ulnar nerve at the elbow, which one of the following is least likely to be a site of compression?

E. The vascular leash of Henry

The vascular leash of Henry is formed by the radial recurrent artery in the antecubital fossa and is a potential site of radial rather than ulnar nerve compression (see Fig. 78-2, *Essentials of Plastic Surgery*, second edition and see the explanation to question 4).

MANAGEMENT OF CUBITAL TUNNEL SYNDROME

13. Which one of the following is correct regarding the management of cubital tunnel syndrome?

E. Results of surgical decompression are quite unpredictable.

The results of ulnar nerve decompression at the elbow are less predictable than those following median nerve decompression at the wrist. There is considerable debate regarding the optimal surgical intervention, with many preferring to perform a simple in situ decompression in the first instance and reserve transposition procedures for recurrent cases. Others are strongly in favor of medial epicondylectomy as the primary surgical procedure. Where epicondylectomy is preferred, a partial bony resection is undertaken, rather than complete resection of the epicondyle, to reduce the risk of valgus instability of the elbow following surgery. Although some patients find splinting of the elbow helpful, this prevents elbow flexion and interferes with activities and is therefore less well tolerated than splinting in carpal tunnel syndrome. In severe ulnar nerve compression, splinting has not been shown to be beneficial, and surgery should not be delayed by a trial of conservative therapy.

ULNAR NERVE COMPRESSION IN GUYON'S CANAL

14. Which one of the following is correct regarding ulnar nerve compression in Guyon's canal?

C. The underlying cause may be an aneurysm of the ulnar artery.

One of the recognized causes of ulnar nerve compression in Guyon's canal is an aneurysm of the ulnar artery, as it can occur in carpenters as a result of repetitive motion (hypothenar hammer syndrome). This is discussed in Chapter 82. However, there are many causes of ulnar tunnel syndrome, including a ganglion, lipoma, fracture of the hook of hamate, and synovial inflammation. Thus plain radiographs, ultrasound with or without Doppler imaging, and even CT/MRI are important to determine the specific cause before surgery, as the management may involve more than a simple decompression. If there is an aneurysm, the involved segment of the artery will be resected and replaced with a vein graft, so the patient must be warned about a donor site scar and the possibility of ischemic complications.

Guyon's canal can be readily decompressed at the same time as a carpal tunnel release through the same incision. Alternatively, a more ulnar incision can be used but does not have to be.

Ulnar nerve compression in Guyon's canal may present with mixed or isolated motor or sensory signs due to the branching pattern of the nerve at this site (see Fig. 78-5, *Essentials of Plastic Surgery*, second edition). In zone I, the ulnar nerve has not yet bifurcated and there will be motor and sensory disturbance. In zone II, the deep motor branch is affected in isolation. In zone III, only the superficial sensory branch to the hypothenar skin and ulnar one and a half digits are affected. Zone III compression is the least common (see Fig. 78-5, *Essentials of Plastic Surgery*, second edition).

UPPER LIMB COMPRESSION SYNDROMES

15. For the following scenarios, the best options are as follows:
   A. **A patient presents with pain and paresthesia over the dorsoradial aspect of the distal forearm and hand but has no motor symptoms or signs.**
      e. **Wartenberg's syndrome**
      In this scenario, the findings are in keeping with superficial radial nerve compression, such as in Wartenberg's syndrome (see the explanation to question 11).
   B. **A patient presents with weakness and pain during finger and wrist extension but has no discernible sensory deficit.**
      f. **Posterior interosseous syndrome**
      In this scenario, the patient has the specific motor signs of a posterior interosseous nerve palsy. The posterior interosseous nerve is a continuation of the radial nerve in the forearm and supplies the extensor muscles to the wrist and digits. It may be injured during trauma such as a deep laceration or radial head dislocation. It may be caused by traction neuritis or inflammation because of rheumatoid arthritis. It can occur in muscular young men because of external compression from muscle bulk or can be a result of another soft tissue mass such as a lipoma. Investigations should include plain films and soft tissue imaging with MRI or ultrasound. Treatment may be nonoperative or operative, depending on the cause.
   C. **An elderly patient complains that his little finger sticks out all the time and his grip on his walking stick is weak.**
      b. **Cubital tunnel syndrome**
      In this scenario, the patient is exhibiting Wartenberg's sign, which has nothing to do with Wartenberg's syndrome. Wartenberg's sign is abduction of the little finger caused by intrinsic muscle weakness that leaves the abducting force of the EDM unopposed. The weak grip is also in keeping with ulnar nerve palsy; the most common cause would be cubital tunnel syndrome.

REFERENCES

1. Wright TW, Glowczewskie F Jr, Cowin D, et al. Ulnar nerve excursion and strain at the elbow and wrist associated with upper extremity motion. J Hand Surg Am 26:655-662, 2001.
2. Papanicolaou GD, McCabe SJ, Firrell J. The prevalence and characteristics of nerve compression symptoms in the general population. J Hand Surg Am 26:460, 2001.
3. Atroshi I, Gummesson C, Ornstein E, et al. Carpal tunnel syndrome and keyboard use at work: a population-based study. Arthritis Rheum 56:3620-3625, 2007.
4. Dellon AL. Patient evaluation and management considerations in nerve compression. Hand Clin 8:229-239, 1992.
5. Upton AR, McComas AJ. The double crush in nerve entrapment syndromes. Lancet 1973 2(7825):359-362, 1973.
6. Sood MK, Burke FD. Anterior interosseous nerve palsy. A review of 16 cases. J Hand Surg Br 22:64-68, 1997.

79. Brachial Plexus

See *Essentials of Plastic Surgery*, second edition, pp. 934-950.

BRACHIAL PLEXUS ANATOMY

1. Which one of the following statements is correct?
    A. The roots of the brachial plexus are C5-T1 and are found between the middle and posterior scalene muscles.
    B. The three trunks are upper, middle, and lower and are found in the anterior triangle of the neck.
    C. The cords are named according to their position in relation to the axillary vein (lateral, posterior, and anterior).
    D. The lateral cord contains contributions from C5, C6, and C7 and is the only cord forming the musculocutaneous/myocutaneous nerve.
    E. The medial cord contains contributions from C7, C8, and T1 and is the only cord forming the median nerve.

PERIPHERAL NERVE BRANCHES FROM THE BRACHIAL PLEXUS

2. For each of the following descriptions, select the correct nerve from the options listed. (Each option may be used once, more than once, or not at all.)
    A. This nerve arises from the C5 nerve root and supplies the rhomboids.
    B. This nerve is the first branch arising from the posterior cord.
    C. This nerve arises from the trunks of the plexus and supplies the infraspinatus muscle.

    Options:
    a. Suprascapular
    b. Long thoracic
    c. Dorsal scapular
    d. Upper subscapular
    e. Lower subscapular
    f. Nerve to subclavius

ERB'S POINT

3. Which one of the following is most suggestive of a brachial plexus injury at Erb's point?
    A. Weakness of the small muscles of the hand
    B. Horner's syndrome in association with upper limb weakness
    C. Loss of elbow and wrist extension
    D. Loss of elbow flexion and shoulder external rotation
    E. Arm weakness following forced elevation with traction

THE MEDIAL CORD

4. Which one of the following movements most specifically tests medial cord function?
    A. Elbow flexion
    B. Wrist flexion
    C. Little finger abduction
    D. Thumb abduction
    E. Forearm pronation

NERVE ROOT INJURIES

5. Which one of the following statements is correct?
A. A root avulsion is a postganglionic injury.
B. Intact paracervical muscles suggests a preganglionic injury.
C. A C5-6 avulsion may result in Horner's syndrome.
D. It is easier to repair a preganglionic than postganglionic injury.
E. Wallerian degeneration does not occur in a preganglionic injury.

BRACHIAL PLEXUS BIRTH PALSY

6. Which one of the following statements is correct regarding brachial plexus birth injury?
A. The Western incidence in the United States is 1 per 100,000 term births.
B. Most cases present with lower nerve root (C8-T1) injuries (Klumpke's palsy).
C. Shoulder dystocia is one of the most common risk factors.
D. Spontaneous recovery is rare following these injuries.
E. Exploration is recommended if no biceps function is observed by 1 month.

MECHANISM OF INJURY IN BRACHIAL PLEXUS

7. Which one of the following statements is correct?
A. Traumatic brachial plexus injuries are most often caused by deep lacerations or crush injuries.
B. Open injuries are less common than closed but are often associated with vascular injury.
C. A violent shoulder abduction greater than 90 degrees is likely to cause injury to C6-7.
D. Violent lateral neck flexion and shoulder depression most commonly leads to weakness of the FCU and the intrinsic hand muscles.
E. Open injuries represent a contraindication to immediate repair because of the risk of infection.

ASSESSING BRACHIAL PLEXUS INJURIES

8. When examining a patient with a suspected brachial plexus injury, which one of the following is correct?
A. Weak digital flexion and extension suggests a T1 nerve root lesion.
B. Weak rhomboids and serratus anterior suggest injury distal to the upper trunk.
C. Examining pectoralis major contraction assesses both the posterior and lateral cords.
D. A fractured clavicle makes a proximal trunk injury more likely than cord or branch injury.
E. Paralysis of the latissimus dorsi may indicate a posterior cord injury.

GRADING MUSCLE POWER

9. You assess a patient who has sustained an upper trunk brachial plexus injury. On examination he is able to flex the elbow horizontally when resting on a table but is unable to elevate his forearm off the table during flexion. What is the British Medical Research Council grade for the biceps in this patient?
A. 1
B. 2
C. 3
D. 4
E. 5

ELECTROPHYSIOLOGIC TESTING

10. Several electrophysiologic tests may be helpful in the care of brachial plexus injuries. **Which one of the following statements is correct?**
    A. Although intraoperative nerve testing is possible, it is not necessary if direct visualization and palpation of the nerves is undertaken.
    B. Somatosensory evoked potentials are detected through the scalp and help to rule out preganglionic injury.
    C. Motor evoked potentials are detected through the paraspinous muscles and help to rule out postganglionic injury.
    D. Electromyography is useful within the first 3 weeks to give a baseline assessment of function.
    E. The combined presence of sensory nerve action potentials (SNAPs), normal peripheral sensory conduction velocity, and paralyzed muscles implies a postganglionic injury.

ORDER OF RECONSTRUCTION

11. *When managing a patient with a brachial plexus injury, which one of the following is usually the first priority?*
    A. Shoulder abduction
    B. Wrist flexion
    C. Elbow flexion
    D. Wrist extension
    E. Finger flexion

TREATMENT OPTIONS FOLLOWING BRACHIAL PLEXUS INJURY

12. *For each of the following scenarios, select the most appropriate option from the list. (Each option may be used once, more than once, or not at all.)*
    A. An otherwise healthy newborn baby is brought to your clinic with the classic signs of an upper trunk Erb-Duchenne palsy. The parents want an early intervention.
    B. A 27-year-old man presents with no recovery clinically or on EMG studies 6 months after a C5-7 injury that includes serratus anterior and rhomboid weakness from a motorcycle accident. You plan to restore elbow flexion as the first priority.
    C. A 60-year-old woman presents 10 years after a complete brachial plexus injury from a horseback riding accident. She is well known to the pain team and is struggling with her shoulder brace and with discomfort attributed to the weight of the arm.

    Options:
    a. Observation for a further 2 months
    b. Observation for a further 6 months
    c. Immediate exploration and repair
    d. Nerve transfer
    e. Nerve grafting
    f. Neurotization
    g. Joint fusion
    h. Insert plexus catheter for local anesthetic infusion
    i. Amputation

NERVE TRANSFERS

13. Which one of the following is the preferred choice for restoring shoulder stability in brachial plexus palsy?
A. Spinal accessory nerve onto suprascapular nerve
B. Intercostal nerves onto suprascapular nerve
C. Thoracodorsal nerve onto axillary nerve
D. Medial pectoral nerve onto axillary nerve
E. Thoracodorsal nerve onto long thoracic nerve

MANAGING THE SHOULDER IN BRACHIAL PLEXUS INJURIES

14. Which one of the following is correct regarding the management of brachial plexus birth injuries?
A. Botulinum toxin injections to rotator cuff contractures may be useful.
B. Plain radiographs are important to monitor deformity of the glenohumeral joint.
C. Spinal accessory to suprascapular nerve transfer is contraindicated.
D. The Waters' classification relates to the degree of plexus injury.
E. Shoulder capsular release should be avoided in obstetric brachial plexus injury.

Answers

BRACHIAL PLEXUS ANATOMY
1. **Which one of the following statements is correct?**
   D. The lateral cord contains contributions from C5, C6, and C7 and is the only cord forming the musculocutaneous/myocutaneous nerve.
   The musculocutaneous nerve is also known as the myocutaneous nerve which supplies the biceps, coracobrachialis, and brachialis muscles. It also supplies sensation to the upper limb through the lateral cutaneous nerves of the arm and forearm, respectively.
   The brachial plexus comprises roots, trunks, divisions, cords, and terminal branches, and typically arises from C5-T1, but may be supplemented by significant contributions from C4 or T2 nerve roots. The roots pass between the anterior and middle scalene muscles (not the middle and posterior) and split into trunks as follows: C5-6 become the upper trunk, C7 the middle trunk, and C8-T1 the lower trunk. The three trunks lie in the posterior triangle of the neck and each split into anterior and posterior divisions. The upper and middle trunk anterior divisions form the lateral cord, while the lower trunk anterior division forms the medial cord. All three posterior divisions combine to form the posterior cord. The cords are named in relation to the axillary artery, not the vein. The lateral and medical cords subsequently rejoin to form the median nerve. The medial cord is formed by the C8 and T1 roots only, and although it is a significant contributor to the median nerve, this nerve also receives a major contribution from the lateral cord (C5-7).

PERIPHERAL NERVE BRANCHES FROM THE BRACHIAL PLEXUS
2. **For the following descriptions, the best options are as follows:**
   A. This nerve arises from the C5 nerve root and supplies the rhomboids.
   c. Dorsal scapular
   B. This nerve is the first branch arising from the posterior cord.
   d. Upper subscapular
   C. This nerve arises from the trunks of the plexus and supplies the infraspinatus muscle.
   a. Suprascapular
   Knowledge of the branches of the brachial plexus is important. There are two nerves arising from the roots. These are the long thoracic and dorsal scapular nerves, which innervate the serratus anterior and rhomboids/levator scapulae, respectively. There are two nerves arising from the trunks: the suprascapular nerve and nerve to subclavius, which innervate the supraspinatus/infraspinatus and subclavius muscles, respectively. There are no nerve branches that arise directly from the divisions of the brachial plexus.

ERB'S POINT
3. **Which one of the following is most suggestive of a brachial plexus injury at Erb's point?**
   D. Loss of elbow fixation and shoulder external rotation
   Erb's point represents the anatomic site where the C5 and C6 nerve roots converge to form the upper trunk and is also the point where the suprascapular nerve arises. Injury at this level typically produces loss of shoulder abduction and external rotation, along with loss of elbow flexion. The classic appearance of an Erb's palsy reflects this, i.e., the arm hangs with the shoulder internally

rotated and the elbow extended. This is sometimes termed a "waiter's tip deformity" and may also include more prominent loss of wrist extension when there is an associated C7 injury. The upper trunk ± C7 pattern of injury is the most common overall and occurs in both obstetric and adult traumatic plexus injury. Weakness of the small muscles of the hand and upper eyelid ptosis with constriction of the pupil are features of lower nerve root injury with damage to the stellate ganglion (C8-T1). This pattern of injury is more typical of the scenario in option E. Elbow and wrist extension are predominantly C7 functions.

THE MEDIAL CORD

4. Which one of the following movements most specifically tests medial cord function?

C. Little finger abduction

The medial cord contributes to the median nerve along with the lateral cord, but it is the only cord contributing to the ulnar nerve, therefore assessing movement in an ulnar innervated muscle such as the abductor digit minimi will test the medial cord most reliably. Elbow flexion is provided predominantly by the biceps and brachialis, with initiation assisted by brachioradialis. These muscles are innervated by the musculocutaneous and radial nerves, respectively. Therefore there is medial and posterior cord involvement with this action. Wrist flexion is provided by the FCU and the FCR which are innervated by the median and ulnar nerves, respectively. It will therefore not usually discriminate between the medial and lateral cords. Thumb abduction is median nerve innervated through the abductor pollicis brevis, as is forearm pronation, which is provided by the pronator quadratus and teres.

NERVE ROOT INJURIES

5. Which one of the following statements is correct?

E. Wallerian degeneration does not occur in a preganglionic injury.

In a preganglionic injury the cell bodies in the dorsal root ganglia are still in continuity with the axons, therefore there is no Wallerian degeneration. This is why somatosensory evoked potentials are preserved. Root avulsions are preganglionic injuries and may be accompanied by signs of proximal injury such as paracervical muscle paralysis or Horner's syndrome (C8 or T1 avulsion affecting sympathetic supply). Preganglionic injuries are not amenable to direct repair or grafting.

BRACHIAL PLEXUS BIRTH PALSY

6. Which one of the following statements is correct regarding brachial plexus birth injury?

C. Shoulder dystocia is one of the most common risk factors.

The U.S. incidence of obstetric brachial plexus injury is reported as 1.5 per 1000 live births, and the most common presentation is Erb-Duchenne palsy with C5-6 upper root pathology. The mechanism of injury is commonly shoulder dystocia, in which the fetus becomes stuck and the advancing head is forced into lateral flexion away from the shoulder (which is restrained at the pelvic inlet). Other common associations include breech birth, forceps delivery, and vacuum extraction. Gestational diabetes and macrosomia are also risk factors. Spontaneous recovery is common, and in some studies 50% have achieved a full recovery by 6 months and the remainder made a partial recovery. Exploration should be considered after 3 months if biceps and deltoid functions are still absent.[1,2,3]

MECHANISM OF INJURY IN BRACHIAL PLEXUS

7. Which one of the following statements is correct?
   B. Open injuries are less common than closed but are often associated with vascular injury.
   Brachial plexus injuries are most commonly closed injuries resulting from excessive traction, but these may also occur with open injuries such as gunshot or stab wounds. Violent shoulder abduction is most likely to cause a lower or complete plexus injury. Violent downward shoulder traction with lateral neck flexion will tend to cause an upper plexus injury and would usually spare the FCU and intrinsic muscle innervation.
   Although less common, open injuries are the strongest indication for immediate exploration and repair. The likelihood of an associated vessel injury is high, particularly with sharp penetrating wounds. These wounds should be formally explored, with assessment and repair of the plexus and other key structures. Only in heavily contaminated or infected wounds or gunshot injuries is delayed repair usually indicated. The argument for delayed repair of the plexus after debridement of gunshot injuries is that there is often a complex multilevel injury with profound tissue edema in an extensive zone of injury, therefore a delay allows edema and neurapraxia to settle and for multiple sites of nerve injury to appear more obvious on inspection and intraoperative neurophysiological testing.

ASSESSING BRACHIAL PLEXUS INJURIES

8. When examining a patient with a suspected brachial plexus injury, which one of the following is correct?
   E. Paralysis of the latissimus dorsi may indicate a posterior cord injury.
   The latissimus dorsi is supplied by the posterior cord, along with the deltoid, subscapularis, teres major, and all the muscles innervated by the radial nerve. A T1 lesion will usually produce weak intrinsic muscle function in the hand and a sensory deficit affecting the medial forearm. Digital flexion and extension may be affected if C8 is also injured. As discussed in question 2, the rhomboid muscles are supplied by the dorsal scapular nerve, which arises early from the C5 nerve root prior to formation of the upper trunk. The nerve to serratus anterior (long thoracic nerve of Bell) arises from the C5-7 nerve roots. Paralysis of these muscles is indicative of a root-level injury, because they would be preserved if the injury occurred at trunk level or distally.
   The pectoralis major is supplied by the medial and lateral pectoral nerves, from the medial and lateral cords of the plexus, respectively, and not by the posterior cord. A fractured clavicle in association with neurologic disturbance is usually associated with injuries to the divisions, cords, or branches that lie near to this bone.

GRADING MUSCLE POWER

9. You assess a patient who has sustained an upper trunk brachial plexus injury. On examination he is able to flex the elbow horizontally when resting on a table but is unable to elevate his forearm off the table during flexion. ***What is the British Medical Research Council grade for the biceps in this patient?***
   B. 2
   The British Medical Research Council grade has five categories (Table 79-1). Because this patient is unable to flex the arm against gravity they have an MRC power grading of 2. This is one of the important classification systems to remember, especially with respect to brachial plexus

assessment. The MRC grade can be used to document changes in function following injury and treatment.

Table 79-1 *British Medical Research Council Grading System*

Grade	Degree of Strength
1	Muscle contracts, but part does not move
2	Movement with gravity eliminated
3	Movement through full range of motion against gravity
4	Movement through full range of motion against resistance
5	Normal strength

ELECTROPHYSIOLOGIC TESTING

10. Several electrophysiologic tests may be helpful in the care of brachial plexus injuries. **Which one of the following statements is correct?**

B. Somatosensory evoked potentials are detected through the scalp and help to rule out preganglionic injury.

Intraoperative nerve testing is an important adjunct to inspection and palpation of the plexus, as it can be difficult to come to an accurate diagnosis; for example, in recovering injuries, neuroma in continuity, and in distinguishing preganglionic and postganglionic injuries. Somatosensory and motor evoked potentials (SSEP and MEPs) can be used intraoperatively to determine preganglionic and postganglionic injury. Both SSEP and MEP are detected through the contralateral scalp and their presence rules out preganglionic injury. Not all surgeons use these tests, but most would use a nerve stimulator in combination with clinical inspection and palpation for "empty" or "hard" segments of nerve. A stimulator is also helpful in assessing potential donor nerves for transfer, such as the phrenic and accessory nerves. The muscular changes associated with denervation take a few weeks to develop, 3 to 6 weeks is usually allowed before initial EMG testing.

ORDER OF RECONSTRUCTION

11. When managing a patient with a brachial plexus injury, which one of the following is usually the first priority?

C. Elbow flexion

The first priority in managing a patient with a brachial plexus palsy is to achieve elbow flexion so that hand-to-mouth transfer is possible. Achieving shoulder stability is the next most important priority, since this will support proper elbow function. Once these areas have been addressed, wrist extension and finger flexion can be considered.

TREATMENT OPTIONS FOLLOWING BRACHIAL PLEXUS INJURY

12. For the following scenarios, the best options are as follows:
    A. **An otherwise healthy newborn baby is brought to your clinic with the classic signs of an upper trunk Erb-Duchenne palsy. The parents want an early intervention.**
       a. **Observation for a further 2 months**
          In this scenario, it is appropriate to start with observation, since most obstetric brachial plexus palsies will improve without surgery. Active range of movement scores at 3 months can serve as a useful predictor of which patients might benefit from surgery. The parents should be taught by a physiotherapist to maintain passive joint range of motion while awaiting recovery. Regular follow-up will help to ensure that passive joint ranges are maintained and that signs of recovery are picked up. If there is no sign of deltoid and biceps recovery by the 3-month visit, then intervention is usually warranted.
    B. **A 27-year-old man presents with no recovery clinically or on EMG studies 6 months after a C5-7 injury that includes serratus anterior and rhomboid weakness from a motorcycle accident. You plan to restore elbow flexion as the first priority.**
       d. **Nerve transfer**
          In this scenario, the findings are in keeping with a root injury due to the involvement of the rhomboid and serratus anterior muscles. At 6 months there is still a window of opportunity to reinnervate some of the shoulder girdle and elbow flexors before permanent loss of motor endplates occurs. In a C5-7 palsy, a nerve transfer is a good option, and the favored donor for elbow flexion is a motor branch to FCU from the ulnar nerve transferred to branches of the musculocutaneous (myocutaneous) nerve. An alternative is to transfer two or three intercostal nerves to the musculocutaneous nerve, although achieving sufficient length to transfer without nerve grafts can be challenging.[4]
    C. **A 60-year-old woman presents 10 years after a complete brachial plexus injury from a horseback riding accident. She is well known to the pain team and is struggling with her shoulder brace and with discomfort attributed to the weight of the arm.**
       g. **Joint fusion**
          In this scenario, there will be established instability at the shoulder. A shoulder fusion may ameliorate some of this patient's symptoms by better supporting the weight of the limb, but this may cause other difficulties as a result of the fixed position of the joint. If the patient has some scapula control, this may actually allow a degree of active limb positioning. Amputation is occasionally indicated, but it is important to recognize that it may not resolve her pain. Local anesthetic catheters can help some patients with chronic pain after plexus injuries, but this should be a joint undertaking with the pain team and will not necessarily alter the heavy dragging sensation from the weight of the arm.

NERVE TRANSFERS

13. **Which one of the following is the preferred choice for restoring shoulder stability in brachial plexus palsy?**
    A. **Spinal accessory nerve onto suprascapular nerve**
       While all of the above transfers are used in various scenarios by different surgeons, the dominant first choice transfer to stabilize the shoulder is the SAN to SSN transfer. It can be readily performed at the time of plexus exploration through the same approach, or it can be performed through a posterior approach. In addition to shoulder stability, this transfer tries to restore some abduction and external rotation and can be supplemented by additional transfers, such as the triceps branch of the radial nerve onto the axillary nerve.

MANAGING THE SHOULDER IN BRACHIAL PLEXUS INJURIES

14. *Which one of the following is correct regarding the shoulder in brachial plexus birth palsy injuries?*

A. Botulinum toxin injections to rotator cuff contractures may be useful.

Infants with BPBP may develop shoulder weakness, contracture, or joint deformity. Internal rotation contractures are common and caused by weakness of the infraspinatus and teres minor muscles leading to unopposed internal rotation forces. Treatment options for the shoulder include contracture release, muscle rebalancing through transfers, such as latissimus dorsi transfer. Formal joint reduction may be required in dislocations, but thankfully this scenario is uncommon.

Botulinum toxin injections are commonly used to treat a range of pediatric spasticity problems, and these are thought to be helpful by some surgeons as part of the management of rotator cuff contractures. Daily physiotherapy should be undertaken by parents to prevent shoulder contractures developing in the first place and to avoid secondary deformity of the growing glenoid fossa and humeral head. They are given as a standard treatment in nonsurgical and surgical care of these patients, but are particularly important to maintain the benefits following tendon lengthening/transfer procedures or capsular release.

BPAP patients also have glenohumeral joint dysplasia and this is assessed using the Waters' classification which grades the degree of abnormality at the glenohumeral joint. Plain radiographs are not particularly helpful in young children, because there is a large cartilaginous component to the immature glenohumeral joint that is better assessed by a skilled ultrasonographer or MRI/CT.[5]

If the trapezius, the rhomboids, and the serratus anterior are functioning, there can be good movement of the scapula, which can allow some compensation for poor shoulder movement. Subscapularis lengthening and greenstick fracture of the coronoid process can sometimes be helpful in the management of obstetric brachial plexus palsy when a severe internal rotation joint contracture is present. This may be in combination with a limited capsular release; however, care must be taken not to destabilize the glenohumeral joint. The spinal accessory nerve is a useful donor for transfer in both adults and children.

REFERENCES

1. Waters PM. Pediatric brachial plexus palsy. In Wolfe SW, Hotchkiss RN, Pederson WC, et al, eds. Green's Operative Hand Surgery, ed 6. Philadelphia: Elsevier, 2010.
2. Shenaq SM, Kim JY, Armenta AH, et al. The surgical treatment of obstetric brachial plexus palsy. Plast Reconstr Surg 113:54E-67E, 2004.
3. Hale HB, Bae DS, Waters PM. Current concepts in the management of brachial plexus birth palsy. J Hand Surg Am 35: 322-331, 2010.
4. Merrell GA, Barrie KA, Katz DL, et al. Results of nerve transfer techniques for restoration of shoulder and elbow function in the context of a meta-analysis of the English literature. J Hand Surg Am 26:303-314, 2001.
5. Pearl ML. Shoulder problems in children with brachial plexus birth palsy: evaluation and management. J Am Acad Orthop Surg 17:242-254, 2009.

80. Nerve Injuries

See *Essentials of Plastic Surgery*, second edition, pp. 951-963.

NERVE ANATOMY

1. **Which one of the following directly surrounds the axons within a peripheral nerve?**
   - A. Schwann cell
   - B. Perineurium
   - C. Epineurium
   - D. Mesoneurium
   - E. Endoneurium

ABERRANT NERVE ANATOMY

2. **Which one of the following anatomic abnormalities could account for the ability to abduct some of the fingers, despite complete median and ulnar nerve transection at the wrist?**
   - A. Martin-Gruber anastomosis
   - B. Riche-Cannieu anastomosis
   - C. Froment-Rauber anastomosis
   - D. Berretini connection
   - E. Double crush phenomenom

NERVE INJURY

3. **After a peripheral nerve has been divided, which one of the following processes is responsible for guiding the regenerating axon to the correct distal nerve stump?**
   - A. Chromatolysis
   - B. Neurotropism
   - C. Wallerian degeneration
   - D. Neurotrophism
   - E. Axonal sprouting

MUSCLE DENERVATION

4. **Following complete transection of the ulnar nerve at the elbow, which one of the following is true with regard to muscle denervation?**
   - A. The denervated forearm and intrinsic muscles require 75% of their motor end plates to retain function.
   - B. Following direct repair, the ulnar nerve should regenerate at a rate of 3 mm/day.
   - C. If the intrinsics are not reinnervated within 6 months, they are unlikely to regain normal function.
   - D. Outcome of muscle reinnervation after ulnar nerve repair is consistent across different age groups.
   - E. Optimal hand function should be achieved when the forearm muscles are reinnervated within 3 months of injury.

CLASSIFICATION OF NERVE INJURIES

5. **What is the main clinical relevance of the Sunderland classification of nerve injury?**
   A. It describes the injury mechanism.
   B. It describes the chronicity of injury.
   C. It describes outcomes according to age.
   D. It dictates surgical management.
   E. It provides prognostic information.

DIAGNOSIS OF ABNORMAL SENSATION

6. **When assessing a patient in clinic for two-point sensory discrimination to the fingertip, which one of the following is true?**
   A. 6 mm represents a normal static two-point discrimination.
   B. 8 mm represents a normal dynamic two-point discrimination.
   C. Semmes-Weinstein monofilaments should be used for the test.
   D. It is important to cross over the digit during each test.
   E. This assessment forms part of a standard nerve conduction test.

PRIMARY NERVE REPAIR

7. **You are repairing a sharply divided digital nerve 1 week after injury. Which one of the following is correct?**
   A. A direct repair should still be possible at this stage.
   B. Fascicular repair will give a superior result to epineurial repair.
   C. An 8 mm deficit is better repaired directly in flexion than with a nerve graft.
   D. Trimming the nerve ends should be avoided to preserve length.
   E. There is no need to apply a splint after digital nerve repair.

MANAGING A NERVE GAP

8. You have a patient with a 4 cm gap in the ulnar nerve above the elbow following debridement of a gunshot injury 1 week ago. **Which one of the following is correct?**
   A. Anterior transposition of the nerve to gain length is contraindicated.
   B. One sural nerve would provide sufficient cable grafts for this defect.
   C. This is a good indication for a vascularized nerve transfer.
   D. Neurotization will give as good a functional outcome as grafting.
   E. This defect is too small to justify using a synthetic conduit.

OPTIONS FOR SURGICAL REPAIR

9. *For each of the following clinical scenarios, select the most appropriate nerve repair technique from the options listed. (Each option may be used once, more than once, or not at all.)*
   A. Repair of a complete transverse division of a digital nerve sustained with a motorized cutting disc
   B. Repair of a complete transverse ulnar nerve transection (junction of the mid and distal thirds of the forearm) sustained during a fall onto broken glass
   C. Repair of the radial nerve at midhumeral level 2 weeks after debridement of necrotizing fasciitis that has left a 6 cm nerve gap

   Options:
   a. Direct perineural repair
   b. Direct epineural repair
   c. Direct group fascicular repair
   d. Mobilization and direct epineural repair
   e. Nerve grafting with lateral antebrachial cutaneous nerve
   f. Nerve grafting with posterior interosseous nerve
   g. Nerve grafting with sural nerve

OUTCOMES FOLLOWING NERVE INJURY

10. *Which one of the following is correct regarding the outcome following nerve injury?*
    A. Peripheral and central nerve injury outcomes are broadly similar.
    B. Median nerve repairs tend to gain superior results to that of the ulnar nerve.
    C. Excision of a neuroma is best carried out early, about 6 weeks after repair.
    D. Interpositional autologous vein grafts give good results in motor nerve repair.
    E. After an initial delay, nerve recovery occurs at approximately 2 inches per month.

11. *When assessing for motor and sensory nerve recovery following injury, what grading represents a return to normal function?*
    A. M0, S0
    B. M3, S3
    C. M4, S4
    D. M5, S5
    E. M5, S4

Answers

NERVE ANATOMY

1. **Which one of the following directly surrounds the axons within a peripheral nerve?**
   E. Endoneurium

   The structure of a peripheral is shown in Fig. 80-1. The basic structure of a nerve comprises a series of axons which are grouped together to form fascicles. Groups of fascicles together form a complete nerve. The axons are covered by a loose gelatinous collagen matrix called endoneurium. This has minimal tensile strength. Schwann cells surround individual myelinated axons in many peripheral nerves and help insulate the nerve and increase conduction speed. Groups of axons arranged into fascicles are collectively surrounded by perineurium. This is a connective tissue layer with selective permeability that is thin but dense with high tensile strength. The bundles of fascicles are covered by epineurium which represents the outer layer of the nerve. This contains collagen and elastin fibers and is surrounded by a thin loose areolar tissue called mesoneurium. Nerve repair is most commonly performed by suturing the epineurium to reconstitute complete external nerve continuity (an epineural repair). In some cases, grouped fascicular repair is performed instead. In this case, sutures are placed in the perineurium. When nerve injury occurs, a predictable set of processes are initiated. These are described in Fig. 80-2.

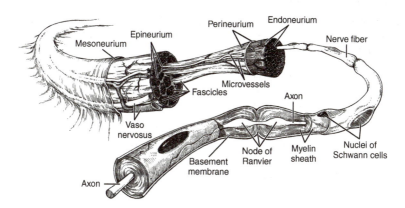

Fig. 80-1 Nerve anatomy. Nerves are formed from multiple axons running in parallel. Axons are grouped together in bundles to form fascicles. Multiple fascicles collectively form the nerve.

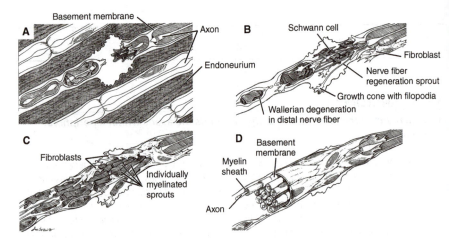

Fig. 80-2 Nerve regeneration. **A,** When a myelinated axon is injured, degeneration occurs distally and for a variable distance proximally. **B,** Multiple regenerating fibers sprout from the proximal axon, forming a regenerating unit. A growth cone at the tip of each regenerating fiber samples the environment and advances the growth process distally. **C,** Schwann cells eventually myelinate the regenerating fibers. **D,** Because it is from a single nerve fiber, a regenerating unit that contains several fibers is formed, and each fiber is capable of functional connections.

ABERRANT NERVE ANATOMY

2. Which one of the following anatomic abnormalities could account for the ability to abduct some of the fingers, despite complete median and ulnar nerve transection at the wrist?
   C. Froment-Rauber anastomosis

   The Froment-Rauber anastomosis is a rare condition in which there is a connection between the posterior interosseous nerve (or superficial radial nerve) and the ulnar nerve motor branches innervating the dorsal interossei. This could explain why a patient could still have residual finger abduction following median and ulnar nerve division. According to Guo et al,[1] Froment[2] first described the distal continuation of the PIN, and Rauber[3] later reported a similar finding. Spinner[4] subsequently referred to this anomalous connection as the Froment-Rauber nerve.

   The Riche-Cannieu and Martin-Gruber anastomoses involve motor connections between the ulnar and median nerves and could mask injury when one but not both nerves is divided. The Berretini connection is a sensory connection between the ulnar and median nerves, so it would not affect ulnar motor nerve function.

   Double crush phenomenon refers to an anatomic arrangement where nerve entrapment at one location can predispose an individual to symptoms of clinical nerve compression at another site along that nerve with only minimal compression required to produce symptoms. An example is ulnar nerve compression at the elbow which may give symptoms at the wrist in Guyon's canal, despite minimal compression at the distal site. In such cases, patients often benefit from decompression of the most simple site to treat in the first instance, followed by review of symptoms. Treatment may no longer be required at the other sites of compression, as overall nerve function is often improved and the other sites become asymptomatic (see Chapter 78).

NERVE INJURY

3. After a peripheral nerve has been divided, which one of the following processes is responsible for guiding the regenerating axon to the correct distal nerve stump?

B. Neurotropism

Neurotropism is a process where a chemotactic gradient attracts a regenerating axon toward the correct end target at the distal nerve stump. Initially around half of axonal sprouts will make an incorrect connection and this is subsequently modified such that correct realignment is achieved. Groups of damaged axonal endings form a growth cone and these ends grow towards the distal nerve ends guided by the neurotropic factors.

Neurotrophism is also important in nerve regrowth but more precisely refers to the nutritional support provided to axons connecting with the correct nerve stump. Factors include nerve growth factor (NGF), insulin-like growth factor (IGF), and epidermal growth factor (EGF). When a nerve is divided, the distal stump undergoes degeneration and this is termed Wallerian degeneration. Although the nerve is not present, the damaged Schwann cells and macrophages form a neural tube and organize into bands called bands of Bunger. This process forms a scaffold or conduit for nerve repair. Proximal to the injury a process called chromatolysis occurs with axon degeneration. These processes help explain the rationale for nerve repair as when nerves are repaired, the main objective is to return continuity to the damaged nerve such that the natural repair process can proceed and nerve regeneration can occur along the correct path. When incorrect alignment and excess scarring occur, a neuroma will form with disorganized and "confused" nerve ends resulting in pain and dysfunction.

MUSCLE DENERVATION

4. Following complete transection of the ulnar nerve at the elbow, which one of the following is true with regard to muscle denervation?

E. Optimal hand function should be achieved when the forearm muscles are reinnervated within 3 months of injury.

Following denervation, muscles undergo atrophy and fibrosis. For optimal functional outcome, a denervated muscle should be reinnervated within 3 months of injury. Functional reinnervation usually remains possible for up to 1 year but thereafter reinnervation is less likely and after 2 or 3 years it is no longer possible. Nerve regeneration occurs at a rate of 1 mm/day (not 3 mm/day) following repair, which equates to around 1 inch per month. Therefore, if the ulnar nerve is repaired at the elbow in an adult, it is likely to take at least a year for the regenerating nerve to reach the intrinsic muscles. Consequently, complete reinnervation of the muscles is unlikely and hand function will be impaired. Denervated muscles require 25% (not 75%) of their motor endplates to be intact and these are lost at a rate of 1% per week. Outcomes following nerve repair vary across ages with younger adults and children having the best outcomes. In a situation where a muscle is expected to remain denervated for a prolonged time, it may be possible to use a temporary nerve supply to maintain motor endplate function. This forms the basis of the babysitter procedure used in facial nerve injury. In this procedure part of the hypoglossal nerve is used to innervate the facial muscles while a cross-face nerve graft is placed to regenerate from the contralateral side.[5]

CLASSIFICATION OF NERVE INJURIES

5. Which is the main clinical relevance of the Sunderland classification of nerve injury?
   E. It provides prognostic information.
   The Sunderland classification for nerve injury contains five grades, 1 through 5, and the grade of injury is clinically important as it corresponds to prognosis. A 1st degree injury is expected to have complete return of function within days or months. This is where the axon has retained continuity with an intact endoneurium. In contrast, a 5th degree injury involves complete transection of all nerve structures and will have a marked reduction in functional return even after satisfactory repair. The original classification system by Seddon had three categories; neuropraxia, axonotmesis, and neurontmesis. Sunderland[5,6] later expanded this classification into five grades by subclassifying neurontmesis into three further grades (3rd, 4th, and 5th degree). Mackinnon and Dellon[7] later added a sixth category which represents a mixed nerve injury. These classifications do not describe the mechanism or chronicity of injury. Nor do they relate specific outcomes to age, although younger patients typically achieve the best outcomes after nerve injury. These classifications partly guide surgical management in that complete transection of a nerve will be managed surgically and an intact nerve will not. However, this does not represent the main clinical relevance of the classification systems (Table 80-1).

Table 80-1 *Two Classification Systems of Nerve Injuries*

Seddon	Sunderland	Disrupted Structure	Prognosis
Neurapraxia	1st degree	Axon (minimal)	Complete return in days or months
Axonotmesis	2nd degree	Axon (total, Wallerian degeneration)	Complete return in months
Neurotmesis	3rd degree	Axon, endoneurium	Mild/moderate reduction in function
Neurotmesis	4th degree	Axon, endoneurium, perineurium	Moderate reduction in function
Neurotmesis	5th degree	All structures	Marked reduction in functional return

DIAGNOSIS OF ABNORMAL SENSATION

6. When assessing a patient in clinic for two-point sensory discrimination to the fingertip, which one of the following is true?
   A. 6 mm represents a normal static two-point discrimination.
   Two-point discrimination is a test of nerve density most applicable for nerve injuries and less reliable in compression neuropathies. A normal static two-point value is up to 6 mm for the volar fingertip. A moving two-point discrimination is 2 to 3 mm when testing perpendicular to the digit, moving longitudinally from proximal to distal. Specialized calipers are used to test this and the patient is asked to confirm whether they feel one or two pressure points with the caliper tips set apart at differing distances. It is important to stay on the ulna or radial aspect of the digit without crossing over, otherwise a false result will occur with sensation being due to different digital nerves. Semmes-Weinstein monofilaments are not used for two-point discrimination. They are used to measure pressure thresholds and are most applicable to compression neuropathies and also for complete nerve injuries. They are often used in diabetic patients to assess for protective sensation in the feet. Other tests include vibration thresholds and tinel's sign where tapping over a distal injury produces paresthesia.

Chapter 80 ▪ Nerve Injuries 661

PRIMARY NERVE REPAIR
7. You are repairing a sharply divided digital nerve 1 week after injury. Which one of the following is correct?
A. A direct repair should still be possible at this stage.
Although the nerve ends are less amenable to mobilization in the digits than more proximally, it is unlikely that there will be sufficient retraction or fibrosis to prohibit primary repair during the first week. There is no established advantage of one repair over another when comparing epineurial and fascicular repairs. In the small digital sensory nerves it is accepted practice to use epineurial sutures. Bulging fascicles should be trimmed to allow a neat epineurial repair.

If there is a nerve gap, it is preferable to insert a good quality graft than to perform a tight primary repair ameliorated by flexing the digit. The digit will need to be mobilized within a few weeks, at which point there will be tension across the nerve repair site again before regeneration has occurred. Use of a postoperative extension blocking splint is common following digital nerve repair; however, this should not be used as a substitute for a nerve graft where indicated.

MANAGING A NERVE GAP
8. You have a patient with a 4 cm gap in the ulnar nerve above the elbow following debridement of a gunshot injury 1 week ago. *Which one of the following is correct?*
B. One sural nerve would provide sufficient cable grafts for this defect.
A single sural nerve may provide 30 to 40 cm of suitable nerve graft material; two to five individual nerve grafts might be used in parallel for an ulnar nerve defect (often termed cable grafting). Anterior transposition of the ulnar nerve at the elbow can gain a small amount of additional nerve length and may well be indicated. While the nerve may have suffered additional injury to the 2 cm defect, this procedure may still be appropriate and could actually be helpful if it moves the nerve repair outside the zone of injury. Vascularized nerve grafts are generally reserved for extensively scarred tissues, such as tissues that have undergone radiotherapy. Synthetic conduits perform better over shorter defects and are recommended in defects less than 3 cm in length.

OPTIONS FOR SURGICAL REPAIR
9. For the following scenarios, the best options are as follows:
A. Repair of a complete transverse division of a digital nerve sustained with a motorized cutting disc
   d. Mobilization and direct epineural repair
   When a digital nerve is cleanly transected, such as with a sharp blade, direct repair should be possible. When transected with a thicker blade, such as a motorized cutting disc or wood saw, the width of the blade will cause a loss of nerve length that will require mobilization of the nerve proximally and distally to achieve direct closure. In some cases, nerve grafting may still be required and the posterior interosseus nerve can be a good donor choice.
B. Repair of a complete transverse ulnar nerve transection (junction of the mid and distal thirds of the forearm) sustained during a fall onto broken glass
   c. Direct group fascicular repair
   When performing direct nerve repair, there is no proven advantage in perineural repair over epineural repair in most cases, although for nerve grafting and nerves with a small number of fascicles individual fascicular repair may be considered (see Fig. 80-2, *Essentials of Plastic Surgery,* second edition). When repairing nerves that have obvious motor and sensory components with consistent topology, such as the ulnar nerve in the distal forearm, repairing groups of fascicles may be helpful to approximate motor and sensory divisions correctly.

C. *Repair of the radial nerve at midhumeral level 2 weeks after debridement of necrotizing fasciitis that has left a 6 cm nerve gap*
   g. **Nerve grafting with sural nerve**
      For small nerve gaps in the upper limb, selection of a local graft donor site is preferable; so for radial nerve repair, the lateral antebrachial cutaneous nerve is a good choice and provides 5 to 8 cm graft length. In the scenario described, the defect is already 6 cm and will require further sharp debridement before graft inset. The multiple lengths of nerve graft required will necessitate sural nerve harvest, which can provide 30 to 40 cm of graft.

OUTCOMES FOLLOWING NERVE INJURY

10. *Which one of the following is correct regarding the outcome following nerve injury?*
    B. **Median nerve repairs tend to gain superior results to that of the ulnar nerve.**
       When looking at outcomes following injuries at wrist level, patients with median nerve divisions tend to show better reinnervation than those with ulnar nerve injuries. Results in patients with proximal radial nerve injuries tend to be fairly poor and early tendon transfer may be indicated, as discussed in Chapter 71. Peripheral nerve recovery is quicker and achieves a superior final result than central nerve recovery injury.

       A neuroma may not be evident at 6 weeks, and there may be other reasons for pain and irritation at the site of repair at this early stage, such as scar hypersensitivity. Interpositional vein grafts can collapse centrally, obstructing nerve regeneration. They are not commonly used for important motor nerve repairs. As discussed in question 3, nerve regeneration advances at around 1 inch per month (1 mm per day), not 2 inches per month.

11. *When assessing for motor and sensory nerve recovery following injury, what grading represents a return to normal function?*
    E. **M5, S4**
       The British medical research council (MRC) grading system is a useful and globally accepted approach to classify nerve function. Highet and Dellon have modified this to relate more specifically to nerve recovery following injury (Box 80-1).

       Motor recovery has six grades ranging from M0 (no muscle contraction) to M5 (complete recovery). Sensory recovery also has six grades but these range from S0 (no sensory recovery) to S4 (complete recovery with two-point discrimination 2 to 6 mm), with S3 being split into two different grades designated S3 and S3+. This terminology allows comparison of results and accurate communication between clinicians regarding outcome following injury.[7]

Box 80-1 HIGHET'S METHOD OF END-RESULT EVALUATION AS MODIFIED BY DELLON ET AL

Motor Recovery

M0	No contraction
M1	Return of perceptible contraction on both proximal muscles
M2	Return of perceptible contraction in both proximal and distal muscles
M3	Return of function in both proximal and distal muscles to degree that all important muscles are sufficiently powerful to act against gravity
M4	Return of function as with stage M3; in addition, all synergistic and independent movements possible
M5	Complete recovery

Sensory Recovery

S0	Absence of sensory recovery
S1	Recovery of deep cutaneous pain sensibility within autonomous area of nerve
S2	Return of some degree of superficial cutaneous pain and tactile sensibility with autonomous area of nerve
S3	Return of superficial cutaneous pain and tactile sensibility throughout autonomous area, with disappearance of any previous overresponse
S3+	Return of sensibility as with stage S3; in addition, discrimination within autonomous area (7-15 mm)
S4	Complete recovery (2-point discrimination, 2-6 mm)

In the hand, proximal muscles are defined as extrinsic and distal muscles are intrinsic.

REFERENCES

1. Guo BY, Ayyar DR, Grossman JA. Posterior interosseus palsy with an incidental Froment-Rauber nerve presenting as a pseudoclaw hand. Hand (N Y) 6:344-347, 2011.
2. Froment JBF. Traité D'Anatomie Humaine. Paris: Mequignon-Marvis, 1846.
3. Rauber A. Vater'sche Köper der Bänder–und Periostnerven. Munich: Inauug Diss, 1865.
4. Spinner M. Injuries to the Major Branches of Peripheral Nerves of the Forearm, ed 2. Philadelphia: WB Saunders, 1978.
5. Sunderland S. A classification of peripheral nerve injuries producing loss of function. Brain 74:491-516, 1951.
6. Sunderland S. The anatomy and physiology of nerve injury. Muscle Nerve 13:771-784, 1990.
7. Mackinnon SE, Dellon AL. Surgery of the Peripheral Nerve. New York: Thieme, 1988.

81. Hand Infections

See *Essentials of Plastic Surgery*, second edition, pp. 964-980.

SURGICAL PRINCIPLES

1. When undertaking surgical drainage of an infected upper limb, **which one of the following is true?**
   A. An Esmarch bandage is recommended to fully exsanguinate the limb.
   B. Minimal access incisions are preferable, as wounds will need to be left open.
   C. Arm tourniquets should be avoided, as bacteremia occurs following release.
   D. Incisions crossing flexion creases should be avoided, as they may cause contractures.
   E. Immobilization in a splint for 48 to 72 hours postoperatively is generally recommended.

PARONYCHIA

2. A patient presents with a swollen and inflamed digit worse over the distal phalanx and is given a diagnosis of acute paronychia. **Which one of the following is true regarding this condition?**
   A. It is a common infection affecting the pulp space.
   B. Incision and drainage is the first-line treatment.
   C. Management usually requires removal of the nail plate.
   D. Eponychial marsupialization is often required.
   E. *Staphylococcus aureus* is the most likely pathogen.

PRESENTATION WITH A PAINFUL, SWOLLEN FINGERTIP

3. A 30-year-old man presents to the clinic with a swollen, red, painful index pulp and nail fold. It began spontaneously 2 days ago as a burning sensation. Clear fluid is evident under some small superficial blisters that only appeared this morning. He is generally fit and well, takes no regular medication, and is not a nail biter. **Which one of the following is the best course of action in this case?**
   A. Admit for 24 to 48 hours of intravenous antibiotic therapy with elevation of the hand.
   B. Admit for surgical incision and drainage under local anesthetic.
   C. Debride and cleanse the finger in the clinic with a prescription for broad-spectrum oral antibiotics.
   D. Apply a simple dressing and follow up in 24 to 48 hours.
   E. Take a scraping of the wound bed for urgent microbiologic analysis and a prescription for acyclovir.

VOLAR/DEEP SPACE ABSCESSES

4. A female patient presents with an acute upper limb infection 3 days after sustaining mild trauma to the little finger. She now has exquisite tenderness in the thumb and little fingers that is worse during flexion. The remaining digits are spared. *Which one of the following hand spaces is associated with this clinical presentation?*
A. Thenar space
B. Midvolar space
C. Parona's space
D. Hypothenar space
E. Interdigital web space

FLEXOR TENOSYNOVITIS

5. A 45-year-old man presents with a 48-hour history of a hot, swollen, painful left middle finger. He works as a builder and accidentally stabbed himself in the palm 3 days ago with a screwdriver. His middle finger has a fusiform shape and is held in a flexed position. He cannot tolerate passive digital extension or direct, gentle pressure over the volar aspect of the digit. A small bead of pus is expressed at the site of his original injury. *Which one of the following is correct regarding this patient?*
A. This case demonstrates all of Kanavel's cardinal signs of flexor sheath infection.
B. The patient can be adequately managed with high-dose antibiotics and splinting.
C. The infection is likely to be polymicrobial and will require at least two antibiotic types.
D. He does not have any specific risk factors for poor outcomes following flexor sheath infection.
E. Minimal access incisions alone should be adequate for surgical management.

MANAGEMENT OF A "FIGHT BITE"

6. A patient is seen for washout of a wound following a punch injury. There is a 1 cm transverse dorsal wound over the right ring finger MP joint with evidence of pus and surrounding cellulitis. His hand is very swollen, and he is unable to fully extend the ring and middle fingers. Plain radiographs show no evidence of fracture or foreign body. *Which one of the following is correct?*
A. The wound edges require debridement, but wound extension should be avoided to prevent joint exposure.
B. After thorough irrigation with saline, any damage to the extensor tendon should be repaired immediately.
C. It is not necessary to formally explore the MP joint in this case, given the radiologic findings.
D. Even if the wound is debrided and irrigated adequately, it should not be closed directly.
E. The hand should be splinted with the MP joints at 20 degrees to relax the joint capsule.

ANIMAL BITES

7. Which one of the following is correct regarding animal bites?
A. Dog bites represent 25% of all reported animal bites in the developed world.
B. Patients are usually bitten by animals not known to them.
C. Cat bites are more likely to become infected than dog bites.
D. Adults are more commonly bitten by animals than children.
E. Infection from *Pasteurella multocida* occurs exclusively in cat bites.

SEPTIC ARTHRITIS

8. In a patient with a suspected septic arthritis in the hand, which one of the following is true?
A. Representative joint fluid samples are best obtained through the area of erythema.
B. Synovial fluid analysis with WBC >10,000 cm^3 is diagnostic.
C. The presence of articular cartilage will prevent development of osteomyelitis.
D. Crystalline arthropathy is best differentiated on plain radiographs.
E. In a young child this may represent secondary spread of another infection.

GAS GANGRENE

9. A patient presents with a rapidly progressing soft tissue infection of the upper limb. There is obvious crepitus within the soft tissues and overlying cellulitis with swelling. A diagnosis of gas gangrene is suspected. **Which one of the following organisms is most likely to be involved?**
A. *Clostridium perfringens*
B. *Staphylococcus aureus*
C. *Streptococcus* spp
D. *Eikenella corrodens*
E. *Bacteroides fragilis*

BIOFILMS

10. Why are bacterial biofilms so difficult to treat?
A. They usually coexist with fungal spores.
B. The bacteria have altered genetics.
C. The bacteria have low adherence to synthetic structures.
D. The bacteria are protected by a polysaccharide matrix.
E. They most commonly involve MRSA.

HIGH-PRESSURE INJECTION INJURIES

11. A patient inadvertently injects an oil-based material into a digit while using a high-pressure tool. **Which one of the following is correct?**
A. The dominant thumb is the most likely digit to be affected.
B. Urgent debridement and decompression is required.
C. Water-based solvents cause similar levels of tissue damage.
D. Risk of subsequent need for amputation is low.
E. Soft tissue damage can be predicted by the size of the entry wound.

DIAGNOSING HAND INFECTIONS

12. For each of the following clinical scenarios, select the most likely infectious etiology. (Each option may be used once, more than once, or not at all.)
    A. A 17-year-old patient develops a hand infection the day after separating her cat from another as they were fighting.
    B. A 50-year-old pet shop owner sustained a superficial glass injury at work while cleaning an aquarium. The wound has since healed, but he has developed painful superficial erythematous nodules nearby.
    C. A 74-year-old avid gardener presents to the clinic with a localized suppurative nodule to the fingertip that has been present for several weeks. He cannot recall any trauma to this finger.

Options:
a. *Candida albicans*
b. *Mycobacterium* spp.
c. *Trichophyton rubrum*
d. *Clostridium perfringens*
e. *Sporothrix schenckii*
f. Group A *Streptococcus* spp.
g. *Pasteurella multocida*
h. *Eikenella corrodens*
i. *Staphylococcus aureus*

Answers

SURGICAL PRINCIPLES
1. When undertaking surgical drainage of an infected upper limb, **which one of the following is true?**
   D. **Incisions crossing flexion creases should be avoided, as they may cause contractures.**
   Some key principles must be considered when surgically managing infections of the upper limb. Incisions should be designed to allow access and minimize subsequent scar complications. In particular, longitudinal incisions across flexion creases should be avoided, as they are likely to lead to scar contractures. As with all hand surgery explorations, incisions should be designed to place scars within skin creases where possible and facilitate good access. For example, Bruner's incisions may be used in the digits, and curvilinear Z-shaped flaps may be used on the volar surface of the forearm. Longitudinal incisions may be well suited to the dorsal aspect of the hand and forearm (Fig. 81-1). Using large access incisions is generally recommended in soft tissue infections to facilitate accurate debridement. Some exceptions include mild flexor sheath infections, which can be irrigated with minimal access incisions (see Fig. 81-5, *Essentials of Plastic Surgery*, second edition).

   It is standard practice to use a tourniquet for incision and drainage of an infected upper limb, as this facilitates a clear, blood-free view of structures during debridement. However, gentle gravity exsanguination is recommended to minimize risk of bacteremia. The Esmarch bandage is a rubber band that is used to wrap the hand and forearm before inflation of a tourniquet. It ensures thorough exsanguination, but is not recommended in infected cases because it may be more likely to cause a bacteremia. Copious irrigation of infected wounds is required and this is often best done with a large saline bag and an intravenous administration set. Following surgery, early active mobilization is optimal to reduce postoperative edema, stiffness, and loss of joint motion.

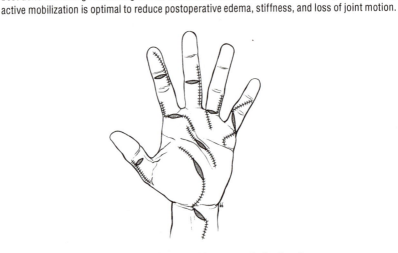

Fig. 81-1 Incision placement for access in the hand.

Chapter 81 ■ Hand Infections   669

PARONYCHIA

2. A patient presents with a swollen and inflamed digit worse over the distal phalanx and is given a diagnosis of acute paronychia. **Which one of the following is true regarding this condition?**
   E. *Staphylococcus aureus* is the most likely pathogen.
   Paronychia is an infection of the soft tissues surrounding the nail and can be acute or chronic. Acute paronychia is generally caused by a bacterial infection with staphylococcus aureus and is associated with nail biting and minor trauma. First-line treatment is oral antibiotics and wound cleaning. In cases unresponsive to conservative management, it is necessary to drain the abscess and/or remove the nail plate. Chronic infections are more likely to be fungal and may require marsupialization in cases resistant to medical management (see Fig. 81-1, *Essentials of Plastic Surgery,* second edition).

PRESENTATION WITH A PAINFUL, SWOLLEN FINGERTIP

3. A 30-year-old man presents to the clinic with a swollen, red, painful index pulp and nail fold. It began spontaneously 2 days ago as a burning sensation. Clear fluid is evident under some small superficial blisters that only appeared this morning. He is generally fit and well, takes no regular medication, and is not a nail biter. **Which one of the following is the best course of action in this case?**
   D. Apply a simple dressing and follow up in 24 to 48 hours.
   The differential diagnosis in this patient is herpetic whitlow or a felon/paronychia. Given the appearance of vesicles, the mild swelling, and the history provided, whitlow is the most likely diagnosis. This condition is generally self-limiting and is caused by infection with herpes simplex virus. Deroofing a vesicle allows a Tzanck smear (microscopic analysis useful for confirming certain viral infections) to be performed for diagnostic purposes, but debridement and release of fluid is not recommended because this can lead to viral spread. In severe cases, usually in immunocompromised patients, viral spread can result in encephalitis. Herpetic whitlow should be treated with application of a dry dressing and avoidance of contact, unless there is concern regarding superimposed bacterial infection (which is not evident in this case). There is no indication here for either antibiotics or antiviral medications in a healthy patient. A secondary bacterial infection would require debridement of purulent vesicles and antibiotics.

VOLAR/DEEP SPACE ABSCESSES

4. A female patient presents with an acute upper limb infection 3 days after sustaining mild trauma to the little finger. She now has exquisite tenderness in the thumb and little fingers that is worse during flexion. The remaining digits are spared. **Which one of the following hand spaces is associated with this clinical presentation?**
   C. Parona's space
   This patient displays signs of a horseshoe abscess (see Fig. 81-4, *Essentials of Plastic Surgery,* second edition). Parona's space is located in the distal forearm between pronator quadratus and FDP tendons. An infection of either the little finger or thumb flexor sheaths can spread by a communication through the ulnar and radial bursae into Parona's space. This explains why a patient can have an injury in the little finger presenting as a thumb flexor sheath infection.
   Other important spaces in the hand that may become infected are the midvolar, hypothenar, thenar, and interdigital spaces. Midvolar infections present with central palm pain and swelling with loss of concavity between thenar and hypothenar eminences. Thenar infections present with associated pain and swelling worse on thumb opposition. Hypothenar space infections are rare and present with pain and swelling on little finger opposition. Collar button abscesses can

form in the interdigital web spaces. They present with loss of web space contour and tenderness within the affected web space.

Any suspected palm space infections require urgent surgical drainage under anesthetic in conjunction with antibiotics. The normal surgical principles apply as discussed in question 1.

FLEXOR TENOSYNOVITIS

5. A 45-year-old man presents with a 48-hour history of a hot, swollen, painful left middle finger. He works as a builder and accidentally stabbed himself in the palm 3 days ago with a screwdriver. His middle finger has a fusiform shape and is held in a flexed position. He cannot tolerate passive digital extension or direct, gentle pressure over the volar aspect of the digit. A small bead of pus is expressed at the site of his original injury. **Which one of the following is correct regarding this patient?**
   A. This case demonstrates all of Kanavel's cardinal signs of flexor sheath infection.
   Kanavel's four cardinal signs of a flexor sheath infection are:
   1. Pain on passive extension of the digit
   2. Fusiform swelling of the digit
   3. Tenderness over the flexor tendon sheath
   4. Partially flexed posture of the digit

   This patient displays all of the four signs, and is quite typical for a more advanced case such as this.

   Some flexor sheath infections can be managed adequately with antibiotics, mobilization, and splinting alone.[1] Such cases are usually mild, are treated early, and do not have an open wound. In contrast, this patient will require urgent surgical drainage because there is pus in the wound and there was an initial penetrating injury, the management of which has already been delayed. Ideally, minimal access incisions are used for flexor sheath washout, but at least a degree of palmar wound extension will be required in this case to explore and debride the initial puncture wound.

   The most common pathogen in flexor sheath infection is *Staphylococcus aureus* alone, rather than a polymicrobial cause. Polymicrobial infections are more common in diabetic and other immune-compromised patients. Treatment would involve a single penicillin-based antibiotic such as amoxicillin with clavulanic acid or floxacillin. He has two risk factors for a poor outcome: age over 43 years, and the presence of subcutaneous pus. Level II evidence has shown a number of other risk factors for poor outcome, which include the presence of diabetes, peripheral vascular or renal disease, and the presence of digital ischemia.[2]

MANAGEMENT OF A "FIGHT BITE"

6. A patient is seen for washout of a wound following a punching injury. There is a 1 cm transverse dorsal wound over the right ring finger MP joint, with evidence of pus and surrounding cellulitis. His hand is very swollen, and he is unable to fully extend the ring and middle fingers. Plain radiographs show no evidence of fracture or foreign body. **Which one of the following is correct?**
   D. Even if the wound is debrided and irrigated adequately, it should not be closed directly.
   Wound closure should generally be avoided in a fight bite and must certainly not be performed if there is frank pus. Any tendon repair should be delayed until the wound is clean, and a monofilament suture is preferred to further reduce the risk of bacterial colonization at the repair site as discussed in Chapter 3. The risk of joint capsule penetration is very high with these injuries, so the capsule should be carefully inspected throughout the range of motion for any breach (see Fig. 81-6, *Essentials of Plastic Surgery*, second edition). Any resting splint should be

as close to the ideal safe position of immobilization as can be achieved in the presence of swelling (i.e., wrist slightly extended, MP joints at approximately 70 degrees of flexion, IP joints straight). The key principles for management of these injuries are as follows:

1. Promptly and thoroughly debride the wound edges and extend the wound to ensure adequate inspection of the tendon and joint capsule. Send specimens for microbiologic analysis.
2. Assess the extensor mechanism and carefully explore the joint capsule throughout the range of motion of the joint (puncture wounds may only become evident when the position of injury is re-created).
3. Thoroughly irrigate the joint and wound (if open or infected).
4. Do not primarily repair the joint capsule or tendon if it is frankly purulent.
5. Leave the wound open but consider closing the wound extensions using a monofilament nonabsorbable suture.
6. Dress the wound with a wick, a low-adherent dressing, gauze, wool, and crepe.
7. Apply a splint with the hand placed in a "safe" position (with the MP joint flexed to 70 degrees, IP joints in extension, and the wrist in mild extension), see Fig. 64-5, *Essentials of Plastic Surgery,* second edition.
8. Continue IV antibiotics and hand elevation, then reassess the wound at 24 hours.

ANIMAL BITES

7. Which one of the following is correct regarding animal bites?
C. Cat bites are more likely to become infected than dog bites.
Dog bites represent 90% of all animal bites, whereas cat bites represent just 5%. Despite this massive difference, cat bites represent three quarters of all infected bites. This is probably because their long, thin teeth are more likely to cause narrow, deep puncture wounds prone to infection. Cat bites need early treatment with antibiotics and washout and can still take a prolonged time to settle. In over two thirds of dog bites, the animal is known to the patient. Children less than 5 years of age are at increased risk of dog bites: half of all dog bites occur in this age group. *Pasteurella multocida* is associated with both cat and dog bites.

SEPTIC ARTHRITIS

8. In a patient with a suspected septic arthritis in the hand, which one of the following is true?
E. In a young child this may represent secondary spread of another infection.
Septic arthritis is infection of the joint space and may represent hematogenous spread from an infective source elsewhere in the body. For this reason, it is important to exclude other sources of infection, particularly in children. Diagnosis involves obtaining joint fluid samples, and these should ideally be obtained without passing the needle through an erythematous area in order to avoid seeding of the joint and to ensure a reliable sample is obtained. Fluid analysis with WBC >50,000 per mm^3 (not 10,000 per cm^3) strongly suggests joint sepsis. This fluid also provides the best evidence to exclude a crystal arthropathy (rather than plain radiographs) such as gout, and some of the fluid should be sent for crystal analysis. An urgent gram stain should also be requested, as this will help guide prompt accurate management which involves urgent joint washout, packing, and antibiotics. Early mobilization with hand therapy input is required. Untreated septic arthritis may quickly invade the articular cartilage and cause irreversible arthritic changes as well as progression to osteomyelitis.

GAS GANGRENE

9. A patient presents with a rapidly progressing soft tissue infection of the upper limb. There is obvious crepitus within the soft tissues and overlying cellulitis with swelling. A diagnosis of gas gangrene is suspected. *Which one of the following organisms is most likely to be involved?*
   A. *Clostridium perfringens*
      Gas gangrene is uncommon in the upper extremity but is a severe life-threatening infection caused by clostridium species. There are more than 60 subtypes of clostridium, but perfringens is most commonly associated with gas gangrene. Clostridia produce multiple toxins which cause local tissue destruction. Management involves rapid diagnosis and early surgical debridement with high-dose antibiotics and general supportive care. Gas gangrene has a high mortality rate (approximately 25%). Necrotizing fasciitis is the main differential diagnosis, and this can be caused by group A streptococci or due to a polymicrobial cause including anaerobes. Many soft tissue infections are caused by staphylococcus infection and they include paronychia, flexor sheath infection, and felon. Eikenella is implicated in some human bites as are streptococcus viridans and bacteriodes.

BIOFILMS

10. Why are bacterial biofilms so difficult to treat?
   D. The bacteria are protected by a polysaccharide matrix.
      Biofilms are extremely relevant to plastic surgery, given the high-volume use of prosthetic devices and also the number of chronic wounds seen. Biofilms are implicated in a variety of infections, as well as capsular contracture following breast implant procedures (see discussion in Chapter 45). Biofilms are particularly difficult to treat because they are strongly adherent to implanted devices and nonviable tissue and form colonies surrounded by exopolysaccharide matrices. This isolates them from surrounding tissues and protects them from host defense mechanisms. The biofilm is often inactive for extended periods of time with no evidence of infection present. It can subsequently become activated to release bacteria, resulting in a planktonic state. As a result, antibiotic concentrations 1000 times higher than normal may be required to penetrate a biofilm. Surgical debridement of chronic wounds and removal of nonviable tissue helps reduce a biofilm, and prosthetic devices are generally exchanged or removed where a biofilm is present and causing infection. Bacterial biofilms are not usually in coexistence with fungal spores and where the genetics of the bacteria are otherwise normal. MRSA has become increasingly common in recent years as a result of antibacterial resistance; however, this is not the main reason why biofilms are difficult to treat.

HIGH-PRESSURE INJECTION INJURIES

11. *A patient inadvertently injects an oil-based material into a digit while using a high-pressure tool. Which one of the following is correct?*
   B. Urgent debridement and decompression is required.
      High-pressure injection injuries can cause significant tissue damage through a small entry wound. Material is inadvertently injected into the digit at high pressure (often as high as 7000 psi). These injuries need urgent surgical management with wound extension, irrigation, and tissue debridement. Both oil-based and water-based solvents can cause significant damage, but oil-based injuries tend to be worse. Risk of amputation is high (up to 50%) after an oil-based, high-pressure injury. The entry wound does not provide much information with regard to severity of tissue damage, so it is easy to underestimate its severity. Debridement often fails to remove all traces of injection material satisfactorily. The most commonly involved digit is the nondominant index finger.

DIAGNOSING HAND INFECTIONS

12. For the following scenarios, the best options are as follows:
   A. A 17-year-old patient develops a hand infection the day after separating her cat from another as they were fighting.

   g. *Pasteurella multocida*

   The patient in scenario A is likely to have an infection from a bite or scratch from one of the cats and the most likely pathogen is *Pasteurella multocida*. As discussed in question 7, she will require treatment with antibiotics and may require formal washout if the infection does not settle.

   B. A 50-year-old pet shop owner sustained a superficial glass injury at work while cleaning an aquarium. The wound has since healed, but he has developed painful superficial erythematous nodules nearby.

   b. *Mycobacterium* spp.

   The patient in scenario B has developed an atypical mycobacterial infection, also known as fish tank granuloma. It is caused by *Mycobacterium marinum*. Treatment is likely to require surgical debridement and antibiotics for an extended time.

   C. A 74-year-old avid gardener presents to the clinic with a localized suppurative nodule to the fingertip that has been present for several weeks. He cannot recall any trauma to this finger.

   e. *Sporothrix schenckii*

   The patient in scenario C most likely has a soft tissue fungal infection acquired while gardening. This is typically sustained from contact with rose thorns, moss, or other plants. Treatment usually involves a prolonged course of an oral antifungal agent.

   Candida albicans is a fungal infection commonly seen in immunocompromised patients and diabetics that has a tendency to affect moist environments. It is treated with nystatin, miconazole, or ketoconazole. *Trichophyton rubrum* represents another fungal infection that causes onychomycosis. This is treated with oral terbinafine. Group A *Streptococcus* spp. can cause an aggressive, rapidly progressing soft tissue infection in previously fit individuals. Early recognition is required as is prompt treatment with high-dose penicillin antibiotics in the first instance. *Eikenella corrodens* is a common pathogen in human bite injuries and should be treated with amoxicillin and clavulanic acid.

REFERENCES

1. Pang HN, Teoh L, Yam A, et al. Factors affecting the prognosis of pyogenic flexor tenosynovitis. J Bone Joint Surg Am 89:1742-1748, 2007
2. Steer AC, Lamagni T, Curtis N, et al. Invasive group a streptococcal disease: epidemiology, pathogenesis and management. Drugs 72:1213-1227, 2012.

82. Benign and Malignant Masses of the Hand

See *Essentials of Plastic Surgery*, second edition, pp. 981-994.

GANGLION CYSTS

1. Your resident sees a patient in clinic and diagnoses a ganglion cyst. **Which one of the following is correct regarding ganglion cysts?**
   A. They are the most common soft tissue tumor in the upper limb and have an equal sex distribution.
   B. Transillumination with a penlight and plain radiographs are required for diagnosis.
   C. Surgical excision should be performed under local anesthetic in almost all adult patients.
   D. The radiovolar aspect of the wrist is the most common site for ganglia in children.
   E. Flexor tendon sheath ganglia are confirmed by their movement on digital flexion.

2. **Which one of the following ligaments is most commonly associated with ganglion cysts at the wrist in adults?**
   A. Radiolunate
   B. Scapholunate
   C. Radiocapitate
   D. Scaphotriquetral
   E. Radioscaphoid

GIANT CELL TUMORS OF THE TENDON SHEATH

3. A patient is referred with a suspected diagnosis of a giant cell tumor of the tendon sheath. **Which one of the following statements is correct?**
   A. It is most likely to affect the little finger.
   B. The patient is most likely to be under 25 years of age.
   C. Hand function is unlikely to be affected.
   D. Previous injury may be a predisposing factor.
   E. Recurrence after surgical excision is unlikely.

FINGERTIP ABNORMALITIES

4. For each of the following scenarios, select the most likely diagnosis from the options listed. (Each option may be used once, more than once, or not at all.)
   A. A 28-year-old hairdresser presents with a nontender 5 mm soft tissue swelling to the right middle finger pulp.
   B. A 78-year-old retired schoolteacher presents with a tender soft tissue swelling at the nail base and DIP joint of the right ring finger.
   C. A 46-year-old woman presents with an 8-week history of a pigmented area to the little finger nail bed. It is nontender and unaffected by temperature, and there is no history of trauma.

   Options:
   a. Glomus tumor
   b. Mucous cyst
   c. Basal cell carcinoma
   d. Squamous cell carcinoma
   e. Inclusion dermoid cyst
   f. Giant cell tumor
   g. Melanoma

SIGNS OF SOFT TISSUE SARCOMA

5. You are working in the sarcoma clinic, and a 34-year-old patient is referred to you with a soft tissue mass in the volar compartment of the proximal forearm. It has been present for 16 months, measures 4 cm in diameter, is fixed by resisted elbow flexion, and is nontender. **Which one of the following represents the most significant concern regarding this lesion?**
   A. The size
   B. The lack of pain
   C. The duration of symptoms
   D. The depth of the mass
   E. The patient's age

DIAGNOSING SOFT TISSUE SARCOMA

6. A young adult patient is referred to the clinic with a rapidly enlarging, painful soft tissue mass in the left midforearm. **Which one of the following is the preferred method for obtaining an initial tissue diagnosis in this case?**
   A. Fine-needle aspiration cytology
   B. Incisional biopsy
   C. Excisional biopsy
   D. Core needle biopsy
   E. Marginal excision

IMAGING IN SOFT TISSUE SARCOMA

7. A patient is referred to the clinic with a suspicious mass in the right deltoid region. It has doubled in size over the past month. **Which one of the following is the best imaging modality to use for this patient?**
   A. High-resolution CT
   B. Isotope bone scan
   C. MRI
   D. Ultrasound
   E. PET scan

MANAGEMENT OF SOFT TISSUE SARCOMAS

8. A 42-year-old patient has a confirmed high-grade sarcoma involving the triceps muscle. It measures 2 cm in diameter and there are no metastases. **Which one of the following is the most appropriate management?**
A. Marginal excision of tumor mass and postoperative radiotherapy
B. Wide excision and regular follow-up
C. Radical compartmentectomy and observation
D. Wide excision with postoperative radiotherapy
E. Primary forequarter amputation and radiotherapy

BENIGN BONE LESIONS

9. A 26-year-old woman presents with a fracture of the left ring finger proximal phalanx sustained while washing dishes. She is otherwise fit and well. A plain radiograph shows a well-demarcated, round, lytic lesion with some areas of calcification within the proximal phalanx. **What is the most likely diagnosis?**
A. Nora's lesion
B. Periosteal chondroma
C. Enchondroma
D. Maffucci's syndrome
E. Ollier's disease

MALIGNANT BONE TUMORS

10. **Which one of the following is the most common primary malignant bone tumor in the hand?**
A. Ewing's sarcoma
B. Chondrosarcoma
C. Osteosarcoma
D. Malignant giant cell tumor
E. Osteoblastoma

CLINICAL SCENARIOS

11. For each of the following scenarios, select the most likely diagnosis from the options listed. (Each option may be used once, more than once, or not at all.)
  A. A 43-year-old builder presents with a small soft tissue swelling over the volar aspect of the right wrist. This has developed over 8 months. He complains of altered sensation in the little finger and pain in the ulnar digits while working, especially in cold weather.
  B. A 37-year-old woman presents with a 9-month history of a nontender swelling over the dorsum of the wrist. Examination shows a hard, fixed 1 cm swelling overlying the middle finger CMC joint.
  C. A 28-year-old man who is fit and well complains of night pain affecting his ring finger. There is little to see on examination and no history of injury, although ibuprofen has been helpful.

Options:
a. Giant cell tumor
b. Ulnar artery aneurysm
c. Ganglion cyst
d. Neurofibroma
e. Carpal boss
f. Chondrosarcoma
g. Osteoid osteoma
h. Lipoma

Chapter 82 ▪ Benign and Malignant Masses of the Hand   677

Answers

GANGLION CYSTS

1. Your resident sees a patient in clinic and diagnoses a ganglion cyst. **Which one of the following is correct regarding ganglion cysts?**
   D. The radiovolar aspect of the wrist is the most common site for ganglia in children.
   Ganglion cysts are the most common benign mass in the hand and are two or three times more common in females. Diagnosis is based on history and clinical examination and may be enhanced by transillumination using a penlight. Radiographs should be obtained to exclude joint pathology or soft tissue calcification, but these do not usually help diagnose a ganglion. Ultrasonography may be of use where there is doubt about the nature and extent of a probable ganglion cyst.

   Many ganglia, such as mucous cysts, can comfortably be excised under local anesthesia, but excision of wrist ganglia is more commonly performed under regional block or general anesthesia to aid tourniquet tolerance. Furthermore, volar wrist ganglia are often intimately related to the radial artery and need to be excised with care in a controlled environment. Flexor sheath ganglia usually occur at the A1 or A2 pulleys and do not move with the tendon as they are fixed to the pulley/sheath.

2. **Which one of the following ligaments is most commonly associated with ganglion cysts at the wrist in adults?**
   B. Scapholunate
   More than two thirds of all wrist ganglia in adults are found on the dorsal aspect of the wrist between the third and fourth extensor compartments. They are most often associated with the scapholunate ligament.

GIANT CELL TUMORS OF THE TENDON SHEATH

3. A patient is referred with a suspected diagnosis of a giant cell tumor of the tendon sheath. **Which one of the following statements is correct?**
   D. Previous injury may be a predisposing factor.
   Giant cell tumors of the tendon sheath are also called pigmented villonodular synovitis (PVNS). They are most common between the fourth and sixth decades of life. The radial three digits are most frequently affected, and disease may be a reaction to injury. Continued growth will usually interfere with hand function. Treatment is with marginal excision to preserve function, but recurrence rates are high because of close margins or satellite lesions. Adjunctive radiotherapy is sometimes used in recurrent tumors or following incomplete surgical excision.

FINGERTIP ABNORMALITIES

4. For the following scenarios, the best options are as follows:
   A. A 28-year-old hairdresser presents with a nontender 5 mm soft tissue swelling to the right middle finger pulp.
      e. Inclusion dermoid cyst
      Inclusion dermoid cysts are commonly seen in the palms and fingertips of patients with occupations that predispose them to penetrating injuries. The penetrating injury causes implantation of epidermal cells into the dermis. Treatment is surgical excision.

B. A 78-year-old retired schoolteacher presents with a tender soft tissue swelling at the nail base and DIP joint of the right ring finger.
b. **Mucous cyst**
   Mucous cysts are small ganglia that originate from the DIP joint and are associated with osteoarthritis. They may be associated with nail grooving and osteophytes. Treatment is with surgical excision of the cyst and adjacent osteophytes.

C. A 46-year-old woman presents with an 8-week history of a pigmented area to the little finger nail bed. It is nontender and unaffected by temperature, and there is no history of trauma.
g. **Melanoma**
   Pigmentation of the nail is concerning in the absence of trauma and warrants urgent biopsy to exclude a subungual melanoma. Discoloration (often red/blue tinged) in the presence of exquisite tenderness is more likely to be caused by a glomus tumor, which is a benign tumor of the arteriovenous anastomosis involved in regulation of cutaneous circulation. Basal cell and squamous cell carcinomas can affect the hand, particularly in immunocompromised patients, or those who have had significant sun exposure. Squamous cell carcinomas typically present as keratinized structures with an ulcerated base. Formal biopsy is advocated in cases where diagnosis is uncertain.

SIGNS OF SOFT TISSUE SARCOMA

5. You are working in the sarcoma clinic, and a 34-year-old patient is referred to you with a soft tissue mass in the volar compartment of the proximal forearm. It has been present for 16 months, measures 4 cm in diameter, is fixed by resisted elbow flexion, and is nontender. *Which one of the following represents the most significant concern regarding this lesion?*
   D. **The depth of the mass**
   This may well be a benign mass such as a lipoma; however, the most concerning feature of this lesion is the tissue depth. Because it is fixed on elbow flexion, this suggests it involves the volar muscle compartment. Being deep to the fascia is one of the key criteria of concern for soft tissue sarcomas. The other red flags are size greater than 5 cm, pain, and rapid growth. The more of these features that coexist, the more likely it is that malignancy is present. In general, the single most important concern is rapid growth of the lesion (i.e., weeks to months).[1]

DIAGNOSING SOFT TISSUE SARCOMA

6. A young adult patient is referred to the clinic with a rapidly enlarging, painful soft tissue mass in the left midforearm. *Which one of the following is the preferred method for obtaining an initial tissue diagnosis in this case?*
   D. **Core needle biopsy**
   Patients with suspected soft tissue sarcomas should undergo triple assessment in a specialist clinic. This involves a history, examination, imaging, and biopsy. Where timing allows, it can be helpful to obtain imaging before biopsy to preserve soft tissue appearances (e.g., on MRI), or imaging may be used to guide biopsies of deeper lesions. The recommended approach to obtaining a tissue biopsy is to take several core biopsies, because this maximizes diagnostic yield.[1] If the lesion is superficial or small, then incisional or excisional biopsies may occasionally be considered. When a biopsy is obtained, it must be planned in such a way that the biopsy tract can be completely removed during the subsequent tumor excision; hence, biopsies are generally better performed by the treating surgical team. Fine-needle aspiration cytology is not

recommended as a primary diagnostic modality, although it may be useful in confirming disease recurrence.[1] Furthermore, it only provides cells for analysis, rather than formal tissue subtyping.

IMAGING IN SOFT TISSUE SARCOMA

7. A patient is referred to the clinic with a suspicious mass in the right deltoid region. It has doubled in size over the past month. *Which one of the following is the best imaging modality to use for this patient?*
   ### C. MRI
   An MRI scan is the preferred initial imaging modality for patients with suspected soft tissue sarcoma, both for identifying the nature and extent of the lesion and to aid surgical planning. CT or ultrasound may also be useful. Once the diagnosis has been confirmed, a high-resolution staging CT scan should be performed to exclude metastases. Isotope bone scans and PET scans are not currently recommended as routine diagnostic or staging investigations.[1]

MANAGEMENT OF SOFT TISSUE SARCOMAS

8. A 42-year-old patient has a confirmed high-grade sarcoma involving the triceps muscle. It measures 2 cm in diameter and there are no metastases. *Which one of the following is the most appropriate management?*
   ### D. Wide excision with postoperative radiotherapy
   Excision margins in soft tissue sarcoma are defined as[1]:
   Intralesional: Margins run through the tumor and therefore the tumor remains.
   Marginal: Surgical planes run through the pseudocapsule (local recurrence rates are high because of tumor satellites).
   Wide: The surgical plane is in normal tissue but in the same compartment as the tumor (local recurrence rates are generally low).
   Radical: The tumor is removed, including affected compartments, and there is a minimal risk of local recurrence.
   A wide excision and radiotherapy gives maximal preservation of function while minimizing local recurrence. Chemotherapy is usually used in a metastatic disease or specific tumor types.

BENIGN BONE LESIONS

9. A 26-year-old woman presents with a fracture of the left ring finger proximal phalanx sustained while washing dishes. She is otherwise fit and well. A plain radiograph shows a well-demarcated, round, lytic lesion with some areas of calcification within the proximal phalanx. *What is the most likely diagnosis?*
   ### C. Enchondroma
   The presence of a pathologic fracture and this radiologic appearance are suggestive of an enchondroma. The presence of multiple enchondromas is called *Ollier's disease,* and when combined with vascular malformations, is termed *Maffucci's syndrome.* Nora's lesion was described by Nora and is also known as *bizarre parosteal osteochondromatous proliferation* (BPOP).[2] It is a rare lesion affecting the tubular bones of the hand (proximal and middle phalanges and metacarpals). It is thought to be a reactive lesion and develops as an exophytic outgrowth from the cortical surface. It contains bone, cartilage, and fibrous tissue. Typical presentation involves development of an obvious tender mass over a few months. Periosteal chondromas are also rare and represent surface lesions arising from the periosteum of the tubular bones. They typically present as painful but slow-growing masses.

MALIGNANT BONE TUMORS

10. Which one is the following is the most common primary malignant bone tumor in the hand
   B. Chondrosarcoma
   Chondrosarcoma is the most common primary malignant bone tumor in the hand and may develop de novo or within a benign lesion such as an osteochondroma. It usually occurs in the epiphyseal regions of the phalanges or metacarpals and presents as a destructive bony lesion which is often slow growing.
   Ewing's sarcoma, osteosarcoma, and malignant giant cell tumors are less common in the hand. Osteoblastoma is usually considered benign, although an aggressive variant has been described.

CLINICAL SCENARIOS

11. For the following scenarios, the best options are as follows:
   A. A 43-year-old builder presents with a small soft tissue swelling over the volar aspect of the right wrist. This has developed over 8 months. He complains of altered sensation in the little finger and pain in the ulnar digits while working, especially in cold weather.
   b. Ulnar artery aneurysm
   This patient has symptoms of ulnar nerve compression close to Guyon's canal. This can occur as a result of lesions such as a lipoma or a ganglion cyst. However, pain on working in cold weather suggests an ischemic component to the compression. Palpation of a pulsatile mass would strongly support the diagnosis of an aneurysm. This condition is commonly seen in manual laborers, such as carpenters, and results from repetitive trauma to the ulnar artery at the wrist (hypothenar hammer syndrome). Treatment involves resection, ligation, or interposition vein grafting.

   B. A 37-year-old woman presents with a 9-month history of a nontender swelling over the dorsum of the wrist. Examination shows a hard, fixed 1 cm swelling overlying the middle finger CMC joint.
   e. Carpal boss
   Carpal bosses are often confused with ganglion cysts at the wrist, but some key differences are that ganglia may fluctuate in size, are generally softer, compressible, and may be sited more proximally.

   C. A 28-year-old man who is fit and well complains of night pain affecting his ring finger. There is little to see on examination and no history of injury, although ibuprofen has been helpful.
   g. Osteoid osteoma
   Osteoid osteomas are uncommon tumors that typically affect the distal phalanx in young adult patients. They are particularly associated with night pain and this is often relieved by NSAID use. Chondrosarcoma can present with a mass (often close to the MP joint) that is usually painful and tends to occur in older individuals. Imaging is important in further characterizing bony lesions.

REFERENCES

1. Grimer R, Judson I, Peake D, et al. Guidelines for the management of soft tissue sarcomas. Sarcoma 2010:506182, 2010.
2. Nora FE, Dahlin DC, Beabout JW. Bizarre parosteal osteochondromatous proliferations of the hands and feet. Am J Surg Pathol 7:245-250, 1983.

83. Dupuytren's Disease

See *Essentials of Plastic Surgery*, second edition, pp. 995-1002.

ETIOLOGIC FACTORS AND EPIDEMIOLOGY OF DUPUYTREN'S DISEASE
1. **Which one of the following is correct regarding Dupuytren's disease?**
   A. It occurs almost exclusively in white males over the age of forty.
   B. Excess alcohol intake has no association with its development.
   C. Inheritance is normally autosomal recessive with variable penetrance.
   D. The middle and ring fingers are the most commonly affected digits.
   E. No clear correlation exists between the use of vibration tools and cord development.

DUPUYTREN'S DIATHESIS
2. A 38-year-old patient presents to clinic with palpable nontender lumps in both palms affecting the ring finger and thumb. They have been present for 6 months and are now limiting his ability to fully open his hands. His father and grandfather had similar problems, and he would like to discuss treatment options with you. **Which one of the following is correct?**
   A. All of the features of Dupuytren's diathesis are present.
   B. This is a typical age of onset for Dupuytren's contracture.
   C. If he has sisters, they are unlikely to be affected.
   D. His risk of recurrence after treatment is high.
   E. Dorsal knuckle pads would be unusual in this patient.

STRUCTURES AFFECTED BY DUPUYTREN'S DISEASE
3. **Which one of the following structures is typically spared in Dupuytren's contracture?**
   A. Cleland's ligament
   B. Grayson's ligament
   C. Spiral cord
   D. Lateral digital sheet
   E. Natatory ligament

CORD COMPONENTS IN DUPUYTREN'S DISEASE
4. Your resident is presenting a case of Dupuytren's disease to you in clinic and states that the patient has a "spiral cord" on examination. **Which one of the following structures does not form part of the spiral cord?**
   A. Lateral digital sheet
   B. Grayson's ligament
   C. Landsmeer's ligament
   D. Pretendinous band
   E. Spiral band

INDICATIONS FOR SURGERY

5. **Which one of the following is most likely to be an indication for surgical intervention in Dupuytren's disease?**
   A. A palpable spiral cord in a straight finger
   B. The presence of Garrod's pads
   C. A PIP joint contracture of 10 degrees
   D. An MP joint contracture of 20 degrees
   E. A negative Hueston's test

COLLAGENASE INJECTIONS FOR DUPUYTREN'S CONTRACTURE

6. A patient comes to clinic having read about "a new enzyme injection therapy" for Dupuytren's disease. He has unilateral disease with palpable pretendinous cords affecting the ring and little fingers. The flexion contractures are 40 degrees at the MP joint and 10 degrees at the PIP joint. **Which one of the following is correct regarding collagenase injections for this patient?**
   A. Even if full correction is achieved, he has a 70% chance of recurrence within 3 years.
   B. Each cord will require two office visits, and each digit is normally treated separately.
   C. He is very unlikely to develop a skin tear following treatment.
   D. He will almost certainly develop antibodies to *Streptococcus histolyticus* spp.
   E. His risk of flexor tendon rupture is approximately 5% following treatment.

THE IP JOINTS IN DUPUYTREN'S DISEASE

7. **When planning a limited fasciectomy for a finger with a PIP joint contracture, which one of the following is correct?**
   A. If a boutonniere deformity is present it is likely that the PIP joint correction will be maintained.
   B. A lazy-S volar incision is the preferred approach.
   C. Contracture of the accessory collateral ligaments and volar plate at the MP joint is common.
   D. Correction of a PIP joint contracture may be limited by tolerance of the neurovascular bundles.
   E. In severe PIP joint contracture, aggressive joint release gives a better long-term result than fasciectomy alone.

TREATMENT OPTIONS FOR DUPUYTREN'S CONTRACTURE

8. A 55-year-old man has Dupuytren's contractures affecting the ring and little fingers of his right hand. Both MP joints have contractures of 45 degrees and the ring finger PIP joint has a contracture of 20 degrees. There are pretendinous and spiral cords. **Which one of the following statements is correct?**
   A. Reported recurrence rates after radical fasciectomy are less than 10% at 5 years.
   B. The risk of neurovascular injury during surgery is minimal, given the anatomy of his disease.
   C. Needle fasciotomy may achieve complete correction, but recurrence would be more likely than with fasciectomy.
   D. Because both MP and PIP joints are affected, a primary dermofasciectomy is recommended.
   E. The PIP joint is unlikely to be fully corrected with limited fasciotomy.

Answers

ETIOLOGIC FACTORS AND EPIDEMIOLOGY OF DUPUYTREN'S DISEASE

1. Which one of the following is correct regarding Dupuytren's disease?

E. No clear correlation exists between the use of vibration tools and cord development.

Dupuytren's disease is a benign fibroproliferative disorder that occurs in the palmar fascia leading to nodules, cords, and contractures of the fingers. There is no proven correlation with vibration tools or other manual work in development of Dupuytren's disease, although there are theories that a possible microtrauma mechanism may act to direct myofibroblast contracture.

The link between alcohol intake and Dupuytren's disease has been questioned over the years; however, a recent review by Hindocha et al[1] concluded that alcohol excess is associated with disease that is more likely to require surgical correction than conservative management, although the mechanism for this is unclear. A previous study by this group has shown that excess alcohol intake was associated with an increased severity of disease.[2]

The inheritance of Dupuytren's disease is thought to be autosomal dominant (not recessive) with variable penetrance. As better epidemiological data emerge, it is recognized that while white men of Northern European descent are most commonly affected, the disease is also regularly encountered in women and in other ethnic groups such as Japanese individuals. There appears to be both a genetic and environmental influence on this. The ring and little fingers (not the middle and ring) are most commonly affected, followed by the middle finger. The thumb and index finger can be affected but this is less common.

DUPUYTREN'S DIATHESIS

2. A 38-year-old patient presents to clinic with palpable nontender lumps in both palms affecting the ring finger and thumb. They have been present for 6 months and are now limiting his ability to fully open his hands. His father and grandfather had similar problems, and he would like to discuss treatment options with you. Which one of the following is correct?

D. His risk of recurrence after treatment is high.

The presence of multiple Dupuytren's diathesis factors in a patient such as this man increases the risk of recurrent disease by up to approximately 70%, compared with a baseline recurrence risk of 20 to 25% in patients without diathesis factors.[3] The initial description of Dupuytren's diathesis by Hueston included four factors[4]:
   1. Ethnicity
   2. Family history
   3. Bilateral disease
   4. Ectopic lesions (outside the palm)

The scenario only gives two of these factors. He may develop ectopic disease, such as dorsal knuckle pads (Garrod's pads) and may also be affected by plantar or penile fibromatosis.

Subsequent to Hueston's description, additional items have been added by Hindocha et al[3] who suggested two new factors: male sex and age at onset less than 50 years (for which this patient meets both criteria). These authors also proposed that the family history should include one or more affected siblings/parents and that only ectopic lesions in the knuckles (Garrod's pads) should count. Finally, because inheritance is autosomal dominant, any of his siblings including sisters, are also at risk, although penetrance of the phenotype is variable.

STRUCTURES AFFECTED BY DUPUYTREN'S DISEASE

3. **Which one of the following structures is typically spared in Dupuytren's contracture?**
   A. Cleland's ligament
   Dupuytren's disease affects much of the palmar fascia, but Cleland's ligaments are usually spared in this condition. These fascial bands pass dorsal to the neurovascular bundles in the fingers from the periosteum and flexor tendon sheath to the lateral skin (see Fig. 59-1, *Essentials of Plastic Surgery*, second edition for the components of the retinacular system of the digits).
   Grayson's ligament passes transversely from the volar aspect of the flexor tendon sheath to the skin. It functions to prevent bowstringing of the neurovascular bundle. In Dupuytren's disease it is often tightly adherent to the bundle, making dissection more challenging. The natatory ligaments are found just deep to the skin, extending transversely between the web spaces and, when involved in Dupuytren's disease, may restrict both MP joint abduction and PIP joint extension. The lateral digital sheet is located lateral to the neurovascular bundles within the digit and, when involved in Dupuytren's disease, can restrict PIP and DIP joint function.

CORD COMPONENTS IN DUPUYTREN'S DISEASE

4. Your resident is presenting a case of Dupuytren's disease to you in clinic and states that the patient has a "spiral cord" on examination. **Which one of the following structures does not form part of the spiral cord?**
   C. Landsmeer's ligament
   The presence of a spiral cord can complicate the surgical management of Dupuytren's disease as the neurovascular bundle can become distorted, spiraling around the disease as it tightens up. Spiral cords may cause flexion contractures of the PIP joint. The common components of a spiral cord are:
   - Lateral digital sheet
   - Pretendinous band
   - Spiral band
   - Grayson's ligament
   - Natatory ligaments (included by many, but not all, authors)

   Landsmeer's ligament is not part of the spiral cord. It is also known as the oblique retinacular ligament and originates on the volar aspect of the middle phalanx and inserts on the dorsal aspect of the distal phalanx. It helps to coordinate PIP joint and DIP joint motion.

INDICATIONS FOR SURGERY

5. **Which one of the following is most likely to be an indication for surgical intervention in Dupuytren's disease?**
   C. A PIP joint contracture of 10 degrees
   Established flexion contractures of the PIP joint are the most difficult to correct because the volar structures shorten when the joint is left in flexion for a prolonged time. The MP joint is far more forgiving, as the collateral ligaments are taut when the joint is flexed (i.e., the "safe" position for splinting) (see Chapter 65, question 4, *Question and Answer* and Fig. 65-4, *Essentials of Plastic Surgery*, second edition). MP joint contractures greater than 30 degrees and any PIP joint contracture are commonly quoted as indications for surgery, although lesser contractures may be sufficiently troubling to warrant treatment, so the decision is tailored to the individual. Garrod's pads are rarely an indication for surgery, but may be if they are symptomatic. A positive Hueston's test is where the hand cannot be placed flat on a tabletop and may be an indication for surgery if there are functional problems.

Chapter 83 ▪ Dupuytren's Disease   685

COLLAGENASE INJECTIONS FOR DUPUYTREN'S CONTRACTURE

6. A patient comes to clinic having read about "a new enzyme injection therapy" for Dupuytren's disease. He has unilateral disease with palpable pretendinous cords affecting the ring and little fingers. The flexion contractures are 40 degrees at the MP joint and 10 degrees at the PIP joint. *Which one of the following is correct regarding collagenase injections for this patient?*
B. Each cord will require two office visits, and each digit is normally treated separately.
Collagenase injection for the treatment of Dupuytren's disease has recently become popular. The treatment involves injecting collagenase into a palpable cord and then allowing it to weaken before physically breaking the cord by external manipulation 24 to 48 hours later. Current recommendations are that one cord should be treated at a time. Two visits is the minimum per cord, assuming that one injection and one manipulation is sufficient. Some cords require more than one injection, and 35% (not 70%) of those who achieve full extension at the initial treatment have some degree of recurrence at three years.[5] All patients must be warned about skin tears, as these are common but heal quickly with nonsurgical management.

The collagenase used in Dupuytren's contracture is a blend of two clostridial collagenases, AUX I and AUX II, from *Clostridium histolyticum* (not *Streptococcus*). *Streptococcus pyogenes, Staphylococcus aureus,* and *Clostridium perfringens* all produce hyaluronidase (rather than collagenase) as a mechanism of penetrating soft tissues. Methods of producing hyaluronidase (hyalase) have led to its use in local anesthesia and correction of hyaluronic acid facial fillers as discussed in Chapter 88.

All patients will have developed antibodies to the injection by their second injection, but this has not been associated with any adverse outcomes. Subsequent tendon rupture is extremely rare, with three reports in 2600 injections performed within the Collagenase Option for Reduction of Dupuytren's (CORD) clinical trials.[6]

THE IP JOINTS IN DUPUYTREN'S DISEASE

7. *When planning a limited fasciectomy for a finger with a PIP joint contracture, which one of the following is correct?*
D. Correction of a PIP joint contracture may be limited by tolerance of the neurovascular bundles.
Following a severe, prolonged contracture, the neurovascular bundles may be restricted and unable to tolerate full extension of the digit. The risk of vascular compromise is also increased in revisional surgery.

Although aggressive release of a contracted PIP joint capsule may give improved correction of the finger intraoperatively, this may be at the expense of joint stability, or result in a loss of flexion if care is not taken. Loss of flexion may be more troublesome than loss of extension for most functional activities. Many surgeons advocate careful serial release of the accessory collateral ligaments and volar plate to improve correction, but many would advise against a forced capsulotomy. The reported outcomes are mixed, with some series demonstrating greater early loss of correction with joint release, but comparable outcomes to fasciectomy alone in the longer term.[7,8]

A lazy-S incision is not recommended (see Fig. 83-1, *Essentials of Plastic Surgery,* second edition), and problems with the MP joint volar plate or ligaments would be highly unusual. A boutonniere deformity indicates a central slip altercation and a PIP joint correction is unlikely to be maintained.

TREATMENT OPTIONS FOR DUPUYTREN'S CONTRACTURE

8. A 55-year-old man has Dupuytren's contractures affecting the ring and little fingers of his right hand. Both MP joints have contractures of 45 degrees and the ring finger PIP joint has a contracture of 20 degrees. There are pretendinous and spiral cords. *Which one of the following statements is correct?*

C. Needle fasciotomy may achieve complete correction, but recurrence would be more likely than with fasciectomy.

There are variable recurrence rates reported worldwide following treatment of Dupuytren's disease, and confusion arises because there is debate about whether any recurrence of disease is included in outcome figures, or whether only recurrent disease requiring further treatment should be included.[9,10] Despite these variations, it is generally accepted that needle fasciotomy shows earlier recurrence than fasciectomy. However, the trade-off of greater downtime after fasciectomy means that many surgeons and patients find needle fasciotomy preferable. Some surgeons do report comparable outcome figures with extensive needle fasciotomy. Reported recurrence rates after limited fasciectomy are in the order of 21% at five years, compared with 85% for needle fasciotomy.[11]

Dermofasciectomy is usually reserved for cases with extensive skin involvement or for aggressive or recurrent disease. It is most often required over the proximal phalanx. Wounds are closed with skin grafts or left to heal by secondary intention. Radical fasciectomy involves extensive resection of volar and digital fascia including diseased and nondiseased tissue. It does not decrease the recurrence rate and carries higher rates of complication than limited fasciectomy. In this scenario, the PIP joint contractures are mild and a full correction is likely whichever technique is performed.

REFERENCES

1. Hindocha S, McGrouther DA, Bayat A. Epidemiological evaluation of Dupuytren's disease incidence and prevalence rates in relation to etiology. Hand (N Y) 4:256-269, 2009.
2. Hindocha S, Stanley JK, Watson JS, et al. Revised Tubiana's staging system for assessment of disease severity in Dupuytren's disease—preliminary clinical findings. Hand (N Y) 3:80-86, 2008.
3. Hindocha S, Stanley JK, Watson S, et al. Dupuytren's diathesis revisited: evaluation of prognostic indicators for risk of disease recurrence. J Hand Surg Am 31:1626-1634, 2006.
4. Hueston JT. Dupuytren's Contracture. Edinburgh: E & S Livingstone, 1963.
5. Peimer CA, Blazar P, Coleman S, et al. Dupuytren contracture recurrence following treatment with collagenase clostridium hystolyticum (CORDLESS study): 3-year data. J Hand Surg Am 38:12-22, 2013.
6. Hurst LC, Badalamente MA, Hentz VR, et al. Injectable collagenase clostridium histolyticum for Dupuytren's contracture. N Engl J Med 361:968-979, 2009.

7. Weinzweig N, Culver JE, Fleegler EJ. Severe contractures of the proximal interphalangeal joint in Dupuytren's disease: combined fasciectomy with capsuloligamentous release versus fasciectomy alone. Plast Reconstr Surg 97:560-566, 1996.
8. Ritchie JF, Venu KM, Pillai K, et al. Proximal interphalangeal joint release in Dupuytren's disease of the little finger. J Hand Surg Br 29:15-17, 2004.
9. Crean SM, Gerber RA, Le Graverand MP, et al. The efficacy and safety of fasciectomy and fasciotomy for Dupuytren's contracture in European patients: a structured review of published studies. J Hand Surg Eur 36:396-407, 2011.
10. Werker PM, Pess GM, van Rijssen AL, et al. Correction of contracture and recurrence rates of Dupuytren contracture following invasive treatment: the importance of clear definitions. J Hand Surg Am 37:2095-2105, 2012.
11. van Rijssen AL, ter Lindan H, Werker PM. Five-year results of a randomized clinical trial on treatment in Dupuytren's disease: percutaneous needle fasciotomy versus limited fasciectomy. Plast Reconstr Surg 129:469-477, 2012.

84. Rheumatoid Arthritis

See *Essentials of Plastic Surgery*, second edition, pp. 1003-1016.

PATHOPHYSIOLOGY OF RHEUMATOID ARTHRITIS
1. **Which one of the following tissues is primarily affected in rheumatoid arthritis?**
   A. Articular cartilage
   B. Periosteum
   C. Bone
   D. Tendon
   E. Synovium

DIAGNOSING RHEUMATOID ARTHRITIS
2. You see a 50-year-old woman in clinic with a 4-week history of bilateral wrist and elbow joint stiffness that is worse in the morning. She is a nonsmoker and is otherwise fit and well. Recent blood tests show her to be seronegative for rheumatoid factor. **Which one of the following is correct?**
   A. She meets the criteria for a diagnosis of rheumatoid arthritis.
   B. Her blood test result excludes a diagnosis of rheumatoid arthritis.
   C. Her risk of developing rheumatoid arthritis is double that of an equivalent male.
   D. Her smoking history is not relevant to a diagnosis of rheumatoid disease
   E. Joint space narrowing on plain radiographs will confirm her diagnosis.

DEFORMITIES IN RHEUMATOID ARTHRITIS
3. **When you examine a patient with rheumatoid arthritis, which one of the following would you expect to observe?**
   A. Weakness of the radial sagittal bands
   B. Ulnar deviation of the wrist
   C. Radial deviation at the MP joints
   D. Dorsal subluxation at the MP joints
   E. Firm subcutaneous swellings over the DIP joints

SITES INVOLVED IN RHEUMATOID ARTHRITIS AT THE WRIST
4. **Which one of the following is usually only seen at the wrist in the later stages of rheumatoid arthritis?**
   A. Degenerative change of the scaphoid waist
   B. Scapholunate ligament disruption
   C. Radiocarpal joint involvement
   D. Ulnar styloid involvement
   E. Distal radioulnar joint degenerative change

SWAN NECK DEFORMITY

5. Which one of the following is correct regarding the swan neck deformity in rheumatoid arthritis?
A. The clinical appearance includes PIP joint flexion with DIP joint hyperextension.
B. Abnormal PIP joint anatomy is the primary cause.
C. It is often caused by central slip attenuation with lateral band subluxation.
D. Function is more significantly impaired than with a boutonniere deformity.
E. Initial treatment involves the use of a sublimis tendon sling to stabilize the PIP joint.

MP JOINT DEFORMITY

6. Which one of the following is not usually implicated in causing the characteristic deviation seen at the MP joints in rheumatoid patients?
A. Radial deviation of the carpus
B. Pinch forces between the finger and thumb
C. Attenuation of the radial sagittal bands
D. Ulnar subluxation of the extensor tendons
E. Tightness of the flexor tendons

THUMB DEFORMITY IN RHEUMATOID ARTHRITIS

7. What is the most common examination finding in the thumb of a rheumatoid patient?
A. MP joint hyperextension
B. IP joint flexion
C. Radial abduction of the metacarpal
D. Ulnar abduction of the metacarpal
E. Adduction of the metacarpal

MANAGING RHEUMATOID MEDICATIONS PERIOPERATIVELY

8. You are planning to replace all four digital MP joints with silicone prostheses in a patient with rheumatoid arthritis. *Which one of the following medications should be stopped during the perioperative period?*
A. Methotrexate
B. Naproxen
C. Sulfasalazine
D. Etanercept
E. Prednisolone

COMMON PROCEDURES IN RHEUMATOID ARTHRITIS

9. Which one of the following is correct for patients with rheumatoid arthritis?
A. Trigger finger should be treated with surgical division of the A1 pulley.
B. Carpal tunnel syndrome should be treated with a standard approach.
C. Tenosynovectomy can reduce tendon rupture and is increasingly common.
D. A Mannerfelt lesion may be treated with an FDS tendon transfer.
E. EPL rupture is the first sign of Vaughn-Jackson syndrome and requires EIP transfer.

MANAGEMENT OF MP JOINT DEFORMITIES

10. *When correcting severe MP joint deformities in a patient with rheumatoid arthritis, which one of the following is commonly required as part of the procedure?*
- A. Radial collateral release
- B. Cross-intrinsic transfer
- C. Radial sagittal band release
- D. Ulnar sagittal band imbrication
- E. Pyrocarbon MP joint arthroplasty

UNSALVAGEABLE JOINTS IN RHEUMATOID ARTHRITIS

11. *When addressing advanced wrist and DRU joint deformities in rheumatoid arthritis, which one of the following is correct?*
- A. The Sauve-Kapandji procedure increases the risk of ulnar carpal translocation.
- B. The ulna stump may be unstable following both Darrach and Sauve-Kapandji procedures.
- C. The Darrach procedure relies on good bone stock for success.
- D. When bone stock is poor, a plate is preferable to a Steinmann pin for wrist fusion.
- E. Radioscapholunate arthrodesis may be helpful if the midcarpus is degenerate.

AUTOIMMUNE DISEASES AFFECTING THE HANDS

12. A 40-year-old woman presents with severe arthritis changes affecting both hands. She has pits in her fingernails. ***What is the most likely diagnosis?***
- A. Systemic lupus erythematosus
- B. Rheumatoid arthritis
- C. Psoriatic arthritis
- D. Scleroderma
- E. Osteoarthritis

Answers

PATHOPHYSIOLOGY OF RHEUMATOID ARTHRITIS

1. *Which one of the following tissues is primarily affected in rheumatoid arthritis?*
   E. Synovium
   Rheumatoid arthritis is a chronically progressive, systemic autoimmune inflammatory disease that primarily affects the synovium. Synovium is a thin layer of tissue that lines the articular surface of joints and tendon sheaths. It has two main functions. The first is to act as a selectively permeable membrane to control entry and exit of factors to the joint. The second is to produce substances that lubricate the joint, e.g., synovial fluid.

   In certain disease processes, such as rheumatoid arthritis and de Quervain's tenosynovitis, there is an abnormal inflammatory response within the synovium. The synovium produces matrix metalloproteinases, collagenases, and cathepsins, which in turn cause damage to the cartilage, bone, and periosteum. The end result is a thickened, inflamed synovium called pannus, with erosion of adjacent soft tissues such as tendon, joint capsule, and ligament, as well as bone.

DIAGNOSING RHEUMATOID ARTHRITIS

2. You see a 50-year-old woman in clinic with a 4-week history of bilateral wrist and elbow joint stiffness that is worse in the morning. She is a nonsmoker and is otherwise fit and well. Recent blood tests show her to be seronegative for rheumatoid factor. ***Which one of the following is correct?***
   C. Her risk of developing rheumatoid arthritis is double that of an equivalent male.
   The risk for females developing rheumatoid arthritis is two or even three times that of males. The diagnosis of rheumatoid arthritis requires that four of seven key criteria are met and that symptoms have been present for at least 6 weeks. The criteria are as follows:
   1. Morning stiffness in joints
   2. Soft tissue swelling at three or more joints
   3. Symmetrical involvement of joints
   4. Involvement of metacarpophalangeal (MP), proximal interphalangeal (PIP), or wrist joints
   5. Rheumatoid nodules
   6. Seropositive for rheumatoid factor (RF)
   7. Typical radiographic findings

   Therefore, although she has three of the key symptoms, she would need one further feature for the diagnosis, and her symptoms would need to persist for at least another 2 weeks. *Note that a patient being rheumatoid factor negative does **not** exclude a diagnosis of rheumatoid arthritis.* Only 70% to 80% of patients are seropositive, and some may develop positivity later in the disease. There does appear to be an epidemiologic association between smoking and caffeine intake and rheumatoid arthritis. Joint space narrowing is one of the radiologic features of rheumatoid arthritis, but this is also seen in other forms of arthritis and joint spaces are sometimes increased because of swelling in early disease.

DEFORMITIES IN RHEUMATOID ARTHRITIS

3. **When you examine a patient with rheumatoid arthritis, which one of the following would you expect to observe?**
    A. **Weakness of the radial sagittal bands**
    Some of the common features of established rheumatoid arthritis in the hand are:
    - Attenuation or rupture of the radial sagittal bands of the EDC mechanism over the MP joint
    - Radial deviation of the wrist
    - Ulnar deviation at the MP joints
    - Volar subluxation of the MP joints
    - Rheumatoid nodules around the olecranon and ulnar proximal forearm or other pressure points
    - Swan neck and boutonniere finger deformities
    - Synovitis with visible swellings from pannus (e.g., around extensor compartments at the wrist)
    - Firm swellings over the DIP joint are more characteristic of osteoarthritis.

SITES INVOLVED IN RHEUMATOID ARTHRITIS AT THE WRIST

4. **Which one of the following is usually only seen at the wrist in the later stages of rheumatoid arthritis?**
    C. **Radiocarpal joint involvement**
    Early sites of involvement around the wrist in rheumatoid arthritis include the scaphoid waist, scapholunate ligament, ulnar styloid, and DRU joint. Late changes occur at the radiocarpal joint and midcarpus. Other late findings include erosion of the volar rim of radius, volar subluxation of the carpus, ulnar translocation and radial deviation of carpus, and dorsal prominence of the ulna with carpal supination (caput ulnae).

SWAN NECK DEFORMITY

5. **Which one of the following is correct regarding the swan neck deformity in rheumatoid arthritis?**
    D. **Function is more significantly impaired than with a boutonniere deformity.**
    When stiff or fixed, swan neck deformities are much more debilitating than boutonniere deformities. With a boutonniere, patients can grip and pinch. With a swan neck, these motions are difficult or impossible. The swan neck deformity involves PIP joint hyperextension with DIP joint flexion (see Fig. 84-2, *Essentials of Plastic Surgery,* second edition). It can occur secondary to joint abnormalities of the DIP, PIP, or MP joints. This is in contrast to a boutonniere deformity, which involves PIP joint flexion with DIP joint hyperextension and is always secondary to a PIP joint abnormality.
    Both boutonniere and swan neck deformities can occur secondary to pannus erosion that weakens joint support. The swan neck deformity can occur from extensor tendon rupture at the

DIP joint (leading to a mallet deformity), rupture of the volar plate at the PIP joint, or rupture of the FDS tendon insertion. Alternatively, a swan neck deformity can begin at the MP joint secondary to volar subluxation and intrinsic muscle tightening. Central slip attenuation (resulting from pannus erosion) with lateral band subluxation describes the process underlying a boutonniere deformity in rheumatoid.

Initial treatment for a swan neck deformity is with a splint, and rebalancing surgery is only considered if this fails and the PIP joint remains supple. Surgical interventions include using a slip of the FDS tendon or one lateral band to prevent PIP joint hyperextension, and may require intrinsic muscle release. PIP joint fusion in a more functional position may also be helpful.

MP JOINT DEFORMITY

6. Which one of the following is not usually implicated in causing the characteristic deviation seen at the MP joints in rheumatoid patients?

E. Tightness of the flexor tendons

The characteristic finding at the MP joints in rheumatoid arthritis is ulnar deviation with volar subluxation. Tightness of the flexor tendons is not usually implicated in this deformity. If, however, an A1 pulley release is performed then the flexor tendon angle of approach will drift ulnarward and further exacerbate the ulnar deformity caused by other factors. Tightness of the intrinsics is implicated in the volar subluxation rather than the flexor tendons.

There are a number of contributory factors in ulnar deviation at the MP joint. All of the factors (A through D) are collectively important. Radial deviation of the carpus alters the angle of approach of the extensor tendons to the MP joints, while pinch forces between the thumb and fingers also push them in an ulnar direction. Pannus stretches and erodes the joint capsule (which tends to erode most dorsoradially because of the other forces in action); the same factors similarly damage the radial sagittal bands and collateral ligaments. The extensor tendons then sublux ulnarward into the valleys between the metacarpal heads, further increasing the deforming forces and pulling the digits ulnarward.

THUMB DEFORMITY IN RHEUMATOID ARTHRITIS

7. What is the most common examination finding in the thumb of a rheumatoid patient?

C. Radial abduction of the metacarpal

The most common thumb abnormality in a rheumatoid patient is a boutonniere deformity, which is also termed a Z-deformity. This involves MP joint flexion with IP joint hyperextension and radial abduction of the metacarpal. It occurs because of dorsal pannus erosion leading to rupture of the EPB insertion and volar subluxation of the EPL.

The other findings described are in keeping with a swan neck deformity which is also seen in rheumatoid patients, although less commonly in the thumb. This involves MP joint hyperextension, IP joint flexion, and adduction contracture of the metacarpal secondary to CMC joint subluxation. This process occurs secondary to volar pannus erosion through the joint capsule and MP joint volar plate (Fig. 84-1).

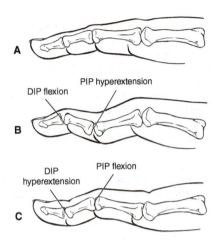

Fig. 84-1 Characteristic swan neck and boutonniere deformities. **A,** Normal. **B,** Swan neck. **C,** Boutonniere deformity.

MANAGING RHEUMATOID MEDICATIONS PERIOPERATIVELY

8. You are planning to replace all four digital MP joints with silicone prostheses in a patient with rheumatoid arthritis. *Which one of the following medications should be stopped during the perioperative period?*
   D. Etanercept
   Pharmacologic agents used in rheumatoid arthritis can be broadly classified as NSAIDs (e.g., naproxen and indomethacin), steroids (e.g., prednisolone) and disease-modifying antirheumatoid drugs (DMARDs). DMARDs are further subdivided into conventional (e.g., methotrexate, sulfasalazine, and gold) and biologic (e.g., etanercept and infliximab).
   As a general guide, most rheumatoid medications can be continued safely during the perioperative period for relatively small procedures like MP joint replacement. However, there is an exception with the biological DMARDS, which should be stopped for 2 to 4 weeks before and after surgery (depending on the drug's half-life). The injectable biologic agents are anti-TNF-alpha agents and their use is associated with increased gram-positive infection.[1] If in doubt, you should discuss the perioperative management of rheumatoid medications with the patient's rheumatologist, because stopping medications can lead to a rheumatoid flare.

COMMON PROCEDURES IN RHEUMATOID ARTHRITIS

9. *Which one of the following is correct for patients with rheumatoid arthritis?*
   D. A Mannerfelt lesion may be treated with an FDS tendon transfer.
   A *Mannerfelt lesion* is a spontaneous rupture of the FPL tendon observed in the rheumatoid hand. It is usually caused by osteophytes around the scaphoid, which must be debrided at the time of reconstruction to reduce the risk of recurrent attrition. The FPL is usually reconstructed with an index FDS transfer, tendon graft, or arthrodesis of the thumb IP joint.
   Trigger finger and carpal tunnel syndrome are treated differently in rheumatoid patients, because the underlying cause is usually tenosynovitis.
   Carpal tunnel syndrome can result from a mass effect of thick tenosynovitis/pannus within the carpal tunnel and should be treated with an extended carpal tunnel release and synovectomy.

Trigger finger results from focal tenosynovitis or a rheumatoid nodule within the sheath or tendon. It should also be treated with synovectomy. Division of the A1 pulley will increase the likelihood of ulnar deviation at the MP joints, as discussed earlier, and should be avoided. Although early tenosynovectomy can reduce the risk of tendon rupture, it is less commonly required nowadays because of the improved medical control of rheumatoid arthritis.

The term *Vaughn-Jackson syndrome* refers to spontaneous attrition rupture of the extensor tendons, starting with the little finger (not the thumb) and progressing with sequential rupture from ulnar to radial. Isolated EPL rupture may be treated with EIP transfer, but again it is vital that the underlying friction points are excised and covered with capsular flaps where possible to prevent recurrence.

MANAGEMENT OF MP JOINT DEFORMITIES

10. When correcting severe MP joint deformities in a patient with rheumatoid arthritis, which one of the following is commonly required as part of the procedure?

B. Cross-intrinsic transfer

As discussed in previous questions, the typical deformity at the MP joint level in rheumatoid is ulnar deviation, with volar subluxation. This can be corrected with the following maneuvers:
- Intrinsic muscle release to allow MP joint extension
- Cross-intrinsic transfer: the tight intrinsic tendon on the ulnar side is sutured to the radial side of the adjacent digit to correct ulnar deviation
- Ulnar-sided sagittal band (which is tight) is released: this helps to centralize the subluxed extensor tendon
- The radial-sided sagittal band (which is attenuated) is tightened: this helps to centralize the subluxed extensor tendon
- The radial collateral ligament is tightened or reconstructed: this helps to correct the ulnar deviation

If the joint surface is preserved, an arthroplasty is not required. However, if the joint surface requires replacement, it is important to complete careful soft tissue rebalancing, since typical flexible silicone prostheses will not be strong enough to realign the joint alone, and deviating forces across a prosthesis will also encourage erosion of arthroplasty stems through soft bone. Silicone prosthesis are preferred to pyrocarbon in rheumatoid MP joints.

UNSALVAGEABLE JOINTS IN RHEUMATOID ARTHRITIS

11. When addressing advanced wrist and DRU joint deformities in rheumatoid arthritis, which one of the following is correct?

B. The ulna stump may be unstable following both Darrach and Sauve-Kapandji procedures.

The Sauve-Kapandji procedure fuses the detached ulnar head to the distal radius, with the aim of relieving pain from a degenerative DRU joint and restoring prosupination, while stabilizing the TFCC and ulnar wrist joint and reducing the risk of ulnarward carpal translocation[2] (see Fig. 84-4, *Essentials of Plastic Surgery*, second edition). The Darrach procedure involves excision of the ulnar head and may increase the risk of carpal translocation, despite preservation of the TFCC remnants and ulnar collateral ligament of the wrist.[3] Since there is no element of fusion or fixation in a Darrach procedure, bone stock is not as important as in many other wrist procedures in rheumatoid arthritis. The distal ulna stump may be unstable following both, potentially leading to pain.

During wrist fusion, a common technique is to insert a Stanley or Steinmann pin (with a single trochar tip) through from the third metacarpal head, along the shaft, through the carpus, and into the radius. This technique has been in use since the 1960s, and since then several different pins have been used. The original general purpose Steinmann pins have been modified by Stanley et al.[4] Some surgeons insert the pin between the metacarpals, although this is less common. Although plating techniques (often using precontoured compression plates) are also available for wrist fusion, these require good bone stock for adequate purchase and are less frequently used in rheumatoid arthritis than in osteoarthritis.

Radioscapholunate arthrodesis is only of use if the midcarpal joint surfaces are preserved.

AUTOIMMUNE DISEASES AFFECTING THE HANDS

12. A 40-year-old woman presents with severe arthritis changes affecting both hands. She has pits in her fingernails. *What is the most likely diagnosis?*

C. Psoriatic arthritis

Nail pitting is a feature of psoriatic arthritis, which is a seronegative arthropathy. The skin may be minimally affected, with some patients only reporting mild scalp psoriasis rather than florid plaques. The arthritic changes can be severe, with marked dissolution of bone leading to arthritis mutilans. The DIP joints are more often involved than in rheumatoid arthritis.

Nail pitting is not a feature of the other conditions listed. Systemic lupus erythematosus is a multisystem disease found in young women. Hand findings include joint problems without cartilage destruction and with normal joint spaces retained. The hallmark of this condition is ligamentous and volar plate laxity with tendon subluxation. The visual deformity is similar to rheumatoid arthritis but with preservation of joint surfaces. Scleroderma is another multisystem disease that can affect the hand. Key features include fingertip ulceration, Raynaud's phenomenon, and sclerodactyly. The small vessel vasculitis can result in fingertip ulceration, chronic wounds, and amputations. Contractures usually result from skin and soft tissue changes, with MP joint hyperextension and PIP joint flexion contractures both common. Osteoarthritis tends to present with pain, swelling, stiffness, and deformity in the small joints of the hand. Characteristic findings include Heberden's nodules near the DIP joint and Bouchard nodes near the PIP joint (see Chapter 85).

REFERENCES

1. Dixon WG, Watson K, Lunt M, et al. Rates of serious infection, including site-specific and bacterial intracellular infection, in rheumatoid arthritis patients receiving anti-tumor necrosis factor therapy: results from the British Society for Rheumatology Biologics Register. Arthritis Rheum 54:2368-2376, 2006.
2. Vincent KA, Szabo RM, Agee JM. The Sauve-Kapandji procedure for reconstruction of the rheumatoid distal radioulnar joint. J Hand Surg Am 18:978-983, 1993.
3. Lee SK, Hausman MR. Management of the distal radioulnar joint in rheumatoid arthritis. Hand Clin 21:577-589, 2005.
4. Stanley JK, Gupta SR, Hullin MG. Modified instruments for wrist fusion. J Hand Surg Br 11:245-249, 1986.

85. Osteoarthritis

See *Essentials of Plastic Surgery*, second edition, pp. 1017-1025.

CLINICAL HISTORY
1. **When taking a history from a patient with osteoarthritis of the hands, which one of the following would be unusual?**
   A. Pain that is worse in the morning
   B. Perceived weakness of grip
   C. Pain that affects sleeping patterns
   D. Increased discomfort with joint loading and movement
   E. Involvement of the IP joint and wrist

PLAIN RADIOGRAPHS IN OSTEOARTHRITIS
2. **Which one of the following tends to be an early finding of osteoarthritis on plain radiographs?**
   A. Joint space narrowing
   B. Joint space widening
   C. Joint subluxation
   D. Subchondral sclerosis/eburnation
   E. Osteophytes and periarticular erosions

IMAGING FOR OSTEOARTHRITIS OF THE THUMB
3. **Which one of the following radiographic views gives a true anteroposterior image of the thumb?**
   A. Waters' view
   B. Bett's view
   C. Robert's view
   D. Eaton stress view
   E. Towne's view

JOINT INVOLVEMENT WITH OSTEOARTHRITIS
4. **Which one of the following first ray joints is most commonly affected by osteoarthritis?**
   A. DIP joint
   B. PIP joint
   C. MP joint
   D. CMC joint
   E. STT joint

EXAMINATION OF THE OSTEOARTHRITIC HAND
5. **When examining a patient with osteoarthritis of the hand, where would you expect to find Heberden nodes?**
   A. DIP joint
   B. PIP joint
   C. MP joint
   D. Overlying the metacarpal
   E. At the wrist

THUMB CMC JOINT OSTEOARTHRITIS

6. A 60-year-old woman has a 1-year history of increasing pain at the base of her dominant thumb. She takes a regular analgesia and has tried wearing a custom thermoplastic splint, but these have not significantly helped her symptoms. Radiographs show Eaton grade IV arthritic changes affecting the thumb base. **What is the next most likely step in management for this patient?**
   A. Perform image-guided steroid injection to the CMC and ST joints.
   B. Perform CMC joint arthroplasty.
   C. Perform CMC joint fusion.
   D. Perform a standard trapeziectomy.
   E. Perform a trapeziectomy with LRTI.

MANAGING THUMB CMC JOINT OSTEOARTHRITIS

7. Select the most appropriate management for each of the following scenarios. (Each option may be used once, more than once, or not at all.)
   A. A 23-year-old woman presents with painful subluxing first CMC joints without degenerative changes.
   B. A 35-year-old rugby player presents with Eaton grade II posttraumatic first CMC joint osteoarthritis that only responded for 6 weeks to an image-guided steroid injection.
   C. A 65-year-old woman undergoing a trapeziectomy has significant degeneration of the distal scaphoid articulation with no metacarpal base collapse after resection.

   Options:
   a. Image-guided first CMC joint steroid injection
   b. Trapeziectomy alone
   c. Trapeziectomy plus LRTI
   d. First CMC joint fusion
   e. Volar beak and intermetacarpal ligament reconstruction
   f. First metacarpal osteotomy
   g. Pyrocarbon arthroplasty

MP JOINT OSTEOARTHRITIS

8. In a young patient with severe osteoarthritis in the middle finger MP joint following trauma, which one of the following interventions is most likely to provide him with the best result, assuming that his range of motion is 0 to 90 degrees in this joint?
   A. Steroid injection
   B. Silastic arthroplasty
   C. Arthrodesis
   D. Pyrocarbon arthroplasty
   E. Ray amputation

PIP JOINT OSTEOARTHRITIS

9. Which one of the following is most likely to fail in painful osteoarthritis of the dominant index finger PIP joint?
   A. Denervation of the PIP joint
   B. Silastic arthroplasty
   C. Arthrodesis–plating
   D. Pyrocarbon arthroplasty
   E. Arthrodesis–tension band technique

DIP JOINT OSTEOARTHRITIS

10. Which one of the following is correct regarding DIP joint osteoarthritis?
A. Severe deformity is always symptomatic.
B. It is frequently associated with Notta's nodes.
C. Joint fusion is commonly indicated.
D. It rarely presents with deformity of the nail plate.
E. Ideal fusion angles are less than for the PIP joint.

Answers

CLINICAL HISTORY

1. **When taking a history from a patient with osteoarthritis of the hands, which one of the following would be unusual?**
   A. Pain that is worse in the morning
   The pain experienced by patients with osteoarthritis (OA) of the upper limb is variable. It can be constant or intermittent and ranges from a dull ache to a sharp pain. Pain typically occurs with joint loading and repetitive movement, and it is often better in the morning and worse at night. This is in contrast to rheumatoid arthritis which tends to be more painful in the morning. OA frequently affects sleep patterns, and this is often a key factor in determining when surgical intervention is warranted. Subjective weakness is common and may result in part from pain and a reduced range of motion. It may be further exacerbated by the fact that many patients, particularly those with first CMC joint arthritis, also have carpal tunnel syndrome.

PLAIN RADIOGRAPHS IN OSTEOARTHRITIS

2. **Which one of the following tends to be an early finding in osteoarthritis on plain radiographs?**
   B. Joint space widening
   The classic radiographic features of osteoarthritis are joint space narrowing, subchondral sclerosis, and osteophyte formation (see Fig. 85-1, *Essentials of Plastic Surgery,* second edition). However, the earliest signs are actually joint space widening, secondary to inflammation. In advanced cases, joint subluxation may also occur. Periarticular erosions are associated with rheumatoid arthritis. Progressive subchondral sclerosis can lead to eburnation, which is the degeneration of bone into a hard, ivorylike mass and is seen in osteoarthritis. It explains why breaking up the trapezium during a trapeziectomy can sometimes seem to be disproportionately difficult.

IMAGING FOR OSTEOARTHRITIS OF THE THUMB

3. **Which one of the following radiographic views gives a true anteroposterior image of the thumb?**
   C. Robert's view
   For patients with suspected osteoarthritis of the first CMC joint, plain radiographs of the hand and wrist in the AP, lateral, and oblique planes are commonly ordered. Further views can sometimes be helpful; for example, Robert's view is a true AP view of the thumb and is taken with the hand in hyperpronation and the dorsum of the thumb against the cassette, which allows visualization of all four trapezoidal articulations. Eaton stress views are taken with the thumbs pressed together and may be useful to assess increased CMC joint laxity. Bett's/Gedda's view is a PA taken in pronation and flexion that gives a true lateral view of the trapezio-metacarpal joint. The other trapezial articulations are also clearly demonstrated. Waters' and Towne's views are both craniofacial radiographs used in assessment of facial trauma injuries (see Chapter 30).

JOINT INVOLVEMENT WITH OSTEOARTHRITIS

4. Which one of the following first ray joints is most commonly affected by osteoarthritis?

D. CMC joint

Although the DIP joint is the joint most commonly affected by osteoarthritis in the upper limb, the most commonly affected joint in the first ray is the CMC joint. When considering treatment for first CMC joint arthritis, it is important to look at the scaphoid-trapezium-trapezoid (STT) joint at the same time, because there may be disease between the scaphoid and trapezoid that could lead to persistent pain after trapeziectomy if it is not addressed.

EXAMINATION OF THE OSTEOARTHRITIC HAND

5. When examining a patient with osteoarthritis of the hand, where would you expect to find Heberden nodes?

A. DIP joint

Heberden nodes are found at the DIP joint in patients with osteoarthritis, while Bouchard nodes are located over the PIP joint. They both represent strong markers for IP joint osteoarthritis and have a familial trait. They were traditionally thought to represent osteophytes, but may actually represent traction spurs due to repetitive loading. They are sometimes painful, although often asymptomatic. They can also be associated with ganglia and mucous cysts. Other characteristic findings in the osteoarthritic hand include swelling and deviation of the digits, particularly at the IP joints and sometimes at the MP joints. There is usually a reduction in both active and passive joint motion with ligament instability.[1]

THUMB CMC JOINT OSTEOARTHRITIS

6. A 60-year-old woman has a 1-year history of increasing pain at the base of her dominant thumb. She takes a regular analgesia and has tried wearing a custom thermoplastic splint, but these have not significantly helped her symptoms. Radiographs show Eaton grade IV arthritic changes affecting the thumb base. What is the next most likely step in management for this patient?

A. Perform image-guided steroid injection to the CMC and ST joints.

This woman has radiographically advanced disease according to Eaton's classification and is likely to need surgical intervention at some point in the future. However, symptoms do not always correlate with radiologic findings, and nonoperative measures should be explored fully in the first instance. The next step in her management is to trial one or more intraarticular steroid injections, and image guidance can be very helpful in ensuring accurate steroid placement (particularly in the presence of subluxation and osteophyte formation).

Eaton's classification may be used to grade the radiographic changes observed in osteoarthritis and originally included four grades (Table 85-1). Grade IV disease involves degenerative destruction of both the first CMC joint and the scaphotrapezial (ST) joint. In this scenario, surgery that only addresses the CMC joint will not resolve the patient's symptoms; therefore neither CMC joint arthroplasty nor CMC joint fusion is appropriate for this woman. The likely surgical procedure of choice would be a trapeziectomy, and if this is performed, the remaining interface between the scaphoid and trapezoid must be inspected, since there is a likelihood of arthritic changes here, too, that can lead to persistent pain if left untreated. There is no consistent evidence that ligament reconstruction and tendon interposition (LRTI) is superior to simple trapeziectomy alone.

Table 85-1 Eaton's Radiographic Stages of CMC Joint Degeneration[2]

Stage	Radiographic Findings
I	Normal articulations with widening of joint space suggestive of an effusion, less than a third CMC joint subluxation
II	Slight narrowing of the thumb CMC joint, minimal subchondral sclerosis, debris/osteophytes <2 mm diameter, more than a third CMC joint subluxation
III	As per stage II, increased sclerosis, subchondral cysts, debris/osteophytes >2 mm diameter
IV	As per stage III, with narrowed ST joint demonstrating sclerosis and cysts
V	Pantrapezial arthritis

CMC, Carpometacarpal; ST, scaphotrapezial.

MANAGING THUMB CMC JOINT OSTEOARTHRITIS

7. For the following scenarios, the best options are as follows:
   A. A 23-year-old woman presents with painful subluxing first CMC joints without degenerative changes.
   e. **Volar beak and intermetacarpal ligament reconstruction**
   First CMC joint instability can occur in young healthy females who may present with painless but visible joint subluxation on thumb loading. Radiographs at rest may be normal, but on pushing the thumbs together during imaging, the dynamic changes may be revealed. Sometimes pain can prevent good stress-view imaging in more severe cases. In first CMC joint laxity, reconstruction of the joint capsule and volar ligamentous support using a partial FCR sling has shown good results in many patients, although the procedure is not recommended in the presence of Eaton grade II-IV arthritis, as the joint surface is not addressed.[3] Some authors have also described good results in patients with early joint changes using extension osteotomy of the metacarpal to alter joint biomechanics.[4]

   B. A 35-year-old rugby player presents with Eaton grade II posttraumatic first CMC joint osteoarthritis that only responded for 6 weeks to an image-guided steroid injection.
   d. **First CMC joint fusion**
   Patients with isolated first CMC joint degenerative changes can respond well to CMC joint fusion, and if a steroid injection has only been effective for 6 weeks despite image guidance to ensure accuracy, then further steroid injections are not going to be of sufficient benefit.

   C. A 65-year-old woman undergoing a trapeziectomy has significant degeneration of the distal scaphoid articulation with no metacarpal base collapse after resection.
   b. **Trapeziectomy alone**
   During a trapeziectomy, the degree of metacarpal collapse should be assessed after removal of the trapezium. If there is an endpoint on loading the thumb axially without abutment against the scaphoid, there is no definitive evidence that a ligament reconstruction with or without a tendon interposition procedure is likely to give additional benefit.[5]

   Pyrocarbon hemi-arthroplasty may be considered an option in some patients with severe CMC joint osteoarthritis. Implant survival rates of 80% have been reported[6] and favorable results in stage III and early stage IV have also been described.[7]

MP JOINT OSTEOARTHRITIS

In a young patient with severe osteoarthritis in the middle finger MP joint following trauma, which one of the following interventions is most likely to provide him with the best result, assuming that his range of motion is 0 to 90 degrees in this joint?

D. Pyrocarbon arthroplasty

The MP joints are not commonly affected by OA, unless as in this case, the condition is as a result of trauma. The best surgical option is arthroplasty, especially as joint range of motion is preserved. Given that this patient is young, a pyrocarbon arthroplasty is preferable to a silastic joint. The latter are reserved for older patients with poor soft tissue stability and lower physical demands. They are commonly used in rheumatoid arthritis. Arthroplasty is the last resort and even a ray amputation is likely to provide a superior result. Steroid injection is only likely to give a very limited, short-term response for this patient, given the extent of his joint disease.

PIP JOINT OSTEOARTHRITIS

Which one of the following is most likely to fail in painful osteoarthritis of the dominant index finger PIP joint?

B. Silastic arthroplasty

While arthrodesis and steroid injections are widely employed, arthroplasty for the PIP joint is less common. Patient selection and technical excellence are critical for successful pyrocarbon arthroplasty and index finger disease is a good indication for this option. A silicone or silastic implant is unlikely to be able to withstand the lateral stresses through the dominant index finger during pinch and key grips. For these reasons, many surgeons would choose arthrodesis over arthroplasty for the border digits. Good results have been reported following denervation procedures for some small joint arthritis.[8,9]

DIP JOINT OSTEOARTHRITIS

10. Which one of the following is correct regarding DIP joint osteoarthritis?

E. Ideal fusion angles are less than for the PIP joint.

If fusion is performed, the joint is usually fixed in 0 to 10 degrees of flexion, although more angulation is sometimes preferred in the index finger (see Fig. 85-3, *Essentials of Plastic Surgery*, second edition). This is in contrast to the PIP joint, which is fused between 20 and 40 degrees of flexion, depending upon the digit and functional requirements. The DIP joint is the most commonly affected joint in osteoarthritis but is frequently asymptomatic and does not often require surgical intervention, other than for excision of a mucous cyst. Nail deformity is often seen in DIP joint osteoarthritis in conjunction with a mucous cyst.

REFERENCES

1. Alexander CJ. Heberden's and Bouchard's nodes. Ann Rheum Dis 58:675-678, 1999.
2. Eaton RG, Glickel SZ. Trapeziometacarpal arthritis: staging as a rationale for treatment. Hand Clin 3:455-471, 1987.
3. Freedman DM, Eaton RG, Glickel SZ. Long-term results of volar ligament reconstruction for symptomatic basal joint laxity. J Hand Surg Am 25:297-304, 2000.
4. Parker WL, Linscheid RL, Amadio PC. Long-term outcomes of first metacarpal extension osteotomy in the treatment of carpal-metacarpal osteoarthritis. J Hand Surg Am 33:1737-1743, 2008.

5. Lane LB, Henley DH. Ligament reconstruction of the painful, unstable, nonarthritic thumb carpometacarpal joint. J Hand Surg Am 26:686-691, 2001.
6. Lorea P, Ezzedine R, Marchesi S. Denervation of the proximal interphalangeal joint: a realistic and simple procedure. Tech Hand Up Extrem Surg 8:262-265, 2004.
7. Loréa PD. First carpometacarpal joint denervation: anatomy and surgical technique. Tech Hand Up Extrem Surg 7:26-31, 2003.
8. Martinez de Aragon JS, Moran SL, Rizzo M, et al. Early outcomes of pyrolytic carbon hemiarthroplasty for the treatment of trapezial-metacarpal arthritis. J Hand Surg Am 34:205-212, 2009.
9. Badia A, Sambandam SN. Total joint arthroplasty in the treatment of advanced stages of thumb carpometacarpal joint osteoarthritis. J Hand Surg Am 31:1605-1614, 2006.

86. Vascular Disorders of the Hand and Wrist

See *Essentials of Plastic Surgery*, second edition, pp. 1026-1052.

UPPER EXTREMITY ANEURYSMS

1. *Which one of the following is true regarding upper extremity aneurysms?*
   A. Mycotic aneurysms are most often idiopathic.
   B. False aneurysms involve all three layers of the arterial wall.
   C. Most aneurysms of the upper limb occur secondary to trauma.
   D. True aneurysms are more common in the hand than false aneurysms.
   E. On radiologic imaging, false aneurysms have a fusiform shape.

ARTERIAL EMBOLI

2. A patient presents with evidence of a spontaneous acute arterial obstruction to the left upper limb. The hand and forearm are cool, pale, and painful. No distal pulses are palpable. *Which one of the following represents the standard approach to treatment?*
   A. Embolectomy and intraarterial urokinase
   B. Percutaneous intraarterial urokinase and a calcium channel blocker
   C. Intravenous heparin therapy and embolectomy
   D. Intravenous heparin therapy, embolectomy, and subsequent warfarin therapy
   E. Low-molecular-weight heparin and embolectomy

RAYNAUD'S DISEASE

3. A 50-year-old woman presents with a diagnosis of Raynaud's disease managed by her general practitioner. For the past 5 years she has had episodes in cold weather where her fingers become pale, then blue, before turning bright red. *Which one of the following is correct regarding this woman's condition?*
   A. She will also have signs of systemic sclerosis.
   B. Her diagnosis forms part of a systemic autoimmune condition.
   C. The age at which she first experienced symptoms is typical of this condition.
   D. She is likely to have been prescribed nifedipine by her own doctor.
   E. Vasospasm and hyperemia will be limited to the hands and feet.

THORACIC OUTLET SYNDROME

4. *Which one of the following statements is correct regarding neurologic thoracic outlet syndrome?*
   A. The most common cause is a cervical rib.
   B. Males and females are equally affected.
   C. Clinical examination is commonly unremarkable.
   D. Adson's test is a reliable provocative test.
   E. Surgery is always performed through an anterior approach.

HEMANGIOMAS

5. **Which one of the following statements is true of hemangiomas?**
   A. They are most often present at birth.
   B. All will eventually spontaneously involute.
   C. They are the most common tumor type in the hand.
   D. They are a type of vascular malformation.
   E. They do not normally require surgical intervention.

ARTERIOVENOUS MALFORMATIONS

6. **Which one of the following statements is correct regarding arteriovenous malformations?**
   A. They develop in utero during the first trimester.
   B. Their cause is well understood.
   C. Most malformations are familial.
   D. Females are more commonly affected than males.
   E. Malformations are clinically evident at birth.

GLOMUS TUMORS

7. **When examining a patient with a suspected glomus tumor, which one of the following is most likely to be true?**
   A. A consistent finding is a solitary painless lesion on the digit.
   B. Attempts to elicit Love's sign should be routinely used to confirm the diagnosis.
   C. Digital pain can be abolished by inflation of a blood pressure cuff.
   D. Abnormal skin color changes from white to blue then red are characteristically observed.
   E. The condition will be limited to the hand.

CLINICAL SCENARIOS

8. A right-hand-dominant, self-employed carpet fitter presents to clinic with cold intolerance and pain to the right little and ring fingers. Examination reveals early signs of ulceration to these digits. **Which one of the following represents the most likely diagnosis?**
   A. True aneurysm
   B. False aneurysm
   C. Venous thrombosis
   D. Glomus tumor
   E. Raynaud's phenomenon

9. A 54-year-old woman presents to clinic with a history of cold hypersensitivity and paroxysmal pain affecting the index fingertip. Examination shows a slight blue discoloration to the nail bed. **What is the most likely diagnosis?**
   A. Venous thrombosis
   B. Autoimmune vasculitis
   C. Hemangioma
   D. Lymphangioma
   E. Glomus tumor

10. A 7-year-old girl falls from a tree and sustains a left supracondylar humeral fracture. Her left hand is cold and pale before and after a closed fracture reduction. **Which one of the following is the next step in managing this patient?**
    A. Arteriography
    B. Doppler ultrasound
    C. Repeat plain radiographs
    D. MR angiography
    E. Urgent return to the operating room

DIAGNOSIS OF VASCULAR LIMB DISORDERS

11. *For each of the following clinical scenarios, select the most likely diagnosis from the list of options. (Each option may be used once, more than once, or not at all.)*
    A. *A 30-year-old left-hand-dominant soldier presents with a 3-month history of dull aching and swelling in the left arm. The pain is exacerbated by activity and the arm fatigues easily.*
    B. *A 26-year-old athlete has been working out at the gym and notices that his right arm has become swollen and purple with distended veins.*
    C. *A 36-year-old man presents to the clinic with a history of calf pain when walking. Examination reveals cool, pale feet with palpable pulses. His upper limbs are unaffected, but digital tar staining is evident.*

Options:
a. Buerger's disease
b. Arterial thrombosis
c. Venous thrombosis
d. True aneurysm
e. False aneurysm
f. Raynaud's disease
g. Thoracic outlet syndrome
h. Glomus tumor
i. Autoimmune vasculitis

Answers

UPPER EXTREMITY ANEURYSMS

1. Which one of the following is true regarding upper extremity aneurysms?
   C. Most aneurysms of the upper limb occur secondary to trauma.
   Most upper extremity aneurysms are caused by trauma and they are classified as either true or false according to the layers of the arterial wall involved. True aneurysms are less common than false aneurysms and involve all three layers of the arterial wall. They typically occur secondary to blunt trauma. False aneurysms are far more common and typically result from arterial perforation. Mycotic aneurysms are most commonly, though not exclusively, seen in intravenous drug users after injection with a dirty needle. They are not usually idiopathic and can also be caused by septic emboli. Radiologic imaging can differentiate between true and false aneurysms, which are fusiform or saccular-shaped, respectively.

ARTERIAL EMBOLI

2. A patient presents with evidence of a spontaneous acute arterial obstruction to the left upper limb. The hand and forearm are cool, pale, and painful. No distal pulses are palpable. *Which one of the following represents the standard approach to treatment?*
   D. Intravenous heparin therapy, embolectomy, and subsequent warfarin therapy
   The standard treatment for acute arterial obstruction is immediate intravenous heparin therapy in combination with an embolectomy using a Fogarty catheter. Subsequent anticoagulation treatment with either warfarin or low-molecular-weight heparin is required to prevent recurrence. Other newer medical therapies may be available including Rivaroxaban. Percutaneous intraarterial thrombolysis of the distal upper extremity is not standard practice but has been shown to be effective in select cases. When this is performed, both a thrombolytic agent such as urokinase and a calcium channel blocker are used to achieve simultaneous vasodilation and thrombolysis.
   Management of emboli secondary to penetrating trauma such as catheter-related brachial artery occlusions, are managed differently because many patients will continue to have compromised circulation even once the thrombosis is removed. In these cases it may be necessary to perform open repair of the involved artery with primary resection and repair, or an interposition vein graft. Long-term anticoagulation is not required in such cases.

RAYNAUD'S DISEASE

3. A 50-year-old woman presents with a diagnosis of Raynaud's disease managed by her general practitioner. For the past 5 years she has had episodes in cold weather where her fingers become pale, then blue, before turning bright red. *Which one of the following is correct regarding this woman's condition?*
   D. She is likely to have been prescribed nifedipine by her own doctor.
   Raynaud's disease and Raynaud's phenomenon are distinctly different, although the terms are often used interchangeably. Raynaud's disease is a condition that involves vasospasm alone, and this is most commonly treated with nifedipine, a calcium channel blocker. Raynaud's phenomenon

refers to reversible ischemia of peripheral arterioles in association with another illness, which is most commonly autoimmune. The most common association with Raynaud's phenomenon is scleroderma. In Raynaud's disease one or more body parts have intense vasospasm with associated pallor and often cyanosis, followed by a hyperemic phase. Fingers are most commonly affected, but the nose, ears, and toes may also be involved. Raynaud's disease can occur at any age, although commonly begins in the second or third decade and is not the typical age of first presentation in this case. Raynaud's disease tends to present later in adult life. *(Note that some texts refer to Raynaud's disease as primary Raynaud's and Raynaud's phenomenon as secondary Raynaud's.)*

THORACIC OUTLET SYNDROME

4. Which one of the following statements is correct regarding neurologic thoracic outlet syndrome?
C. Clinical examination is commonly unremarkable.

Clinical examination findings are usually normal in thoracic outlet syndrome (TOS). Although cervical ribs are involved in most arterial cases, they are rarely present in venous and neurologic cases. The most common site of neurologic compression is the scalene triangle (between the anterior scalene, middle scalene, and upper border of the first rib) and many patients have congenital fibromuscular bands in this region. Females are more commonly affected by TOS than males, and this difference is most apparent in neurologic TOS, with a ratio of 3.5:1.

Adson's test assesses the radial pulse during compression of the subclavian artery with positional change but is unreliable, since patients without TOS may have considerable positional pulse variation.[1] Surgical decompression may be performed through axillary, anterior supraclavicular, or posterior subscapular approaches.

HEMANGIOMAS

5. Which one of the following statements is true of hemangiomas?
E. They do not normally require surgical intervention.

Hemangiomas are a type of vascular tumor that may arise in utero or during the first few weeks of life. They are therefore classified as either infantile or congenital, depending on the time of first presentation. They are distinctly different from vascular malformations.[2] Classic infantile lesions show three phases of growth, with first appearance as a vascular papule followed by rapid growth then involution. By age seven, approximately 70% of infantile hemangiomas have spontaneously involuted, but not all subtypes do so. Congenital hemangiomas are mature at birth and are classified by their natural history as either rapidly involuting (RICH) or noninvoluting (NICH). Because most hemangiomas involute, surgical intervention is not usually required. Problematic hemangiomas, such as those that ulcerate or occlude orifices, may be treated with either surgery, sclerotherapy, laser therapy, or beta blocker medication.

ARTERIOVENOUS MALFORMATIONS

6. Which one of the following statements is correct regarding arteriovenous malformations?
A. They develop in utero during the first trimester.

Vascular malformations are inborn errors in embryonic development that occur between weeks 4 and 10 of intrauterine growth. The causes are not well understood and most occur spontaneously. Males and females are equally affected, and although all malformations are present at birth, they may not be clinically evident. For example, a triggering stimulus during puberty or pregnancy can precipitate the first clinical signs of the malformation.

GLOMUS TUMORS

7. When examining a patient with a suspected glomus tumor, which one of the following is most likely to be true?
C. Digital pain can be abolished by inflation of a blood pressure cuff.

Hildreth's sign is observed in patients with glomus tumors of the hand, when pain is abolished on exsanguination of the limb and inflation of a blood pressure cuff. There is supporting evidence to show the efficacy of this test in diagnosis of glomus tumors, with sensitivity and specificity above 90%.[3]

Glomus tumors are benign vascular lesions containing cells from the glomus apparatus involved in thermoregulation that commonly affect the nail bed and fingertip. They often present as a bluish discoloration under the nail plate, with or without nail ridging. Although lesions are often painful and solitary, this is not always the case and multiple painful or painless lesions may be present.

Love's sign is elicited when point pressure is applied to the nail bed with a pinhead at the site of the tumor, resulting in intense pain. There are usually enough other signs to make a diagnosis without performing this test, which is clearly unpleasant for the patient.

The skin color changes described are more characteristic of those described by patients themselves with Raynaud's disease, where the hand passes through a series of vascular changes: white (pallor), blue (cyanosis), and red (hyperemia). Although most cases of glomus tumor (75%) are found in the hand, the condition is not exclusively seen in this site. They may be present in the toes or in extracutaneous sites such as bone and the gastrointestinal tract. Following examination, further imaging with ultrasound or MRI may be useful. Treatment is with surgical excision.[4,5]

CLINICAL SCENARIOS

8. A right-hand-dominant, self-employed carpet fitter presents to clinic with cold intolerance and pain to the right little and ring fingers. Examination reveals early signs of ulceration to these digits. *Which one of the following represents the most likely diagnosis?*
A. True aneurysm

This patient has hypothenar hammer syndrome where repetitive blunt trauma leads to a true aneurysm (not false) of the ulnar artery in the area of Guyon's canal. This typically occurs in upholsterers and carpet layers. The trauma results in tunica media damage followed by the aneurysm formation and then eventual arterial thrombosis (not venous). If neglected, the digits can ulcerate and it may be necessary to replace the damaged segment of artery with a vein graft.

Venous thrombosis typically presents with a swollen upper limb with signs of venous congestion such as skin discoloration. Glomus tumors are discussed in questions 7 and 9, and Raynaud's phenomenon is discussed in question 3. Neither of these conditions would present as in this scenario.

9. A 54-year-old woman presents to clinic with a history of cold hypersensitivity and paroxysmal pain affecting the index fingertip. Examination shows a slight blue discoloration to the nail bed. *What is the most likely diagnosis?*
   E. Glomus tumor
   This woman has the typical features of a glomus tumor, which is a benign vascular lesion commonly affecting the fingertip. The glomus apparatus contains an AV shunt that contributes to temperature regulation. The classic triad observed with glomus tumors is cold hypersensitivity, paroxysmal pain, and pinpoint tenderness (see question 7).

10. A 7-year-old girl falls from a tree and sustains a left supracondylar humeral fracture. Her left hand is cold and pale before and after a closed fracture reduction. *Which one of the following is the next step in managing this patient?*
    E. Urgent return to the operating room
    This patient has sustained a common childhood fracture that risks damage to the brachial artery both during the initial injury and during fracture reduction. Loss of arterial flow can occur due to direct compression of the artery within the fracture site or secondary to arterial thrombosis following intimal damage. A persistent abnormality after fracture reduction requires urgent investigation and warrants operative exploration. Brachial artery thrombectomy ± arterial repair or vein grafting should be anticipated. No further imaging is required in this case, but noninvasive Doppler studies may be helpful in documenting abnormal perfusion in the injured extremity, where there remains uncertainty about distal perfusion. Arteriography is best avoided in children because of the risk of iatrogenic damage.

DIAGNOSIS OF VASCULAR LIMB DISORDERS

11. *For the following scenarios, the best options are as follows:*
    A. *A 30-year-old left-hand-dominant soldier presents with a 3-month history of dull aching and swelling in the left arm. The pain is exacerbated by activity and the arm fatigues easily.*
       g. Thoracic outlet syndrome
       The patient in this scenario is most likely to have thoracic outlet syndrome with an arterial component. This would explain the exercise-induced ischemic pain he is experiencing and the time frame over which the problems have been present. The swelling suggests a concomitant venous component to the compression.
    B. *A 26-year-old athlete has been working out at the gym and notices that his right arm has become swollen and purple with distended veins.*
       c. Venous thrombosis
       The patient in this scenario has evidence of acute onset venous thrombosis of the upper limb. This is called *effort vein thrombosis* when associated with vigorous upper limb exercise, as in this case, and can cause an acute venous thoracic outlet obstruction.
    C. *A 36-year-old man presents to the clinic with a history of calf pain when walking. Examination reveals cool, pale feet with palpable pulses. His upper limbs are unaffected, but digital tar staining is evident.*
       a. Buerger's disease
       The patient in this scenario demonstrates features of Buerger's disease, which include intermittent claudication of the lower limbs, poor lower limb perfusion, and sparing of the upper limbs in a young person who smokes heavily.

REFERENCES

1. Plewa MC, Delinger M. The false-positive rate of thoracic outlet shoulder maneuvers in healthy subjects. Acad Emerg Med 5:337-342, 1998.
2. Mulliken JB, Glowacki J. Classification of pediatric vascular lesions. Plast Reconstr Surg 70:120-121, 1982.
3. Giele H. Hildreth's test is a reliable clinical sign for the diagnosis of glomus tumors. J Hand Surg Br 27:157-158, 2002.
4. Vasisht B, Watson HK, Joseph E, et al. Digital glomus tumors: a 29-year experience with a lateral subperiosteal approach. Plast Reconstr Surg 114:1486-1489, 2004.
5. Al-Qattan MM, Al-Namla A, Al-Thunayan A, et al. Magnetic resonance imaging in the diagnosis of glomus tumours of the hand. J Hand Surg Br 30:535-540, 2005.

Part VII

Aesthetic Surgery

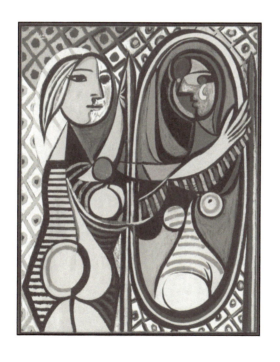

© 2015 Estate of Pablo Picasso / Artists Rights Society (ARS), New York.

87. Facial Analysis

See *Essentials of Plastic Surgery*, second edition, pp. 1055-1064.

SKIN QUALITY

1. A patient is referred to clinic unhappy with their facial appearance. The referring practitioner has assessed this patient using the Glogau classification. **What key information will this provide regarding the patient?**
- A. Their response to sun exposure
- B. Their age and gender
- C. Their degree of photoaging
- D. Their prior treatment
- E. Their required treatment

THE FIBONACCI RATIO

2. When discussing aesthetically pleasing facial proportions, the Fibonacci ratio is often quoted. **Which one of the following numbers represents this "golden ratio"?**
- A. 1:1.33
- B. 1:1.62
- C. 1:2.33
- D. 1:2.62
- E. 1:4.33

FACIAL CANONS OF DIVINE PROPORTION

3. *According to the classical description of facial canons, which one of the following statements is correct?*
- A. The horizontal midpoint of the head is the nasal base.
- B. The length of the ear equals the length of the nose.
- C. The nasal width is one third of the facial width.
- D. The nose occupies one quarter of the facial height.
- E. The mouth has twice the width of the nose.

ASSESSMENT OF THE FACE FROM THE FRONTAL VIEW

4. *When considering the "ideal" facial proportions in the frontal view, which one of the following is correct?*
- A. The lateral and medial canthi can be used to divide the face into vertical thirds.
- B. The width of the mouth and the vertical stomion-to-menton distance are equal.
- C. The distance between the medial canthi should approximate the width of the mouth.
- D. Facial width at the malar level is similar to the vertical distance from the anterior hairline to the menton.
- E. The upper lip vermilion marks the vertical midpoint of the lower third of the face.

ASSESSMENT OF THE FACE FROM THE LATERAL VIEW

5. **When considering the "ideal" facial proportions in the lateral view, which one of the following is correct?**
   A. The facial profile is usually divided into horizontal fifths.
   B. The vertical hairline-to-menton distance is approximately three times the mandibular angle to the menton distance.
   C. The lower lip should project 2 mm further than the upper lip.
   D. The nasolabial angle is normally more acute in female patients.
   E. The ear lobule and nasal base lie at similar horizontal levels.

ANALYSIS OF THE UPPER EYELID

6. **When assessing a white patient with normal upper eyelid anatomy in forward gaze, which one of the following is expected?**
   A. A neutral intercanthal axis
   B. An intercanthal distance of 38 mm
   C. Vertical eye opening greater than 15 mm
   D. Upper lid level with the upper limbus
   E. A supratarsal fold 10 mm from the lash line

FACIAL PROPORTIONS

7. **When considering the relative proportions of the face, which one of the following normally has the same measurement as intercanthal distance?**
   A. Eye width
   B. Ear width
   C. Nose width
   D. Mouth width
   E. Chin width

ANALYSIS OF THE NOSE

8. **When assessing the aesthetics of a white nose, which one of the following is correct?**
   A. Deviation is best assessed by drawing a line from the radix to the supratip break.
   B. Nasal length is most accurately measured from the radix to the columella base.
   C. Tip rotation may appear increased secondary to a prominent caudal septum.
   D. Tip projection should be approximately one third of the nasal length.
   E. The dorsal nasal line lies more anteriorly in females in the lateral view.

ANALYSIS OF THE EXTERNAL EAR

9. **When assessing a patient with normal ears, which one of the following would be expected?**
   A. Posterior inclination of 40 degrees from the vertical in the lateral view
   B. Slight projection of the helix beyond the antihelix in the anterior view
   C. The top of ear sited level with the superior brow in the lateral view
   D. Lateral inclination of 5 degrees from the vertical in the anterior view
   E. An ear height to width ratio of 3:1 in the lateral view

Answers

SKIN QUALITY

1. A patient is referred to clinic unhappy with their facial appearance. The referring practitioner has assessed this patient using the Glogau classification. **What key information will this provide regarding the patient?**
   C. Their degree of photoaging
   When assessing a patient's face during a cosmetic consult, assessment of photoaging is vital, as this can affect treatment selection and outcome following treatment. Photoaging forms a key part of the Glogau classification system.[1] See Table 87-2, *Essentials of Plastic Surgery,* second edition, which considers many of the key signs of photoaging including degree of wrinkling, scarring, pigmentary changes, and actinic damage. It also considers the requirement for make-up and the age group, but not gender or specific patient age. It does not provide information on prior or required treatment, although this would be a useful addition. The ideal classification system should guide treatment and facilitate comparison of results of different treatments between patient groups.

   There are some other useful classification systems other than the Glogau system. These include the Fitzpatrick,[2,3] Shiffman,[4] and Ellenbogen[5] systems.

   There are two different Fitzpatrick classifications relevant to photoaging. The most commonly used system assesses different skin types, ranging from I to VI, with white individuals representing types I to III and those with darker skin tones representing types IV to VI. This system is often used as a measure of patients' susceptibility to sun damage with respect to skin cancer.[2] There is also a separate Fitzpatrick classification (not the same author) for wrinkles that has three grades ranging from fine to deep wrinkles.[3]

   The Shiffman[4] classification is used to assess facial aging and considers four factors: tear trough depth, cheek fat loss, nasolabial fold depth, and jowl prominence. The Ellenbogen classification considers aspects of the neck that change with age: the cervicomental angle, the inferior mandibular border, the presence of subhyoid depression, and the visibility of thyroid cartilage and sternocleidomastoid.[5,6]

THE FIBONACCI RATIO

2. When discussing aesthetically pleasing facial proportions, the Fibonacci ratio is often quoted. **Which one of the following numbers represents this "golden ratio"?**
   B. 1:1.62
   The Fibonacci sequence is a set of numbers starting with a 1 or 0. The number sequence proceeds as 1, 2, 3, 5, 8, 13 ... where two consecutive numbers add up to form the next number. The so-called "golden ratio" between a given number and the preceding number is 1:1.62. (e.g. 13/8 = 1.62). This ratio, termed *Phi,* is characteristic of forms with aesthetically pleasing proportions and is highly relevant to relative facial proportions. Many examples are found in

nature; a good example is the external ear, which displays a spiral pattern conforming to Fibonacci ratios (Fig. 87-1).

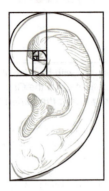

Fig. 87-1 The external ear, demonstrating the Fibonacci spiral.

FACIAL CANONS OF DIVINE PROPORTION

3. *According to the classical description of facial canons, which one of the following statements is correct?*
   B. The length of the ear equals the length of the nose.
   The facial canons of proportion were formulated and documented by artists of the Renaissance (Fig. 87-2). According to these descriptions, the length of the ear and nose are equal. The head can be divided into equal horizontal halves or quarters and the face can be divided into equal horizontal thirds. The horizontal midpoint of the head is the nasal bridge and not the nasal base. Nasal width at the alar base is one quarter of the facial width. The mouth is 1.5 times the width of the nasal base.

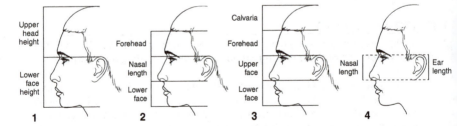

Fig. 87-2 Neoclassical canons. **1,** The head can be divided into equal halves at a horizontal line through the eyes. **2,** The face can be divided into equal thirds, with the nose occupying the middle third. **3,** The head can be divided into equal quarters, with the middle quarters being the forehead and nose. **4,** The length of the ear is equal to the length of the nose.

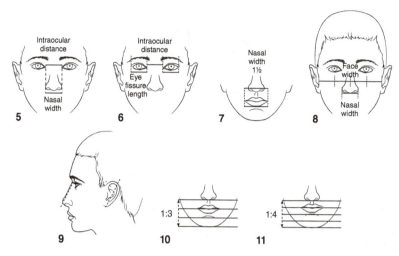

Fig. 87-2, cont'd **5,** The distance between the eyes is equal to the width of the nose. **6,** The distance between the eyes is equal to the width of each eye (the face width can be divided into equal fifths). **7,** The width of the mouth is 1½ times the width of the nose. **8,** The width of the nose is one fourth the width of the face. **9,** The nasal bridge inclination is the same as the ear inclination. **10,** The lower face can be divided into equal thirds. **11,** The lower face can be divided into equal quarters.

ASSESSMENT OF THE FACE FROM THE FRONTAL VIEW

4. When considering the "ideal" facial proportions in the frontal view, which one of the following is correct?
   B. The width of the mouth and the vertical stomion-to-menton distance are equal.
   Facial proportions, angles, and contours vary with race, age, and sex, but there are certain measurements considered to represent aesthetic ideals. The width of the mouth and the vertical distance between the stomion and menton should be equal in a patient with a normal chin (Fig. 87-3, see also Fig. 87-2, *Essentials of Plastic Surgery*, second edition).
   The lateral and medial canthi can be used to divide the face into vertical fifths (not thirds). It is the distance between the medial limbus of each cornea and not the distance between the medial canthi that equates to the mouth width. Mouth width is approximately 1.5 times the width of the intercanthal distance. Facial width at the malar level is similar to the vertical distance from the brows (not the anterior hairline) to the menton. The lower lip vermilion (not the upper) marks the vertical midpoint of the lower third of the face.

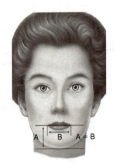

Fig. 87-3 Stomion to menton *(A)* and the width of the mouth *(B)* are equidistant.

ASSESSMENT OF THE FACE FROM THE LATERAL VIEW

5. When considering the "ideal" facial proportions in the lateral view, which one of the following is correct?
   E. The ear lobule and nasal base lie at similar horizontal levels.

The facial profile can be divided into horizontal thirds by drawing transverse lines at the nasal base and nasal root. The desired lip-chin complex relationship is an upper lip that projects approximately 2 mm more than the lower lip. In women, the chin lies slightly posterior to the lower lip. The lower third of the face can be further subdivided into upper third and lower two thirds by drawing a transverse line at the level of the oral commissure (not the upper lip vermilion). The vertical hairline to menton distance is approximately twice (not three times) the mandibular angle to the menton distance (Fig. 87-4).

The nasolabial angle is measured by drawing a straight line through the most anterior and posterior points of the nostrils on lateral view. Where this line bisects with a perpendicular line to the natural horizontal facial plane is the nasolabial angle. Women tend to have more obtuse nasolabial angles than men (95 to 100 degrees compared with 90 to 95 degrees). The ear lobule and nasal base lie at similar horizontal levels.

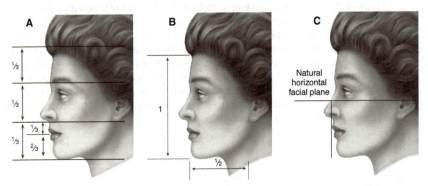

Fig. 87-4 A, Horizontal thirds. **B,** Distance from the mandibular angle to menton is half the distance from the hairline to the menton. **C,** Desired lip-chin complex relationship.

ANALYSIS OF THE UPPER EYELID

6. When assessing a white patient with normal upper eyelid anatomy in forward gaze, which one of the following is expected?
E. A supratarsal fold 10 mm from the lash line

When assessing the normal upper eyelid, the skin quality, fat herniation, and soft tissues should all be assessed. The supratarsal fold is between 7 and 11 mm above the lash line. There is usually a tilt to the intercanthal axis with the lateral canthus sited higher than the medial canthus. A normal intercanthal distance is 31 to 33 mm; however, a slightly increased distance (33 to 36 mm) may be considered attractive. Vertical eye opening is normally around 10 mm and the upper eyelid should sit just below (not at the same level as) the upper limbus.

FACIAL PROPORTIONS

7. When considering the relative proportions of the face, which one of the following normally has the same measurement as intercanthal distance?
A. Eye width

Many facial structures share similar proportions. The intercanthal distance is a good example of this, with a number of other measurements being equal to it. These include eye width, alar base width, nasal projection and the vertical distance between the infraorbital rim and the nasal base. Ear width is not equivalent to these distances. However, the ear does share some proportions with other facial components, for example, ear length is the same as nasal length and ear width is approximately half of ear length in most individuals. Nose width is a nonspecific measurement, as the nose differs in width from root to alar base. The alar base width is the widest part of the nose and this does match the intercanthal distance. The nasal body width is normally 80% of the nasal base width. Mouth and chin widths are essentially the same as one another and are usually 1.5 times the width of the nose at its widest point (i.e., alar base). When any of these typical distances do not match, it is important to identify why this is the case. For example, alar flaring or lack of nasal tip projection can increase the alar base width. Ethnicity also affects these measurements, for example, black patients tend to have broader nasal bridges and more alar flaring.

ANALYSIS OF THE NOSE

8. When assessing the aesthetics of a white nose, which one of the following is correct?
C. Tip rotation may appear increased secondary to a prominent caudal septum.

Tip rotation is determined by the degree of the nasolabial angle. The nasolabial angle is measured by drawing a straight line through the most anterior and posterior points of the nostrils on lateral view, and noting the point this bisects with a perpendicular line to the natural horizontal facial plane. The angle between these lines represents the nasolabial angle and varies from 90 to 100 degrees, depending on gender and race (Fig. 87-5).

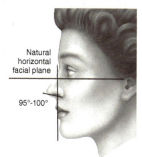

Fig. 87-5 Nasolabial angle.

It is important to be aware of other factors that may give the appearance of increased tip projection. For example, a prominent caudal septum can give this appearance, even when the nasolabial angle is within normal range. Understanding these principles is key to rhinoplasty, which is further discussed in Chapter 96. Also, a nose with a high dorsum without a supratip break will appear less rotated than one with a low dorsum and supratip break, even though the degree of rotation is the same.

Nasal deviation is best assessed by drawing a plumb line from the midglabellar point to the menton. This line should bisect the nasal bridge, nasal tip, and Cupid's bow (Fig. 87-6).

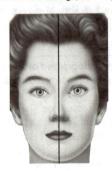

Fig. 87-6 Deviation of the nose is evaluated by drawing a line from the midglabella to the menton.

Nasal length is the distance from the radix to the tip and should be 1.5 times nasal tip projection (see Fig. 87-5, *Essentials of Plastic Surgery,* second edition). The dorsal nasal line typically lies 2 mm posterior to and parallel with a line connecting the nasofrontal angle with the desired tip projection. In men it lies slightly more anteriorly.

ANALYSIS OF THE EXTERNAL EAR

9. **When assessing a patient with normal ears, which one of the following would be expected?**
   B. **Slight projection of the helix beyond the antihelix in the anterior view**
   Understanding of external ear aesthetics is critical to ear reconstruction and correction of ear deformities such as prominent ear. In the anterior view, the helix should be slightly more prominent (approximately 5 mm) than the antehelical fold (Fig. 87-7).

   Overcorrection of the prominent ear can leave the antihelix as the most prominent part of the ear, resulting in an unnatural appearance and increased risk of development of pressure damage to the ear that may result in *chondrodermatitis nodularis helicis*. The ear usually measures 5 to 6.5 cm high and 2 to 3.5 cm wide. The ratio of width to height is usually 55% to 60%. The ear is normally placed with its superior aspect level with the upper eyelid and just below the lateral-most part of the eyebrow and around 5 to 6 cm posterior to the lateral orbital rim. It is inclined posteriorly in the lateral view about 20 degrees. It is inclined laterally from the scalp in the anterior view (20 to 30 degrees) and this means that the top of the ear is about 1.5 to 2 cm from the scalp.[7]

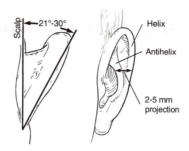

Fig. 87-7 Normal ear aesthetics.

REFERENCES

1. Glogau RG. Aesthetic and anatomic analysis of the aging skin. Semin Cutan Med Surg 15:134-138, 1996.
2. Fitzpatrick TB. The validity and practicality of sun-reactive skin types I through VI. Arch Dermatol 124:869, 1988.
3. Fitzpatrick RE, Goldman MP, Satur et al. Pulsed carbon dioxide laser resurfacing of photo-aged facial skin. Arch Dermatol 132:395-402, 1996.
4. Shiffman MA, Mirrafati SJ, Lam SM, eds. Simplified Facial Rejuvenation. New York: Springer, 2008.
5. Ellenbogen R, Karlin V. Visual criteria for success in restoring the youthful neck. Plast Reconstr Surg 66:826-837, 1980.
6. O'Brien M. Plastic & Hand Surgery in Clinical Practice—Classifications and Definitions. New York: Springer, 2009.
7. Janis JE, Rohrich, RJ, Gutowski, KA. Otoplasty. Plast Reconstr Surg 115:60e-72e, 2005.

88. Nonoperative Facial Rejuvenation

See *Essentials of Plastic Surgery*, second edition, pp. 1065-1098.

ACTINIC DAMAGE
1. **Which one of the following statements is relevant to the Fitzpatrick skin type classification?**
   A. The degree of wrinkling
   B. The use of make-up
   C. The presence of actinic damage
   D. The response to sun exposure
   E. The age of the patient

CHRONOLOGIC AGING
2. **Which one of the following is most likely to be increased in aging skin?**
   A. Epidermal thickness
   B. Dermal thickness
   C. The number of fibroblasts
   D. The amount of collagen and elastin
   E. The ratio of collagen type III to I

Laser and Light Resurfacing

WAVELENGTHS OF DIFFERENT RESURFACING MODALITIES
3. **Which one of the following resurfacing modalities uses a wavelength of 2940 nm and is a popular tool for ablative resurfacing?**
   A. Fractionated CO_2
   B. CO_2 laser
   C. Er:YAG
   D. Nd:YAG
   E. IPL

4. **Which one of the following laser modalities has a variant with a higher wavelength developed to use water as a target chromophore in order to achieve a more effective nonablative facial rejuvenation?**
   A. Nd:YAG
   B. Er:YAG
   C. Fractional resurfacing
   D. Fractionated CO_2
   E. IPL

CHROMOPHORES IN REJUVENATION THERAPY

5. Which one of the following resurfacing modalities uses blue dye as a target chromophore?

A. CO_2
B. Er:YAG
C. IPL
D. Nd:YAG
E. Fractional photothermolysis

CO_2 LASER

6. You are planning to use CO_2 laser resurfacing in your aesthetic practice. Which one of the following is correct regarding its use in resurfacing?

A. It is a particularly effective treatment that is mainly indicated for superficial rhytids.
B. A major strength of this technique is the minimal downtime after treatment.
C. The target chromophore is collagen at a wavelength of 10,600 nm.
D. It represents the best treatment option for patients with skin dyschromias.
E. The clinical endpoint is evidenced by pale yellow coloration to the skin.

LASER AND LIGHT REJUVENATION TECHNIQUES

7. For each of the following clinical scenarios, select the most likely previous rejuvenation therapy undertaken from the options listed. (Each answer may be used once, more than once, or not at all.)

A. You see a 37-year-old white man in your office who underwent laser resurfacing under the care of another clinician for acne scarring 12 months ago. He remembers the healing time to be quite extensive, with scabbing at the scar sites, and he is now concerned about obvious pale patches that are visible on both cheeks.

B. You are obtaining a history from a 45-year-old woman who previously underwent laser rejuvenation treatment with another physician. She is unable to recall which type of laser was used but states that she heard a popping sound during the treatment received under local anesthetic and sedation.

C. You see a 51-year-old woman who underwent a series of four treatments at weekly intervals for patches of facial dyschromia. She is delighted with the excellent results and wishes to consider other rejuvenation techniques.

Options:
a. Er:YAG laser
b. Nd-YAG laser
c. CO_2 laser
d. Intense pulsed light
e. Fractional photothermolysis

SELECTION OF LASER/LIGHT THERAPIES FOR FACIAL REJUVENATION

8. For each of the following clinical scenarios, select the best rejuvenation therapy from the options listed. (Each option may be used once, more than once, or not at all.)
   A. A 65-year-old retired woman wishes to have a face-lift procedure. She has Fitzpatrick type III skin with deep rhytids affecting her forehead and periorbital and perioral areas. She stopped smoking 5 years ago.
   B. A 33-year-old woman has fine, static rhytids developing in the crow's-feet and forehead regions. She has pale skin with mild dyschromia. The patient works in the media and has a hectic schedule. She has been receiving Botox injections as a preventive therapy for 12 months and requests minimal downtime for any treatments.
   C. A 45-year-old head teacher has requested facial rejuvenation at the start of the summer vacation. She has Fitzpatrick skin type IV and deep facial rhytids. She dislikes hospitals and wants a minimum number of treatments. She needs to be able to return to work after 4 weeks and does not want people to know she has received treatment.

Options:
   a. Er:YAG laser
   b. Nd-YAG laser
   c. CO_2 laser
   d. Intense pulsed light
   e. Fractional photothermolysis

TREATMENT OF FACIAL RHYTIDS WITH ABLATIVE LASER THERAPY

9. You see a 68-year-old man who has Fitzpatrick type IV skin and thick, deep static rhytids in the forehead, crow's-feet, and midface. He has lived and worked in hot climates for many years and has considerable actinic damage. He has recurrent cold sores. His wife has undergone resurfacing with Er:YAG laser therapy and is pleased with the results. Accordingly, he is now interested in having this treatment. **When discussing this treatment for this patient, which one of the following is correct?**
   A. Treatment can be begun immediately once a treatment decision is made.
   B. He could achieve similarly good results with a deep chemical peel or CO_2 laser treatment.
   C. He has a 20% approximate risk of developing posttreatment hypopigmentation.
   D. Erythema duration will be less than with a CO_2 laser for the same depth of resurfacing.
   E. He would not be at risk of developing milia or hypertrophic scarring because of his age.

INTENSE PULSED LIGHT (IPL)

10. A 37-year-old pregnant woman is concerned about her facial appearance. She has pale, thin skin with small areas of telangectasia, dyschromia, and poor general texture. She has read about IPL treatment and wonders whether this will be a suitable treatment for her condition. **Which one of the following is correct regarding IPL in this setting?**
    A. She would require a pretreatment regimen before undergoing therapy.
    B. The limitations of this treatment would not be able to address her skin problems.
    C. A major benefit of this treatment is that it can be completed in a single session.
    D. Use of this treatment modality is currently contraindicated for this patient.
    E. If more than one treatment is required, these can be performed on successive days.

Chemical Peels

PRETREATMENT FOR CHEMICAL PEELS

11. A 50-year-old woman comes to the clinic requesting facial rejuvenation with a chemical peel. She has Fitzpatrick type II thick, oily skin with moderate wrinkling and laxity and minimal dyschromia. She smokes 10 cigarettes per day and currently has no specific skin care regimen. *Which one of the following is incorrect regarding a pretreatment regimen for this woman?*
A. Smoking cessation and avoidance of sun exposure are key to the treatment plan.
B. Daily skin care should include a buffing grain cleanser, an alpha-hydroxy acid toner, and a vitamin A conditioning lotion.
C. Inclusion of a monthly glycolic acid peel should be considered before treatment.
D. Tretinoin should be prescribed in conjunction with high factor sunscreen.
E. She requires prescription of a tyrosinase inhibitor to minimize posttreatment hyperpigmentation.

ALPHA-HYDROXY ACID PEELS (AHA)

12. A patient has been using glycolic acid peels at home with modest effects and now wishes to know what benefits an office-based approach may offer her. *What is the main benefit of an office-based approach to glycolic acid peels?*
A. Multiple coats of the peeling agent can be applied in a single session.
B. Different acids can be combined to enhance effectiveness.
C. A local anesthetic is administered.
D. Higher concentrations of acid can be used.
E. The peel can be safely left on for a longer duration.

JESSNER'S SOLUTION

13. *Which one of the following is correct regarding Jessner's solution?*
A. It is used solely as a superficial peel.
B. The solution includes salicylic, trichloroacetic, and lactic acids.
C. The number of coats has little effect on penetration depth.
D. It should be neutralized with water after creation of a light frost.
E. It works in a different manner than that of alpha-hydroxy acids.

TRICHLOROACETIC ACID PEELS

14. *What is the clinical endpoint of a deep trichloroacetic acid (TCA) peel?*
A. A foggy white frost
B. A foggy white frost on an erythematous base
C. An epidermal slide
D. An intense white to yellow blanch
E. The accordion sign

PHENOL PEELS

15. *What has been proposed to be the main active ingredient in a Baker-Gordon phenol peel?*
A. Phenol
B. Emulsifying agent
C. Croton oil
D. Septisol
E. Acetic acid

16. **What is the main risk when using high concentration phenol peels?**
    A. Anaphylactic reaction
    B. Full-thickness dermal injury
    C. Respiratory collapse
    D. Gastrointestinal cramps
    E. Cardiac arrhythmias

Botulinum Toxin and Injectable Fillers

BOTULINUM TOXIN

17. Botulinum toxins are derived from the bacterium *Clostridium botulinum*. **Which one of the following statements is correct regarding their use in facial aesthetics?**
    A. Toxin subtypes A and B are commercially available for facial rejuvenation.
    B. All subtypes work through direct interaction with a protein called *SNAP-25*.
    C. Subtypes A and B have FDA approval for use in bunny lines and perioral wrinkles.
    D. Units are measured in mouse units and are comparable between different manufacturers.
    E. Toxins cause temporary chemodenervation by preventing binding and release of acetylcholine.

ADMINISTRATION OF BOTOX FOR FACIAL REJUVENATION

18. You are preparing some Botox for a 30-year-old woman who has requested treatment for her frown line (glabellar) region. It is her first experience with Botox injections. **Which one of the following is correct?**
    A. A standard dilution should be 4 units/ml in water for injection.
    B. Reconstitution involves firmly shaking the bottle to mix it fully.
    C. The product should be used within 4 hours of reconstitution.
    D. A typical starting dose for this woman would be 20 units.
    E. Four to six injections should be used, each placed above the orbital rim.

CONSTITUENTS OF DIFFERENT FILLERS

19. For each of the following descriptions of fillers used in facial rejuvenation, select the most likely trade name from the options listed. (Each option may be used once, more than once, or not at all.)
    A. *A hyaluronic acid derivative with midsized particles*
    B. *A calcium hydroxyapatite synthetic injectable*
    C. *A synthetic filler containing poly-L-lactic acid*

    Options:
    a. Radiesse
    b. Perlane
    c. Juvéderm Ultra Plus
    d. Artefill
    e. Sculptra
    f. Restylane

HYALURONIC ACID

20. You are using a hyaluronic acid derivative as an injectable filler in your cosmetic practice. **Which one of the following is true of this filler?**
    A. A pretreatment skin test is normally required.
    B. Further tissue expansion following injection is unlikely.
    C. Effectiveness decreases with repeated injections.
    D. Incorrectly placed product is difficult to correct.
    E. Injections are painful and best combined with lidocaine.

USE OF ARTEFILL AS AN INJECTABLE FILLER

21. Your colleague has been advising you of his recent successful outcomes using Artefill. *Which one of the following is correct regarding use of this product?*
A. It is a temporary filler that will require top-up injections.
B. It contains absorbable polymethylacrylate beads that often cause granuloma formation.
C. It contains collagen that provides the increased volume at the injection site.
D. It should be avoided in the glabellar and periorbital regions.
E. The first-line treatment of problematic irregularities after Artefill is surgical excision.

USE OF POLY-L-LACTIC ACID (SCULPTRA)

22. A woman comes to your practice for an injectable filler consultation. On the telephone, she advised the nurse that her main concern was superficial upper lip rhytids that were previously treated with hyaluronic acid. You were anticipating using this filler again and had prepared some, along with a range of 20- to 27-gauge needles. When she arrives, you find that the main issue is deep nasolabial folds, and she is dissatisfied that the improvement from her previous injection was relatively short lived. Therefore she is interested in a longer-lasting improvement. She has been reading about Sculptra while in the waiting area and asks if this can be used. *Which one of the following limits your use of Sculptra in this case?*
A. The nature of the defect
B. The lack of preparation time
C. The availability of needles
D. A lack of skin pretesting
E. The longevity of Sculptra

NONOPERATIVE FACIAL REJUVENATION

23. *For each of the following clinical scenarios, select the most suitable injectable treatment option. (Each option may be used once, more than once, or not at all.)*
A. A 33-year-old woman with early dynamic crow's-feet rhytids.
B. A 46-year-old man with fine static rhytids of the forehead and lip.
C. A 62-year-old man with deep nasolabial folds who requests a longer-lasting result.

Options:
a. Dysport 12-30 units
b. Botox 12-30 units
c. Xeomin 40-60 units
d. Juvéderm Ultra Plus
e. Perlane
f. Sculptra
g. Belotero Balance

COMPLICATIONS FOLLOWING INJECTABLE FILLERS

24. A nurse attends your office having undergone injectable filler treatment at another clinic while on vacation. She is concerned about the appearance of a blue discoloration at the injection site and wonders whether this is connected with the injection or a possible vascular lesion. *What is the most likely filler substance she has had injected?*
A. Juvéderm
B. Zyderm
C. Sculptra
D. Radiesse
E. Artefill

Answers

ACTINIC DAMAGE
1. Which one of the following statements is relevant to the Fitzpatrick skin type classification?
   D. The response to sun exposure
   The Fitzpatrick skin type classification describes the likely response to sun exposure with six grades and is most relevant to the risk of skin cancer development. It also describes the skin type/ethnicity of the patient ranging from white, to brown and black skin types. It is relevant to both an aesthetic consult and one for potential skin cancer given the photoaging effects of UV light.[1]

   Fitzpatrick skin type classification
   Class I: never tans, burns easily, fair skin
   Class II: usually burns, tans minimally
   Class III: burns moderately, tans moderately
   Class IV: tans moderately and easily burns minimally
   Class V: rarely burns, dark brown skin
   Class VI: never burns, dark brown or black skin

   The Fitzpatrick classification of facial wrinkling is different and considers perioral and periorbital wrinkling with three classes based on depth of wrinkles and degree of elastosis. This may be a useful system more specifically for an aesthetic assessment.[2]

   Fitzpatrick classification of facial wrinkling
   Class I: fine wrinkles and mild elastosis
   Class II: fine to moderate wrinkles and moderate elastosis
   Class III: fine to deep wrinkles and severe elastosis

   The other descriptors (A, B, C, and E) form part of the Glogau classification, which can be used to describe features of photoaging. There are four categories ranging from mild to severe. Each of these is linked to a typical age range and clinical findings that detail the degree of wrinkles, evidence of actinic sun damage, scarring, and make-up use. Patients are classified into age brackets according to the degree of photoaging (see Table 88-1, *Essentials of Plastic Surgery*, second edition). This is most applicable to the assessment of patients before facial rejuvenation.[3]

CHRONOLOGIC AGING
2. Which one of the following is most likely to be increased in aging skin?
   E. The ratio of collagen type III to I
   In aging skin, the ratio of collagen types changes with an increase in the ratio of type III to type I. Many other changes occur in the skin with increased age and include dermal and epidermal thinning with less well-organized stratum corneum. There are also fewer fibroblasts, mast cells, and blood vessels, as well as a reduction in the total number of collagen and elastin fibers.[4] Dermal thickness decreases approximately 6% per decade and is increased by sun exposure and

Chapter 88 ▪ Nonoperative Facial Rejuvenation 731

smoking. These skin changes are further compounded by gravitational forces that cause deep wrinkles as facial fat descends and the dynamic forces from mimetic muscles that cause rhytids in the overlying skin. Approaches to improve skin quality include actinic damage prevention by using sun block and daily skin care, while reducing sun exposure and smoking. Techniques to address changes once they have developed include laser resurfacing and chemical peels.

Laser and Light Resurfacing

WAVELENGTHS OF DIFFERENT RESURFACING MODALITIES

3. Which one of the following resurfacing modalities uses a wavelength of 2940 nm and is a popular tool for ablative resurfacing?
   C. Er:YAG

   Er:YAG works at a wavelength of 2940 nm with a chromophore of water. It works as an ablative laser resurfacer. CO_2 and fractionated CO_2 are also ablative resurfacing modalities with a chromophore of water but with a wavelength of 10,600 nm. IPL can work at different wavelengths between 500 and 1300 nm, depending on settings. It can target different chromophores and works as a nonablative tool. Nd:YAG works at a wavelength of 1064 nm and targets tissues nonspecifically to act as a nonablative resurfacer. Downtime is reduced with nonablative modalities at the expense of such dramatic improvements in longer term appearance.

4. Which one of the following laser modalities has a variant with a higher wavelength developed to use water as a target chromophore in order to achieve a more effective nonablative facial rejuvenation?
   A. Nd:YAG

   The normal wavelength for Nd:YAG is 1064 nm. At this wavelength energy is nonspecifically absorbed by target tissues. Various proteins appear to be the main target. Blood vessels, red blood cells, collagen, and melanin are also sensitive. A 1320 nm wavelength version of this laser has been produced and marketed specifically for nonablative facial rejuvenation. At this wavelength the laser targets dermal water.

   A key point to note when using this laser, however, is that a cooling agent must be placed on the epidermis to prevent blistering.

   As discussed in question 2, Er:YAG and CO_2 are both ablative lasers that also target water as the chromophore. Fractional resurfacing and IPL are both nonablative modalities. Although water is one of the chromophores for IPL, this is not technically a laser technique.

CHROMOPHORES IN REJUVENATION THERAPY

5. Which one of the following resurfacing modalities uses blue dye as a target chromophore?
   E. Fractional photothermolysis

   Fractional photothermolysis is a technique that involves the application of blue dye to the skin to act as the target chromophore. The dye is laid down in a "pixilated" manner such that when the laser contacts the skin, heat is only passed through the dye covered zones, leaving the surrounding skin untreated. This reduces the amount of tissue damage present at any given time and means that patients have a reduced downtime with less severe side effects. Because only a proportion of the total skin surface is treated, the clinical improvement is less than with more aggressive techniques.

CO_2 LASER

6. You are planning to use CO_2 laser resurfacing in your aesthetic practice. **Which one of the following is correct regarding its use in resurfacing?**
   E. The clinical endpoint is evidenced by pale yellow coloration to the skin.
   When using the CO_2 laser, the clinical endpoint for treatment is evidenced by a pale yellow color of the skin which represents the midreticular dermis. The effectiveness of CO_2 laser ablation can reduce with each pass, as vaporization decreases and thermal injury increases because of the reduced tissue water content after the initial pass. The depth of ablation is affected by both the number of passes and the amount of cooling time between them. Shortening the cooling time too far will result in less ablation and increased thermal damage to the tissues. Obtaining good results with the CO_2 laser requires experience and understanding of these principles.

   CO_2 laser is one of the first and longest used ablative laser types in facial rejuvenation and tends to be used for deeper rhytids. For superficial rhytids, more gentle techniques are used, because a major disadvantage of the CO_2 laser is a downtime of a few weeks.

   Although the aim of laser resurfacing is to tighten dermal collagen, this is not the target chromophore. The target chromophore is water, and the laser wavelength is 10,600 nm. Skin dyschromias are not treated with the CO_2 laser and may even be accentuated by postprocedure erythema.

LASER AND LIGHT REJUVENATION TECHNIQUES

7. For the following scenarios, the best options are as follows:
   A. You see a 37-year-old white man in your office who underwent laser resurfacing under the care of another clinician for acne scarring 12 months ago. He remembers the healing time to be quite extensive, with scabbing at the scar sites, and is now concerned about obvious pale patches that are visible on both cheeks.
      c. CO_2 laser
      This man has hypopigmentation following facial rejuvenation therapy. This is the most common adverse reaction after CO_2 laser resurfacing, leading to obvious demarcation lines between treated and untreated areas—in this case, the cheek and surrounding region. This complication tends to be most pronounced in fair-skinned individuals. Consequently, some people advocate using the CO_2 laser only when the entire face will be treated. Other treatments such as Er:YAG can also cause hypopigmentation, but it is less common with this laser type.
   B. You are obtaining a history from a 45-year-old woman who previously underwent laser rejuvenation treatment with another physician. She is unable to recall which type of laser was used but states that she heard a popping sound during the treatment received under local anesthetic and sedation.
      a. Er:YAG laser
      This woman has undergone treatment with Er:YAG laser. This ablative laser represents an alternative to CO_2 and produces a popping sound as ablated desiccated tissue is ejected when hit by the laser.
   C. You see a 51-year-old woman who underwent a series of four treatments at weekly intervals for patches of facial dyschromia. She is delighted with the excellent results and wishes to consider other rejuvenation techniques.
      e. Fractional photothermolysis
      This patient is most likely to have undergone fractional photothermolysis, a treatment with minimal downtime that requires multiple sessions at weekly intervals. This treatment is particularly useful for treating dyschromias.

Chapter 88 ■ Nonoperative Facial Rejuvenation 733

SELECTION OF LASER/LIGHT THERAPIES FOR FACIAL REJUVENATION

8. For the following scenarios, the best options are as follows:

A. A 65-year-old retired woman wishes to have a face-lift procedure. She has Fitzpatrick type III skin with deep rhytids affecting her forehead and periorbital and perioral areas. She stopped smoking 5 years ago.

  c. CO_2 laser

  This woman has deep rhytids and will have significant downtime after her face-lift procedure. She is less likely to require a short downtime because she has retired. Combining this resurfacing procedure at the time of surgery is generally safe and time efficient, since she is already having a general anesthetic and an overnight hospital stay. Alternatively, she could have Er:YAG treatment.

B. A 33-year-old woman has fine, static rhytids developing in the crow's-feet and forehead regions. She has pale skin with mild dyschromia. The patient works in the media and has a hectic schedule. She has been receiving Botox injections as a preventive therapy for 12 months and requests minimal downtime for any treatments.

  e. Fractional photothermolysis

  Because this patient is young, has minor skin imperfections, and requires minimal downtime, IPL or fractional photothermolysis are her best options. Fractional photothermolysis is probably a better option and would fit in well with this woman's lifestyle.

C. A 45-year-old head teacher has requested facial rejuvenation at the start of the summer vacation. She has Fitzpatrick skin type IV and deep facial rhytids. She dislikes hospitals and wants the minimal number of treatments. She needs to be able to return to work after 4 weeks and does not want people to know she has received treatment.

  a. Er:YAG laser

  This woman has a window of 4 to 6 weeks to fully recover from treatment. She requires a more aggressive treatment, given her deep facial rhytids. If she does not want people to know that she has undergone a procedure, the Er:YAG rather than the CO_2 laser would be a better option, since this will provide a deep peel in a single setting with a reepithelialization time of less than 1 week. Visible erythema should have resolved within 4 weeks.

TREATMENT OF FACIAL RHYTIDS WITH ABLATIVE LASER THERAPY

9. You see a 68-year-old man who has Fitzpatrick type IV skin and thick, deep static rhytids in the forehead, crow's-feet, and midface. He has lived and worked in hot climates for many years and has considerable actinic damage. He has recurrent cold sores. His wife has undergone resurfacing with Er:YAG laser therapy and is pleased with the results. Accordingly, he is now interested in having this treatment. When discussing this treatment for this patient, which one of the following is correct?

  B. He could achieve similarly good results with a deep chemical peel or CO_2 laser.

  Treatment for this gentleman should not be begun immediately, since he would benefit from pretreatment with hydroxyquinone and tretinoin for 4 to 6 weeks. These stimulate faster healing and help to prevent posttreatment hyperpigmentation. He should also receive antiviral prophylaxis 7 to 10 days before treatment. There is debate whether Er:YAG provides comparable results to those with the CO_2 laser. The benefits of Er:YAG are that water absorption is much more efficient than with the CO_2 laser, leading to reduced heat diffusion in surrounding tissues. The depth of penetration is also less than with a CO_2 laser. Although the downtime is reduced with

Er:YAG compared with CO_2, this may be simply because the treatment is less aggressive and the overall clinical effects are less. When the depth of CO_2 and Er:YAG resurfacing is identical, no difference in duration of erythema is seen. Use of a deep peel will probably provide a comparable result. His risk of postoperative hypopigmentation is not more than 12%.

INTENSE PULSED LIGHT (IPL)

10. A 37-year-old pregnant woman is concerned about her facial appearance. She has pale, thin skin with small areas of telangectasia, dyschromia, and poor general texture. She has read about IPL treatment and wonders whether this will be a suitable treatment for her condition. *Which one of the following is correct regarding IPL in this setting?*
    D. **Use of this treatment modality is currently contraindicated for this patient.**
    IPL is a useful treatment for facial rejuvenation, because it can provide consistent results and is very versatile. The target chromophore can be altered by using different wavelengths. Depending on the selected setting, melanin, hemoglobin, or water can be targeted. This woman's skin problems should be amenable to IPL therapy, and there is no requirement for a pretreatment regimen. However, IPL is contraindicated in pregnancy. A typical course of treatment is every other week for four to seven sessions and these can be performed in the office with a local anesthetic.

Chemical Peels

PRETREATMENT FOR CHEMICAL PEELS

11. A 50-year-old woman comes to the clinic requesting facial rejuvenation with a chemical peel. She has Fitzpatrick type II thick, oily skin with moderate wrinkling and laxity and minimal dyschromia. She smokes 10 cigarettes per day and currently has no specific skin care regimen. *Which one of the following is incorrect regarding a pretreatment regimen for this woman?*
    E. **She requires prescription of a tyrosinase inhibitor to minimize posttreatment hyperpigmentation.**
    Use of a pretreatment regimen before performing a chemical peel is essential to prevent complications and optimize outcomes. Tyrosinase inhibitors such as hydroquinone are indicated for use in patients with Fitzpatrick type III through VI skin or with pigment dyschromias to reduce melanin production. This may prevent hyperpigmentation after the peel. Because this patient has pale skin and minimal pigment dyschromia, hydroquinone is not required.

    A standard approach to the pretreatment regimen includes smoking cessation and minimizing sun exposure. A daily skin care program should include a buffing cleanser, an alpha hydroxy acid toner, and a vitamin A conditioner. Tretinoin is a synthetic retinoic acid that can stimulate collagen synthesis, exfoliate the stratum corneum, and increase glycosaminoglycan deposition. It does cause increased photosensitivity, so it must be used in conjunction with a sunscreen. This woman has significant photoaging and may benefit from other additional pretreatments, such as microdermabrasion, IPL, or glycolic acid peels.

ALPHA-HYDROXY ACID PEELS (AHA)

12. A patient has been using glycolic acid peels at home with modest effects and now wishes to know what benefits an office-based approach may offer her. **What is the main benefit of an office-based approach to glycolic acid peels?**
D. Higher concentrations of acid can be used.

AHAs are naturally occurring acids found in citrus fruits. They are used as superficial peel agents and cause exfoliation. They are available as over-the-counter preparations and prescription-only preparations, depending on their concentration and pH values. Higher concentrations of acid will provide a deeper peel. The FDA has limited AHAs for over-the counter-sale to those of maximum 10% concentration (with a pH of greater than 3.5), because more concentrated acids can cause epithelial necrosis instead of exfoliation. Therefore the benefits of an office-based approach are that a higher concentration of acid may be used to achieve a greater response.

JESSNER'S SOLUTION

13. **Which one of the following is correct regarding Jessner's solution?**
D. It should be neutralized with water after creation of a light frost.

Jessner's solution includes resorcinol, salicylic acid, lactic acid, and ethanol. It does not contain trichloroacetic acid (TCA) but is useful as a pretreatment for a TCA peel. In its own right it is a useful peel agent that can provide superficial or intermediate depth treatments, depending on the number of coats applied. It works in a similar way to AHAs (as a keratolytic). After application it should form a light frost, and this should then be neutralized with water.

TRICHLOROACETIC ACID PEELS

14. **What is the clinical endpoint of a deep trichloroacetic acid (TCA) peel?**
D. An intense white to yellow blanch

TCA peels are useful for providing intermediate to deep peels, but in concentrations greater than 45% they risk irregular penetration and scarring. Their effectiveness can be optimized by careful skin preparation. This includes washing and degreasing the skin, mechanically removing surface debris, and applying three or four coats of Jessner's solution. The endpoint for a TCA peel depends on the required depth. An intermediate peel is a foggy white frost on an erythmatous base. A second endpoint is an epidermal slide, which is produced if a cotton tip applicator is applied to the surface of the skin. This is also known as the *accordion sign*. When a deep peel is reached, the epidermal slide will disappear and be replaced by an intense white or yellow blanch.

PHENOL PEELS

15. **What has been proposed to be the main active ingredient in a Baker-Gordon phenol peel?**
C. Croton oil

The Baker-Gordon peel includes phenol, tap water, liquid soap (Septisol), and croton oil. Some authors, such as Hetter,[5,6] believe that the true active ingredient in these peels is the croton oil and that minute changes in the concentration of croton oil can cause very different results. The soap is an emulsifying agent that acts as a surfactant to lower surface tension. There is no acetic acid in the preparation.

16. **What is the main risk when using high concentration phenol peels?**
E. Cardiac arrhythmias

Phenol has been used as a peeling agent for many years to provide a medium depth peel by the action of protein coagulation. It is a high-risk agent to use, as it is rapidly absorbed through the skin and can lead to renal failure and liver toxicity. It has a direct action on the myocardium which can lead to cardiac arrhythmias. For this reason patients undergoing a phenol peel require careful cardiac monitoring.[7]

Botulinum Toxin and Injectable Fillers

BOTULINUM TOXIN

17. Botulinum toxins are derived from the bacterium *Clostridium botulinum*. **Which one of the following statements is correct regarding their use in facial aesthetics?**

E. Toxins cause temporary chemodenervation by preventing binding and release of acetylcholine.

There are seven subtypes of botulinum toxin, but only two are commercially available (A and B). All of the subtypes cause chemodenervation by blocking the action of acetylcholine at the neuromuscular junction. Type A works on the SNAP-25 protein; and type B, on the synaptobrevin protein. Both of these proteins act at the SNARE complex. Only type A is intended for use in facial aesthetics, while type B is for use in cervical dystonia. FDA approval for botulinum toxin A is for glabellar rhytids or blepharoptosis (depending on brand) so other uses are off-label.

The units of different botulinum toxin preparations are not uniformly comparable, although they are derived from the effects on laboratory mice. One unit is sufficient to cause death in 50% of a specific strain of mouse with intraperitoneal injection. Botox (Onabotulinumtoxin A, Allergan, Santa Barbara, CA) and Xeomin (Incobotulinumtoxin A, Merz Pharmaceuticals, Greensboro, NC) units are roughly equivalent. Between 2 and 2.5 Dysport (Abobotulinumtoxin A, Medicis Aesthetics, Scottsdale, AZ) units are equivalent to a single Botox unit.[8]

The difference in units between products arises from differences in the specifics of the assays used and this has the potential to cause confusion when changing from Botox or Xeomin to Dysport in clinical practice.

ADMINISTRATION OF BOTOX FOR FACIAL REJUVENATION

18. You are preparing some Botox for a 30-year-old woman who has requested treatment for her frown line (glabellar region). It is her first experience with Botox injections. **Which one of the following is correct?**

D. A typical starting dose for this woman would be 20 units.

Botox is available in 100 and 200 unit vials and is typically diluted with normal saline to provide 4 units per 0.1 ml. Reconstitution should be performed gently to avoid damage to the product. It should be clear following reconstitution. Consensus suggests it may be stored for up to 6 weeks, providing it is stored at 4° C. A typical starting dose would be 20 units placed via 4-6 injections. The central injection is placed below the superior orbital rim but the lateral ones must be placed above.[9,10] (Fig. 88-1).

Fig. 88-1 Injection points for glabellar complex and vertical forehead lines.

Chapter 88 ■ Nonoperative Facial Rejuvenation   737

CONSTITUENTS OF DIFFERENT FILLERS

19. *For the following descriptions, the best options are as follows:*
A. *A hyaluronic acid derivative with midsized particles*
   f. Restylane
   Hyaluronic acid derivatives are useful temporary fillers commonly used in facial rejuvenation. They are available in different particle sizes (small, medium, and large) for use in different size and depths of defect. Juvéderm, Restylane, and Perlane are all types of hyaluronic acid, but Perlane and Juvéderm Ultra Plus contain large particles.

B. *A calcium hydroxyapatite synthetic injectable*
   a. Radiesse
   This calcium hydroxyapatite filler was originally used in maxillofacial defects and vocal cord insufficiency. Now it has approval for use as a soft tissue filler.

C. *A synthetic filler containing poly-L-lactic acid*
   e. Sculptra
   Poly-L-lactic acid is the synthetic absorbable substance used to produce Vicryl sutures and absorbable implants such as endotine. Sculptra is a nonpermanent filler used to augment soft tissue deformities and deep facial rhytids. Artefill is a composite filler discussed in more detail in question 21.

HYALURONIC ACID

20. You are using a hyaluronic acid derivative as an injectable filler in your cosmetic practice. *Which one of the following is true of this filler?*
E. Injections are painful and best combined with lidocaine.

Hyaluronic acid filler is very popular for facial rejuvenation procedures. Since its FDA approval in 2003, its use has supplanted collagen as the synthetic filler of choice. There are many advantages of using hyaluronic acid as a filler, but injections can be painful so topical and or injectable local anesthetic agents should be used. There is no species specificity and therefore no immunological activity, meaning skin tests are not required. However, after injection, patients should apply ice packs for the first 24 hours and take antihistamines to settle local reactions.

Hyaluronic acid is a normal component of a ground substance responsible for dermal hydration, so it absorbs water following injection resulting in further expansion. Injections initially last 6 to 9 months and subsequent injections actually last longer with lesser volumes usually required. Hyaluronic acid fillers are readily available, reliable to use, and have the added benefit of being reversible if placed incorrectly. This is achieved by injection of hyaluronidase at the previously injected site.

USE OF ARTEFILL AS AN INJECTABLE FILLER

21. Your colleague has been advising you of his recent successful outcomes using Artefill. *Which one of the following is correct regarding use of this product?*
D. It should be avoided in the glabellar and periorbital regions.

Artefill is a permanent filler composed of collagen-covered polymethylmethacrylate (PMMA) beads and may require a top-up injection. The PMMA beads are permanent and rarely cause granuloma formation. The injected collagen acts as a temporary transport vehicle only and is absorbed during the first 6 weeks post injection. Long-term volume increases are achieved by secondary formation of connective tissue around the beads. Artefill is best used in the nasolabial folds and deep marionette lines, and should be used with caution in thin skin or areas liable to thin with age such as the periorbital and glabellar areas. First-line treatment of irregularities discovered soon after injection is steroid injection to soften the tissues. Surgical resection is only required in persistent problematic irregularities.

USE OF POLY-L-LACTIC ACID (SCULPTRA)

22. A woman comes to your practice for an injectable filler consultation. On the telephone, she advised the nurse that her main concern was superficial upper lip rhytids that were previously treated with hyaluronic acid. You were anticipating using this filler again and had prepared some, along with a range of 20- to 27-gauge needles. When she arrives, you find that the main issue is deep nasolabial folds, and she is dissatisfied that the improvement from her previous injection was relatively short lived. Therefore she is interested in a longer-lasting improvement. She has been reading about Sculptra while in the waiting area and asks if this can be used. **Which one of the following limits your use of Sculptra in this case?**
    B. The lack of preparation time
    As discussed in question 19, Sculptra is a synthetic polymer that would be a good option in this case. It is biodegradable, biocompatible, immunologically inert, and does not require a skin test. It contains poly-L-lactic acid, which initiates a foreign body reaction and is ultimately replaced with collagen.
    Sculptra requires injection with a needle of at least 26 gauge given its viscous nature, and may be combined with local anesthetic. It can provide longer-lasting rhytid correction than hyaluronic acid, typically lasting for up to 2 years. The limiting factor in this case is the lack of preparation time, since it must be reconstituted at least 2 hours before injection and preferably overnight.

NONOPERATIVE FACIAL REJUVENATION

23. For the following scenarios, the best options are as follows:
    A. A 33-year-old woman with early dynamic crow's-feet rhytids.
    b. Botox 12-30 units
    This patient could benefit from chemodenervation of the orbicularis oculi muscle; the options include Xeomin, Dysport, and Botox. A suggested starting dose for crow's-feet Botox injection is 12 to 30 units. Since Xeomin units are roughly equivalent, the same dose can be used. The approximate dosing conversion for Botox to Dysport is 2.5:1, so a starting dose would be 30-75 units.
    B. A 46-year-old man with fine static rhytids to the forehead and lip.
    g. Belotero Balance
    This patient could benefit from a filler injection. As the lines are superficial, a small to medium particle hyaluronic acid derivative would be suitable. Juvéderm Ultra Plus and Perlane contain large particles. Belotero Balance contains medium-sized particles.
    C. A 62-year-old man with deep nasolabial folds who requests a longer-lasting result.
    f. Sculptra
    This patient could benefit from a Sculptra injection, as the nasolabial folds are deep. An alternative would be to use a large particle hyaluronic acid such as Perlane or Juvéderm Ultra Plus, but the effects would not last so long.

COMPLICATIONS FOLLOWING INJECTABLE FILLERS

24. A nurse attends your office having undergone injectable filler treatment at another clinic while on vacation. She is concerned about the appearance of a blue discoloration at the injection site and wonders whether this is connected with the injection or a possible vascular lesion. **What is the most likely filler substance she has had injected?**

    A. Juvéderm

    This woman is most likely to have undergone injection of hyaluronic acid (Juvéderm). Injection of this filler too superficially can lead to a bluish discoloration. This is described as the *Tyndall effect*, also known as Tyndall scattering, and is observed when light is reflected by small particles that are in suspension. It is named after the nineteenth century physicist John Tyndall. As this is a temporary filler, the problem will be self-limiting, but could be treated with an injection of hyaluronidase if the patient is not prepared to wait.

REFERENCES

1. Fitzpatrick TB. The validity and practicality of sun-reactive skin types I through VI. Arch Dermatol 124:869, 1988.
2. Fitzpatrick RE, Goldman MP, Satur et al. Pulsed carbon dioxide laser resurfacing of photo-aged facial skin. Arch Dermatol 132:395-402, 1996.
3. Glogau RG. Aesthetic and anatomic analysis of the aging skin. Semin Cutan Med Surg 15:134-138, 1996.
4. Sauermann K, Clemann S, Jaspers S, et al. Age related changes of human skin investigated with histiometric measurements by confocal laser scanning microscopy in vivo. Skin Res Technol 8:52-56. 2002.
5. Hetter GP. An examination of the pheno-croton oil peel. IV. Face peel results with different concentrations of phenol and croton oil. Plast Reconstr Surg 105:1061-1083; discussion 1084-1087, 2000.
6. Hetter GP. An examination of the phenol-croton oil peel: I. Dissecting the formula. Plast Reconstr Surg 105:227-239; discussion 249-251, 2000.
7. Truppman ES, Ellenby JD. Major electrocardiographic changes during chemical face peeling. Plast Reconstr Surg 63:44-48, 1979.
8. Carruthers J, Stubbs HA. Botulinum toxin for benign essential blepharospasm, hemifacial spasm and age-related lower eyelid entropion, Can J Neurol Sci 14:42-45, 1987.
9. Carruthers J, Fagien S, Matarasso SL; Botox Consensus Group. Consensus recommendations on the use of botulinum toxin type a in facial aesthetics. Plast Reconstr Surg 114(6 Suppl):1S-22S, 2004.
10. Lorenc ZP, Kenkel JM, Fagien S, et al. Consensus panel's assessment and recommendations on the use of 3 botulinum toxin type A products in facial aesthetics. Aesthet Surg J 33(1 Suppl):35S-40S, 2013.

89. Fat Grafting

See *Essentials of Plastic Surgery*, second edition, pp. 1099-1110.

GENERAL PRINCIPLES OF FAT GRAFTING
1. **Which one of the following statements is correct regarding fat grafting?**
   A. It involves the transfer of free autografts of vascularized adipose tissue.
   B. It provides predictable results when used to correct soft tissue contour deformities.
   C. It transfers adipocytes and their surrounding stroma in a single setting.
   D. Only mature adipocytes are able to survive the grafting process.
   E. Preadipocytes are immature fat cells that are poorly tolerant of ischemia.

CLINICAL INDICATIONS
2. A 48-year-old woman is considering fat grafting to the left breast following a wide local excision of a 2 cm breast tumor and subsequent chemoradiotherapy. She dislikes the appearance of the left breast, which has a contour defect with puckered scarring. **In addition to addressing the volume deficiency, what is the main secondary benefit of fat grafting in this patient?**
   A. Tumor recurrence risk will be reduced
   B. Tumor surveillance will be simplified
   C. Breast skin quality will be improved
   D. Wound healing will be enhanced
   E. Postoperative swelling will be avoided

3. You see a woman in clinic who has undergone breast construction with a free DIEP flap. The lateral part of the flap did not survive and the patient is now lacking lateral and upper pole fullness. **When discussing risks and benefits of fat grafting to the breast, which one of the following statements is correct?**
   A. Overcorrection of the deficit in the OR should be avoided.
   B. Multiple fat transfer procedures are likely to be required.
   C. External tissue expansion with the Brava system is needed.
   D. A traditional corrective surgical approach cannot address this problem.
   E. Reconstruction will be unaffected by subsequent fluctuations in weight.

BENEFITS OF FAT GRAFTING
4. You are running a clinic for facial deformity and see patient who is interested in fat grafting. He has been taking antiretroviral medications for many years and has been receiving synthetic facial fillers to improve his malar fullness. His CD4 count is normal and his BMI is 20. **In this case, which one of the following is likely to be the greatest challenge of fat grafting?**
   A. Increased risk of rejection
   B. Availability of donor tissue
   C. Low immune status
   D. Unnatural appearance
   E. High donor site morbidity

FAT HARVEST

5. You are performing fat transfer on a patient following breast reconstruction surgery and want to maximize the viability of the fat cells during harvest. **Which one of the following approaches to harvest has traditionally been associated with improved fat cell viability?**
A. Ultrasound-assisted liposuction
B. Power-assisted liposuction
C. Manual harvest with a large-bore cannula
D. Use of tumescent infiltration with epinephrine and lidocaine
E. Use of the central, lower abdomen as a donor site

FAT PROCESSING

6. You are setting up a new practice in fat transfer and have visited a number of units using the technique. You are uncertain which type of fat processing technique to use and consult the literature. **Which approach to fat processing has been shown to have the best graft retention in in vivo studies?**
A. Centrifugation
B. Washing
C. Sedimentation
D. Straining
E. Cotton-gauze rolling

7. When using the Coleman approach to fat processing, which one of the following is correct?
A. The lipoaspirate is spun in a centrifuge for 3 minutes at 3000 rpm.
B. The middle layer of the lipoaspirate is discarded after centrifugation.
C. The lipoaspirate is washed in sterile water before injection.
D. Sedimentation and straining of the aspirate through a wire basket is performed.
E. The lipoaspirate is gently rolled in absorbent gauze before injection.

FAT INJECTION

8. When injecting fat into the face using the Coleman technique, **which one of the following is correct?**
A. Fat should be injected with 10 ml syringes and a 25-gauge cannula.
B. Small deposits of fat should be placed during advancement of the cannula.
C. Pickle fork-style cannulas should be used in most settings.
D. A cross-hatching technique should be used to evenly distribute fat grafts.
E. External digital manipulation should be avoided.

CLINICAL TECHNIQUES

9. A 25-year-old woman with a body mass index of 30 has small breasts and is interested in enhancing her breast volume without using prosthetic implants. A combined fat transfer and external expansion technique is planned. **Which one of the following is true?**
A. External expansion with the Brava system is started 4 weeks before surgery.
B. Optimal fat retention is achieved where smaller volumes of fat are injected per stage.
C. Graft survival is marginally improved by the use of external expansion with the Brava system.
D. Fat should be injected into the breast parenchyma but not into the pectoralis major.
E. Fat transfer has now largely replaced the need for prosthetic augmentation.

POSTOPERATIVE CARE

10. **Which one of the following should be avoided during the first week after fat transfer?**
    A. Elevation and ice
    B. Compression garments
    C. Gentle massage
    D. Resumption of daily activities
    E. Anticoagulant medication

POSTOPERATIVE FOLLOW-UP

11. You see a 45-year-old woman 3 months after she underwent fat grafting as a primary breast augmentation procedure. She is feeling very well following her surgery and has been inspired to lose a further 10 pounds. **When examining her, which one of the following is correct?**
    A. There should be no residual swelling.
    B. Her final result should be evident.
    C. Mammography at this stage would be compromised.
    D. About three quarters of the transferred volume will remain.
    E. Firm, palpable areas may represent fat necrosis.

Chapter 89 ■ Fat Grafting   743

Answers

GENERAL PRINCIPLES OF FAT GRAFTING

1. **Which one of the following statements is correct regarding fat grafting?**
   C. It transfers adipocytes and their surrounding stroma in a single setting.
   Fat grafting involves transfer of nonvascularized but viable fat cells from one location to another within the same individual. Although fat grafting is generally successful in many circumstances, the results can be unpredictable in terms of volume maintenance. It does transfer fat and stroma in a single setting, although it usually requires multiple stages to achieve satisfactory clinical results, especially when larger contour defects are treated. Both mature adipocytes and preadipocytes can be transferred, but of the two cell types, preadipose cells are more resilient to ischemia and can continue to differentiate and proliferate after regaining a blood supply.

CLINICAL INDICATIONS

2. **A 48-year-old woman is considering fat grafting to the left breast following a wide local excision of a 2 cm breast tumor and subsequent chemoradiotherapy. She dislikes the appearance of the left breast, which has a contour defect with puckered scarring. In addition to addressing the volume deficiency, what is the main secondary benefit of fat grafting in this patient?**
   C. Breast skin quality may be improved
   One of the main advantages of fat transfer is its beneficial effects on irradiated skin and soft tissue. Although the precise mechanism is not fully understood, fat grafting can soften the skin and allow it to become more pliable. Skin complexion and scar appearance can also be improved. Histologic and electron micrographic evaluation after fat transfer show progressive regeneration of tissue ultrastructure with a reduction in epidermal thickening, vascular density, and fibrosis. Often, after the first lipofilling procedure, improvements in skin appearance are the most obvious visible benefit. There is no evidence to suggest that tumor recurrence is affected by fat grafting. Concerns have been raised as to whether injection of stem cells places patients at an increased (not decreased) risk of developing further tumors, but this has not been substantiated. Some authorities suggest that fat transfer may make tumor surveillance more difficult rather than more simple due to micro calcification on mammogram, but it should not interfere with detection providing the evaluation is performed by an experienced radiologist. Moderate bruising and swelling to both donor and recipient sites are inevitable following fat grafting, so patients must be aware of this preoperatively.

3. **You see a woman in clinic who has undergone breast construction with a free DIEP flap. The lateral part of the flap did not survive and the patient is now lacking lateral and upper pole fullness. When discussing risks and benefits of fat grafting to the breast, which one of the following statements is correct?**
   B. Multiple fat transfer procedures are likely to be required.
   Use of fat injection (lipomodeling) for refining autologous breast reconstruction has become standard practice for many breast reconstructive surgeons, particularly for correction of superior and medial pole deficiencies. Correction in this scenario is possible with fat transfer but will require multiple stages and achieving a perfect contour is challenging. The patient's body habitus will affect outcome, and in thin patients obtaining sufficient volume for transfer can be

a challenge. This is exacerbated by the fact that the anterior abdominal wall has already been harvested for the main flap, leaving little fat excess present in this area. Often the flanks are a useful source for fat harvest in these patients. Other suitable donor sites include the thighs and upper central abdomen.

Because up to half of the transferred fat may not survive, it is standard practice to overcorrect defects in the OR where possible. Quite large volumes of fat (200 to 300 cc) should be placed at multiple levels within the flap to improve graft take. External expansion with the Brava system is not routinely used in this scenario, although it could be. It is most commonly indicated for use in primary breast augmentation where a combination of fat transfer and the Brava system may improve outcomes.[1,2]

Although fat transfer is a useful technique in revision reconstructive cases, its limitations must be recognized. Where large deformities are present, standard surgical approaches may be more helpful to inset or contour the flap. In some cases, where the lateral defect is large, further flap reconstruction with a thoracodorsal artery perforator flap (TDAP) or partial latissimus dorsi flap (LD) may be indicated. A caveat of fat transfer is that fluctuations in weight will affect the recipient area. However, the same is also true of transferred vascularized tissues such as TRAM and DIEP flaps, so patients should be advised of this before surgery.[3]

BENEFITS OF FAT GRAFTING

4. You are running a clinic for facial deformity and see a patient who is interested in fat grafting. He has been taking antiretroviral medications for many years and has been receiving synthetic facial fillers to improve his malar fullness. His CD4 count is normal and his BMI is 20. *In this case, which one of the following is likely to be the greatest challenge of fat grafting?*
   B. Availability of donor tissue

   Fat transfer has many advantages over synthetic fillers, including low material cost, ready availability, a natural appearance, excellent biocompatibility, permanence, low donor site morbidity, and the ability to contour donor sites where required. In patients with HIV and subsequent lipodystrophy as a result of taking antiretroviral medications, there is often insufficient fat available for harvest, and these individuals might require a synthetic alternative. Some HIV patients can develop fat excess in the posterior neck (buffalo hump appearance) and central regions. In these cases it may be possible to use these areas for harvest.

FAT HARVEST

5. You are performing fat transfer on a patient following breast reconstruction surgery and want to maximize the viability of the fat cells during harvest. *Which one of the following approaches to harvest has traditionally been associated with improved fat cell viability?*
   C. Manual harvest with a large-bore cannula

   Atraumatic harvesting, handling, and transfer of fat are key to maximizing fat cell viability during fat grafting. Consequently, minimizing pressure by using a large-bore cannula (e.g., 3, 4, or 5 mm) and low pressure should be beneficial. For this reason, the Coleman technique involves the use of 10 cc syringes for harvest. There is debate regarding the benefits of assisted techniques for fat harvest, such as power-assisted or ultrasound-assisted liposuction,[4] and traditionally these had been associated with decreased viability. Recent evidence has shown high levels of fat cell viability after harvest with ultrasound-assisted liposuction that was at least comparable with or possibly superior to manual harvest.[5] Use of a tumescent infiltrate with epinephrine or local anesthetic does not improve viability, although it can reduce bleeding and facilitate ease of harvest. Some evidence suggests that local anesthetics may actually decrease fat cell viability.[6]

FAT PROCESSING

6. You are setting up a new practice in fat transfer and have visited a number of units using the technique. You are uncertain which type of fat processing technique to use and consult the literature. **Which approach to fat processing has been shown to have the best graft retention in in vivo studies?**
   ### E. Cotton-gauze rolling
   The aim of fat processing after harvest is to remove unwanted fluid, cells, and debris from the lipoaspirate, while causing minimal damage to the fat cells. There are different techniques used to achieve this, including centrifugation, sedimentation, straining, rolling, and washing. Cotton-gauze rolling has been reported as having the highest graft retention *in vivo*.[7] This technique involves pouring the lipoaspirate from the syringe onto a nonstick absorbent gauze, which is then gently rolled with an instrument handle in order to remove aqueous and oil layers.

   A comparative study by Rose et al[8] compared the other three main processing techniques (centrifugation, washing, and sedimentation) and showed that the number of viable fat cells maintained was highest when sedimentation was used. However, this team did not then assess the outcomes after injection with the different processing techniques. Whether this would translate into a clinical outcome benefit therefore remains unproven. Based on current clinical data, outcomes appear similar irrespective of processing technique, so in your practice you should select that which you are most familiar with until stronger evidence is available.

7. **When using the Coleman approach to fat processing, which one of the following is correct?**
   ### A. The lipoaspirate is spun in a centrifuge for 3 minutes at 3000 rpm.
   As discussed in question 6, there are a number of approaches to fat processing after harvest. The Coleman[9] technique uses the centrifugation approach. Centrifugation involves spinning fat in small syringes at speeds of approximately 3000 rpm for up to 3 minutes. This process will separate the harvest into three layers: top (oil), middle (fat cells), and bottom (blood/infiltrate). The middle layer must therefore be kept, as this represents the fat used for grafting. Centrifugation for longer than this is not recommended, as further separation does not occur and fat cells may be damaged.

   When using a washing technique, a number of different solutions may be used including normal saline, 5% glucose, or sterile water. Given the available evidence, saline is preferred compared with water and is common practice. In theory, washing cells in sterile water risks causing cell lysis because of the osmolarity difference. This difference is traditionally related to red blood cells but may also apply to fat cells. Rubin and Hoefflin[10] have an interesting and somewhat controversial "survival of the fittest" view on fat preparation. They use sterile water to wash the fat preparation and combine this with centrifugation at 6000 rpm, reporting satisfactory clinical results. They believe that stressing fat cells before injection results in only the most resilient cells reaching the injection stage. In general, most authorities work to minimize trauma to the fat cells (not increase it) during processing and this would be a more conventional approach.

   Sedimentation, decanting, and straining are not part of the Coleman technique, but are thought to represent the least traumatic method of fat processing. The main disadvantage is that this increases processing time and risks prolonged exposure of fat cells to the air, which in turn may lead to desiccation. Handling of the fat is also increased so it may risk damage. As described in question 6, cotton-gauze rolling is an alternative low trauma method of fat processing, again not part of the Coleman technique. A potential benefit is that the stromal component is largely retained.

FAT INJECTION

8. When injecting fat into the face using the Coleman technique, which one of the following is true?
   D. A cross-hatching technique should be used to evenly distribute fat grafts.
   When performing fat grafting, it is important to place fat in a crosshatched pattern using long radial passes from multiple directions. This helps to avoid placing an excess of fat in a single place or line. Injection in the face with the Coleman technique involves placement of small aliquots of fat in different tissue layers using 1 cc syringes and a 17-gauge blunt-tipped cannula 7 to 9 cm long. These are used to minimize trauma to the fat grafts and provide for accurate placement of small fat units; 10 cc syringes are used for harvest only. Fat should be placed on withdrawal, not advancement of the cannula. The pickle fork cannula is only used in areas of scarring and fibrosis where it is useful to break down the tissues and create a space for the fat grafts to sit. External digital manipulation is used to flatten clumps and minor irregularities during fat injection.

CLINICAL TECHNIQUES

9. A 25-year-old woman with a body mass index of 30 has small breasts and is interested in enhancing her breast volume without using prosthetic implants. A combined fat transfer and external expansion technique is planned. **Which one of the following is true?**
   A. External expansion with the Brava system is started 4 weeks before surgery.
   The Brava system is an external tissue expander that has shown promising results when combined with fat transfer for primary breast augmentation. The expander is worn for 4 weeks before fat injection and for one week after. Graft survival can be substantially higher when external tissue expansion is used (82% compared to 55%).[1,2] Fat survival is also improved when injected into muscle, so placement of fat in the pectoralis major as well as the breast parenchyma is often performed. Long-term fat retention is improved when larger fat volumes are injected at each stage. While fat transfer has become very popular, it has not replaced the need for prosthetic breast augmentation which still remains much more commonly performed.

POSTOPERATIVE CARE

10. Which one of the following should be avoided during the first week following fat transfer?
   C. Gentle massage
   Massage of the recipient area following fat transfer should be avoided for at least one week following surgery as this risks displacement of the grafts. Compression garments should be worn at all times for a few weeks after surgery at both donor and recipient sites. Edema and bruising may be reduced by application of cool packs. Surgery is generally performed in an outpatient setting. Normal activities of daily living can be resumed early in the postoperative phase and full activities can be resumed after a few weeks. Anticoagulant medication can often be continued throughout the perioperative period or restarted the day after surgery, depending on the indication and medication type.

POSTOPERATIVE FOLLOW-UP

11. You see a 45-year-old woman 3 months after she underwent fat grafting as a primary breast augmentation procedure. She is feeling very well following her surgery and has been inspired to lose a further 10 pounds. ***When examining her, which one of the following is correct?***

E. Firm palpable areas may represent fat necrosis.

The swelling following lipomodeling typically lasts for up to 6 months. At 3 months the final outcome is unlikely to be apparent. Mammography should not be compromised with an experienced radiologist, but given her age, mammography should have been performed preoperatively and is unlikely to be required at this stage.[11] Fat transfers are affected by weight changes and behave as they would have at the donor site. Therefore as this patient has lost weight, the transferred fat will also be affected and it is unlikely that three quarters of the transferred volume will remain.

REFERENCES

1. Khouri RK, Eisenmann-Klein M, Cardoso E, et al. Brava and autologous fat transfer is a safe and effective breast augmentation alternative: results of a 6-year, 81-patient, prospective multicenter study. Plast Reconstr Surg 129:1172-1187, 2012.
2. Del Vecchio DA, Bucky LP. Breast augmentation using preexpansion and autologous fat transplantation: a clinical radiographic study. Plast Reconstr Surg 127:2441-2450, 2011.
3. Delay E, Garson S, Tousson G, et al. Fat injection to the breast: technique, results, and indications based on 880 procedures over 10 years. Aesthet Surg J 29:360-376, 2009.
4. Keck M, Kober J, Riedl O, et al. Power assisted liposuction to obtain adipose-derived stem cells: impact on viability and differentiation to adipocytes in comparison to manual aspiration. J Plast Reconstr Aesthet Surg 67:e1-e8, 2014.
5. Schafer ME, Hicok KC, Mills DC, et al. Acute adipocyte viability after third-generation ultrasound-assisted liposuction. Aesthet Surg J 33:698-704, 2013.
6. Keck M, Zeyda M, Gollinger K, et al. Local anesthetics have a major impact on viability of preadipocytes and their differentiation into adipocytes. Plast Reconstr Surg 126:1500-1505, 2010.
7. Fisher C, Grahovac TL, Schafer ME, et al. Comparison of harvest and processing techniques for fat grafting and adipose stem cell isolation. Plast Reconstr Surg 132:351-361, 2013.
8. Rose JG Jr, Lucarelli MJ, Lemke BN, et al. Histologic comparison of autologous fat processing methods. Ophthal Plast Reconstr Surg 22:195-200, 2006.
9. Coleman SR. Structural Fat Grafting. St Louis: Quality Medical Publishing, 2004.
10. Rubin A, Hoefflin S. Fat purification: survival of the fittest. Plast Reconstr Surg 109:1463-1464, 2002.
11. Ihrai T, Georgiou C, Machiavello JC, et al. Autologous fat grafting and breast cancer recurrences: retrospective analysis of a series of 100 procedures in 64 patients. J Plast Surg Hand Surg 47:273-275, 2013.

90. Hair Transplantation

See *Essentials of Plastic Surgery*, second edition, pp. 1111-1121.

HAIR ANATOMY

1. **Which one of the following is true with respect to the anatomy of scalp hair?**
   A. Scalp hairs are unusual in that they have a mesodermal origin.
   B. An average scalp contains approximately 200,000 follicular units.
   C. An average scalp contains approximately 350,000 individual hairs.
   D. The total number of hairs is unaffected by natural hair color.
   E. Bald scalps have as many hair follicles as nonbald scalps.

PHYSIOLOGY OF HAIR GROWTH

2. **Which one of the following is correct regarding hair growth?**
   A. It involves four key phases.
   B. Most hairs are usually in the telogen phase.
   C. The catagen phase is the longest phase.
   D. Length of the anagen phase is sex dependent.
   E. On average, 20 to 30 hairs are shed daily.

ALOPECIA INCIDENCE

3. **In which race is alopecia most common?**
   A. Whites
   B. Blacks
   C. American Indians
   D. Asians
   E. Equal across races

MALE PATTERN BALDNESS

4. A 20-year-old man presents with male pattern baldness. His maternal grandfather lost his hair at a similar age. **Which one of the following is correct regarding his condition?**
   A. The fact that his maternal grandfather also lost his hair is likely to be a coincidence.
   B. His condition will be due to an excess of dihydroxytestosterone.
   C. He can expect his condition to take a fairly severe course.
   D. Treatment with 5-alpha reductase may be beneficial.
   E. His circulating testosterone will be significantly elevated.

CLASSIFICATION OF MALE PATTERN BALDNESS

5. The Norwood classification is commonly used with reference to male pattern baldness. **What is the clinical relevance of this classification?**
   A. It describes the anatomic location of hair loss.
   B. It describes the physiologic causes of hair loss.
   C. It describes the age of onset of hair loss.
   D. It describes the treatment algorithm for hair loss.
   E. It describes the outcome after surgery for hair loss.

CLINICAL PRESENTATION OF HAIR LOSS

6. For each of the following clinical scenarios, select the most likely option from those listed below. (Each option may be used once, more than once, or not at all.)

   A. A 12-year-old patient presents with a single round bald patch on the scalp with no history of trauma. He has no other obvious signs or symptoms, but his mother has a similar condition.

   B. A young male adult patient presents with progressive hair loss to the vertex and frontotemporal areas. He is generally fit and well. His brothers are similarly affected.

   C. A young woman with learning difficulties and mental illness presents with itchiness of the scalp and recent onset patchy baldness without signs of head lice or inflammation. Examination shows evidence of broken hairs in the scalp.

   Options:
   a. Traumatic alopecia
   b. Cicatricial alopecia
   c. Androgenic alopecia
   d. Alopecia areata
   e. Lichenplanopilaris

PHARMACOLOGIC MANAGEMENT OF HAIR LOSS

7. You are considering prescribing finasteride for a patient with significant hair loss. **Which one of the following is correct regarding this treatment?**
   A. It is a topical treatment for hair loss used twice daily.
   B. Side effects such as lethargy and rash are common.
   C. It should be reserved for the treatment of early hair loss in women.
   D. It is particularly effective at treating the temporal region.
   E. The major caveat is that lifelong use is required.

LASER THERAPY IN HAIR LOSS

8. When using laser therapy for the management of hair loss, which one of the following is correct?
   A. Its discovery as a modality of treating hair loss was purely accidental.
   B. The FDA has approved laser devices for use in hair loss based on studies demonstrating efficacy.
   C. Large multicenter studies have consistently shown improved hair growth.
   D. Common wavelengths are between 500 and 600 nm, such as KTP and pulsed dye lasers.
   E. The mechanism of action is well understood and involves production of dermal inflammation and increased blood flow.

NORMAL HAIR DENSITY

9. When planning a hair transplant procedure, it is important to be aware of the volume of hairs in the normal individual and the density that will appear satisfactory. *What is the normal density of scalp hairs per square centimeter in an average individual?*
   A. 40
   B. 100
   C. 200
   D. 350
   E. 400

SURGICAL MANAGEMENT OF HAIR LOSS

10. When treating moderate frontotemporal hair loss in a 28-year-old male with hair transplants, which one of the following donor sites should be used?
    A. Parietal
    B. Temporal
    C. Vertex
    D. Upper occipital
    E. Lower occipital

11. Which technique of harvesting in hair transplantation may provide the best donor site appearance with the least obvious scarring?
    A. Strip excision
    B. Triple-blade knife
    C. Quadruple-blade knife
    D. Follicular unit extraction
    E. Laser harvest

12. You are undertaking hair transplantation for a patient with frontotemporal recessions. Which one of the following is true regarding this procedure?
    A. The new anterior hairline should start 5 cm above the glabella.
    B. Slit minigrafts will provide the most natural appearance.
    C. Angles selected for hair placement should reflect the anatomic location.
    D. Mixing both slit and hole grafts should be avoided in this area.
    E. Micrografts should be used in preference to minigrafts.

POSTOPERATIVE CARE

13. Which one of the following should be part of the typical postoperative care following hair transplant?
    A. A single overnight stay in the hospital.
    B. A head bandage left undisturbed for two weeks.
    C. Daily hair washing with a pouring technique.
    D. Resumption of normal hair washing at day five.
    E. Two weeks of antibiotic cover.

Answers

HAIR ANATOMY
1. *Which one of the following is true with respect to the anatomy of scalp hair?*
   E. Bald scalps have as many hair follicles as nonbald scalps.
   Although counterintuitive, there are the same number of hair follicles in a bald scalp as there are in a normal hair-bearing scalp. The difference is that the follicles do not remain in the normal growth cycle within the bald scalp. Scalp hair originates from both ectodermal and mesodermal origins, as do hairs on the rest of the body. A normal scalp contains around 100,000 to 150,000 individual hairs. A follicular unit typically contains two hairs, so there are usually around 50,000 to 75,000 follicular units. The follicular unit is relevant to hair transplant, as single or multiple units are grafted during this process. Single follicular units containing one or two hairs are termed micrografts and those containing more hairs are termed minigrafts. The total number of scalp hairs is influenced by natural hair color, with blondes having more hairs and redheads having fewer hairs.

PHYSIOLOGY OF HAIR GROWTH
2. *Which one of the following is correct regarding hair growth?*
   D. Length of the anagen phase is sex dependent.
   The process of hair growth has three, not four, phases: anagen, catagen, and telogen. The anagen phase is the active growth phase, and 90% of hairs are usually produced in this phase. It is the longest phase, lasting about 3 years in men and 5 to 8 years in women. The catagen phase (degradation phase) is the shortest, at 2 or 3 weeks, and prepares hairs for shedding by separation of the base from the dermal papilla. The telogen phase is the resting phase and lasts 3 to 4 months. Approximately 10% of hair is in this phase and within it, 50 to 100 hairs are lost daily. Concurrent shortening of the anagen phase and lengthening of the telogen phase results in hair thinning and the subsequent development of baldness.[1]

ALOPECIA INCIDENCE
3. *In which race is alopecia most common?*
   A. Whites
   There is a difference in the incidence of alopecia across races, although the mechanism of male pattern baldness remains the same in all groups (see question 4 for further information regarding the mechanism). Whites are most commonly affected, followed by Asians and blacks. The lowest incidence is seen in American Indians. The reason for these apparent racial differences is not known and may reflect both genetic and environmental factors. In the United States around 35,000,000 men and 21,000,000 women are affected by scalp hair loss. Onset typically commences in the third and fourth decades, with half of patients affected by age fifty.[2,3]

MALE PATTERN BALDNESS

4. A 20-year-old man presents with male pattern baldness. His maternal grandfather lost his hair at a similar age. *Which one of the following is correct regarding his condition?*

C. He can expect his condition to take a fairly severe course.

Male pattern baldness that occurs at such a young age tends to be more severe in terms of extent and speed of hair loss. Male pattern baldness can be inherited in an X-linked autosomal dominant fashion, therefore coming from the maternal grandfather. So it is no coincidence that the patient's grandfather is also affected. Not all cases will be inherited this way, however, as there is evidence for several non-X-linked autosomal dominant (variable penetrance) routes of inheritance.

The mechanism of hair loss in male pattern baldness is thought to be due to the effects of dihydroxytestosterone (DHT) on the growth cycle of scalp hair follicles. However, it is not necessarily an excess of DHT that is responsible. A normal DHT can cause alopecia if the hair follicles are abnormally sensitive to its effects. Likewise, testosterone levels do not need to be elevated to cause androgenic alopecia. Testosterone is normally converted to DHT by the enzyme 5-alpha reductase which is found within the cells of susceptible hair follicles and skin. Therefore an excess of any of these substances can be responsible for the effects observed in androgenic alopecia, and it is most likely that this patient has both normal testosterone and DHT levels. Treatment with 5-alpha reductase inhibitors, but not 5-alpha reductase itself, may be helpful in some cases in order to reduce the amount of DHT.

CLASSIFICATION OF MALE PATTERN BALDNESS

5. The Norwood classification is commonly used with reference to male pattern baldness. *What is the clinical relevance of this classification?*

A. It describes the anatomic location of hair loss.

The Norwood classification[2] is very commonly used and describes the anatomic location and extent of male pattern baldness. It has seven subtypes (I through VII) ranging from mild to severe. It is difficult and unnecessary to memorize the precise details of the classification for daily practice. However, the underlying principles and extremes are worth knowing because male pattern baldness tends to follow relatively predictable patterns in terms of anatomic areas affected. It typically begins affecting only the hairline and frontotemporal areas (type I) and progressively affects the frontotemporal regions and the vertex. Type VII is the most extreme, affecting the hairline, vertex, and frontotemporal areas. Some patients first present with vertex baldness only. Within this classification there is no subtype for either a normal scalp and hairline or complete baldness. The physiologic causes, age of onset, treatment, and outcomes are not part of this classification system either (Fig. 90-1).

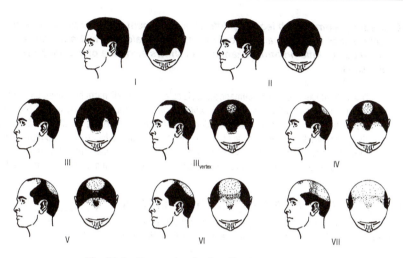

Fig. 90-1 Norwood male classification of alopecia.

CLINICAL PRESENTATION OF HAIR LOSS

5. *For the following scenarios, the best options are as follows:*
   A. *A 12-year-old patient presents with a single round bald patch on the scalp with no history of trauma. He has no other obvious signs or symptoms, but his mother has a similar condition.*
      d. **Alopecia areata**
         Alopecia areata is a condition in which hair is lost from small areas of the body, particularly the scalp. It is an inherited condition that can present at any age. It can affect the entire scalp in more extreme cases (alopecia totalis) or even the entire body (alopecia universalis).[4]
   B. *A young male adult patient presents with progressive hair loss to the vertex and frontotemporal areas. He is generally fit and well. His brothers are similarly affected.*
      c. **Androgenic alopecia**
         This patient has androgenic alopecia or male pattern baldness, which involves the conversion of healthy, thick terminal hairs to clear, microscopic vellus hairs.

C. *A young woman with learning difficulties and mental illness presents with itchiness of the scalp and recent onset patchy baldness without signs of head lice or inflammation. Examination shows evidence of broken hairs in the scalp.*

a. **Traumatic alopecia**

This patient has sustained traumatic alopecia as a result of self-harm by pulling out sections of her hair. This condition is called *trichotillomania*, and affected individuals feel compelled to pull their hair. This compulsive disorder may affect up to 4% of the population.[4] Cicatricial alopecia refers to a diverse range of conditions that destroy the hair follicle and replace them with scarring. This normally results in permanent hair loss. *Lichenplanopilaris* refers to hair loss in patients with the inflammatory condition *Lichen planus* that progresses to affect the scalp.

PHARMACOLOGIC MANAGEMENT OF HAIR LOSS

7. You are considering prescribing finasteride for a patient with significant hair loss. **Which one of the following is correct regarding this treatment?**

E. **The major caveat is that lifelong use is required.**

Finasteride is a 5-alpha-reductase inhibitor that has been used to treat benign prostatic hypertrophy and male pattern baldness. It is an oral (not topical) medication taken once daily. It is most effective on the vertex and frontal region in male pattern baldness and less effective in the temporal region. Side effects are uncommon. The major caveat is that it must be used indefinitely to maintain a response.

Topical solutions of 2% and 5% minoxidil are also used as treatment for baldness. Minoxidil is an antihypertensive medication that causes vasodilation that can also stimulate hair growth. Minoxidil may be useful in both men and women, but at present there is no strong evidence to show a measurable improvement in female hair loss with finasteride.

LASER THERAPY IN HAIR LOSS

8. When using laser therapy for the management of hair loss, which one of the following is correct?

A. **Its discovery as a modality of treating hair loss was purely accidental.**

Laser was originally found to be effective in treating hair loss when used on laboratory mice to initiate skin cancer. The FDA has approved the use of laser, but this is based on safety rather than efficacy. Large placebo-controlled trials are lacking. Some smaller studies have shown a benefit of laser on hair growth. The mechanism of action is not well understood. Common lasers used are within the red/infrared spectrum with wavelengths of between 600 and 900 nm.

NORMAL HAIR DENSITY

9. When planning a hair transplant procedure, it is important to be aware of the volume of hairs in the normal individual and the density that will appear satisfactory. **What is the normal density of scalp hairs per square centimeter in an average individual?**

C. **200**

The average number of scalp hairs per unit centimeter is 200. This equates to around 100,000 to 150,000 total hairs. A good visual result can be achieved with a density of around 50 hairs per unit centimeter. This equates to around 25 follicular units per unit centimeter. In order to treat large areas of hair loss, a few thousand grafts may be required to achieve the required hair density and this is one of the main reasons why the procedure is so time consuming to perform.

SURGICAL MANAGEMENT OF HAIR LOSS

10. When treating moderate frontotemporal hair loss in a 28-year-old male with hair transplants, *which one of the following donor sites should be used?*
   E. Lower occipital

   In general the most popular site for hair harvest is the occipital region. This is commonly used because the donor follicles have decreased or absent DHT and are therefore not influenced by hormonal factors usually associated with hair loss. In addition, providing that the hair is kept above a certain length, the donor scar can be well hidden in this area. The precise level of harvest from the occiput will vary according to age and extent of alopecia. In younger patients such as this man, the donor site is at the junction of the middle and caudal thirds of the vertical distance between the posterior upper healthy fringe and lower hairline (Fig. 90-2).

   In older patients the harvest site is placed higher at the midpoint of the healthy fringe and lower hairline. In this patient, who already has frontotemporal hollowing, temple grafts should be avoided. The vertex and parietal regions are not common donor site areas.

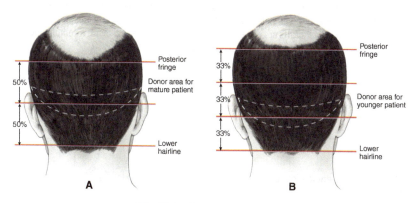

Fig. 90-2 Donor site locations.

11. Which technique of harvesting in hair transplantation may provide the best donor site appearance with the least obvious scarring?
   D. Follicular unit extraction

   There are a number of ways to harvest hair for hair transplantation and the factors that must be considered include speed of harvest, risk of damage to follicular units, and donor site scarring. Traditional harvest techniques involve taking a strip of hair (strip excision) with a standard scalpel as a full-thickness graft and then splitting this into smaller mini and micro grafts for transfer. Triple-blade and quadruple-blade knives have been developed so that 2 mm parallel incisions can be made more quickly and accurately to harvest thinner strips of hair-bearing skin. A laser can be used to harvest the skin as an alternative to a blade but appears to offer no advantages.

   Because of the problems with donor site scarring, the technique of follicular unit extraction has been developed. This is a technique that involves harvesting single follicular units individually using a small diameter punch (less than 1 mm diameter). The advantage of this technique is that linear harvest scars are avoided and instead the harvested areas heal by secondary intention with no visible scarring. The limitations of the technique are that it is blind so it risks inadvertent transection of the follicle, it is slow and is technically demanding. It may be best suited to treatment of smaller areas in patients who are keen to wear their hair short.[5]

12. You are undertaking hair transplantation for a patient with frontotemporal recessions. Which one of the following is true regarding this procedure?

C. Angles selected for hair placement should reflect the anatomic location.

In order to achieve a natural look after hair transplant surgery, the hairline must be re-created carefully and the grafts should be placed in different formations. The angle of orientation is critical to get right and this varies according to anatomic location. At the anterior hairline, angles of 45 to 60 degrees should be used for hair placement. Posterior to the hairline, the angles should be increased to 75 or 80 degrees. In general, the hairs should be placed to reflect the direction of hair growth if they are to look natural (Fig. 90-3).

The anterior hairline should start 7 to 9 cm above the glabella and the lateral extent should be in line with the lateral canthus. Grafts can be micro (containing one or two hairs) or mini (containing three to eight hairs). Ideally a combination of these should be used. Grafts may be placed into small slits or holes. Placing smaller grafts in slits is a good approach, as this is simple and preserves adjacent hair follicles. However, slits do not allow larger grafts to spread out and may give a tufted appearance. In this instance it may be preferable to place these in holes instead of slits. In general, a mixture of micrografts and minigrafts should be used. For example, at the anterior hairline finer grafts are placed first with larger grafts behind them. A combination of slits and holes is probably best to obtain a natural result.

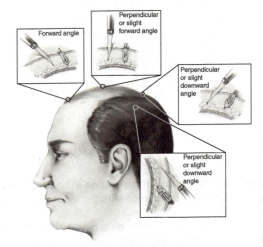

Fig. 90-3 Natural angles in hairline design.

POSTOPERATIVE CARE

13. Which one of the following should be part of the typical postoperative care following hair transplant?

C. Daily hair washing with a pouring technique.

Following a hair transplant it is important to wash the hair early, but this must be done with a pouring technique using a light mix of shampoo with warm water and no scalp massage, which may risk inadvertent removal of the grafts. Normal hair washing can be resumed after 2 weeks once the grafts have taken. The head should be wrapped in a turban with a nonstick base layer such as Telfa. Hair transplant is performed as an outpatient procedure but it takes a significant length of time to perform, so ensure that patients are well hydrated and fed before discharge. They should be accompanied home by a friend or family member. A follow-up appointment should be made for 1 week. There is no reason for patients to have a 2-week course of antibiotics after this surgery.

REFERENCES

1. Orentriech N, Durr NP. Biology of scalp hair growth. Clin Plast Surg 9:197-205, 1982.
2. Norwood OT. Male pattern baldness: classification and incidence. South Med J. 68:1359-1365, 1975.
3. Norwood OT, Shiell RC, eds. Hair Transplant Surgery, ed 2. Springfield, IL: Charles C Thomas, 1984.
4. Messenger AG, McKillop J, Farrant P, et al. British Association of Dermatologists' guidelines for the management of alopecia areata 2012. Br J Dermatol 166:916-926, 2012.
5. Dua A, Dua K. Follicular unit extraction hair transplant. J Cutan Aesthet Surg 3:76-81, 2010.

SUGGESTED READING

Walter P. Unger, Ronald Shapiro, Robin Unger, Mark Unger. Hair Transplantation, ed 5. Philadelphia: CRC Press, 2010.

91. Brow Lift

See *Essentials of Plastic Surgery*, second edition, pp. 1122-1131.

ANATOMY OF THE FOREHEAD AND BROW

1. **Which one of the following statements is correct regarding brow anatomy?**
   A. The corrugator supercilii has both oblique and vertical heads.
   B. The procerus is the sole muscle responsible for creation of oblique glabellar lines.
   C. The corrugator supercilii would be completely denervated by division of the frontal branch.
   D. The frontalis is the main brow elevator and is encased within the galeal sheath.
   E. The orbicularis oculi is a significant contributor to glabellar rhytids.

2. *A patient attends clinic to consider brow and periorbital rejuvenation. He is concerned about wrinkles to the brow and eyes that occur during animation. You discuss the merits of botulinum toxin therapy. For each of the following anatomic areas, select the main target muscle for botulinum toxin therapy in order to eliminate the rhytids. (Each answer may be used once, more than once, or not at all.)*
   A. Vertical glabellar rhytids
   B. Transverse forehead rhytids
   C. Lateral orbital rhytids

   Options:
   a. Frontalis
   b. Corrugator oblique head
   c. Corrugator transverse head
   d. Depressor supercilii
   e. Procerus
   f. Orbital orbicularis oculi
   g. Preseptal orbicularis oculi

3. The sentinel vein can be a source of bleeding during an endoscopic brow lift and should be visualized intraoperatively. **What anatomic landmark is particularly useful to guide its location?**
   A. Medial canthus
   B. Midbrow
   C. Glabella
   D. Lateral canthus
   E. Superior orbital ridge

AESTHETIC ASSESSMENT OF THE BROW

4. You assess a 43-year-old beautician who is considering surgical rejuvenation of the brow. When evaluating this woman, you notice she has very thin eyebrows that taper laterally and sit just above the supraorbital ridge. Her anterior hairline is on the vertical aspect of the forehead. **Which one of the following statements is correct?**
   A. Her eyebrows may be artificially lowered, confounding your assessment.
   B. A brow to hairline distance of 5 cm would indicate a low hairline.
   C. The highest point of her eyebrow should be at its midpoint in the frontal view.
   D. A high hairline is likely in this case, given the clinical description.
   E. The description of her eyebrow position is normal for a young woman.

Chapter 91 ▪ Brow Lift 759

5. **During assessment of the brow and periorbital region in a white patient, which one of the following vertical distances should normally be approximately 1.5 cm (measured in the midpupillary line during a forward gaze)?**
   A. Brow to the superior orbital rim
   B. Brow to the mid pupil
   C. Brow to the upper lash
   D. Brow to the supratarsal crease
   E. Brow to the lower lash

6. A patient is concerned regarding deep transverse brow rhytids that are present at rest. ***How would these best be treated?***
   A. Botulinum toxin injection
   B. Injection of hyaluronic acid filler
   C. Combined botulinum toxin and hyaluronic acid filler
   D. Combined botulinum toxin and laser resurfacing
   E. Surgical muscle weakening and soft tissue redraping

SURGICAL APPROACHES TO BROW LIFT

7. **When undertaking an open coronal approach for brow elevation, which one of the following should be avoided in order to minimize the appearance of a postoperative bald patch or visible scarring?**
   A. Placement of the incision a few centimeters behind the anterior hairline
   B. Beveling the incision at 45 degrees through the skin
   C. Meticulous hemostasis at the skin edges with electrocautery
   D. Closure of the galea with deep sutures combined with skin staples
   E. Avoiding excessive skin resection, particularly in the midline

8. You assess a frail 75-year-old man who underwent excision of a basal cell carcinoma from the left temple with a local flap technique 3 months earlier. Histologic analysis confirms the excision margins are complete. On examination, there is obvious left-sided brow ptosis and loss of transverse forehead rhytids. He is distressed by a degree of visual obstruction by the upper eyelid since the procedure. ***Which one of the following is the next most appropriate step in management?***
   A. Wait six months and review.
   B. Plan for an endoscopic brow lift under general anesthetic.
   C. Plan for a transblepharoplasty brow lift under local anesthetic and sedation.
   D. Plan for an upper eyelid blepharoplasty under local anesthetic and sedation.
   E. Plan for a direct brow lift under local anesthetic.

9. **Which one of the following is correct when performing an endoscopic brow lift?**
   A. Access should be achieved using just two paramedian incisions placed at the hairline.
   B. Central dissection should proceed in the subcutaneous plane.
   C. Lateral dissection should pass deep to the deep temporal fascia.
   D. Release of the periorbital septa and associated adhesions should be performed.
   E. Fixation should be achieved using screws rather than sutures or custom-designed products.

10. **Which one of the following procedures is best avoided in patients with a high hairline and high forehead?**
    A. Direct brow lift
    B. Coronal brow lift
    C. Endoscopic brow lift
    D. Temporal brow lift
    E. Transpalpebral brow lift

11. **What does the elastic band principle refer to with respect to brow lift?**
    A. That brow ptosis will normally recur after a brow lift.
    B. That the soft tissues of the brow have elastic properties.
    C. That fixation in a brow lift should use flexible fixation devices.
    D. That the lift is best when the suspension point is close to the brow.
    E. That the lift is best when the suspension point is further from the brow.

POSTOPERATIVE COMPLICATIONS AFTER BROW LIFT

12. You assess a patient 6 months after performing an endoscopic brow-lift procedure. She has paresthesias at the scar within the hairline. **Which nerve is most likely affected?**
    A. Superficial branch of the supratrochlear nerve
    B. Deep branch of the supratrochlear nerve
    C. Superficial branch of the supraorbital nerve
    D. Deep branch of the supraorbital nerve
    E. Deep branch of the lesser occipital nerve

Answers

ANATOMY OF THE FOREHEAD AND BROW
1. *Which one of the following statements is correct regarding brow anatomy?*
   D. The frontalis is the main brow elevator and is encased within the galeal sheath.
   The frontalis originates at the galea and inserts into the supraorbital dermis and orbicularis oculi to act as the main brow elevator. The galea is an aponeurotic layer that connects the frontalis and the occipitalis muscles over the top of the scalp. It splits into two sheaths around the frontalis, with the deeper layer extending to the periosteum at the supraorbital rim. This attachment needs to be released during a brow lift.

   When closing scalp wounds, such as following an open brow technique, repair of the galeal layer can help reduce skin tension across the wound. It is also a useful layer in more general plastic surgery, as it can be resected to provide deep clearance in skin tumor excision or used in reconstruction of scalp defects as a local flap. In order to enable the frontalis to have mobility to elevate the brow, there is a loose areolar plane beneath the deeper galeal layer and the periosteum. This plane is termed the scalping layer.

   The corrugator supercilii has two heads (oblique and transverse, not vertical), which are innervated by the zygomatic and frontal branches of the facial nerve, respectively. Therefore division of the frontal branch will only denervate part of the muscle. Procerus, corrugator, and depressor supercilii muscles all contribute to oblique glabellar lines. Orbicularis oculi has three parts: the pretarsal, preseptal, and orbital. The orbital is responsible for forced eye closure and it has a medial and a lateral component. Although the medial portion can cause medial brow depression, it is not a significant contributor to glabellar rhytids. The lateral portion may give rise to crow's-feet.

2. *For the following anatomic areas, the best options are as follows:*
   A. Vertical glabellar rhytids
   c. Corrugator transverse head
   As discussed in question 1, corrugator supercilii has two heads, oblique and transverse, and is responsible for creating oblique and vertical glabellar rhytids. It is the transverse head that is predominantly responsible for the vertical lines apparent on frowning, as this passes from the superomedial orbital rim to attach into the dermis in the middle third of the eyebrow, thereby moving the brow medially. The corrugator can be palpated and often visualized when asking a patient to frown. It is a target site for botulinum toxin to reduce vertical glabellar lines. Starting injections using a total of 20 to 40 units of Botox are placed just above the orbital rim at the medial third of the brow. A midline injection in the glabellar area will target the procerus (Fig. 91-1).

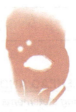

Fig. 91-1 Injection points for glabellar complex and vertical forehead lines.

B. Transverse forehead rhytids
a. Frontalis
As discussed in question 1, the frontalis is the main brow elevator. Its fibers are vertically oriented so contraction lifts the brow and results in transverse brow rhytids. Four to eight injections should be placed into the muscle at least 2 cm above the brow to reduce the risk of brow ptosis. Starting doses are between 10 and 30 units total (Botox). Central injections should be avoided, as they can result in a "quizzical" eyebrow appearance with elevation of the lateral brow and central depression.

C. Lateral orbital rhytids
f. Orbital orbicularis oculi
The orbicularis oculi has three components: pretarsal, preseptal, and orbital (see Chapters 35 and 92). The orbital components are responsible for voluntary movements and cause tight closure of the eye and slight brow depression. The orbital component is subdivided into medial and lateral portions. The lateral portion is responsible for lateral orbital rhytids also known as crow's-feet. These may also be treated with Botox therapy by injecting between 12 and 30 units total at points 1 cm lateral to the bony orbit. Injections must be above the zygomatic arch to avoid inadvertent paralysis of the zygomaticus muscle leading to lip or cheek ptosis (Fig. 91-2).

Fig. 91-2 Injection points for crow's-feet.

3. The sentinel vein can be a source of bleeding during an endoscopic brow lift and should be visualized intraoperatively. **What anatomic landmark is particularly useful to guide its location?**
   D. Lateral canthus
      The sentinel vein is the medial (and larger) of two communicating zygomaticotemporal veins that connect the superficial and deep venous systems in the brow. It is usually located 1.5 cm above and lateral to the lateral canthus. It is just lateral to the temporal crest and is itself a useful anatomic landmark, as it represents a key area for release of the periorbital septa and adhesions. It is also related to the frontal branch of the facial nerve which passes a centimeter above the vein and is therefore a useful guide to avoid injury to this nerve branch. It is important to locate and preserve this vein during a brow lift to avoid bleeding that would obscure the operative view and may lead to a subsequent hematoma formation (Fig. 91-3).

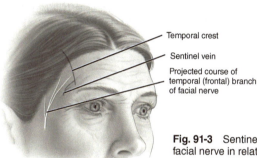

Fig. 91-3 Sentinel vein and frontal branch of facial nerve in relation to the temporal crest.

AESTHETIC ASSESSMENT OF THE BROW

4. You assess a 43-year-old beautician who is considering surgical rejuvenation of the brow. When evaluating this woman, you notice she has very thin eyebrows that taper laterally and sit just above the supraorbital ridge. Her anterior hairline is on the vertical aspect of the forehead. **Which one of the following statements is correct?**
   E. The description of her eyebrow position is normal for a young woman.
      When assessing a patient's brow during an aesthetic consultation, the brow position at rest and during activation should be assessed. The position of the hairline is also important to ascertain. Although the description of her eyebrow position is normal, women may have an artificially elevated brow either from chemodenervation or from plucking. The brow should form a curve with the medial and lateral ends sitting at the same vertical level. The arch should peak at the junction of the middle and lateral thirds. A high hairline in females is indicated either by a measured distance of greater than 5 cm from the brow to hairline or by an anterior hairline sited on the oblique part of the forehead. This is relevant to correctional surgery, particularly endoscopic brow lifting.

5. **During assessment of the brow and periorbital region in a white patient, which one of the following vertical distances should normally be approximately 1.5 cm (measured in the midpupillary line during a forward gaze)?**
   D. Brow to the supratarsal crease
   The vertical distance from the brow to the supratarsal crease (where the levator muscle inserts into the dermis of the upper eyelid) in the midpupillary line is approximately 1.5 cm. Other key measurements in the midpupillary line are as follows:
   - Visible pretarsal upper lid skin: 3 to 6 mm
   - Supratarsal crease to upper lash line 8 to 10 mm
   - Brow to the superior orbital rim: 10 mm
   - Brow to the midpupil: 25 mm
   - Brow to the anterior hairline: 5 to 6 cm

   Knowledge of these distances is clinically relevant when assessing patients for brow lift and eyelid rejuvenation surgery. Knowledge of the distance from the upper lash line to the supratarsal crease is important when planning incisions for upper lid blepharoplasty (Fig. 91-4).

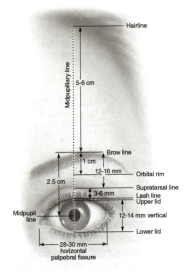

Fig. 91-4 Aesthetic measurements.

6. **A patient is concerned regarding deep transverse brow rhytids that are present at rest. *How would these best be treated?***
   E. Surgical muscle weakening and soft tissue redraping
   Management of rhytids is an important part of brow and periorbital rejuvenation. Rhytids may be classified as static or dynamic and superficial and deep. Static rhytids are present at rest and are due to sustained muscle hyperactivity. They may be partially improved with surgical or chemical muscle weakening but, if deep, as in this case, they will require surgical redraping of the soft tissues. Superficial static rhytids may be improved with fillers such as hyaluronic acid, or resurfacing techniques such as laser or chemical peels as discussed in Chapter 88.

Dynamic rhytids are only present during animation and are often amenable to botulinum toxin injections. They can also be improved more permanently with surgical weakening during brow-lift procedures.

SURGICAL APPROACHES TO BROW LIFT

7. When undertaking an open coronal approach for brow elevation, which one of the following should be avoided in order to minimize the appearance of a postoperative bald patch or visible scarring?
   C. Meticulous hemostasis at the skin edges with electrocautery
   Surgery to the scalp can result in hair loss around the incision site, which can be distressing for patients and signposts the fact that patients have undergone treatment. There are a number of techniques that may minimize visible scalp hair loss. It is important to minimize use of electrocautery on the skin edges, as this damages hair follicles. Raney clips are small U-shaped clips that are temporarily placed at the skin edge to gently compress vessel ends and minimize intraoperative bleeding. They are commonly used in neurosurgery and may be useful for coronal approaches to brow lift. Minimizing tension during closure is also important, as excessive tension results in scar stretch and risk of wound dehiscence, each of which result in a more obvious scar with alopecia. For this reason, skin resection should be conservatively performed and the galea should be closed to reduce tension across the skin edges. As discussed in Chapter 3, staples are useful for scalp closure, as they minimize tissue ischemia. Buried dermal sutures may strangulate the hair follicles and should generally be avoided in the hair-bearing scalp. Placement of the scar is important to help camouflage, although it has no direct effect on the area of hair loss. Beveling the skin incision to either avoid follicle damage or encourage growth through the scar should help disguise a scar. Use of a zigzag incision can have similar benefits.

8. You assess a frail 75-year-old man who underwent excision of a basal cell carcinoma from the left temple with a local flap technique 3 months earlier. Histologic analysis confirms the excision margins are complete. On examination, there is obvious left-sided brow ptosis and loss of transverse forehead rhytids. He is distressed by a degree of visual obstruction by the upper eyelid since the procedure. Which one of the following is the next most appropriate step in management?
   E. Plan for a direct brow lift under local anesthetic.
   This patient has signs and symptoms of frontal nerve injury following his skin cancer excision. Because this is affecting his vision, surgical intervention is warranted. Given his age, previous scarring, and current symptoms, a direct brow lift would be the most suitable procedure for him. This technique has a reliable outcome, is quick and simple to perform, can be achieved under local anesthetic, and has minimal risk of complications.

9. Which one of the following is correct when performing an endoscopic brow lift?
   D. Release of the periorbital septa and associated adhesions should be performed.
   A key part of performing an endoscopic brow lift is to ensure that the periorbital septa and adhesions are adequately released. If this is not performed then the brow cannot be fully elevated, as the soft tissue attachments to bone at the supraorbital rim will limit its upward movement.

   Common approaches to endoscopic brow lift involve three incisions placed behind the anterior hairline. A small central incision is combined with two lateral incisions placed in the temple region. Some surgeons prefer to use two additional paramedian incisions as well. Once the midline incision has been made down through galea, dissection can proceed centrally, either subperiosteally or subgaleally in the "scalping" plane. Both of these approaches provide relatively avascular planes that are easily elevated, but choice of plane will differ according to surgeon's preference. (The subcutaneous plane should be avoided, as it is slow and tedious to dissect and is the wrong plane to achieve either adequate soft tissue release or muscle resection.) Where a subperiosteal dissection is used, initial dissection can be performed blindly using a periosteal elevator to within a few centimeters of the supraorbital rim. The temporal dissection is performed just above the deep temporal fascia (not below), as this safely preserves the frontal branch of the facial nerve. The central and temporal planes of dissection are then joined up, and the endoscope can be used to complete the dissection to the supraorbital rim with direct visualization of the supraorbital and supratrochlear sensory nerves. If required, the glabellar musculature can then be weakened by incising the periosteum and performing partial muscle resection/denervation. There is no proven benefit of fixation with screws over other products.[1]

10. **Which one of the following procedures is best avoided in patients with a high hairline and high forehead?**
    C. **Endoscopic brow lift**
    An endoscopic brow lift is a very useful technique but should be avoided in patients with both a high hairline and a high forehead, particularly when the hairline is situated on the oblique part of the forehead in the lateral view. This is because it is technically difficult to advance the scope around the curvature of the forehead and achieve adequate reach to safely release the supraorbital attachments. The best candidates for endoscopic approaches to brow lift are patients with short, flat foreheads with nonreceding thick hairlines and normal skin. Poor candidates are those with a high convex forehead, a high receding hairline with thin hair, thick skin, and deep rhytids with true excess skin on the forehead and brow.[1]

11. **What does the elastic band principle refer to with respect to brow lift?**
    D. **That the lift is best when the suspension point is close to the brow.**
    The elastic band principle has clinical relevance to brow-lift procedures as it states that the further away the suspension point is from the brow, the lift will be less effective.[1]
    Therefore placement of the fixation point should, in theory, be kept as close to the brow as possible. For this reason, a transpalpebral approach may be ideal, as the fixation will be close to the brow. When performing an open coronal or endoscopic approach, fixation is usually just behind the hairline. However, there is no consensus on the best site of fixation or best device for fixation in brow-lift procedures. Furthermore, some surgeons debate whether fixation is even required, given the rebalancing of soft tissues that occurs following the procedure. In practice, maintaining fixation as close to the brow as possible is probably beneficial, given the underlining biomechanical principles.
    Recurrence of brow ptosis can occur after brow lift and patients must be made aware of this preoperatively. The soft tissues of the brow do have elastic properties, but this is not described by the elastic band principle. Rigid fixation devices (not flexible) are used in brow lifts such as endotine devices, screws, and sutures with or without cortical drill holes.

POSTOPERATIVE COMPLICATIONS AFTER BROW LIFT

12. You assess a patient 6 months after performing an endoscopic brow-lift procedure. She has paresthesias at the scar within the hairline. **Which nerve is most likely affected?**
    D. **Deep branch of the supraorbital nerve**
    The forehead and scalp are supplied by the bilateral supraorbital nerves. These nerves divide into superficial and deep branches. The superficial branch enters the frontalis muscle 2 to 3 cm

above the rim and then supplies the forehead. The deep branch supplies the scalp posterior to the hairline and runs laterally up to 0.5 to 1.5 cm medial to the temporal crest. Transection of the deep branch can result in postoperative scalp paresthesias.[2]

REFERENCES

1. Nahai F, ed. The Art of Aesthetic Surgery: Principles & Techniques, ed 2. St Louis: Quality Medical Publishing, 2011.
2. Flowers FS, Caputy GC, Flowers SS. The biomechanics of brow and frontalis function and its effect on blepharoplasty. Clin Plast Surg 20:255-268, 2003.

92. Blepharoplasty

See *Essentials of Plastic Surgery*, second edition, pp. 1132-1148.

MUSCLES OF THE EYELID AND GLOBE

1. **Correctly identify the anatomic components of the eyelid and extraocular region on the diagram below (Fig. 92-1). Five of the nine options will be used.**

    Options:
    a. Levator palpebrae superioris
    b. Superior rectus muscle
    c. Inferior rectus muscle
    d. Superior oblique muscle
    e. Müller's muscle
    f. Inferior oblique muscle
    g. Pretarsal orbicularis oculi
    h. Preseptal orbicularis oculi
    i. Preorbital orbicularis oculi

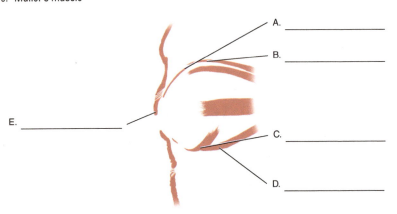

Fig. 92-1 Anatomy of the eyelid.

COMPONENTS OF THE EYELID

2. Correctly identify the anatomic components of the eyelid and extraocular region on the diagram (Fig. 92-2). Six of the nine options will be used.

Options:
a. Superior orbital rim
b. Arcus marginalis
c. Levator aponeurosis
d. Retroorbicularis oculi fat (ROOF)
e. Suborbicularis oculi fat (SOOF)
f. Conjunctiva
g. Tarsal plate
h. Capsulopalpebral fascia
i. Postseptal fat pad

A. _____
B. _____
C. _____
D. _____

E. _____
F. _____
G. _____

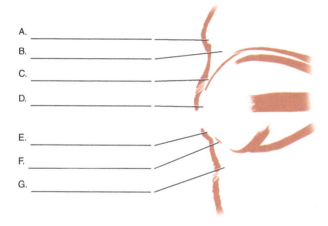

Fig. 92-2

3. When asking a patient to keep their eyes tightly closed against resistance, which muscle is chiefly responsible?
A. Inferior rectus
B. Superior rectus
C. Pretarsal orbicularis
D. Preseptal orbicularis
E. Orbital orbicularis

4. You are undertaking an upper lid blepharoplasty and have removed the skin and underlying orbicularis muscle as a single composite. What is most likely the next layer of tissue?
A. Muscle
B. Fascia
C. Fat
D. Fibrous tissue
E. Mucosa

5. Which muscle of the eye has its vector of pull altered by Whitnall's ligament?
A. Superior oblique
B. Inferior oblique
C. Levator palpebrae superioris
D. Orbicularis oculi
E. Superior rectus

6. **Which one of the following structures is responsible for causing subtle downward migration of the lower eyelid when asking a patient to look down at the floor?**
   A. Capsulopalpebral fascia
   B. Orbital septum
   C. Lockwood's ligament
   D. Orbicularis oculi
   E. Arcus marginalis

7. You see a patient in clinic before blepharoplasty surgery and note that there is a very subtle ptosis on the left side. On further examination, you also notice that the pupil is slightly smaller on this side. The patient is still able to elevate the eyelid. **Which muscle is primarily affected?**
   A. Superior oblique
   B. Superior rectus
   C. Levator palpebrae superioris
   D. Müller's muscle
   E. Pretarsal orbicularis

ORBITAL FAT

8. **How does orbital fat differ from fat in other anatomic locations?**
   A. Larger cell size
   B. Less saturated
   C. More lipoprotein lipase
   D. More metabolically active
   E. Less affected by diet

FAT COMPARTMENTS OF THE EYELIDS

9. **What separates the medial and middle postseptal fat compartments in the upper eyelid?**
   A. Lateral rectus muscle
   B. Inferior oblique muscle
   C. Superior rectus muscle
   D. Superior oblique muscle
   E. Lacrimal gland

PREOPERATIVE ASSESSMENT

10. **When examining the normal eye during an aesthetic assessment, which one of the following measurements is most likely?**
    A. A palpebral fissure measuring 12 by 28 mm
    B. 12 mm of visible pretarsal skin
    C. A vertical lash line to supratarsal crease distance of 17 mm
    D. A negative canthal tilt
    E. A vertical brow-to-midpupil distance of 15 mm

ASIAN EYELID ANATOMY

11. Asians have different aesthetic eyelid features compared with white individuals. **Which one of the following is a common feature of the Asian eyelid?**
    A. A high supratarsal crease
    B. An increased tarsal height
    C. Descent of the preaponeurotic fat
    D. Absence of the eyelashes
    E. Dermal connection with the levator

DEFORMITIES OF THE EYELIDS

12. A 24-year-old woman presents with a history of recurrent bilateral swelling in the periorbital region. She has concerns regarding the appearance of her eyes, which have thin, puffy upper and lower eyelid skin. **Which one of the following is the most likely diagnosis?**
    A. Blepharoptosis
    B. Blepharochalasis
    C. Steatoblepharon
    D. Dermatochalasis
    E. Pseudoblepharoptosis

PREOPERATIVE PLANNING

13. **Which one of the following preoperative test findings suggests a high risk of developing scleral show and ectropion following blepharoplasty?**
    A. A negative Bell's phenomenon
    B. A negative vector globe position
    C. A positive Schirmer's test
    D. A positive brow compensation test
    E. A positive vector globe position

14. You are assessing a patient's upper eyelid during a cosmetic consultation and note a lateral fullness to the lid. **What is the most likely procedure to benefit this condition?**
    A. Fat transfer
    B. Excision of ROOF
    C. Excision of postseptal fat
    D. Septal redraping
    E. Lacrimal glandulopexy

15. You see a 50-year-old woman who is eager to proceed with upper and lower eyelid rejuvenation surgery. She is generally fit and well and states she has not undergone any recent surgery. You make a plan with her for upper and lower blepharoplasty surgery in 1 month. At the end of the consultation you are finalizing the date, and she mentions that this will fit nicely with her planned corrective laser eye surgery and time off from work. **How would this statement alter your management plan?**
    A. Cancel the surgery.
    B. Proceed with surgery as planned.
    C. Postpone the surgery for 1 year after the laser correction.
    D. Postpone the surgery for 6 weeks after the laser correction.
    E. Assess her status in the office once her laser treatment is complete.

TECHNIQUES FOR EYELID CORRECTION

16. For each of the following clinical scenarios, select the most suitable surgical option from the list. (Each answer may be used once, more than once, or not at all.)
    A. You see a 66-year-old man with prominent lower eyelid bags. He has an excess of skin, fat, and muscle with improvement of his festoon on forcible eye closure (positive squinch test).
    B. You see a 50-year-old woman with marked ectropion, a positive snap test, mild scleral show, 5 mm of anterior lid distraction, but satisfactory skin volume.
    C. You see a 34-year-old woman with a mild excess of lower lid skin, fine crow's-feet, and good soft tissue lid volume.

    Options:
    a. Kuhnt-Szymanowski procedure
    b. Lateral canthoplasty
    c. Lower lid pinch blepharoplasty
    d. Loeb procedure with canthopexy
    e. Skin and muscle excision blepharoplasty with septal reset
    f. Transconjunctival blepharoplasty

17. A 22-year-old Asian model attends clinic keen to have surgery on her eyelids in order to have a more white appearance. **Which one of the following adjuncts to blepharoplasty would be most beneficial for her?**
    A. Tarsal fixation
    B. Tarsal shortening
    C. Lid tightening
    D. Fat grafting
    E. Septal reset

EARLY COMPLICATIONS AFTER BLEPHAROPLASTY

18. A 59-year-old patient undergoes upper and lower blepharoplasties with postseptal fat removal and is initially well on postoperative rounds. An hour later you are called to see the patient, who has described decreased clarity of vision on the left side with increasing eye pain. On examination, there is mild left-sided proptosis and ecchymosis with reduced eye movement. The direct pupillary light response is diminished, but the consensual reflex is maintained. **Which one of the following actions should you perform first?**
    A. Lie the patient flat.
    B. Give oral mannitol.
    C. Apply topical acetazolamide.
    D. Remove the sutures.
    E. Perform medial cantholysis.

Answers

MUSCLES OF THE EYELID AND GLOBE

1. For the following image (Fig. 92-3), the anatomic components of the eyelid are as follows:

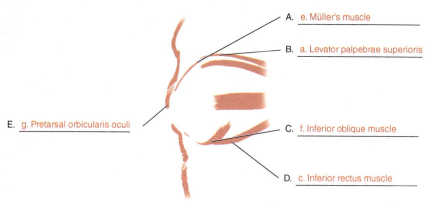

- A. e. Müller's muscle
- B. a. Levator palpebrae superioris
- C. f. Inferior oblique muscle
- D. c. Inferior rectus muscle
- E. g. Pretarsal orbicularis oculi

Fig. 92-3 Anatomy of the eyelid.

COMPONENTS OF THE EYELID

2. For the following image (Fig. 92-4), the anatomic components of the eyelid are as follows:

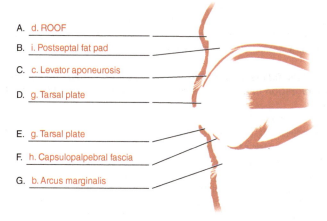

- A. d. ROOF
- B. i. Postseptal fat pad
- C. c. Levator aponeurosis
- D. g. Tarsal plate
- E. g. Tarsal plate
- F. h. Capsulopalpebral fascia
- G. b. Arcus marginalis

Fig. 92-4

3. **When asking a patient to keep their eyes tightly closed against resistance, which muscle is chiefly responsible?**
   E. Orbital orbicularis
   The orbicularis oculi is a sphincter muscle surrounding the eye aperture. It has three portions orbital, preseptal, and pretarsal which relate to the underlying structures. The functions of each are different. For example, the orbital part is under voluntary control and causes tight closure of the eye and medial brow depression. It is the outermost part and lies superficial to the corrugators and procerus. It is innervated by the frontal and zygomatic branches. The preseptal part is involved in both voluntary and involuntary actions including blinking. The pretarsal part is involuntary and also assists with blinking. It is primarily innervated by the zygomatic branch. The superior and inferior recti are both extraocular muscles involved in movement of the globe, causing elevation and depression, respectively. They are innervated by the oculomotor nerve CN III and work in conjunction with the other extraocular muscles to coordinate eye movement.

4. You are undertaking an upper lid blepharoplasty and have removed the skin and underlying orbicularis muscle as a single composite. **What is most likely the next layer of tissue?**
   C. Fat
   The eyelid is comprised of anterior and posterior lamella. The anterior lamella contains the skin and orbicularis oculi. The posterior lamella contains the tarsus and conjunctiva. The septum between them is sometimes referred to as the middle lamella. When undertaking an upper eyelid blepharoplasty, the next layer after orbicularis will be fat and this is termed the retroorbicularis oculi fat layer or ROOF. It is clinically relevant, as it may be a cause of upper eyelid hooding and puffiness. Excision of this fat may well be indicated to reduce fullness. This must not be confused with the preseptal fat compartments, which are accessed by incising the septum beneath the ROOF layer.

5. **Which muscle of the eye has its vector of pull altered by Whitnall's ligament?**
   C. Levator palpebrae superioris
   The levator palpebrae superioris (LPS) is the key upper eyelid elevator. It originates from the lesser wing of sphenoid and inserts into the upper eyelid dermis and upper tarsus. It is innervated by the oculomotor nerve CN III. The natural vector of pull of this muscle would be posterior, given the attachments. Whitnall's ligament is a fascial condensation that translates this posterior vector into a superior vector. This allows LPS to provide 10 to 15 mm of upper eyelid excursion. The superior and inferior oblique muscles are involved in movement of the globe assisting with abduction and adduction, respectively. The superior rectus causes elevation of the globe.

6. **Which one of the following structures is responsible for causing subtle downward migration of the lower eyelid when asking a patient to look down at the floor?**
   A. Capsulopalpebral fascia
   The capsulopalpebral fascia is the lower eyelid equivalent of the levator muscle. It originates from the inferior oblique muscle fascia and inserts on the septum below the tarsus. In contrast to the levator muscle, it has only a subtle action on the lower eyelid, resulting in a couple of millimeters migration only (Fig. 92-5). Lockwood's ligament is a hammocklike structure that supports the globe; it is part of the tarsoligamentous complex shown in Fig. 92-5.

   The tarsoligamentous complex is a connective tissue framework supporting the eyelids and globe. It also includes the upper and lower tarsal plates and the medial and lateral canthal ligament complexes. The orbital septum is an extension of orbital periosteum that extends from the orbital rim to the eyelid retractors. The *arcus marginalis* is the fibrous attachment of the eyelid to the inferior orbital rim. It is released during some lower eyelid blepharoplasty techniques, but it does not cause downward migration of the eyelid.

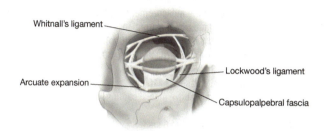

Fig. 92-5 The capsulopalpebral fascia is shown as it originates from the inferior fascia and inserts on the inferior portion of the tarsus and orbital septum.

7. **You see a patient in clinic before blepharoplasty surgery and note that there is a very subtle ptosis on the left side. On further examination, you also notice that the pupil is slightly smaller on this side. The patient is still able to elevate the eyelid. Which muscle is primarily affected?**
   D. Müller's muscle
   Müller's muscle is a component of the upper eyelid. It is a small muscle responsible for 2 to 3 mm of eyelid elevation. It originates from the levator palpebrae superioris and is essentially the deep continuation of this muscle where it inserts on the superior edge of the tarsus. It has sympathetic innervation and when denervated, results in a subtle ptosis on the affected side. This clinical appearance is classically seen as a triad of features due to loss of sympathetic function known as Horner's syndrome. It includes upper eyelid ptosis, meiosis (pupillary constriction), and anhidrosis (loss of sweating on the affected side).

ORBITAL FAT

8. *How does orbital fat differ from fat in other anatomic locations?*
   E. Less affected by diet
   Orbital fat is physiologically different from normal body fat and is minimally affected by diet. In addition, the fat cells are smaller, the fat is more saturated, and it is less metabolically active and has less lipoprotein lipase.

FAT COMPARTMENTS OF THE EYELIDS

9. *What separates the medial and middle postseptal fat compartments in the upper eyelid?*
   D. Superior oblique muscle
   The upper lid has two postseptal fat compartments: middle and medial (the lacrimal gland occupies the lateral compartment; see Fig. 92-4, *Essentials of Plastic Surgery,* second edition). These are separated by the trochlea of the superior rectus muscle. In contrast, the lower lid has three fat compartments and the lateral and central compartments are separated by the inferior oblique muscle. The compartments are relevant to blepharoplasty, since they can be manipulated during the procedure. In some cases, the fat within the compartments can cause excessive bulkiness to the eyelids and is therefore removed or cauterized during blepharoplasty. In the lower eyelid, redraping of the fat may also be undertaken.

PREOPERATIVE ASSESSMENT

10. When examining the normal eye during an aesthetic assessment, which one of the following measurements is most likely?
A. A palpebral fissure measuring 12 by 28 mm

There is individual variation in the measurements of the eyelids and brow. However, in most individuals, there are some standard measurements usually quoted during forward gaze[1] (see Fig. 92-5, *Essentials of Plastic Surgery,* second edition):
- Palpebral fissure: 12 to 14 mm vertically, 28 to 30 mm horizontally
- Visible pretarsal skin: 3 to 6 mm
- Lash line to supratarsal crease: 8 to 10 mm
- Lateral canthus: 1 to 2 mm above medial canthus (i.e., negative canthal tilt)
- In the midpupillary line:
    Anterior hairline to brow: 5 to 6 cm
    Brow to orbital rim: 1 cm
    Brow to supratarsal crease: 12 to 16 mm
    Brow to midpupil: 2.5 cm

ASIAN EYELID ANATOMY

11. Asians have different aesthetic eyelid features compared with white individuals. Which one of the following is a common feature of the Asian eyelid?
C. Descent of the preaponeurotic fat

The Asian eyelid is distinctly different from other races. The key differences are descent of the preaponeurotic fat and absence of the supratarsal fold. This gives the upper eyelid a fuller and less well-defined appearance. In addition, the tarsus is also shorter (see Fig. 92-6, *Essentials of Plastic Surgery,* second edition). Absence of the eyelashes is termed madarosis. It is associated with multiple conditions ranging from skin conditions such as eczema, through autoimmune diseases such as lupus and scleroderma, to malignancies such as sebaceous gland and squamous cell carcinomas. It is not specifically related to a particular racial group.

DEFORMITIES OF THE EYELIDS

12. A 24-year-old woman presents with a history of recurrent bilateral swelling in the periorbital region. She has concerns regarding the appearance of her eyes, which have thin, puffy upper and lower eyelid skin. Which one of the following is the most likely diagnosis?
B. Blepharochalasis

Blepharochalasis is a condition with thin, excessive upper and lower eyelid skin caused by repeated bouts of painless edema. It most often occurs before the age of 20 and is refractory to antihistamines and steroids. Dermatochalasis refers to an excess of upper eyelid skin. Steatoblepharon is a condition where fat protrudes through a lax septum. Blepharoptosis is drooping of the upper eyelid (see Chapter 93, *Essentials of Plastic Surgery,* second edition). Pseudoblepharoptosis is an appearance of ptosis with a normal lid position, commonly due to a ptotic brow and excess brow skin.

PREOPERATIVE PLANNING

13. Which one of the following preoperative test findings suggests a high risk of developing scleral show and ectropion following blepharoplasty?
B. A negative vector globe position

Understanding the concept of positive and negative vectors in blepharoplasty is critical in decision-making for surgery. This term refers to the relationship of the lower eyelid to the orbital rim. It considers the anterior projection of the globe compared with the most anteriorly projecting portion of the lateral orbital rim.

A **prominent** eye is described as having a *negative* vector, where the anterior portion of the globe is anterior to the orbital rim. In this case, a lower eyelid blepharoplasty risks development of downward "clothes lining" of the lower eyelid below the inferior limbus (i.e., the lower lid becomes too tight and slides under the globe, leading to a low eyelid with scleral show and ectropion).

A **deep-set** eye has a *positive* vector and in mild cases this does not represent a problem for a standard lower lid blepharoplasty, because tightening the lower lid will tend to act as a snug hammock for the globe. In more severe cases, patients will need lower and deeper lateral canthal anchoring, however, because a standard canthal position would cause upward "clothes lining" of the lower lid with narrowing of the eye fissure and a reduction in the size of the lateral scleral angle.[1]

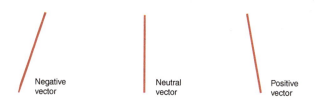

Fig. 92-6 Globe vectors.

Eye prominence and vector assessment can be formally measured using a Hertel exophthalmometer. With this tool a normal globe prominence should be 16 to 18 mm. A prominent eye would be 19 mm or more, and a deep-set eye would be 15 mm or less.[1]

The Bell's phenomenon is a natural protective reflex and refers to upward movement of the globe during eye closure. Where this is absent the patient is at increased risk of dry-eye symptoms with postoperative lagopthalmus. Schirmer's test assesses the lacrimal function and, if positive, indicates that dry eye is present preoperatively. Blepharoplasty should be avoided in these patients.

It is vital to test for compensated brow ptosis before blepharoplasty, as this needs to be addressed before blepharoplasty, otherwise it is likely that the problem will not be corrected and may even be exacerbated. In addition, excess skin may be removed, and once brow correction is achieved, there may be insufficient eyelid skin leading to lagopthalmus.

14. You are assessing a patient's upper eyelid during a cosmetic consultation and note a lateral fullness to the lid. ***What is the most likely procedure to benefit this condition?***
   E. Lacrimal glandulopexy
   Lateral upper-lid fullness is most likely caused by ptosis of the lacrimal gland. The upper eyelid has only two (central and medial) postseptal fat pads, and the lacrimal gland fills the lateral aspect. If the fullness is in the lower lids, then removal of the lateral postseptal fat pad may be indicated. Awareness of the location of the lacrimal gland is vital when performing eyelid surgery, since damage to this structure can lead to a dry-eye condition. Fat transfer is not commonly used in the eyelids, though may be used to improve a tear-trough deformity. Septal redraping is another lower lid technique that may be useful to improve the tear-trough deformity.

15. You see a 50-year-old woman who is eager to proceed with upper and lower eyelid rejuvenation surgery. She is generally fit and well and states she has not undergone any recent surgery. You make a plan with her for upper and lower blepharoplasty surgery in 1 month. At the end of the consultation you are finalizing the date, and she mentions that this will fit nicely with her planned corrective laser eye surgery and time off from work. **How would this statement alter your management plan?**
    E. **Assess her status in the office once her laser treatment is complete.**

    This patient will be at risk of developing dry-eye syndrome following her laser eye surgery. Although there are no strict rules or guidelines, it would be most sensible to defer eyelid correction surgery until after the laser surgery is complete; 6 months is generally thought to be adequate. Given the situation, it would be most appropriate to assess this woman again a few months after her laser eye surgery to review and discuss her options.

TECHNIQUES FOR EYELID CORRECTION

16. *For the following scenarios, the best options are as follows:*
    A. *You see a 66-year-old man with prominent lower eyelid bags. He has an excess of skin, fat, and muscle with improvement of his festoon on forcible eye closure (positive squinch test).*
        e. **Skin and muscle excision blepharoplasty with septal reset**

        This man needs attention to each layer of the lower eyelid with resection of skin, muscle, and fat. This could be achieved through a subciliary skin approach, lower lid blepharoplasty with muscle and skin removal, fat redraping, and lower lid tightening. The Loeb procedure involves fat manipulation by sliding fat out of the lower eyelid compartment into the tear trough. This is best suited to patients with deep tear troughs and excess postseptal fat.

    B. *You see a 50-year-old woman with marked ectropion, a positive snap test, mild scleral show, 5 mm of anterior lid distraction, but satisfactory skin volume.*
        b. **Lateral canthoplasty**

        This woman requires lower eyelid tightening, which can be achieved with either a lateral canthopexy or a canthoplasty. In her case, given the degree of laxity, a canthoplasty is probably preferable. For less tightening, a Kuhnt-Szymanowski procedure would be appropriate.

    C. *You see a 34-year-old woman with a mild excess of lower lid skin, fine crow's-feet, and good soft tissue lid volume.*
        c. **Lower lid pinch blepharoplasty**

        This woman requires minimal intervention and could benefit from a pinch blepharoplasty, which would remove a small amount of lower lid skin only. A transconjunctival approach may be indicated where there is no skin resection required.

17. A 22-year-old Asian model attends clinic keen to have surgery on her eyelids in order to have a more white appearance. **Which one of the following adjuncts to blepharoplasty would be most beneficial for her?**
    A. **Tarsal fixation**

    Tarsal fixation techniques are used to help create a high supratarsal fold. These may be suture or no suture techniques. An example of a suture technique is the anchor blepharoplasty approach described by Flowers,[2,3] which uses a permanent suture passing from the skin to the tarsus and levator. Baker et al[4] used an excise approach without sutures that involved resection of a section of the orbicularis oculi and allowing the skin to scar to the septum.

These techniques are particularly useful in the Asian eyelid which has an absent or short supratarsal crease. They may also be useful in other scenarios including secondary blepharoplasty, men with brow ptosis, and patients with low preoperative eyelid folds.

The Asian eyelid tends to have a shorter tarsus and descent of the aponeurotic fat, so tarsal shortening and fat transfer would not be indicated. Lid tightening is indicated in lax lower eyelids, but this is not a characteristic of the young Asian eyelid. Septal reset is used to improve a tear-trough deformity which is not typically present in the Asian eyelid.

EARLY COMPLICATIONS AFTER BLEPHAROPLASTY

18. A 59-year-old patient undergoes upper and lower blepharoplasties with postseptal fat removal and is initially well on postoperative rounds. An hour later you are called to see the patient, who has described decreased clarity of vision on the left side with increasing eye pain. On examination, there is mild left-sided proptosis and ecchymosis with reduced eye movement. The direct pupillary light response is diminished, but the consensual reflex is maintained. *Which one of the following actions should you perform first?*
D. Remove the sutures.

Patients who undergo blepharoplasty with removal of postseptal fat have a very small but appreciable risk of developing retrobulbar hematoma.[5] This is a clinical emergency that without appropriate treatment within 1 to 2 hours can result in permanent blindness.

The patient above has key signs and symptoms of this condition: proptosis, altered vision and pain, and bruising around the eye. The pathophysiology is similar to that of compartment syndrome where there is an expanding volume (continued bleeding/swelling) held within a fixed space (the bony orbit).

Removal of the sutures should be performed immediately, as this will help to decompress the area. The patient should be placed with the head up (approximately 30 degrees) to help venous drainage and reduce swelling. Other measures also directed at relieving intraorbital pressure can be medical (such as steroids, mannitol, and acetazolamide) or surgical (such as release of the lateral canthus to decompress the globe).

Mannitol and acetazolamide both act to shrink the vitreous humor, thereby reducing intraocular pressure. Mannitol is an osmotic agent that should be given intravenously in boluses. Acetazolamide is a carbonic anhydride inhibitor also administered intravenously (not topically) in 500 mg doses. Lateral cantholysis is required and the patient should be transferred to the OR so release can be performed and the hematoma fully evacuated.

REFERENCES

1. Codner MA, Mejia JD. Lower eyelid blepharoplasty. In Nahai F, ed. The Art of Aesthetic Surgery: Principles & Techniques, ed 2. St Louis: Quality Medical Publishing, 2011.
2. Flowers RS. Upper blepharoplasty by eyelid invagination: anchor blepharoplasty. Clin Plast Surg 20:193-207, 1993.
3. Flowers RS, DuVal C. Blepharoplasty and periorbital aesthetic surgery. In Aston SJ, Beasley RW, Thorne CM, et al, eds. Grabb & Smith's Plastic Surgery, ed 6. Philadelphia: Lippincott Williams & Wilkins, 2006.
4. Baker TJ, Gordon HL, Mosienko P. Upper lid blepharoplasty. Plast Reconstr Surg 60:692-698, 1977.
5. Winterton JB, Patel K, Mizen KD. Review of Management Options for a Retrobulbar Hemorrhage. J Oral Maxillofac Surg 65:296-299, 2007.

93. Blepharoptosis

See *Essentials of Plastic Surgery*, second edition, pp. 1149-1159.

CONGENITAL PTOSIS

1. You see a 6-month-old infant in clinic. His parents are concerned about the appearance of his left eye, as the upper lid sits lower on this side, partially covering the iris. He is otherwise well and developing normally. **Which one of the following is true of his condition?**
   A. It is likely to be present in other close family members.
   B. It probably reflects abnormal levator development.
   C. His upper eyelid excursion is still likely to be normal.
   D. A supratarsal crease would be present on examination.
   E. The appearance is likely to become worse over time.

2. **For each of the following clinical scenarios, select the most likely diagnosis. (Each option may be used once, more than once, or not at all.)**
   A. A young boy is referred to your pediatric clinic with congenital ptosis. His parents have noticed the child's left eyelid consistently elevates while he is eating.
   B. You see a 2-year-old girl whose parents are concerned about her eye appearance. On examination, she has an increased intercanthal distance, bilateral ptosis, and small eyelids.
   C. You see a 3-year-old child in the clinic with a retracted globe and apparent ptosis. In addition, there is poor eye movement with strabismus and an inability to lateralize the globe.

   Options:
   a. Neurofibromatosis
   b. Duane's syndrome
   c. Chronic squinting
   d. Marcus Gunn syndrome
   e. Congenital anophthalmos
   f. Blepharophimosis syndrome

ACQUIRED PTOSIS

3. **What is the most common type of acquired blepharoptosis?**
   A. Physiologic
   B. Neurogenic
   C. Involutional
   D. Mechanical
   E. Traumatic

DIFFERENTIATION OF CONGENITAL AND ACQUIRED PTOSIS
4. When examining a young patient with ptosis of the upper eyelids, which one of the following may be useful to differentiate between congenital and acquired causes?
   A. Strabismus
   B. Amblyopia
   C. Telecanthus
   D. Lagophthalmos
   E. Hypoglobus

DIAGNOSING ABNORMAL UPPER EYELID ANATOMY
5. In an adult patient with a unilateral elevated supratarsal fold, mild ptosis, and an accentuated supratarsal hollow, which one of the following is the most likely diagnosis?
   A. Prior botulinum toxin
   B. Levator dehiscence
   C. Myasthenia gravis
   D. Reduced sympathetic innervation
   E. CN III compression

TECHNIQUE SELECTION FOR BLEPHAROPTOSIS SURGERY
6. Which one of the following is considered the single most important factor when selecting a technique for correction of blepharoptosis?
   A. Lid height position
   B. Duration of ptosis
   C. Degree of ptosis
   D. Amount of lid elevation
   E. Presence of lagopthalmus

SURGICAL MANAGEMENT OF BLEPHAROPTOSIS
7. A 60-year-old patient is seen with a chronic unilateral visual impairment resulting from obstruction from the right upper eyelid. Examination of the affected eye shows severe blepharoptosis, with 8 mm of levator excursion. Which one of the following is the best surgical approach to management?
   A. Müllers muscle–conjunctival resection
   B. Levator advancement
   C. Frontalis suspension
   D. Levator reinsertion
   E. Aponeurosis repair

8. When undertaking surgical correction of upper eyelid ptosis in adult patients, which one of the following is correct?
   A. Undercorrection should be performed when using epinephrine in the local anesthetic.
   B. Correction is best achieved with the use of general anesthetic because of patient compliance difficulties.
   C. When using local anesthetic agents, overcorrection may be required to achieve satisfactory results.
   D. In patients who wear contact lenses, a Schirmer's test must be performed before surgery.
   E. All patients must be counseled about and should receive appropriate management for lagophthalmos.

THE FASANELLA-SERVAT TECHNIQUE
9. You have a patient with blepharoptosis and have decided to perform the Fasanella-Servat technique. Which one of the following is correct regarding this procedure?
   A. It is ideal when levator function is poor.
   B. It involves a transversal skin incision.
   C. It may result in a floppy upper lid.
   D. It has very predictable outcomes.
   E. It is a levator advancement technique.

LEVATOR APONEUROSIS ADVANCEMENT

10. A 58-year-old patient has moderate unilateral upper lid ptosis and a plan is made for advancement of the levator aponeurosis under general anesthesia. Preoperative lid height is 3 mm below the upper limbus and levator excursion is 9 mm. **When performing this surgery, which one of the following is true?**
    A. A transconjunctival approach should be made at the superior tarsal border.
    B. Correction of ptosis will require 6 mm of levator advancement.
    C. The upper lid should be set to lie above the upper limbus.
    D. Using the gapping method, a distance of 9 mm should be used to set advancement.
    E. A single central mattress suture should be used to repair the aponeurosis.

FRONTALIS SUSPENSION

11. A young patient has unilateral blepharoptosis with poor levator function. They are seen by your assistant and scheduled to undergo frontalis suspension. **Which one of the following is true in this case?**
    A. This technique is not well suited to treat this patient's condition.
    B. Surgery would involve resection of the remaining viable Müller's muscle.
    C. Suspension is achieved by direct suturing of the upper tarsus to the frontalis.
    D. Simultaneous surgery to the contralateral eyelid would not normally be required.
    E. Long-term night-time patching and ointment will be required after surgery.

POSTOPERATIVE PROBLEMS AFTER PTOSIS CORRECTION

12. You assess a patient in the clinic after a left unilateral levator aponeurosis advancement. She is satisfied with the improvement gained to the left eye but is concerned that the right eye now appears ptotic. **Which one of the following explains these clinical findings?**
    A. Putterman's test
    B. Schirmer's test
    C. Hering's law
    D. Fasanella's law
    E. Hering's test

Answers

CONGENITAL PTOSIS

1. You see a 6-month-old infant in clinic. His parents are concerned about the appearance of his left eye, as the upper lid sits lower on this side, partially covering the iris. He is otherwise well and developing normally. **Which one of the following is true of this condition?**
   B. It probably reflects abnormal levator development.
   Congenital ptosis is due to developmental dysgenesis in the levator muscle. It is usually noticed shortly after birth and does not have a clear inheritance pattern. It is most often a sporadic, isolated occurrence, although it can be observed in some rare syndromes. Because the levator is poorly formed, upper lid excursion is usually reduced and the supratarsal crease is absent. The condition is not usually progressive, so is unlikely to become worse over time.

2. *For the following scenarios, the best options are as follows:*
   A. A young boy is referred to your pediatric clinic with congenital ptosis. His parents have noticed the child's left eyelid consistently elevates while he is eating.
   d. Marcus Gunn syndrome
   This child displays findings in keeping with trigeminooculomotor synkinesis, also known as Marcus Gunn syndrome. This involves unwanted upper lid elevation during activation of the muscles of mastication, such as when chewing or biting.[1] It occurs in 5% of children with congenital ptosis and is caused by aberrant CN V innervation to the levator muscle. There is also another condition called Inverse Marcus Gunn syndrome that involves unwanted eyelid closure during biting and is an extremely rare acquired condition. A similar condition is Marin-Amat syndrome, which is a rare synkinesis in which eye closure occurs on full opening of the jaw.[2]

   B. You see a 2-year-old girl whose parents are concerned about her eye appearance. On examination, she has an increased intercanthal distance, bilateral ptosis, and small eyelids.
   f. Blepharophimosis syndrome
   This child displays findings in keeping with blepharophimosis syndrome. This rare inherited condition is a complex eyelid malformation characterized by ptosis, blepharophimosis (narrowing of the horizontal aperture), telecanthus, and epicanthus inversus (a skin fold arising from the lower eyelid).

   C. You see a 3-year-old child in the clinic with a retracted globe and apparent ptosis. In addition, there is poor eye movement with strabismus and an ability to lateralize the globe.
   b. Duane's syndrome
   This child shows signs of Duane's syndrome, which is a congenital condition that results in pseudoptosis and strabismus. It is caused by abnormal development of the abducens nerve, and subsequently lateral rectus muscle function is impaired.

Neurofibromatosis (NF1) can be associated with ptosis of the upper eyelid, due to the increased physical bulk of the eyelid because of neurofibroma formation. Lesions may need debulking if they begin to compromise vision, but commonly recur over time following surgery. Other key features of NF1 include café au lait spots, pigmented lesions on the iris (Lisch nodules), optic nerve tumors, and skin nodules.

A squint refers to a misalignment of the eyes and an uncontrolled squint can lead to a lazy eye (amblyopia). It can also give the appearance of a ptotic upper lid. Congenital anophthalmia and microphthalmia refer to maldevelopment of the eye and periorbita that results in either complete or partial absence of these structures. In mild cases, hypoplasia of the lids, globe, and orbital bones can also give the appearance of ptosis.

ACQUIRED PTOSIS

3. **What is the most common type of acquired blepharoptosis?**
   C. Involutional
   Acquired ptosis may be classified as myogenic, neurogenic, traumatic, or mechanical. Involutional ptosis is the most common type of acquired ptosis. It represents a subtype of myogenic ptosis and is caused by stretching of the levator aponeurosis attachments to the tarsal plate. Dermal attachments remain in place. Traumatic causes are the next most common where there is disruption of the levator aponeurosis. Neurogenic causes include CN III palsy and Horner's syndrome. Mechanical causes tend to refer to external physical causes that counteract normal elevation, such as upper lid tumors and excess upper eyelid skin.

DIFFERENTIATION OF CONGENITAL AND ACQUIRED PTOSIS

4. **When examining a young patient with ptosis of the upper eyelids, which one of the following may be useful to differentiate between congenital and acquired causes?**
   D. Lagophthalmos
   Differentiation between congenital and acquired causes of blepharoptosis is usually straightforward, given the timing of symptoms. In the event that the diagnosis is less obvious, it may be useful to differentiate between the two, based on the presence or absence of lagopthalmos on downward gaze. This occurs secondary to levator fibrosis which is more commonly seen in congenital cases.

   Strabismus refers to a misalignment of the eyes as a result of impaired extraocular muscle function. Amblyopia is a lazy eye where there is decreased vision secondary to abnormal visual development in infancy. Telecanthus is an increase in distance between the medial canthi. The interpupillary distance remains normal. Hypoglobus is downward displacement of the eye in the orbit and may give the appearance of ptosis. None of these features specifically help differentiate between congenital and acquired ptosis, although many of them can be associated with congenital ptosis.

DIAGNOSING ABNORMAL UPPER EYELID ANATOMY

5. **In an adult patient with a unilateral elevated supratarsal fold, mild ptosis, and an accentuated supratarsal hollow, which one of the following is the most likely diagnosis?**
   B. Levator dehiscence
   This patient is likely to have dehiscence of the levator palpebrae superioris. The other options may all lead to ptosis, but an elevated fold and supratarsal hollowing are classic signs of levator dehiscence. Botulinum toxin inadvertently placed can lead to isolated temporary brow or lid ptosis. Reduced sympathetic innervation could reduce Müller's muscle function leading to a

subtle ptosis in conjunction with meiosis and anhidrosis (Horner's syndrome). Compression of CN III can cause loss of levator function, also leading to an isolated ptosis. Myasthenia gravis can cause ptosis that is typically worse towards the end of the day.

TECHNIQUE SELECTION FOR BLEPHAROPTOSIS SURGERY

6. Which one of the following is considered the single most important factor when selecting a technique for correction of blepharoptosis?
D. Amount of lid elevation

When assessing patients for surgical correction of blepharoptosis, an assessment should be made of levator function (Fig. 93-1). The amount of lid elevation is graded as mild (more than 10 mm lift), moderate (5 to 10 mm lift), or severe (0 to 5 mm lift), and this is the most important factor in determining surgical management. Naturally, this will be linked to the cause of the ptosis. For example, if there is good elevation in the presence of ptosis, the levator mechanism is probably elongated or stretched.

Other factors which are important in surgical planning include the degree of ptosis and lid height position, which are essentially the same thing. The duration of ptosis is not usually relevant, other than if sudden onset which may suggest a traumatic cause. As discussed in question 4, lagopthalmus is often present in congenital ptosis. Furthermore, it is highly likely to occur after ptosis surgery and can exacerbate dry-eye symptoms.

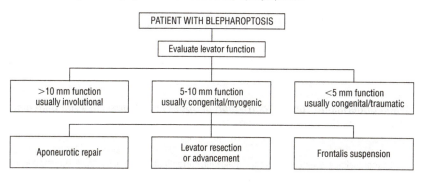

Fig. 93-1 Algorithm for ptosis repair.

SURGICAL MANAGEMENT OF BLEPHAROPTOSIS

7. A 60-year-old patient is seen with a chronic unilateral visual impairment resulting from obstruction from the right upper eyelid. Examination of the affected eye shows severe blepharoptosis, with 8 mm of levator excursion. Which one of the following is the best surgical approach to management?
B. Levator advancement

There are a number of surgical procedures available for the correction of upper eyelid ptosis,[3] but at present there have been no randomized controlled studies comparing the effectiveness of these techniques. McCord et al[4] proposed a treatment algorithm for blepharoptosis based on levator function (see Fig. 93-1). According to this, the patient could have either resection or advancement procedures.

A patient with more than 10 mm of levator function would have aponeurotic repair, and a patient with less than 5 mm of levator elevation would have frontalis suspension.

More recently, Chang et al[5] have undertaken a systematic review of blepharoptosis studies and proposed a treatment algorithm more specifically for involutional blepharoptosis, which would also advocate the use of an advancement procedure for this patient. According to this algorithm (Fig. 93-2), a patient with minimal to moderate ptosis and good levator function would be a candidate for Müllers muscle–conjunctival resection.

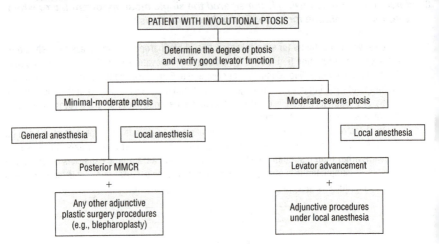

Fig. 93-2 Algorithm for treatment of involutional ptosis. (*MMCR,* Müller's muscle–conjunctival resection.)

8. **When undertaking surgical correction of upper eyelid ptosis in adult patients, which one of the following is correct?**
   E. **All patients must be counseled about and should receive appropriate management for lagophthalmos.**

   Lagophthalmos is very likely to occur following correctional surgery, so patients must be advised about this risk and its potential postoperative management. When undertaking ptosis correction surgery, care must be taken to avoid overcorrection or undercorrection. The use of epinephrine can increase the sympathetic tone to Müller's muscle, so slight overcorrection may be required to take this into account. When using local anesthetic agents, the levator muscles may be paralyzed, so undercorrection may be required. Although a general anesthetic avoids difficulties with patient compliance, where possible, local anesthetic is preferable because it allows assessment of lid position during surgery. Schirmer's test is performed to assess for the presence of dry eye. Patients who regularly wear contact lenses are unlikely to suffer from dry eyes, so this test is not typically indicated for them.

THE FASANELLA-SERVAT TECHNIQUE

9. You have a patient with blepharoptosis and have decided to perform the Fasanella-Servat technique. **Which one of the following is correct regarding this procedure?**
   C. **It may result in a floppy upper lid.**

   The Fasanella-Servat technique is used for mild cases of blepharoptosis in patients with excellent levator function (see Fig. 93-3, *Essentials of Plastic Surgery,* second edition). It involves a transconjunctival approach and thereby avoids a skin scar, but the outcomes can be unpredictable. It is a resection technique, not an advancement technique, and involves resection of Müller's muscle, the tarsus, and the conjunctiva. It can result in a floppy upper lid as a result of the tarsal resection.

LEVATOR APONEUROSIS ADVANCEMENT

10. A 58-year-old patient has moderate unilateral upper lid ptosis and a plan is made for advancement of the levator aponeurosis under general anesthesia. Preoperative lid height is 3 mm below the upper limbus and levator excursion is 9 mm. **When performing this surgery, which one of the following is true?**
   D. Using the gapping method, a distance of 9 mm should be used to set advancement.
   The gapping method is useful for achieving correct advancement when patients undergoing levator aponeurosis advancement are under general anesthesia. The preoperative excursion measurement (9 mm in this case) is used as a guide to set advancement so that the distance between the upper and lower eyelids matches the excursion measurement.
   Levator aponeurosis advancement is indicated for mild to moderate ptosis and is undertaken using a skin incision at the desired supratarsal fold rather than a transconjunctival approach. The upper lid is set according to excursion such that with good excursion, as in this case, the upper lid should be set just below (not just above) the upper limbus. Only if the excursion was poor, should the lid be set above the upper limbus.
   In general a 4:1 ratio of advancement to ptosis correction is required with this technique. Therefore 12 mm of levator advancement (not 6 mm) would probably be needed to achieve correction of the 3 mm ptosis. Although a central lifting suture is used initially to secure the levator to the superior tarsus, this is not sufficient by itself and therefore an additional two sutures are placed, one medial and one lateral to the central suture. In addition, supratarsal crease fixation may be performed (see Fig. 93-4, *Essentials of Plastic Surgery,* second edition).

FRONTALIS SUSPENSION

11. A young patient has unilateral blepharoptosis with poor levator function. They are seen by your assistant and scheduled to undergo frontalis suspension. **Which one of the following is true in this case?**
   E. Long-term night-time patching and ointment will be required after surgery.
   Frontalis suspension can provide 1 cm of excursion with a good result in a straightforward gaze, but will likely produce lagophthalmus during sleep. Therefore night-time patching and ointment will be required to protect the globe. The main indication for this surgery is congenital blepharoptosis with poor excursion, so it is an appropriate technique in this scenario. This surgery does not involve resection of Müller's muscle. This is part of the Putterman conjunctival technique and the external levator resection techniques as described by Beard and Burke, respectively. Suspension is not achieved by direct suturing, instead it requires slips of fascia lata, other fascia, or similar tissue to suspend the upper eyelid to the frontalis (see Fig. 93-7, *Essentials of Plastic Surgery,* second edition). Bilateral suspension is often required, even where there is a unilateral ptosis, in order to achieve good symmetry.[6]

POSTOPERATIVE PROBLEMS AFTER PTOSIS CORRECTION

12. You assess a patient in the clinic after a left unilateral levator aponeurosis advancement. She is satisfied with the improvement gained to the left eye but is concerned that the right eye now appears ptotic. **Which one of the following explains these clinical findings?**
   C. Hering's law
   The levator muscles receive bilateral equal innervation. The presence of severe ptosis on one side will create an impulse for bilateral lid retraction. If, as in this case, a patient undergoes unilateral

correction, the innervation for lid retraction decreases, leading to ptosis on the nonoperated side. This is described in Hering's law.

Hering's test should therefore be performed preoperatively to avoid this occurrence; this involves immobilizing the brow and having the patient maintain a straightforward gaze. The affected upper eyelid is then gently elevated using a cotton-tipped applicator to alleviate the ptosis. The presence of contralateral ptosis should then be assessed. Putterman and Fasanella are both names associated with blepharoptosis surgical techniques, not tests. Schirmer's test is for evaluation of tear production.

REFERENCES

1. Gunn RM. Congenital ptosis with peculiar associated movements of the affected lid. Trans Ophthal Soc UK 3:283-287, 1883.
2. Jethani J. Marin-Amat syndrome: a rare facial synkinesis. Indian J Ophthalmol 55:402-403, 2007.
3. Beard C, Sullivan JH. Ptosis: current concepts. Int Opthalmol 18:53-73, 1978.
4. McCord CD Jr, Codner MA, Hester TR Jr. Eyelid Surgery: Principles and Techniques. Philadelphia: Lippincott-Raven, 1995.
5. Chang S, Lehrman C, Itani K, Rohrich RJ. A systematic review of comparison of upper eyelid involutional ptosis repair techniques: efficacy and complication rates. Plast Reconstr Surg 129:149-157, 2012.
6. McCord CD Jr. Complications of ptosis surgery and their management. In McCord CD Jr, Codner MA, Hester TR, eds. Eyelid Surgery: Principles and Techniques. Philadelphia: Lippincott-Raven, 1995.

94. Face Lift

See *Essentials of Plastic Surgery*, second edition, pp. 1160-1188.

SOFT TISSUE LAYERS OF THE FACE

1. **When performing surgery on the face, directly under which anatomic layer would the main neurovascular structures normally be located?**
   A. Skin
   B. Subcutaneous tissue
   C. SMAS
   D. Mimetic muscles
   E. Deep facial fascia

2. The SMAS is a key structure in rhytidectomy and is continuous with other anatomic fascial planes. **Which one of the following layers is distinct from the SMAS layer?**
   A. Temporoparietal fascia
   B. Superficial cervical fascia
   C. Parotidomasseteric fascia
   D. Frontalis and platysmal fascia
   E. Zygomaticus major fascia

3. **Which one of the following represents the site where the SMAS is both thickest and fixed?**
   A. The parotid
   B. The neck
   C. The temple
   D. The midface
   E. The brow

4. **When performing surgery on the temple, just lateral to the brow, running on which structure would you expect to find the frontal branch of the facial nerve?**
   A. Temporoparietal fascia
   B. Parotidotemporal fascia
   C. Superficial layer of the deep temporal fascia
   D. Deep layer of the deep temporal fascia
   E. Superficial temporal fat pad

FACIAL FAT COMPARTMENTS

5. **Which one of the following is true of the facial fat compartments?**
   A. The bulk of facial fat in the cheek is deep to SMAS.
   B. The nasolabial fat compartment loses most of its volume with increasing age.
   C. The buccal fat pad and the malar fat pad are equivalent.
   D. The malar fat pad is formed by the nasolabial and medial cheek fat compartments.
   E. The SOOF and ROOF both lie superficial to the orbicularis oculi.

789

RETAINING LIGAMENTS OF THE FACE

6. For each of the following descriptions of facial ligaments, select the correct anatomic region from the list. (Each option may be used once, more than once, or not at all.)
   A. McGregor's patch forms part of this ligament that is released during an extended SMAS face lift.
   B. Attenuation of this ligament results in overhang at the nasolabial fold.
   C. Jowls are commonly associated with weakening of this ligament.

Options:
a. Masseteric
b. Zygomatic
c. Mandibular
d. Orbital
e. Maxillary
f. Parotid
g. Temporal

CHANGES IN THE AGING FACE

7. Which one of the following is typically observed in the aging face (Fig. 94-3)?
   A. Deflation and volume loss in the lower face
   B. Fat accumulation in the upper and midface
   C. Retrusion of the anterior maxilla and inferior orbital rim
   D. Cessation of bony growth irrespective of dentition
   E. Soft tissue ptosis at the inferior orbital rim

8. Where on the aging face are the effects of "radial expansion" most apparent?
   A. Glabella
   B. Orbital rim
   C. Nasolabial fold
   D. Neck
   E. Lateral cheek

SENSORY DEFICITS AFTER A FACE LIFT

9. For each of the following clinical scenarios, select the most likely nerve injured. (Each option may be used once, more than once, or not at all.)
   A. A patient has numbness of the lobule of the ear following a SMAS plication face lift.
   B. A patient reports sweating in the left cheek at mealtimes 3 months after undergoing a full face lift with SMASectomy.
   C. A patient has altered sensation in the mastoid region after an extended face-lift procedure.

Options:
a. Lesser auricular
b. Lesser occipital
c. Great auricular
d. Greater occipital
e. Auriculotemporal
f. Zygomaticotemporal

MOTOR DEFICITS AFTER A FACE LIFT

10. For each of the following clinical scenarios, select the most likely nerve injured. (Each option may be used once, more than once, or not at all.)
   A. A patient has temporary shoulder weakness after an extended face and neck lift.
   B. A patient has temporary weakness of the upper lip and cheek after a MACS-lift.
   C. Following a combined face-lift and neck-lift procedure, a patient has a new onset lower lip asymmetry when performing a full smile. He is still able to pucker his lips normally.

   Options:
   a. Marginal mandibular branch of facial nerve
   b. Cervical branch of facial nerve
   c. Frontal branch of facial nerve
   d. Buccal branch of the facial nerve
   e. Zygomatic branch of the facial nerve
   f. Transverse cervical nerve
   g. Spinal accessory nerve

INCISION PLACEMENT

11. You are planning a primary face lift on a 52-year-old man who has a good head of hair and long sideburns. He has descent of the facial soft tissues with only mild skin excess. **Which one of the following incisions should be used?**
    A. A preauricular incision passing behind the tragus
    B. A temporal incision placed behind the anterior hairline
    C. A postauricular incision running vertically 1 cm behind the sulcus
    D. An occipital incision running along the hairline
    E. A retroauricular transverse incision level with the tragus

TECHNIQUES USED IN FACE-LIFT SURGERY

12. **In which plane of dissection would a deep plane face lift be performed?**
    A. Subcutaneous
    B. SubSMAS
    C. Supraperiosteal
    D. Deep fascial
    E. Subperiosteal

13. A patient comes to clinic for a second opinion to discuss face-lift procedures, having been offered Minimal Access Cranial Suspension (MACS-lift) by another clinician. **Which one of the following is true of this procedure?**
    A. It is reliant on the skin for providing soft tissue elevation.
    B. It is usually performed using an endoscopic approach.
    C. It carries a theoretical risk of compression damage to facial nerve branches.
    D. It commonly uses a vector of elevation perpendicular to the nasolabial fold.
    E. It most often involves elevation and resection of the SMAS layer.

14. **What was the main limitation of the face-lift technique originally described by Skoog?**
    A. It had a high risk of skin slough.
    B. It had a short lasting result.
    C. It failed to improve the nasolabial folds.
    D. It required separate dissection of the skin and SMAS layers.
    E. Skin excess was difficult to treat.

15. **What is the main perceived advantage of using a subperiosteal approach to face lifting?**
    A. Technically easier and quicker dissection.
    B. Enhanced manipulation of skin tissue fat compartments.
    C. Avoids the need for endoscopic skills.
    D. Reduced risk of facial palsy.
    E. Targets large skin excesses of the jawline and neck.

THE AGING LIP

16. **Which one of the following changes would be expected when examining the upper lip of an elderly patient during an aesthetic consultation?**
    A. Increased dental show
    B. Increased lip volume
    C. Increased visible vermilion
    D. Decreased commissure width
    E. Decreased dental show

PERIOPERATIVE MANAGEMENT

17. A patient comes to the clinic to discuss a face-lift procedure. She is 40 years old and recently separated from her long-term partner. She smokes 10 cigarettes per day and takes a range of herbal medications. She takes regular analgesics for lower back pain, but no other prescription drugs. **When assessing this woman for a face lift, which one of the following is correct?**
    A. She should consider a consult with your clinical psychologist after surgical treatment.
    B. Neither her prescribed nor over-the-counter remedies will increase her risk of complications.
    C. She would need to undertake smoking cessation before treatment.
    D. Her risk of skin slough would be about 5% if she proceeded with a sub-SMAS face lift.
    E. She is likely to be satisfied with her surgical outcome postoperatively.

18. You are asked to see a patient in recovery after a face lift. On examination, he has visible unilateral swelling overlying the mandibular border and neck. The neck drain is empty. Blood pressure has been well maintained at 125 mm Hg systolic. **What is your next step in management of this patient?**
    A. Give an intravenous dose of Chlorpromazine
    B. Flush and revacuum the drain
    C. Remove sutures and suction hematoma in recovery
    D. Return the patient to the operating room
    E. Observe and reassess in 30 minutes

COMPLICATIONS IN FACE-LIFT SURGERY

19. **When discussing informed consent with a patient for a face lift, which one of the following represents the most common early complication?**
    A. Facial nerve weakness
    B. Infection
    C. Hematoma
    D. Skin slough
    E. Altered sensation to the lobule

20. When planning perioperative care for a patient undergoing a face lift, which one of the following is most likely to lower the risk of hematoma formation?
   A. Insertion of vacuum drains beneath the skin flaps
   B. Use of fibrin glue before closure
   C. Preoperative injection with epinephrine
   D. Tumescent infiltration with saline solution after induction
   E. Administration of a prophylactic dose of low-molecular-weight heparin daily

STIGMATA OF FACE LIFTS

21. A patient is seen before a face lift and is noted to have marked submalar hollowing. *What deformity are they at increased risk of developing after rhytidectomy?*
   A. Lateral sweep
   B. Joker's lines
   C. Smile blocks
   D. Pixie deformity
   E. Hairline distortion

Answers

SOFT TISSUE LAYERS OF THE FACE

1. **When performing surgery on the face, directly under which anatomic layer would the main neurovascular structures normally be located?**
   E. Deep facial fascia
   The soft tissue layers of the face can be conceptualized as a series of concentric layers from superficial to deep (Fig. 94-1). These layers are the skin, subcutaneous tissues, SMAS, mimetic muscles, deep facial fascia, and bone. The neurovascular structures lie just deep to the deep facial fascia and include the facial nerve, parotid duct, and facial vessels. This layer also contains the buccal fat pad. However, it is possible to damage the facial nerve intraoperatively when deep to SMAS and medial to the parotid, as the facial nerve becomes more superficial in this area, so care must be taken during subSMAS dissection.[1]

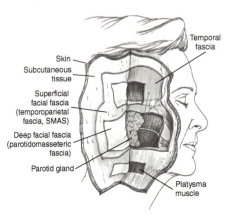

Fig. 94-1   Facial soft tissue layers.

2. The SMAS is a key structure in rhytidectomy and is continuous with other anatomic fascial planes. **Which one of the following layers is distinct from the SMAS layer?**
   C. Parotidomasseteric fascia
   The SMAS is the superficial fascial system of the face and neck, whereas the parotidomasseteric fascia is part of the deep fascial system. The SMAS is highly relevant to face-lift procedures and is often elevated and manipulated to support facial soft tissue structures during rhytidectomy. It is continuous caudally with the platysma and superficial cervical fascia and cranially with the frontalis, galea, and superficial temporal fascia. At its most anterior extent, the SMAS forms the fascia around zygomaticus major, which can be a tethering point during a face lift requiring release. In contrast, the deep fascia which consists of the masseteric fascia, investing fascia of the parotid, deep temporal fascia, and deep cervical fascia, is not normally manipulated during face-lift procedures.

3. **Which one of the following represents the site where the SMAS is both thickest and fixed?**
   A. **The parotid**

   The SMAS has both mobile and fixed components. The fixed SMAS overlies the parotid gland and is thickest in this region. The mobile SMAS lies beyond the parotid over the facial mimetic muscles, facial nerves, and parotid duct. This is clinically relevant to face-lifting techniques where the SMAS is mobilized around the parotid region and elevated in a posterior or vertical direction. The SMAS is then secured in its new position to elevate the face and neck during rhytidectomy.

4. **When performing surgery on the temple, just lateral to the brow, running on which structure would you expect to find the frontal branch of the facial nerve?**
   C. **Superficial layer of the deep temporal fascia**

   Knowledge of the location of the frontal branch of the facial nerve is relevant to many procedures in plastic surgery including face lift, brow lift, and temporal tumor excision. The frontal branch travels along a line from 0.5 cm below the tragus to a point 1.5 cm above the lateral brow (Pitanguy's line). After crossing the zygomatic arch, at the midpoint between the tragus and lateral canthus, it may be identified running on top of the superficial part of the deep temporal fascia. There is often confusion with regards to the fascial layers of the temple but they are fairly simple to remember (Fig. 94-2). There are four fascial layers in this region. The most superficial of which is the temporoparietal fascia. This is also known as the superficial temporal fascia and is continuous with the SMAS. Just deep to this layer is the parotidotemporal fascia which is an additional layer of soft tissue that covers the frontal branch in this area. Beneath this layer is the deep temporal fascia, which comprises both superficial and deep components separated by a fat pad. The temporalis muscle is deep to both of these layers and is adherent to the underlying pericranium. Protection of the frontal branch intraoperatively can be achieved by keeping superficial to the SMAS layer or deep to the deep fascia. When dissection is required in the plane just above the superficial layer of the deep fascia, care must be taken to protect the nerve branch.

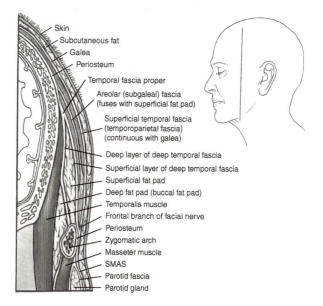

Fig. 94-2 Anatomic layers of the temporal region.

FACIAL FAT COMPARTMENTS

5. Which one of the following is true of the facial fat compartments?
   D. The malar fat pad is formed by the nasolabial and medial cheek fat compartments.

   The malar fat pad is a commonly used term referring to the region of the superficial fat compartments that is thought to play a role in the appearance of the youthful cheek. With age the fat pad descends and loses midface volume, secondarily creating lower-face fullness and deepening of the nasolabial folds. The two primary components of the malar fat pad are the nasolabial and medial cheek fat compartments. The inferior orbital fat compartment can also be considered as part of this fat pad.

   The facial fat compartments are divided into superficial and deep layers and described according to the anatomic region. There is a fairly even split between superficial and deep volume proportions (54% compared to 46%, respectively). The superficial fat compartments of the cheek include the nasolabial, medial, middle, and lateral cheek fat compartments. The deep parts of the cheek are the buccal fat pad and the deep medial compartment. The superficial parts of the periorbital region are the superior, inferior, and lateral compartments. The deep compartments are the SOOF and ROOF which are located beneath orbicularis oculi, not superficial to it. Of all the compartments in the face, the nasolabial one is unusual in that its volume remains fairly consistent through life.[2]

RETAINING LIGAMENTS OF THE FACE

6. For the following descriptions, the best options are as follows:
   A. McGregor's patch forms part of this ligament that is released during an extended SMAS face lift.
      b. Zygomatic
   B. Attenuation of this ligament results in overhang at the nasolabial fold.
      b. Zygomatic
   C. Jowls are commonly associated with weakening of this ligament.
      a. Masseteric

   The retaining ligaments of the face provide support for the facial soft tissues and are implicated in the facial aging process, either from attenuation or tethering. They originate from bone or fascia and include the following:

   Attenuation: Orbitomalar ligamen–tear-trough deformity
   Zygomaticocutaneous ligament: deepening of the nasolabial fold and tear-trough deformity
   Masseteric ligament: jowls and marionette lines
   Tethering: Mandibular ligament–jowls and marionette lines (Fig. 94-3)

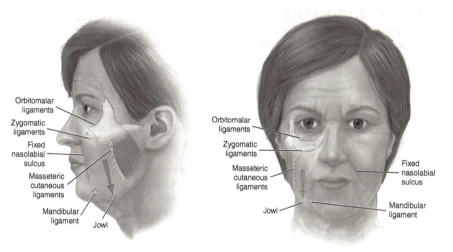

Fig. 94-3 Changes in the aging face.

CHANGES IN THE AGING FACE

7. Which one of the following is typically observed in the aging face?
C. Retrusion of the anterior maxilla and inferior orbital rim

There are a number of changes within the bone and soft tissues during aging. These include retrusion of the anterior maxilla and inferior orbital rim, downward rotation of the facial skeleton with respect to the cranial base, and expansion of the orbital socket volume which leads to a sunken eye appearance and contributes to the tear-trough deformity. The adult facial skeleton continues to grow in dentate patients. In edentulous patients, however, there is a reduction in facial height because of loss of alveolar bone in the mandible and maxilla.

Soft tissue changes include deflation and volume loss in the upper two thirds of the face, while there is accumulation of fat in the lower face and neck. The appearance of these volume changes is exacerbated by descent of the remaining upper tissues from gravity and attenuation of retaining ligaments. There may be an appearance of ptosis along the inferior orbital rim but this is really a pseudoptosis due to the effects of soft tissue volume loss.[3]

8. Where on the aging face are the effects of "radial expansion" most apparent?
C. Nasolabial fold

Radial expansion refers to a process occurring with aging that results in deepening of the nasolabial fold. Repeated animation stretches the retaining ligaments of the face and allows the soft tissues to expand away from the face. This is most apparent at the nasolabial fold during smiling, because the skin of the lip is forced under the subcutaneous fat of the cheek, allowing the soft tissues to prolapse outward from the skeleton.[4]

SENSORY DEFICITS AFTER A FACE LIFT

9. For the following scenarios, the best options are as follows:
   A. **A patient has numbness of the lobule of the ear following a SMAS plication face lift.**
      c. **Great auricular**
         The great auricular nerve lies on the sternocleidomastoid muscle in the subplatysmal plane and is the most often recognized nerve injury after a face lift (up to 7%). Division of the nerve leads to numbness of the lower half of the ear on both the cranial and lateral surfaces.
   B. **A patient reports sweating in the left cheek at mealtimes 3 months after undergoing a full face lift with SMASectomy.**
      e. **Auriculotemporal**
         The auriculotemporal nerve courses with the superficial temporal artery and may be divided during a face lift. If the auriculotemporal nerve is divided, sympathetic reinnervation can occur, causing gustatory sweating (Frey's syndrome).
   C. **A patient has altered sensation of the mastoid region after an extended face-lift procedure.**
      b. **Lesser occipital**
         The lesser occipital nerve supplies the superior third of the ear and mastoid region and is located near the sternocleidomastoid.

         The zygomaticotemporal nerve is a branch of the trigeminal nerve that supplies sensation to the small area of skin in the temple. It is located lateral to the lateral canthus. It may be intentionally avulsed during migraine surgery as discussed in Chapter 20, but is not usually affected in face-lift surgery. The greater occipital nerve supplies the occiput and is also implicated in migraine surgery. It is decompressed rather than used in this situation but is not at risk during face-lift surgery. There is no named lesser auricular nerve.

MOTOR DEFICITS AFTER A FACE LIFT

10. For the following scenarios, the best options are as follows:
    A. **A patient has temporary shoulder weakness after an extended face and neck lift.**
       g. **Spinal accessory nerve**
          The spinal accessory nerve supplies the sternocleidomastoid and trapezius muscles. It usually passes deep to or through the sternocleidomastoid in the anterior neck and is unlikely to be damaged there during a face lift. It is most at risk in the posterior triangle, passing between the sternocleidomastoid and trapezius, where it lies more superficially
    B. **A patient has temporary weakness of the upper lip and cheek after a MACS-lift.**
       d. **Buccal branch of the facial nerve**
          A buccal branch is probably the most commonly injured motor nerve during a face lift, but given the arborization between buccal branches and zygomatic branches, this could often go unnoticed. Temporary weakness is suggestive of a neurapraxia or the effects of local anesthetic and most likely will resolve spontaneously. Injury to one of the zygomatic branches is therefore similarly affected.
    C. **Following a combined face and neck lifting procedure, a patient has a new onset lower lip asymmetry when performing a full smile. He is still able to pucker his lips normally.**
       b. **Cervical branch of facial nerve**
          Both the marginal mandibular and cervical branches of the facial nerve are at risk of injury when the neck is undermined during a face lift. They can have a similar clinical appearance.

Paralysis from the marginal mandibular branch results in an inability to evert the lower lip, indicating depressor labii inferiors (DLI) paralysis. *Platysma pseudoparalysis* is characterized by an asymmetrical lower lip during a "full denture smile." It results from injury to the cervical branches innervating the platysma. Patients typically recover completely from this injury within 6 months.

As discussed in question 4, the frontal branch of the facial nerve is at risk during surgical procedures including face and brow lift. This can result in permanent weakness of the ipsilateral frontalis muscle.

INCISION PLACEMENT

11. You are planning a primary face lift on a 52-year-old man who has a good head of hair and long sideburns. He has descent of the facial soft tissues with only mild skin excess. *Which one of the following incisions should be used?*
    B. A temporal incision placed behind the anterior hairline
    There are four areas of the face-lift scar to consider: temporal, preauricular, postauricular, and occipital. The location of incisions should be individualized for each patient (see Figs. 94-11 through 94-13, *Essentials of Plastic Surgery*, second edition). In situations in which large amounts of skin will be resected, it is best to place incisions at the interface between skin and hair; otherwise, the hairline will be altered, producing an unnatural appearance. In this case, the temporal incision can be placed within the hairline and the occipital incision can be placed high, since minimal skin excision is planned. In women, the preauricular incision should normally be placed passing behind the tragus, but in men, a pretragal approach is better; otherwise, this risks transfer of facial hair onto the tragus. The vertical component of the postauricular incision should run in the sulcus, because it will be well hidden in this site. An occipital hairline incision is best suited to patients with massive skin redundancy in the face and neck.

TECHNIQUES USED IN FACE-LIFT SURGERY

12. *In which plane of dissection would a deep plane face lift be performed?*
    B. SubSMAS
    Face-lift procedures can be categorized by the plane of dissection. Common dissection planes for face lifts are subcutaneous and subSMAS. Less commonly, subperiosteal and supraperiosteal planes are used. The term deep plane refers to a subSMAS dissection and this is performed so that the SMAS can be elevated and resuspended to provide support for redraped soft tissues such as skin, fat, and muscle. The intended benefit is to obtain long-term support for the face lift without reliance on skin fixation alone. Many, but not all deep plane techniques also involve separate subcutaneous dissection, so that skin and SMAS layers can be moved in different vectors. This means that SMAS can be elevated and fixed in a more vertical or diagonally vertical direction, while skin can be elevated and fixed in a more posterior and vertical direction.

13. A patient comes to clinic for a second opinion to discuss face-lift procedures, having been offered Minimal Access Cranial Suspension (MACS-lift) by another clinician. *Which one of the following is true of this procedure?*
    C. It carries a theoretical risk of compression damage to facial nerve branches.
    The MACS-lift is a popular supraSMAS plication technique that uses continuous purse-string sutures placed within the SMAS to elevate the face and neck in a vertical vector. Plication techniques in general are used to tighten the SMAS layer and avoid reliance on skin to hold the required lift. A perceived advantage of SMAS plication compared with other SMAS manipulation techniques is that subSMAS dissection is avoided and therefore the risk of facial nerve damage is decreased. However, risk of facial nerve damage is still present because the SMAS is not

elevated, and therefore the sutures passed to tighten the SMAS are done so blindly in relation to facial nerve branches. Therefore branches of the facial nerve may be inadvertently caught within the suture. Intraoperatively, it is therefore important to recognize any mimetic muscle twitches during passing of this suture, and if there is any doubt that the suture may have contacted or compressed a facial nerve branch, it should be removed and replaced.[5]

MACS stands for "minimal access cranial suspension" because it uses a short scar (not an endoscopic) approach and elevates soft tissues vertically/cranially. A lateral SMASectomy elevates facial tissues parallel to the nasolabial fold and involves excision of a small patch of SMAS over the parotid. Techniques that involve elevation and resection of the SMAS are termed deep plane techniques (see question 12) and include low and high SMAS approaches, where both subcutaneous and subSMAS planes are elevated and SMAS is secured in a posteriovertical direction.

14. **What was the main limitation of the face-lift technique originally described by Skoog?**
    C. It failed to improve the nasolabial folds.
    Skoog described a technique for face lifting in 1974[6] that involved elevation of the skin and SMAS as a single unit, advancing the entire skin-SMAS unit posteriorly onto the cheek and neck. The main limitation of this technique was that it failed to address the nasolabial folds and anterior neck. Hamra[7] later modified this approach to better treat the nasolabial folds. His "composite" technique incorporates the lower lid orbicularis muscle into the single dissected soft tissue unit. Each of these techniques has a robust blood supply to the skin because it is elevated in conjunction with the SMAS, rather than as a separate layer independent of it. Results are long lasting as the SMAS is able to support the elevated soft tissues. Skin excess can be managed as required with these techniques.

15. **What is the main perceived advantage of using a subperiosteal approach to face lifting?**
    D. Reduced risk of facial palsy
    The subperiosteal approach to face lifting involves elevation of the midface periosteum as a single unit and then redraping of the composite face to achieve tissue repositioning. The main perceived advantage is that the facial nerve is protected because dissection is deep to it. A further advantage is that visible scarring can be minimized by using temporal and intraoral approaches. There are however, a number of disadvantages to this technique. First, it is technically difficult and may need to be performed using endoscopic techniques. This can make for a steep learning curve, particularly for surgeons not used to working on the bony facial skeleton. Second, it does not allow for skin and fat excesses to be treated, so it is less effective at managing skin redundancy of the nasolabial folds, jawline, and neck compared with other techniques.[8,9]

THE AGING LIP

16. **Which one of the following changes would be expected when examining the upper lip of an elderly patient during an aesthetic consultation?**
    E. Decreased dental show
    The upper lip becomes longer and less full with increasing age so there is decreased dental show. Because a long upper lip is characteristic of aging, techniques have been developed to address this. The appearance of a long upper lip can be improved using a vermillion advancement technique. However this does leave a visible scar on the lip margin. Alternatively, the lip can be

shortened by using a skin incision at the base of the nose and this can effectively hide the scar at the lip nose interface. Lip volume can be enhanced using fillers such as hyaluronic acid and autologous fat grafting. This also addresses the decreased (not increased) vermillion exposure characteristic of the aging lip. The oral commissure does not specificity alter with age.[9]

PERIOPERATIVE MANAGEMENT

17. A patient comes to the clinic to discuss a face-lift procedure. She is 40 years old and recently separated from her long-term partner. She smokes 10 cigarettes per day and takes a range of herbal medications. She takes regular analgesics for lower back pain, but no other prescription drugs. **When assessing this woman for a face lift, which one of the following is correct?**
   C. She would need to undertake smoking cessation before treatment.
   Smoking is a contraindication to a face lift, and the incidence of skin slough is much higher than 5% among smokers with a subSMAS technique. Therefore patients should be advised to stop smoking before face-lift surgery.
   Because this woman has recently separated from her partner, there is a risk that this is the trigger for her desire to have a face lift, and it may be a poor time for her to proceed with this surgery. She is also relatively young to need or want her first face lift. As with any cosmetic procedure, unrealistic expectations must be assessed, and if that is determined to be the case, surgery should be avoided. A consult with a clinical psychologist preoperatively is strongly advised given the above.
   The risk of bleeding during and immediately after a face lift should be minimized, and many herbal medications such as *Arnica* can increase bleeding. Her regular analgesics may include NSAIDs that can also increase bleeding risk.

18. You are asked to review a patient in recovery after a face lift. On examination, he has visible unilateral swelling overlying the mandibular border and neck. The neck drain is empty. Blood pressure has been well maintained at 125 mm Hg systolic. **What is your next step in management of this patient?**
   D. Return the patient to the operating room
   A hematoma is a common early complication following a face lift. As discussed elsewhere, the risk is higher in men. Although it may be prudent to release the suture line if there is a threatened area of skin, it would be better to promptly return to the operating room to achieve hemostasis and formal evacuation of the hematoma. Measures to avoid rebound hypertension include intravenous chlorpromazine at 1 and 3 hours after surgery. Alternatives include clonidase or labetalol. In this case they are not warranted, as blood pressure is satisfactory and the hematoma has already occurred.

COMPLICATIONS IN FACE-LIFT SURGERY

19. **When discussing informed consent with a patient for a face lift, which one of the following represents the most common early complication?**
   C. Hematoma
   The most common complication during or after a face lift is hematoma. It is most likely to occur within the first 24 hours. The risk can be minimized by meticulous intraoperative hemostasis and careful perioperative blood pressure control. The reported rate is about 2% or 3% in women and 8% in men. Other avenues to reduce this risk are discussed in question 18.

20. When planning perioperative care for a patient undergoing a face lift, which one of the following is most likely to lower the risk of hematoma formation?
D. Tumescent infiltration with saline solution after induction

Jones and Grover[10] reported that tumescent infiltration of around 200 ml per side without epinephrine reduced the rate of postoperative hematomas without significantly increasing wound bleeding or facial edema.

The use of drains will not lower the risk of hematoma formation but can reduce postoperative bruising. Many surgeons use fibrin glue under the skin flaps, but there is no evidence to show that this action actually reduces hematoma occurrence either. Preoperative injection of epinephrine may limit early intraoperative bleeding but could lead to a rebound effect part way through the case. Prophylactic administration of low-molecular-weight heparin may increase postoperative bleeding without decreasing the risk of venous thrombosis.

STIGMATA OF FACE LIFTS

21. A patient is seen before a face lift and is noted to have marked submalar hollowing. What deformity are they at increased risk of developing after rhytidectomy?
B. Joker's lines

Face lifting can lead to unnatural appearances if the lift is performed with incorrect or inappropriate vectors and preexisting deformities may be amplified. For example, Joker's lines were described by Lambros and Stuzin[11] and refer to the appearance of the oral commissure extending onto the cheek following a face lift. This is a potential sequela of performing a face lift in a patient who has submalar hollowing preoperatively. Prevention of this deformity requires careful patient selection and for those with submalar hollowing, a more limited SMAS and skin release in combination with a more subtle vertical lift should be performed. Established joker's lines are difficult to treat but may be improved by fat-transfer procedures.

Hamra introduced the term "lateral sweep" caused by an excess of lateral pull in the lower face without treatment of the midface.[12] This allows natural descent from aging over time to sag over the lateral pleat in the lower face. It can be avoided by using vectors that provide a more vertical lift and avoid excessive lateral tightening, while ensuring that the midface is adequately supported. Smile blocks have been described as hypodynamic cheek mounds that do not move appropriately with animation and these may be improved with fat transfer. A pixie-ear deformity may arise from distortion of the lobule because of excessive tension on the skin flap. It can be minimized by securing SMAS to the postauricular region (mastoid) in order to minimize caudal pull on the lobule. Hairline distortion can generally be avoided by ensuring that skin is not excessively removed and that tension during closure is minimized.

REFERENCES

1. Nahai F, ed. The Art of Aesthetic Surgery: Principles & Techniques. St Louis: Quality Medical Publishing, 2005.
2. Rohrich RJ, Pessa JE. The fat compartments of the face: anatomy and clinical implications for cosmetic surgery. Plast Reconstr Surg 119:2219-2227, 2007.
3. Warren RJ, Aston SJ, Mendelson BC. Face lift. Plast Reconstr Surg 128:747e-764e, 2011.
4. Stuzin JM. Restoring facial shape in face lifting: the role of skeletal support in facial analysis and midface soft-tissue repositioning. Plast Reconstr Surg 119:362-376; discussion 377-378, 2007.
5. Tonnard PL, Verpaele AM. The MACS-Lift: Short-Scar Rhytidectomy. St Louis: Quality Medical Publishing, 2004.

6. Skoog T, ed. Plastic Surgery: New Methods and Refinements. Philadelphia: WB Saunders, 1974.
7. Hamra ST. Composite rhytidectomy. Plast Reconstr Surg 90:1-13, 1992.
8. Tessier P. [Subperiosteal face-lift] Ann Chir Plast Esthet 34:193-197, 1989.
9. Gonyon DL Jr, Barton FE Jr. The aging face: rhytidectomy and adjunctive procedures. Sel Read Plast Surg 11, 2012.
10. Jones BM, Grover R. Avoiding hematoma in cervicofacial rhytidectomy: a personal 8-year quest. Reviewing 910 patients. Plast Reconstr Surg 113:381-387; discussion 388-390, 2004.
11. Lambros V, Stuzin JM. The cross-cheek depression: surgical cause and effect in the development of the "joker line" and its treatment. Plast Reconstr Surg 122:1543-1552, 2008.
12. Hamra ST. Frequent facelift sequelae: hollow eyes and the lateral sweep: cause and repair. Plast Reconstr Surg 102:1658-1665, 1998.

95. Neck Lift

See *Essentials of Plastic Surgery*, second edition, pp. 1189-1202.

ANATOMY OF THE PLATYSMA

1. **Which one of the following is true regarding the platysma?**
   A. The origin is the lower border of the mandible.
   B. It represents a continuation of the deep cervical fascia.
   C. The dominant blood supply arises from the suprasternal artery.
   D. Motor innervation is received from the cervical plexus.
   E. Most commonly, the right and left sides interdigitate.

NERVES OF THE NECK

2. **When performing surgery in the neck, which one of the following statements is true regarding the marginal mandibular nerve?**
   A. It normally travels 1 cm below the lower mandibular border throughout its course.
   B. It can be identified in the supraplatysmal plane as it passes anteromedially across the neck.
   C. Iatrogenic damage is unlikely to occur during neck rejuvenation surgery, as the nerve is away from the operative field.
   D. Inadvertent nerve transection will cause denervation of the platysma, risorius, and lower lip depressors.
   E. The nerve is most at risk of damage within a circle with a 2 cm radius, inferior and posterior to the oral commissure.

3. **On which muscle does the great auricular nerve travel 6 cm inferior to the external auditory canal?**
   A. Platysma
   B. Sternocleidomastoid
   C. Trapezius
   D. Splenius capitus
   E. Posterior scalene

DIGASTRIC MUSCLES

4. **What do the two bellies of digastric have in common?**
   A. The same nerve supply
   B. A similar length
   C. A shared central tendon
   D. An origin on the mandible
   E. An insertion on the mastoid

PREOPERATIVE ASSESSMENT

5. You are assessing a patient in clinic before neck rejuvenation surgery. They are concerned regarding soft tissue overhang beyond the lower border of the mandible, just lateral to the chin. **Tethering of which ligament is responsible for this appearance?**
   A. Mandibulocutaneous
   B. Platysma-auricular
   C. Masseteric-cutaneous
   D. Zygomaticocutaneous
   E. Mandibuloauricular

6. **When examining the neck of a young, healthy patient in clinic, which one of the following should normally be visible?**
   A. The submandibular gland
   B. The thyroid gland
   C. The digastric muscle
   D. The sternocleidomastoid muscle
   E. The hyoid bone

LIPOSUCTION OF THE NECK

7. **When performing suction-assisted liposuction to the neck in a patient with submental fat excess, which one of the following is correct?**
   A. A single-access point should be used.
   B. A 7 mm multihole cannula should be used.
   C. Subplatysmal fat volumes should be cautiously reduced.
   D. Small quantities of aspirate will normally provide satisfactory results.
   E. Drains and compression garments should be used.

SURGICAL APPROACHES TO NECK REJUVENATION

8. **Which one of the following is most commonly performed during correction of the deep plane (deep to the platysma) in neck rejuvenation?**
   A. Full resection of the anterior belly of the digastric muscle
   B. Extracapsular excision of the deep lobe of submandibular gland
   C. Resection of subplatysmal and interplatysmal fat
   D. Excision of suprahyoid fascia to improve the cervical angle
   E. Resection of multiple central lymph nodes

SELECTION OF SURGICAL PROCEDURES IN NECK REJUVENATION

9. **For each of the following clinical scenarios, select the best treatment option from the list. (Each option may be used once, more than once, or not at all.)**
   A. You see a 63-year-old, mildly obese woman with loss of neck contour and jowling. She has a large excess of neck skin and fat with prominent platysmal banding at rest.
   B. You see a 39-year-old woman with excellent skin quality and moderate submental fat excess. She has no platysmal banding at rest, but banding becomes apparent on animation. A skin pinch test reveals no alteration in pinch size on animation.
   C. You see a 55-year-old woman of average build who is concerned about the appearance of her neck contour. On examination, she has no evidence of platysmal banding or skin excess but does have fullness blunting the cervicomental angle and lower border of mandible. A skin pinch test reveals a diminished pinch size during animation.

Options:
a. Botulinum toxin injection only
b. Liposuction only
c. Submental neck lift
d. Submental neck lift with liposuction
e. Short-scar face and neck lift
f. Full-scar face and neck lift

PLATYSMAL PROCEDURES

10. You see a patient after previous surgery to the neck. On examination they have a visible transverse step in the neck and a window shading effect. **Which one of the procedures has most likely been undertaken?**
    A. Platysma flap
    B. Suspension sutures
    C. Corset platysmaplasty
    D. Platysma muscle sling
    E. Percutaneous platysma myotomy

POSTOPERATIVE COMPLICATIONS

11. A patient referred to you has undergone neck rejuvenation at another clinic and is dissatisfied with the appearance of her neck contour. On examination, she has an irregular contour with thin, visible bilateral bulges and adjacent hollowing in the anterior aspect of the neck just below the mandible. **What is the most likely explanation for this appearance?**
    A. Dehiscence of platysma plication
    B. Excessive submental liposuction
    C. Inadequate resection of the submandibular gland
    D. Excessive botulinum toxin use
    E. Excessive resection of the digastric muscles

Answers

ANATOMY OF THE PLATYSMA

1. Which one of the following is true regarding the platysma?
E. Most commonly, the right and left sides interdigitate.

The platysma is a broad, thin muscle situated in the subcutaneous plane of the neck. It originates from the pectoralis and deltoid fascia, with insertions to the mandibular symphysis and SMAS. It receives its main blood supply from the submental artery, which is a branch of the facial artery. The nerve supply is from the facial nerve (cervical branch). Three different anatomic patterns were described by de Castro[1] in 50 patients (Fig. 95-1). Type I was most common (75%), with limited decussation of the muscles for 1 to 2 cm below the mandibular symphysis. In type II, the decussation was more extensive and passed down to the thyroid cartilage. In type III, no decussation was present. Since these original descriptions, an anatomic study was undertaken by Kim et al[2] in 70 Korean patients; this showed that subtypes I and II were equally common (43% each), which may reflect racial differences.

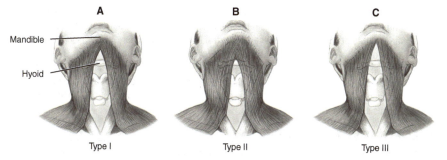

Fig. 95-1 Three anatomic patterns of the neck. **A,** Type I is most common and occurs in 75% of individuals. This type demonstrates a limited decussation of the platysma muscles, extending 1 to 2 cm below the mandibular symphysis. **B,** Type II occurs in 15% and demonstrates decussation of the platysma from the mandibular symphysis to the thyroid cartilage. **C,** Type III occurs in 10% and demonstrates no decussation or interdigitations.

NERVES OF THE NECK

2. When performing surgery in the neck, which one of the following statements is true regarding the marginal mandibular nerve?
E. The nerve is most at risk of damage within a circle with a 2 cm radius, 2 cm inferior and posterior to the oral commissure.

The marginal mandibular nerve is at risk of damage during neck rejuvenation procedures. The danger zone is within a circle with a 2 cm radius, located 2 cm posterior and inferior to the oral commissure overlying the lower border of the mandible. This region corresponds to where the facial vessels cross the lower mandibular border. The marginal mandibular nerve originates from the lower division of the facial nerve and passes close by the tail of the parotid, from lateral to anteromedial in the subplatysmal plane. It is important to remember this, as any subplatysmal dissection in the region of the lower mandibular border can risk iatrogenic damage. It travels close to the lower border of the mandible and most commonly runs above the lower border throughout its course. Before the point at which it crosses the facial vessels, it runs above the inferior border in more than 80% of cases. Beyond the facial vessels, all of its branches are above the inferior border. The marginal mandibular nerve innervates the lower lip depressors, the risorius, and part of orbicularis oris. It does not usually innervate the platysma, as this is innervated by the cervical branches.

3. **On which muscle does the great auricular nerve travel 6 cm inferior to the external auditory canal?**
   B. **Sternocleidomastoid**
   The great auricular nerve is at risk of damage during neck-lift and face-lift surgery. The main danger zone is located within a circle with a 3 cm radius dropped 6.5 cm inferior to the external auditory canal. This corresponds to the midpoint of the sternocleidomastoid muscle and the nerve emerges beneath the sternocleidomastoid just below this site, which is also known as McKinney's point. This nerve supplies sensation to the lobule of the ear and was discussed in Chapter 94, as it is the most commonly injured nerve during a face lift because of its superficial location.

DIGASTRIC MUSCLES

4. **What do the two bellies of digastric have in common?**
   C. **A shared central tendon**
   The digastric muscle is so named because it has two heads. Each of these has a different bony origin (anterior belly originates from the mandibular symphysis; posterior belly originates from the mastoid process), but they share a central tendon. The posterior belly is longer than the anterior belly and together they form the lower border of the submandibular triangle. They originate from different branchial arches (see Table 19-1, *Essentials of Plastic Surgery*, second edition), and so have different motor innervation. The anterior digastric develops from the first arch and has trigeminal innervation. The posterior digastric develops from the second arch and has facial nerve innervation.

PREOPERATIVE ASSESSMENT

5. You are assessing a patient in clinic before neck rejuvenation surgery. They are concerned regarding soft tissue overhang beyond the lower border of the mandible, just lateral to the chin. **Tethering of which ligament is responsible for this appearance?**
   A. **Mandibulocutaneous**
   Tethering of the mandibulocutaneous ligament produces the appearance of jowls. These can be assessed by inspection and palpation near the lower border of the mandible at the lateral edge of the chin. Assessment of jowl volume with the patient supine helps to plan surgical intervention. An excess of soft tissue alone may be treated with liposuction, whereas laxity of the deeper soft tissues will require SMAS-platysma tightening. The masseteric-cutaneous ligament is also relevant to the formation of jowls, as this attenuates with age allowing ptosis of the midfacial tissues.

   The platysma-auricular ligament is also relevant to neck-lift procedures because it marks the posterior extent of the platysma and also the site where the platysma is often anchored to provide elevation of the neck. Weakening of the zygomaticocutaneous ligament causes downward migration of the malar soft tissues and creates redundant skin that hangs over the fixed nasolabial fold.

6. **When examining the neck of a young, healthy patient in clinic, which one of the following should normally be visible?**
   D. The sternocleidomastoid muscle
   When examining a normal neck, the sternocleidomastoid muscle should be visible at its anterior border. Ellenbogen and Karlin[3] classified features of the youthful neck that change with age. Features of a youthful neck involve a visible thyroid cartilage (not the thyroid gland), subhyoid depression (not the hyoid), and the inferior mandibular border. A normal cervicomental angle of between 105 to 120 degrees should also be observed. The submandibular gland and digastric muscle should not be visible. A bulge below the mandibular rim within the submandibular triangle may represent a ptotic or enlarged submandibular gland. Sometimes prominent digastric muscles may be observed bulging below the inferior mandibular border. This may only become apparent following neck rejuvenation.

LIPOSUCTION OF THE NECK

7. **When performing suction-assisted liposuction to the neck in a patient with submental fat excess, which one of the following is correct?**
   D. Small quantities of aspirate will normally provide satisfactory results.
   Neck liposuction carries a risk of overresection of fat, which will lead to suboptimal results. This is difficult to correct, so it is better to slightly underresect. Even small volumes of aspirate can make a significant difference to aesthetics. When undertaking liposuction of the neck, some key principles should be employed. Tumescent infiltration containing epinephrine should be injected before skin preparation and be allowed to take effect for 10 minutes. Three incisions are often required, especially if there is lateral fat to be harvested. (A single submental incision is combined with two postauricular incisions.) This approach facilitates feathering which can be useful to minimize irregularities. Small, flat cannulas (2 to 3 mm) should be used with a single hole facing toward deeper tissues, ensuring that no more than one or two passes are made within a given tunnel. (Multihole cannuale are normally used for infiltration, not harvest, and a 7 mm cannula would be too coarse for the detailed contouring required in the neck.)

   Liposuction is intended to treat subcutaneous fat excess, not subplatysmal fat, which would risk damage to other subplatysmal structures such as blood vessels and nerves. If there is subplatysmal excess, an open approach is required. A drain is not required, but a compression garment should be worn.[4]

SURGICAL APPROACHES TO NECK REJUVENATION

8. **Which one of the following is most commonly performed during correction of the deep plane (deep to the platysma) in neck rejuvenation?**
   C. Resection of subplatysmal and interplatysmal fat
   During the deep plane component of neck rejuvenation, a number of factors may be addressed. Interplatysmal and subplatysmal fat may be performed in addition to subcutaneous defatting. The anterior belly of digastric may also be resected, but this is most commonly performed tangentially to debulk it, rather than completely excise it. Intracapsular piecemeal resection of the superficial (not deep) lobe of submandibular gland may be performed if the gland is large or ptotic. It is unwise to perform an extracapsular dissection, because this risks damage to the facial artery and marginal mandibular nerve. The suprahyoid fascia is occasionally released to improve the cervical angle in patients with a high hyoid. During the resection of interplatysmal and subplatysmal fat, there are often one or two lymph nodes taken with the specimen, but no attempt is made to specifically resect nodes.

SELECTION OF SURGICAL PROCEDURES IN NECK REJUVENATION

9. *For the following scenarios, the best options are as follows:*
   A. **You see a 63-year-old, mildly obese woman with loss of neck contour and jowling. She has a large excess of neck skin and fat with prominent platysmal banding at rest.**
      f. **Full-scar face and neck lift**
         The patient in this scenario has multiple problems to be dealt with. Since she has excess submental fat and platysmal banding, she will require an open submental approach to her neck. This entails resection of fat with platysmal midline plication. She will also require a face lift to address her skin excess and jowls.
   B. **You see a 39-year-old woman with excellent skin quality and moderate submental fat excess. She has no platysmal banding at rest, but banding becomes apparent on animation. A skin pinch test reveals no alteration in pinch size on animation.**
      d. **Submental neck lift with liposuction**
         The patient in this scenario has moderate subcutaneous fat without subplatysmal fat excess. She could be a good candidate for liposuction but will also need to have her platysmal bands treated, because these are likely to become evident at rest following liposuction. For this reason, she should have liposuction combined with an open submental approach.
   C. **You see a 55-year-old woman of average build who is concerned about the appearance of her neck contour. On examination, she has no evidence of platysmal banding or skin excess but does have fullness blunting the cervicomental angle and lower border of mandible. A skin pinch test reveals a diminished pinch size during animation.**
      c. **Submental neck lift**
         The patient in this scenario may also seem a good candidate for liposuction given that she has fat excess without skin excess or platysmal banding. However, she has evidence of subplatysmal fat, and this is not amenable to liposuction. In this case a submental open approach is warranted.

PLATYSMAL PROCEDURES

10. You see a patient after previous surgery to the neck. On examination they have a visible transverse step in the neck and a window shading effect. **Which one of the procedures has most likely been undertaken?**
    D. **Platysma muscle sling**
       The platysma muscle sling technique involves dividing the platysma horizontally across the entire width. This creates a wide gap that is potentially visible. Retraction of the platysma superiorly results in a window shading effect which has diminished the popularity of this procedure (see Fig. 95-11, *Essentials of Plastic Surgery,* second edition).
       Platysmal suspension involves placement of sutures along the inferior madibular border over the superficial fascia on platysma.
       Platysmal flap cervical rhytidectomy involves a sectional myotomy of the medial edge of platysma so that lateral rotation and advancement of flap edges can be achieved.
       Corset platysmaplasty is used to eliminate static paramedian muscle bands and reshape the neck. No muscle resection is performed, but platysma is plicated in the midline (see Figs. 95-10 through 95-12, *Essentials of Plastic Surgery,* second edition).

POSTOPERATIVE COMPLICATIONS

11. A patient referred to you has undergone neck rejuvenation at another clinic and is dissatisfied with the appearance of her neck contour. On examination she has an irregular contour with thin, visible bilateral bulges and adjacent hollowing in the anterior aspect of the neck just below the mandible. ***What is the most likely explanation for this appearance?***

B. Excessive submental liposuction

The appearance described is in keeping with excessive submental liposuction that has left visible prominent digastric muscles (Fig. 95-2). Liposuction should be performed with caution in the neck, as this case illustrates. Only small quantities of aspirate should be harvested and 3 to 5 mm of subcutaneous fat should be left to provide a natural, soft contour. This is a difficult problem to address and may require fat grafting.

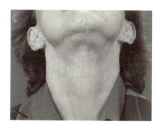

Fig. 95-2 Overaggressive fat removal from the neck and submental area has unmasked platysma bands and prominent digastric muscles.

REFERENCES

1. de Castro CC. The anatomy of the platysma muscle. Plast Reconstr Surg 66:680-683, 1980.
2. Kim HJ, Hu KS, Kang MK, et al. Decussation patterns of the platysma in Koreans. Br J Plast Surg 54:400-402, 2001.
3. Ellenbogen R, Karlin V. Visual criteria for success in restoring the youthful neck. Plast Reconstr Surg 66:826-837, 1980.
4. Nahai F. Neck lift. In Nahai F, ed. The Art of Aesthetic Surgery: Principles & Practices, ed 2. St Louis: Quality Medical Publishing, 2011.

96. Rhinoplasty

See *Essentials of Plastic Surgery*, second edition, pp. 1203-1229.

NASAL ANATOMY

1. **Correctly identify the anatomic components of the nose on the diagram below. Five of the nine options will be used (Fig. 96-1).**

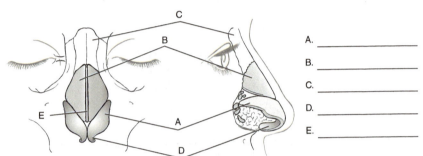

A. _____
B. _____
C. _____
D. _____
E. _____

Fig. 96-1

Options:
a. Nasal bone
b. Upper lateral cartilage
c. Medial crus of lower lateral cartilage
d. Lateral crus of lower lateral cartilage
e. Middle crus of lower lateral cartilage
f. Nasal septum
g. Inferior nasal spine
h. Keystone area
i. Scroll area

2. A patient with unresolving unilateral Bell's palsy is seen in clinic, as they are experiencing problems with nasal obstruction. **Paralysis of which one of the following muscles is most likely to be responsible for their symptoms?**
   A. Nasalis
   B. Depressor septi nasi
   C. Buccinator
   D. Levator labii alaeque nasi
   E. Levator labii superioris

Chapter 96 ■ Rhinoplasty 813

3. A 30-year-old woman attends clinic requesting rhinoplasty. She has two issues: the first is a mild dorsal hump and the second is nasal obstruction on the left side. On examination, you note that her nasal tip frequently drops during animation and on discussion with her and her partner you find that they have noticed this and like the aesthetics this produces. **In this case, what muscle should be specifically preserved to maintain the aesthetics described?**
   A. Levator labii superioris
   B. Levator labii alaeque nasi
   C. Depressor septi nasi
   D. Depressor anguli oris
   E. Depressor labii inferioris

4. **What is the main blood supply to the nasal tip after an open rhinoplasty?**
   A. Lateral nasal
   B. Columellar
   C. Angular
   D. Dorsal nasal
   E. Superior labial

5. **What is the sensory nerve supply to the nasal tip?**
   A. Anterior ethmoid
   B. Posterior ethmoid
   C. Infraorbital
   D. Supratrochlear
   E. Supraorbital

KEY ANATOMIC STRUCTURES IN THE NOSE

6. **For each of the following descriptions, select the most likely answer from the options listed. (Each option may be used once, more than once, or not at all.)**
   A. This structure is formed predominantly by the caudal edge of the lateral crus of the lower lateral cartilage and the nasal septum.
   B. This structure is formed where the bony nasal vault and upper cartilaginous vault meet.
   C. This structure is formed by the caudal edge of the upper lateral cartilage and the nasal septum.

   Options:
   a. Keystone area
   b. Scroll area
   c. External nasal valve
   d. Lower turbinate
   e. Piriform aperture
   f. Internal nasal valve
   g. Lateral crural complex

INTERNAL NASAL STRUCTURES

7. **What structure is formed by the interface between the upper and lower lateral cartilages?**
   A. The lateral crural complex
   B. The medial crural complex
   C. The scroll area
   D. The piriform aperture
   E. The keystone area

EMPTY NOSE SYNDROME

8. **In a patient with "empty nose syndrome," what structure is most likely to have been resected?**
   A. Posterior nasal septum
   B. Anterior nasal septum
   C. Superior turbinate
   D. Inferior turbinate
   E. Lower lateral cartilages

NASAL PHYSIOLOGY

9. **Which one of the following is correct regarding nasal airflow physiology?**
   A. During inhalation, the nostrils and internal nasal valve narrow due to negative pressure generation.
   B. The nasal airway normally contributes less than a quarter of the overall airway resistance.
   C. Constant nasal obstruction is due to a fixed structural abnormality and requires surgical intervention.
   D. Gradual worsening of nasal obstruction warrants further investigation, including endonasal scoping, and possibly biopsy.
   E. Rhinitis medicamentosus should be treated with oxymetazoline (Afrin) and oral antibiotics for 2 months.

TYPES OF GRAFTS USED IN RHINOPLASTY

10. For each of the following descriptions, select the most likely graft from the options above. (Each option may be used once, more than once, or not at all.)
    A. Used to augment the nasofrontal angle and may give an appearance of nasal lengthening
    B. Used to improve internal nasal valve patency or correct inverted-V or open-roof deformities
    C. Used to correct a pinched nasal tip deformity and improve external nasal valve function

    Options:
    a. Dorsal onlay graft
    b. Radix graft
    c. Lateral sidewall onlay graft
    d. Septal extension graft
    e. Spreader graft
    f. Alar rim graft
    g. Alar spreader graft

SURGICAL APPROACHES TO RHINOPLASTY

11. For each of the following descriptions, select the most likely surgical approach to rhinoplasty from the options listed. (Each option may be used once, more than once, or not at all.)
    A. This approach may result in a loss of tip support and projection.
    B. This approach is made below the lower lateral cartilages.
    C. This approach is made between the upper and lower lateral cartilages.

    Options:
    a. Partial transfixion
    b. Intracartilaginous
    c. Intercartilaginous
    d. Transcartilaginous
    e. Marginal
    f. Complete transfixion

NASAL TIP GRAFTS

12. **Which one of the following procedures combines strut and onlay graft techniques to improve tip projection and support?**
    A. Cap graft
    B. Columellar strut
    C. Shield graft
    D. Alar base graft
    E. Umbrella graft

NASAL TIP PROCEDURES

13. You are performing an open rhinoplasty and want to increase tip rotation and projection. **Which one of the following techniques would be most helpful?**
   A. Shortening of the medial crura
   B. Lengthening of the lateral crura
   C. Placement of medial crural septal sutures
   D. Resection of both lateral and medial crura
   E. Placement of medial crural sutures

OSTEOTOMIES IN RHINOPLASTY

14. **Which one of the following is correct regarding osteotomies in rhinoplasty?**
   A. They are rarely required after dorsal hump correction.
   B. Lateral osteotomies should be performed before medial osteotomies.
   C. There are two main types of lateral osteotomy, each with similar indications.
   D. They may be contraindicated in elderly patients and in individuals of some ethnic groups.
   E. They cannot be used to widen the nasal vault.

ALAR DEFORMITIES

15. A patient is seen in clinic with excessive alar flaring. **Which one of the following techniques is most effective at correcting this deformity?**
   A. Full-thickness alar wedge excision
   B. Partial-thickness alar wedge excision
   C. Medial crural suture placement
   D. Lateral crural strut graft
   E. Alar contour graft

NASAL AIRWAY MANAGEMENT

16. You assess a 25-year-old woman who complains of long-term nasal obstruction that is relieved when she moves her cheek laterally. She has a mild septal deviation and a narrow midvault. **Which one of the following interventions is most likely to improve her symptoms?**
   A. Submucosal turbinate resection
   B. Infracture of the inferior turbinate
   C. Closed septoplasty
   D. Insertion of spreader grafts
   E. Placement of a lateral nasal wall graft

MANAGEMENT OF THE DEVIATED NOSE

17. You are performing an open rhinoplasty on a patient with a deviated nose. He has a caudal deformity and an apparent straight tilt to the septum. **Which one of the following should be performed?**
   A. A swinging door flap secured to the nasal spine
   B. Cartilage scoring with batten grafts
   C. Cartilage weakening and spreader grafts
   D. Horizontal mattress sutures to the upper lateral cartilages
   E. Osteotomy and infracture of the nasal bones

18. You see a patient in clinic following closed rhinoplasty. They are concerned about the appearance of their nasal bridge, which is wide and flat just distal to the radix. **What procedure would you ideally use to correct this deformity?**
   A. Hump reduction
   B. Dorsal and sidewall augmentation
   C. Osteotomy and infracture
   D. An A-frame graft
   E. A U-frame graft

19. You see a patient in clinic keen to undergo a rhinoplasty because they are unhappy with the appearance and function of their nose. They have unilateral airway problems, with breathing difficulties at night. They also dislike the appearance of their nose because of a dorsal hump, bulbous tip, and wide alar bases. **What is the main benefit of performing a cephalic trim during rhinoplasty for this patient?**
   A. Improved airway patency
   B. Reduced dorsal hump
   C. Reduced tip rotation
   D. Refinement of the nasal tip
   E. Reduction of alar flaring

Answers

NASAL ANATOMY
1. For Fig. 96-2, the labels are as follows:

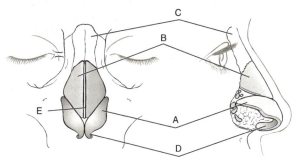

A. d. Lateral crus of lower lateral cartilage

B. b. Upper lateral cartilage

C. a. Nasal bone

D. c. Medial crus of lower lateral cartilage

E. f. Nasal septum

Fig. 96-2

The nose comprises a bony cartilaginous frame with three components: upper, middle, and lower thirds. The upper third is formed by the paired nasal bones and nasal septum, the middle third is formed by the paired upper lateral cartilages and nasal septum, and the lower third is formed by the paired lower lateral cartilages and nasal septum. Having a good understanding of this anatomy is vital to both rhinoplasty and nasal reconstruction surgery. The nasal bones are around 2.5 cm long and are continuous with the frontal processes of the maxilla. They overlap the upper lateral cartilages for around 6 to 8 mm. At this point, the upper lateral cartilages and nasal septum join to form a T-shaped construct. The upper lateral cartilages continue caudally to join with the paired lower lateral cartilages, which also overlap the upper lateral cartilages. The lower lateral cartilages have three different components: lateral, middle, and medial crura. They join with the nasal septum in the midline at the medial crus. The lower lateral cartilages are intimately related to tip projection, rotation, and definition and are usually modified during rhinoplasty. It is important to realize that the nasal alae do not contain cartilage, as the lower lateral cartilage finishes more cranially than the alae. Alar support is instead provided by the fibrous nature and shape of the alar construct. The keystone and scroll areas are discussed further in questions 6 and 7.

2. A patient with unresolving unilateral Bell's palsy is seen in clinic, as they are experiencing problems with nasal obstruction. **Paralysis of which one of the following muscles is most likely to be responsible for their symptoms?**
   D. Levator labii alaeque nasi
   In patients with Bell's palsy, the muscles of facial expression are paralyzed, either temporarily or permanently. A number of muscles will affect nasal obstruction in a facial palsy patient, but the levator labii superioris alaeque nasi muscle is the most important in this regard. It originates from the upper frontal process of the maxilla and inserts into the skin of the lateral nostril and upper lip. It is innervated by the buccal branch of the facial nerve and elevates the medial nasolabial fold and nasal alae. The nasalis has two components that affect nasal airway patency. There are

both compressor and dilator components which cause reduction or enlargement of the nasal alae, respectively. Paralysis of this muscle will therefore also contribute to nasal obstruction in this patient, but less so than the levator labii alaeque muscle. The buccinator muscle pulls the corner of the mouth laterally and compresses the cheek, the levator labii superioris muscle elevates the lip and midportion of the nasolabial fold, and the depressor septi nasi muscle pulls the septum inferiorly.

3. A 30-year-old woman attends clinic requesting rhinoplasty. She has two issues: the first is a mild dorsal hump and the second is nasal obstruction on the left side. On examination, you note that her nasal tip frequently drops during animation and on discussion with her and her partner you find that they have noticed this and like the aesthetics this produces. *In this case, what muscle should be specifically preserved to maintain the aesthetics described?*
   C. Depressor septi nasi
   The depressor septi nasi muscle is a small muscle that arises from the incisive fossa of the maxilla or orbicularis oris and inserts into the nasal septum and part of the nasalis muscle. It acts to depress the nasal septum and tip, acting as an antagonist to the other muscles of the nose. It is innervated by the buccal branch of the facial nerve and is relevant to rhinoplasty because it can accentuate a drooping nasal tip on animation of the upper lip. Many surgeons resect or divide this muscle in certain patients to prevent these effects. Rohrich et al[1] performed an anatomic study of this muscle and found that it is commonly in continuity with the orbicularis oris and they describe a procedure to dissect and transpose this muscle during rhinoplasty in order to improve tip and upper lip appearance in some patients. In the scenario described, the patient has activity of the depressor that is clearly liked by her and her partner. For this reason, preservation of the depressor is indicated in this case.

4. **What is the main blood supply to the nasal tip after an open rhinoplasty?**
   A. Lateral nasal
   Understanding the blood supply to the nasal tip is crucial when undertaking an open rhinoplasty, because inadvertent damage of the lateral nasal artery (for example, during alar base resection) may lead to soft tissue necrosis of the tip.[2] The nose normally receives its blood supply from both the ophthalmic and facial arteries (see Fig. 96-1, *Essentials of Plastic Surgery*, second edition). The ophthalmic artery branches supply the cranial aspect, and the facial artery branches supply the caudal aspect. In most patients the superior labial artery gives rise to the columellar artery, which supplies the nasal tip. After an open rhinoplasty this vessel is divided, so the blood supply becomes dependent upon a branch of the angular artery called the lateral nasal artery, which passes from the nasojugal groove over the alar.

5. **What is the sensory nerve supply to the nasal tip?**
   A. Anterior ethmoid
   Sensory innervation of the external nose is from the trigeminal nerve divisions I and II. The supraorbital and supratrochlear nerves from the ophthalmic division supply the cephalad portion, while the external nasal branch of anterior ethmoid supplies the middle vault and nasal tip.

Chapter 96 ▪ Rhinoplasty 819

KEY ANATOMIC STRUCTURES IN THE NOSE

6. *For the following descriptions, the best options are as follows:*
   A. *This structure is formed predominantly by the caudal edge of the lateral crus of the lower lateral cartilage and the nasal septum.*
      c. **External nasal valve**
   B. *This structure is formed where the bony nasal vault and upper cartilaginous vault meet.*
      a. **Keystone area**
   C. *This structure is formed by the caudal edge of the upper lateral cartilage and the nasal septum.*
      f. **Internal nasal valve**

   The external nasal valve is created primarily by the caudal edge of the lateral crus and nasal septum, with contributions from the ala and nasal sill soft tissues. External valve collapse may be seen with nostril collapse on inspiration. The internal nasal valve is the narrowest portion of the nasal airway and is therefore important in regulating airflow resistance. It is formed by the junction of the caudal border of the upper lateral cartilages and the nasal septum where they form a T shape. The keystone area of the nose refers to the point at which the upper and middle vaults meet (see Fig. 96-1). It usually represents the widest part of the nose.

INTERNAL NASAL STRUCTURES

7. *What structure is formed by the interface between the upper and lower lateral cartilages?*
   C. **The scroll area**

   The scroll area is the region of abutment between the upper and lower lateral cartilages. The lateral crural complex is formed by the lateral crus and accessory cartilage (see Fig. 96-1). There is no named medial crural complex; the piriform aperture (derived from the Latin "piri," meaning pear) is a pear-shaped opening of the skull where the nose is situated.

EMPTY NOSE SYNDROME

8. *In a patient with "empty nose syndrome," what structure is most likely to have been resected?*
   D. **Inferior turbinate**

   Empty nose syndrome describes a situation in which a patient has nasal obstruction and a dry nose following nasal or sinus surgery.[3] Most commonly, it occurs after resection of the inferior turbinate. Symptoms may be delayed for months or years after surgery and are counterintuitive, since there is no physical obstruction present. The turbinates are paired bony structures that regulate and humidify inspired air. The inferior turbinate is the primary turbinate treated in rhinoplasty, and a severely deviated septum may induce the contralateral turbinate to hypertrophy to balance bilateral nasal cavities. A hypertrophied turbinate may be responsible for up to two thirds of airway resistance.

NASAL PHYSIOLOGY

9. *Which one of the following is correct regarding nasal airflow physiology?*
   D. **Gradual worsening of nasal obstruction warrants further investigation, including endonasal scoping, and possibly biopsy.**

   Gradual worsening of an airway obstruction, particularly in smokers or in association with epistaxis, may indicate a neoplasm and warrants further investigation. The nasal airway contributes around half of total nasal obstruction and can significantly reduce airflow when mucosal swelling is present, such as during a cold. During inspiration, the internal nasal valve narrows from negative pressure, but the nostrils usually open to facilitate airflow. Nasal obstruction can be either anatomic or physiologic; constant obstruction is more likely, but not exclusively, caused by a structural problem. Rhinitis medicamentosus is a condition arising secondary to excessive use of nasal congestants such as Afrin. Treatment involves stopping the offending agent and may include antihistamines and steroids.

TYPES OF GRAFTS USED IN RHINOPLASTY

10. For the following descriptions, the best options are as follows:
    A. **Used to augment the nasofrontal angle and may give an appearance of nasal lengthening**
       b. **Radix graft**
          The radix graft involves placing a small piece of cartilage within a soft tissue pocket over the proximal nasal bone. This can help mask deformity or bony deficiency in this region.
    B. **Used to improve internal nasal valve patency or correct inverted-V or open-roof deformities**
       e. **Spreader graft**
          The spreader graft is placed between the septum and upper lateral cartilages and can also help straighten a deviated septum or smooth the dorsal aesthetic lines, as well as open the internal nasal valve.
    C. **Used to correct a pinched nasal tip deformity and improve external nasal valve function**
       g. **Alar spreader graft**
          The alar spreader graft is placed between the lateral crura and vestibular skin to improve nasal valve function. The dorsal onlay graft usually recontours or augments the length of the nasal dorsum, starting just below the radix. Lateral sidewall grafts are used to improve the contour of depressed upper lateral cartilages. The septal extension graft controls projection, rotation, and support of the nasal tip and helps to create a supratip break. The alar rim graft is placed within the intranasal rim to correct notching and retraction (see Figs. 96-8 through 96-14, *Essentials of Plastic Surgery*, second edition).

SURGICAL APPROACHES TO RHINOPLASTY

11. For the following descriptions, the best options are as follows:
    A. **This approach may result in a loss of tip support and projection.**
       f. **Complete transfixion**
    B. **This approach is made below the lower lateral cartilages.**
       e. **Marginal**
    C. **This approach is made between the upper and lower lateral cartilages.**
       c. **Intercartilaginous**
          Rhinoplasty can be performed as an open or closed procedure. Both open and closed rhinoplasty approaches require internal nasal incisions. These are classified as those made through the alar mucosa and those made to the septum. Open rhinoplasty will also require an additional columellar incision. Alar incisions are made between the upper and lower lateral cartilages (intercartilaginous), through the lower lateral cartilage (transcartilaginous/intracartilaginous), or below the lower lateral cartilage (marginal; see Fig. 96-15, *Essentials of Plastic Surgery*, second edition).
          Septal incisions include complete and partial subtypes. During a complete (full) transfixion, the entire septum is incised at the membranous and caudal cartilaginous junction. This releases the tip completely and exposes the nasal spine and depressor septi muscle. It

disrupts the attachments of the medial footplates to the caudal septum and can result in a loss of projection and nasal tip support.

In contrast, a partial transfixion begins caudal to the anterior septal angle and ends just short of the medial crural attachments to the caudal septum.

NASAL TIP GRAFTS

12. *Which one of the following procedures combines strut and onlay graft techniques to improve tip projection and support?*
    E. Umbrella graft

There are many different grafts used to improve the nasal tip appearance or projection. They include strut grafts that support the nasal septum and tip, or onlay grafts that augment it at specific sites. Umbrella grafts include a vertical columellar strut placed between the medial crura, with the addition of a horizontal tip onlay graft. Therefore they increase both tip projection and support.

The cap graft is placed between the tip-defining points and the medial crura. It serves to increase projection or refine the infratip lobule. A columellar strut graft is placed between the medial crura and helps maintain or increase tip projection and aids in shaping the columellar-lobular angle. Shield grafts are placed on the anterior middle crura and extend to the nasal tip to improve tip projection and definition. The alar base graft is placed along the lateral piriform aperture to augment a recessed lip–alar base junction rather than improve the nasal tip itself.

NASAL TIP PROCEDURES

13. You are performing an open rhinoplasty and want to increase tip rotation and projection. *Which one of the following techniques would be most helpful?*
    C. Placement of medial crural septal sutures

Medial crural septal sutures are placed between the medial crura and the septum and are used for correction of a drooping tip or aging nose and help to increase both tip projection and rotation (see Fig. 96-21, *Essentials of Plastic Surgery,* second edition)

The "tripod" model is useful for understanding the relationship between projection and rotation. When the lateral crura are shortened, the tip will be rotated, while projection is decreased. Shortening of the medial crura will derotate and deproject the tip (both options A and B will therefore derotate the tip). Equivalent portions of both medial and lateral crura are resected, the projection is decreased, while the rotation should remain the same (option D).

Medial crural sutures differ from medial crural septal sutures. They involve horizontal mattress sutures placed between the medial crura that unify the lower lateral cartilages and stabilize the columellar strut to resist flaring of the medial crura (see Fig. 96-19, *Essentials of Plastic Surgery,* second edition).

OSTEOTOMIES IN RHINOPLASTY

14. *Which one of the following is correct regarding osteotomies in rhinoplasty?*
    D. They may be contraindicated in elderly patients and in individuals of some ethnic groups.

Osteotomies are useful to allow repositioning of the nasal bones during rhinoplasty. Relative contraindications to their use include elderly patients with thin nasal bones, ethnic noses that are low and broad, and patients who wear heavy glasses.

Osteotomies in rhinoplasty are described as either medial or lateral. They can be used independent of one another or may be combined. Lateral osteotomies are classified by the level at which they are performed in relation to the face of the maxilla (low to low, low to high, or double level; see Figs. 96-33 and 96-34, *Essentials of Plastic Surgery,* second edition). They are commonly used after dorsal hump reduction to correct an open-roof deformity or narrow a wide bony dorsum. Medial osteotomies are used to narrow the bony vault, but may be used to widen it when combined with lateral osteotomies (see Figs. 96-33 and 96-34, *Essentials of Plastic Surgery,* second edition). Medial osteotomies should be performed before lateral osteotomies; otherwise, the bones will have little support, making them a moving target during the medial osteotomies.

ALAR RIM DEFORMITIES

15. A patient is seen in clinic with excessive alar flaring. **Which one of the following techniques is most effective at correcting this deformity?**
    B. **Partial-thickness alar wedge excision**

    Flared alae are best corrected with partial-thickness wedge excisions that preserve the alar base and do not extend into the nasal vestibule (see Fig. 96-36, *Essentials of Plastic Surgery,* second edition). Alar base width reduction is also performed with wedge excisions, but in this case, full-thickness incisions are made (see Fig. 96-37, *Essentials of Plastic Surgery,* second edition). Alar base reduction will alter the alar-cheek junction and may alter the appearance of nasal projection. Medial crural suture placement is used to improve tip definition and provide tip support (see Fig. 96-23, *Essentials of Plastic Surgery,* second edition). Lateral crural strut grafts and alar contour grafts are used to treat alar rim deformities and provide internal alar support (see Fig. 96-35, *Essentials of Plastic Surgery,* second edition). Alar rim deformities are commonly due to excessive lateral crural resection during previous rhinoplasty.

NASAL AIRWAY MANAGEMENT

16. You assess a 25-year-old woman who complains of long-term nasal obstruction that is relieved when she moves her cheek laterally. She has a mild septal deviation and a narrow midvault. **Which one of the following interventions is most likely to improve her symptoms?**
    D. **Insertion of spreader grafts**

    There are a number of structural factors that may lead to nasal obstruction, and management is specific to the cause. This patient displays a positive Cottle's sign, in which lateral displacement of the cheek opens the internal nasal valve and improves airflow. The obstruction is usually caused by a decreased nasal valve angle (less than 15 degrees) or weak upper lateral cartilage where the septum and upper lateral cartilages meet. This is addressed by placing a cartilage graft between the upper lateral cartilages and the septum. Submucosal turbinate resection or outfracture (not infracture) may be helpful if the obstruction has resulted from turbinate hypertrophy. If the lateral nasal wall is weak, strengthening it with lateral grafts may be helpful. A septoplasty can also help correct nasal obstruction, depending on the cause.

MANAGEMENT OF THE DEVIATED NOSE

17. You are performing an open rhinoplasty on a patient with a deviated nose. He has a caudal deformity and an apparent straight tilt to the septum. **Which one of the following should be performed?**
    A. **A swinging door flap secured to the nasal spine**

    Rohrich et al[4] proposed a treatment algorithm for managing patients with deviated noses (Fig. 96-3). Correction is performed through an open rhinoplasty technique and differs, depending on whether deviation is caudal or dorsal and whether the septum is C-shaped, S-shaped, or has a straight tilt. In the case of a straight tilt with the septum incorrectly located, the approach is to

reduce the caudal septum onto the nasal spine and this may require vertical sectioning to create a "swinging door."

If this is insufficient, small wedges of cartilage can also be excised from the convex side of the deviation, with cartilage scoring on the concave side to decrease the cartilage memory and straighten the septum. The caudal septum is sutured to the nasal spine and may be secured using a piece of septal cartilage.

Cartilage scoring with batten grafts may be useful to treat C-shaped or S-shaped **caudal** deformity. Cartilage weakening and spreader grafts may be used to treat C-shaped or S-shaped dorsal deformity. Horizontal mattress sutures to the upper lateral cartilages may be used to control any residual deviation after correction with the other techniques. Ostetomies are generally used to correct a proximal (cranial) bony deviation.

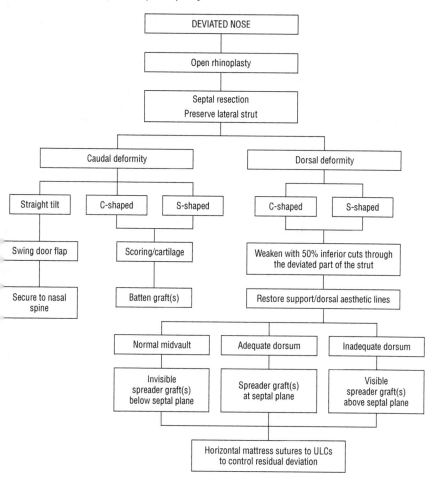

Fig. 96-3 Algorithm for correction of a deviated nose. (*ULCs,* Upper lateral cartilages.)

18. You see a patient in clinic following closed rhinoplasty. They are concerned about the appearance of their nasal bridge, which is wide and flat just distal to the radix. **What procedure would you ideally use to correct this deformity?**
    C. **Osteotomy and infracture**
    This patient has an open-roof deformity of the nasal bridge following their previous rhinoplasty. The open-roof deformity occurs when a dorsal hump is reduced without bringing the nasal bones together in the midline. It may be conceptualized as shaving the top of a triangular prism structure and not folding the open edges back together again. The usual way to correct or prevent an open-roof deformity is to perform osteotomies and infracture of the nasal bones to bring them together and reconstruct the "roof." It is possible to augment an open-roof deformity with a graft but osteotomies are generally preferred, as they correct rather than mask the deformity.

    There are a number of techniques used to augment the nasal dorsum and these include septal, auricular, and costal cartilage grafts. Graft shapes include inverted-V, inverted-U, and A-shaped examples.

19. You see a patient in clinic keen to undergo a rhinoplasty because they are unhappy with the appearance and function of their nose. They have unilateral airway problems, with breathing difficulties at night. They also dislike the appearance of their nose because of a dorsal hump, bulbous tip, and wide alar bases. **What is the main benefit of performing a cephalic trim during rhinoplasty for this patient?**
    D. *Refinement of the nasal tip*
    A cephalic trim refers to removal of some of the lower lateral cartilages along their superior aspect. It may be beneficial in this patient in order to reduce the bulbous nasal tip and refine its appearance. It is also useful for increasing (not decreasing) tip rotation when this is required, but this was not a problem identified in this patient. Sometimes cephalic trims are further augmented with suture techniques in order to refine and support the nasal tip (see Figs. 96-18 through 96-20, *Essentials of Plastic Surgery*, second edition).

    A cephalic trim is unlikely to affect airway patency. Depending on the cause, patency may be improved with manipulation of the septum or nasal valves. Reduction of a dorsal hump removes the prominent nasal septum and nasal bones, as well as the upper lateral cartilages. It does not affect the lower lateral cartilages. Alar flaring is not usually affected by tip work and reduction of alar bases in this case would require a wedge excision.

REFERENCES

1. Rohrich RJ, Huynh B, Muzaffar AR, et al. Importance of the depressor septi nasi muscle in rhinoplasty: anatomic study and clinical application. Plast Reconstr Surg 105:376-383; discussion 384-388, 2000.
2. Rohrich RJ, Gunter JP, Friedman RM. Nasal tip blood supply: an anatomic study validating the safety of the transcolumellar incision in rhinoplasty. Plast Reconstr Surg 95:795-799; discussion 800-801, 1995.
3. Coste A, Dessi P, Serrano E. Empty nose syndrome. Eur Ann Otorhinolaryngol Head Neck Dis 129:93-97, 2012.
4. Rohrich RJ, Gunter JP, Deuber MA, et al. The deviated nose: optimizing results using a simplified classification and algorithmic approach. Plast Reconstr Surg 110:1509-1523, 2002.

97. Genioplasty

See *Essentials of Plastic Surgery*, second edition, pp. 1230-1241.

ANATOMY

1. **Failure to repair which muscle during genioplasty can lead to a "witch's chin" deformity?**
   A. Depressor anguli oris
   B. Depressor labii oris
   C. Mentalis
   D. Geniohyoid
   E. Genioglossus

2. **Which nerve is most at risk of inadvertent injury during a sliding genioplasty?**
   A. Marginal mandibular nerve
   B. Hypoglossal nerve
   C. Mandibular nerve
   D. Inferior alveolar nerve
   E. Mental nerve

OCCLUSION

3. **What is the most common type of malocclusion in North American white individuals?**
   A. Angle class I
   B. Angle class II
   C. Angle class III
   D. Angle class IV
   E. Angle class V

EVALUATION OF SOFT TISSUES

4. **When evaluating chin prominence in clinic, which one of the following structures should normally lie on Riedel's plane?**
   A. Upper lip
   B. Nasal tip
   C. Alar base
   D. Labiomental crease
   E. Modiolus

OSSEOUS GENIOPLASTY

5. **Which one of the following statements is true regarding osseous genioplasty?**
   A. Malocclusion can be corrected with osseous genioplasty.
   B. A large vertical excess of the mandible is best corrected with a jumping genioplasty.
   C. Soft tissue movement during advancement genioplasty parallels skeletal changes predictably.
   D. Complex deficiencies are better treated by prosthetic augmentation.
   E. Shallow labiomental folds are exacerbated by advancing genioplasty techniques.

IMPLANT GENIOPLASTY

6. *What is the main indication for performing an implant genioplasty?*
   A. An isolated mild horizontal chin excess
   B. An isolated mild vertical chin deficiency
   C. An isolated mild vertical chin excess
   D. An isolated mild horizontal chin deficiency
   E. An isolated mandibular asymmetry

7. Implant genioplasty can be undertaken through intraoral or submental approaches. *Which one of the following is a benefit of an intraoral approach?*
   A. A lower infection rate
   B. More precise placement of the implant
   C. Reduced visible scarring
   D. Less chance of mental nerve injury
   E. Reduced operative time

COMPLICATIONS

8. *Which one of the following complications is most commonly observed following genioplasty?*
   A. Hematoma
   B. Infection
   C. Extrusion of implant or metalwork
   D. Lower lip weakness
   E. Lower lip paresthesia

Answers

ANATOMY

1. **Failure to repair which muscle during genioplasty can lead to a "witch's chin" deformity?**
   C. Mentalis
   A witch's chin deformity is present when there is soft tissue ptosis of the chin caudal to the menton that results in an exaggerated submental crease. During an intraoral approach to genioplasty, the mentalis muscle is transected. In order to prevent subsequent ptosis, the mentalis should be reattached to the mandible and repaired during closure. The remaining muscles are relevant to local anatomy of the chin and lower lip but are not specifically relevant to the witch's chin deformity.

2. **Which nerve is most at risk of inadvertent injury during a sliding genioplasty?**
   E. Mental nerve
   The mental nerve is at risk of damage during a sliding genioplasty if the osteotomy is placed too high or if the mental foramen is lower than anticipated. The mental nerve supplies sensation to the lower lip and dentition and it is a continuation of the inferior alveolar nerve which passes through the mandible. The inferior alveolar nerve is a branch of the mandibular division of the trigeminal nerve. These two nerves are too proximal to be at significant risk during genioplasty. The hypoglossal nerve supplies motor function to the tongue but is well protected during a genioplasty. The marginal mandibular nerve is also protected during a genioplasty, as it lies above the lower border of the mandible at this point.

OCCLUSION

3. **What is the most common type of malocclusion in North American white individuals?**
   B. Angle class II
   There are three types of malocclusion as described by Edward Angle. These are numbered I through III, and of these the most common type in North American white individuals is type II. The precise definition for this malocclusion is that the mesiobuccal cusp of the maxillary first molar rests mesial to the buccal groove. This means that the maxillary dentition sits more anterior to the mandibular dentition than normal in the lateral view. A normal occlusion involves the mesiobuccal cusp of the maxillary first molar resting in the buccal groove of the mandibular first molar without any teeth being malrotated or malposed. This means that the maxillary dentition is only slightly anterior to the mandibular dentition in the lateral view. A class I malocclusion is where the mesiobuccal cusp of the first molar sits in the buccal groove of the mandibular first molar but teeth are malposed or malrotated. Class III malocclusion is where the mesiobuccal cusp of the first maxillary molar sites distal to the buccal groove of the mandibular first molar. This means that the mandibular dentition sits anterior to the maxillary dentition in the lateral view. Often, though not always, patients with micrognathia have a class II malocclusion, and those with prognathism have a class III malocclusion. However, this cannot be guaranteed, as occlusion and chin prominence may not always be linked. For this reason, the two must be assessed independently (see Fig. 97-3 and Chapter 32, *Essentials of Plastic Surgery,* second edition).

EVALUATION OF SOFT TISSUES

4. When evaluating chin prominence in clinic, which one of the following structures should normally lie on Riedel's plane?

A. Upper lip

When assessing the profile of a patient before genioplasty, the relationship between the upper and lower lips and pogonion need to be considered. Ideally, the upper lip should be just anterior to the lower lip, and the lower lip just anterior to the soft tissue pogonion.[1] Riedel's plane is a straight line that connects the most prominent parts of the upper and lower lip in lateral view, which on a balanced face should also touch with the soft tissue pogonion (the soft tissue pogonion is the most projected soft tissue point covering the mandible). (See Fig. 97-1 and also see Fig. 87-9, *Essentials of Plastic Surgery,* second edition). (Note there is slight variation between males and females in ideal chin prominence, with the male chin having greater prominence). Chin advancement beyond the lower lip will result in an artificial appearance with poor aesthetics.

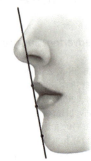

Riedel's plane

Fig. 97-1 Riedel's plane is a simple line that connects the most prominent portion of the upper and lower lip, which on a balanced face should touch the pogonion.

OSSEOUS GENIOPLASTY

5. Which one of the following statements is true regarding osseous genioplasty?

C. Soft tissue movement during advancement genioplasty parallels skeletal changes predictably.

Soft tissue movement during genioplasty follows bony advancement predictably, with a ratio close to 1:1 (the precise amount varies slightly between 0.8:1 and 1:1). However, this ratio does not hold true for posterior repositioning of the chin, which may be reduced. For this reason, outcomes are less predictable for prominent chin correction, and the potential soft tissue effects must be taken into account during preoperative planning.

Osseous genioplasty provides good flexibility for correction of chin deformities in multiple planes, and this represents an advantage over prosthetic techniques.[2] Most commonly, it is used for horizontal (sagittal) advancement but can also be used to increase or decrease vertical deformities and amend symphyseal asymmetries. A jumping genioplasty is indicated for very minor vertical excess correction, but larger excess is better treated by a reduction genioplasty (see Fig. 97-6, *Essentials of Plastic Surgery,* second edition). The labiomental crease should normally be about 4 mm deep in women and 6 mm deep in men.

Deep (not shallow) labiomental folds will be exacerbated by horizontal chin advancement or by shortening the vertical chin height. Therefore, when advancing the chin in patients with a normal or short lower face height, vertical advancement of the chin can be incorporated into the sliding genioplasty to compensate and thus maintain a normal labiomental fold depth. This approach must not be used in patients with long lower faces, and these patients are better served with orthognathic procedures.

IMPLANT GENIOPLASTY

6. *What is the main indication for performing an implant genioplasty?*
D. An isolated mild horizontal chin deficiency

In general, alloplastic augmentation should only be used for patients with relatively mild chin deficiency in the sagittal plane and a shallow labiomental fold. Contraindications include excess horizontal deficiency, vertical deficiency of any severity, mandibular asymmetry, significant microgenia, diabetes, and smoking.

7. Implant genioplasty can be undertaken through intraoral or submental approaches. *Which one of the following is a benefit of an intraoral approach?*
C. Reduced visible scarring

The only advantage of the intraoral approach is that external scars are avoided. However, when undertaking a submental approach the scar can be well hidden beneath the chin. This access can also be useful when combined procedures such as a neck lift or corset platysmaplasty are required (see Chapter 95, *Essentials of Plastic Surgery,* second edition). Infection rates are similar for both intraoral and extraoral approaches to implant genioplasty. Possible benefits of using the submental approach are a more precise implant placement and reduced chances of traction injury to the mental nerve.

COMPLICATIONS

8. *Which one of the following complications is most commonly observed following genioplasty?*
E. Lower lip paresthesia

The most common complication of those listed following genioplasty is a transient lower lip paresthesia which is seen almost universally. This resolves in almost all patients who have solely undergone genioplasty without other combined procedures such as orthognathic surgery, where rates of continued paresthesia are between 15% and 29%.[3,4]

Hematomas are rare and most often occur at the osteotomy site in association with an osseous genioplasty. Infection is less than 5% for implant genioplasty and 3% for osseous genioplasty. Extrusion of implant or metalwork is also rare. Lower lip weakness can occur leading to drooling, but again is usually temporary and not common. The most common complication following genioplasty is a poor aesthetic outcome, but in spite of this, patient satisfaction rates are very high (>90%). Poor aesthetic outcomes include overcorrection, undercorrection, and asymmetry.[1,5]

REFERENCES

1. McCarthy JG, Ruff JG. The chin. Clin Plast Surg 15:125-137, 1988.
2. Rosen HM. Osseous genioplasty. In Thorne CH, ed. Grabb & Smith's Plastic Surgery, ed 6. Philadelphia: Lippincott Williams & Wilkins, 2006.
3. Hoenig JF. Sliding osteotomy genioplasty for facial aesthetic balance: 10 years of experience. Aesthetic Plast Surg 31:384-391, 2007.
4. Lindquist C, Obeid G. Complications of genioplasty done alone or in combination with sagittal split-ramus osteotomy. Oral Surg Oral Med Oral Pathol 66:13-16, 1988.
5. Rosen HM. Aesthetic guidelines in genioplasty: the role of facial disproportion. Plast Reconstr Surg 95:463-469, 1995.

98. Liposuction

See *Essentials of Plastic Surgery*, second edition, pp. 1242-1252.

HISTORICAL DEVELOPMENT IN LIPOSUCTION

1. **Which one of the following changes in practice has been key in the development of current liposuction techniques?**
   A. Introduction of taper-tipped cannulae as standard practice
   B. Evacuation using pressures greater than 1 atmosphere
   C. Phasing out of wetting solutions containing epinephrine
   D. A focus on preserving zones of adherence
   E. A trend towards fat aspiration from the superficial fat layer

ANATOMY RELEVANT TO LIPOSUCTION

2. **Which layer of fat is considered safest to target when performing liposuction on the buttock?**
   A. Superficial
   B. Intermediate
   C. Deep
   D. Cellulite
   E. All areas are equally safe

ZONES OF ADHERENCE

3. **Which one of the following is a zone of adherence only found in male patients?**
   A. Distal iliotibial tract
   B. Gluteal crease
   C. Lateral gluteal depression
   D. Iliac crest
   E. Distal posterior thigh

PHYSICS OF LIPOSUCTION

4. **What is the main benefit of selecting a smaller-diameter cannula for traditional suction-assisted liposuction?**
   A. To reduce the chances of damaging blood vessels
   B. To achieve a more even fat removal
   C. To allow better control of the instrument
   D. To accelerate the process of fat removal
   E. To make the process more comfortable for the operator

WETTING SOLUTIONS

5. You are working as a fellow during your aesthetic fellowship preparing a patient for liposuction to the trunk and abdomen. Your supervisor leaves the operating room to see a sick patient and asks you to begin the infiltration. She estimates the patient requires removal of 400 to 500 cc of fat and wishes to use a tumescent technique.
   What approximate volume of infiltrate should you use?
   A. 250 cc
   B. 500 cc
   C. 750 cc
   D. 1500 cc
   E. 2000 cc

6. **When preparing a typical solution for infiltration in liposuction, what is the most common dilution used for epinephrine?**
   A. 1:200,000
   B. 1:1000
   C. 1:10,000
   D. 1:100,000
   E. 1:1,000,000

7. You are preparing a solution to infiltrate for tumescent liposuction in a patient requiring comprehensive body contouring under local anesthetic and sedation. You plan to target the trunk, thighs, and buttocks. The patient weighs 86 kg and has a BMI of 33. **What is the approximate maximum dose of lidocaine that can be used for this procedure according to work undertaken by Klein?**
   A. 600 mg
   B. 1000 mg
   C. 1600 mg
   D. 3000 mg
   E. 3600 mg

ULTRASOUND-ASSISTED LIPOSUCTION (UAL)

8. You have been trained in the use of suction-assisted liposuction (SAL) and move to a new facility where ultrasound-assisted liposuction (UAL) is being used. **Which one of the following is correct about the UAL technique?**
   A. An oscillating reciprocating cannula is used at rates of 4000 cycles per minute.
   B. It is a four-stage procedure involving subdermal skin stimulation.
   C. The sole mechanism of action is cavitation by collapse of intracellular microbubbles.
   D. It still requires the use of suction-assisted liposuction.
   E. It carries a minimal risk of thermal injury compared with laser-assisted techniques.

POWERED-ASSISTED LIPOSUCTION (PAL)

9. **Which one of the following situations best suits the use of power-assisted liposuction?**
   A. When subtle fine contouring is required
   B. When patients are conscious and low noise is preferable
   C. Where vibration transmission to the surgeon must be avoided
   D. When overlying skin perfusion is felt to be compromised
   E. When large volumes of fibrofatty tissue are to be removed

LASER-ASSISTED LIPOSUCTION

10. **What is the proposed benefit of using laser-assisted liposuction over power-assisted liposuction?**
    A. Faster and less labor intensive
    B. Fewer stages need to be undertaken
    C. Conventional evacuation techniques are not required
    D. The machinery is less expensive
    E. There may be a potential skin-tightening effect

FLUID RESUSCITATION

1. When should a patient receive both maintenance and intravenous crystalloid fluid therapy after liposuction?
A. In all cases
B. In all patients with a BMI greater than 30
C. When the aspirate to infiltrate ratio is 1:1
D. In ASA grade 3 patients
E. When more than 5 L is aspirated

LIPOSUCTION STAGES

2. Which one of the following is true when performing suction-assisted liposuction?
A. The entire process has three stages.
B. There should be a four-minute gap between the first and second stages.
C. The cannula should be progressively moved from superficial to deep.
D. The primary clinical endpoint of the final stage is guided by a pinch test.
E. The port sites must be protected with wet towels.

LIPOSUCTION BY AREA

3. When performing body contouring procedures using liposuction, it is important to have a concept of the "ideal" or "normal" aesthetically pleasing form for both males and females. This may differ according to personal tastes and with racial variations. Which one of the following is not a feature of the ideal female body contour?
A. A flat contour to the lower abdomen
B. Convexity over the hips and thighs
C. Concavity below the rib cage
D. A rounded contour to the lateral buttock crease
E. Shallow convexities to the upper thighs

CLINICAL SCENARIO

4. A 34-year-old woman is seeking lower abdominal recontouring following pregnancy and weight loss. Her weight is stable within 30% of her ideal and she is otherwise fit and well. On examination, she has an excess of fat in the infraumbilical region and loose skin with striae. She has a Pfannestiel scar and significant cellulite. Which one of the following is correct?
A. Liposuction alone is likely to give her a good result.
B. Further weight loss is required before liposuction.
C. She may be better served by an abdominoplasty.
D. Her skin changes will improve with suction-assisted liposuction (SAL).
E. Liposuction is the best modality to address her cellulite.

Answers

HISTORICAL DEVELOPMENT IN LIPOSUCTION

1. **Which one of the following changes in practice has been key in the development of current liposuction techniques?**
   D. A focus on preserving zones of adherence

   A better understanding of natural soft tissue zones of adherence as described by Rohrich et al[1] has led to surgeons tending to preserve these zones during liposuction to avoid undesirable contour changes (Fig. 98-1).

   Current liposuction techniques have been developed from work performed by doctors in France and Italy in the 1970s. They have been regularly practiced in the United States since the early 1980s, following presentation by a French team at the 1982 ASPS conference.

   The first description of liposuction was traced back to the 1920s, and this tragically ended in eventual amputation of the involved lower limb. An Italian father and son team by the name of Fischer were the first to develop liposuction techniques using a blunt hollow cannula attached to a suction source. The Italians' ideas were further developed by surgeons in Paris including Illouz, Fournier, and Otteni, who were instrumental in popularizing the technique in France. Illouz developed the wet infiltration technique to decrease bleeding and ease suctioning. Fournier originally preferred a dry harvesting technique, although later converted to a wet technique. He made further contributions such as refinements to contoured harvesting and postoperative compression, and spent time widely teaching these techniques.

   Liposuction techniques generate variable degrees of negative pressure less than 1 atmosphere pressure. Rodriguez and Condé-Green[2] quantified the degree of negative pressure generated using syringe techniques between -165 mm Hg and -718 mm Hg (a maximum of -0.94 atmospheric pressure).

   The introduction of epinephrine into solutions has been attributed to Hetter, who showed that large decreases in postoperative hematocrit level could be reduced when incorporating epinephrine into the liposuction infiltrate.[3,4] The tumescent approach currently used by many plastic surgeons was later introduced by Klein in the 1980s. Most surgeons recommend caution in using liposuction in the superficial fat plane, as there is a high risk of creating surface irregularities.

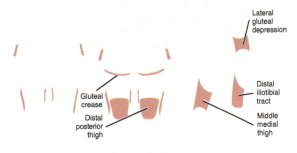

Fig. 98-1 Zones of adherence.

ANATOMY RELEVANT TO LIPOSUCTION

2. Which layer of fat is considered safest to target when performing liposuction on the buttock?
   B. Intermediate

   In general, it is safest to perform liposuction in the intermediate layer, as it is least likely to result in surface irregularities or deep tissue damage. Depth of liposuction is also affected by anatomic area. For example, in most anatomic regions it is safe to liposuction the deep layers of fat; however, in the buttock region it should be avoided. Liposuction in the superficial fat layer must always be done with caution, as there is a risk of creating visible surface irregularities. Cellulite is caused by hypertrophy of the superficial fat within septa that connect the superficial fascial system and the epidermis. It is more appropriately treated with skin-tightening procedures than liposuction.

ZONES OF ADHERENCE

3. Which one of the following is a zone of adherence only found in male patients?
   D. Iliac crest

   Zones of adherence are areas where the superficial fascial system has dense connections with the deep/investing layer of muscle fascia, meaning that the superficial subcutaneous plane is adherent to the muscle fascia.[1,5] There are sex differences in the zones of adherence that result in different effects with weight gain. In men, there is a zone of adherence along the iliac crest and this defines the inferior margin of the flank. In contrast, women carry fat from this area over the iliac crest due to an absence of adherence (Fig. 98-2). The fat is held by the next zone of adherence, which lies with the gluteal depression overlying the greater trochanter.

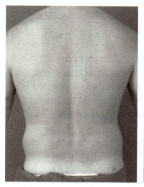 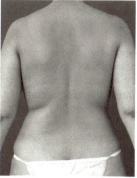

Fig. 98-2 Sex differences in the zones of adherence result in different weight gain effects. Males have a zone of adherence along the iliac crest that women lack.

PHYSICS OF LIPOSUCTION

4. What is the main benefit of selecting a smaller-diameter cannula for traditional suction-assisted liposuction?
   B. To achieve a more even fat removal

   The main benefit of using a smaller-diameter cannula for suction-assisted liposuction is that it helps to ensure even removal of fat. This is at the expense of making the process more work and more time consuming for the operator, as the resistance increases dramatically with a decrease in the cannula diameter. Cannulas are designed with blunt tips to minimize damage to vessels, nerves, and fascia. A larger, blunt cannula is less likely to damage these anatomic structures, but both should tend to move them out of the way. Control is improved when using a shorter cannula, especially for fine work, but this does not directly affect the evenness of fat removal.

WETTING SOLUTIONS

5. You are working as a fellow during your aesthetic fellowship preparing a patient for liposuction to the trunk and abdomen. Your supervisor leaves the operating room to review a sick patient and asks you to begin the infiltration. She estimates the patient requires removal of 400 to 500 cc of fat and wishes to use a tumescent technique. **What approximate volume of infiltrate should you use?**
   D. **1500 cc**
   There are three types of infiltration ratio used for liposuction: wet, superwet, and tumescent. They differ in their volume-to-aspiration ratios. A wet technique involves infiltration of 200 to 300 ml per treated area. A superwet technique involves a 1:1 ratio between infiltrate and planned aspirate. A tumescent technique involves infiltration-to-aspiration ratios of 3:1, so in this case, 1.2 to 1.5 L should be administered.

6. **When preparing a typical solution for infiltration in liposuction, what is the most common dilution used for epinephrine?**
   E. **1:1,000,000**
   Epinephrine is used to induce vasoconstriction in liposuction techniques. It forms an important component of the infiltrate. A typical dilution involves 1 mg of epinephrine diluted in 1 L of normal saline or Hartman's solution. Each 1 mg vial of epinephrine normally has a concentration of 1:1000. Following dilution in the liter bag of saline/Hartman's solution, the epinephrine will be diluted to a final concentration of 1:1,000,000.

7. You are preparing a solution to infiltrate for tumescent liposuction in a patient requiring comprehensive body contouring under local anesthetic and sedation. You plan to target the trunk, thighs, and buttocks. The patient weights 86 kg and has a BMI of 33. **What is the approximate maximal dose of lidocaine that can be used for this procedure according to work undertaken by Klein?**
   D. **3000 mg**
   The maximum dose of subcutaneous lidocaine when using epinephrine is often quoted as 7 mg/kg. In this case, the maximum dose would be just 602 mg for this patient. However, Klein[6] published a paper on the use of far greater doses of lidocaine for tumescent liposuction with no adverse effects. In 1990 he published a study in which plasma concentrations of lidocaine were measured after injection of dilute lidocaine and epinephrine in patients undergoing liposuction. He found that peak doses of lidocaine were reached 12 to 14 hours after injection. He concluded that a combination of lidocaine dilution, epinephrine, and liposuction limits the systemic absorption and potential toxicity of lidocaine in this setting. He estimated a maximum safe dose of 35 mg/kg for tumescent infiltration, and this has been widely accepted in clinical practice. For the patient described in this scenario, this would equate to an absolute maximum of 3010 mg. However, it is recommended that attention be paid to the concentration of lidocaine administered, as well as the overall dose. Concentrations over 0.05% are not recommended in large-volume liposuction infiltration fluid.[7]

Chapter 98 ■ Liposuction 837

ULTRASOUND-ASSISTED LIPOSUCTION (UAL)

8. You have been trained in the use of suction-assisted liposuction (SAL) and move to a new facility where ultrasound-assisted liposuction (UAL) is being used. **Which one of the following is correct about the UAL technique?**
  D. It still requires the use of suction-assisted liposuction.
  UAL was first described by Zocchi in Italy in the 1990s. It works by creating alternating currents with piezoelectric crystals that expand and contract, releasing ultrasonic waves. It is a three-stage process involving infiltration, ultrasound treatment to emulsify fats, then evacuation of fat and final contouring with suction-assisted liposuction. Emulsification is achieved by three mechanisms: micromechanical, thermal, and cavitation. It is a very effective treatment but carries a risk of thermal injury; for this reason, many surgeons prefer not to use it.

  Power-assisted liposuction uses an oscillating reciprocating cannula and may reduce risks of thermal injury while providing a more efficient method compared with standard liposuction. Laser-assisted liposuction involves four phases, one of which is direct dermal stimulation for skin tightening. It has shown promising results, but no prospective trials have shown a benefit over conventional techniques.

POWER-ASSISTED LIPOSUCTION (PAL)

9. *Which one of the following situations best suits the use of power-assisted liposuction?*
  E. When large volumes of fibrofatty tissue are to be removed
  Power-assisted liposuction uses an externally powered cannula that oscillates in a 2 mm reciprocating motion at rates of 4000 to 6000 cycles per minute. The main advantage of this technique is that liposuction is faster and less labor intensive. It is therefore ideal for performing liposuction in larger areas, particularly in fibrofatty tissues and those that have had prior liposuction. The disadvantages are significant noise generation, mechanical vibration transmission to the operator, and the system tends to be more bulky and cumbersome than traditional equipment. It is therefore not well suited to fine-contouring changes. Radiographic dye studies show that UAL, not PAL, reduces the vascular disruption to skin and soft tissues following liposuction. However no form of liposuction is advisable in areas where skin vascularity is compromised.

LASER-ASSISTED LIPOSUCTION

10. *What is the proposed benefit of using laser-assisted liposuction over power-assisted liposuction?*
  E. There may be a potential skin-tightening effect.
  Laser-assisted liposuction involves insertion of a laser fiber through a small skin incision. This may either be housed within the cannula or a stand-alone device. The main proposed advantage of laser-assisted liposuction is that it may produce a skin-tightening effect secondary to heating of the subdermal tissues. However, this is anecdotal and no large prospective studies have proven a difference between laser-assisted and conventional techniques. The process involves four stages with infiltration, application of energy, evacuation, and then subdermal skin stimulation. It therefore is more time and labor intensive than other techniques and the equipment is expensive.

FLUID RESUSCITATION

11. When should a patient receive both maintenance and intravenous crystalloid fluid therapy after liposuction?

E. When more than 5 L is aspirated

Fluid balance must be carefully assessed and managed during the perioperative period for liposuction, as infiltration of large volumes can lead to significant fluid shifts. Only a quarter of the infiltration fluid is removed during suctioning. The remainder is therefore reabsorbed over a 6- to 12-hour period. Most patients can be managed with maintenance fluids alone. The requirement for additional intravenous crystalloid is only for patients who have more than 5 L of aspirate removed. In such patients, the recommended fluid is 0.25 ml of intravenous crystalloid per ml of aspirate over 5 L. As with all guidelines, the actual fluid given must be tailored to the patient's parameters such as blood pressure, urine output, and tissue characteristics.

LIPOSUCTION STAGES

12. Which one of the following is true when performing suction-assisted liposuction?

D. The primary clinical endpoint of the final stage is guided by a pinch test.

The process of suction-assisted liposuction has two main stages: infiltration and evacuation/contouring. There should be a 10-minute gap between the two stages to allow for the epinephrine effects on vasoconstriction to occur. The endpoint to stage one is uniform blanching and skin turgor. In stage two, the cannula should be moved from deep to superficial. When using UAL, this is reversed. The primary clinical endpoint of the final stage is guided by the final contour appearance and the symmetry of pinch test results. When using UAL, port sites must be protected and wet towels are used to cool the area. However, this is not applicable to standard SAL.

LIPOSUCTION BY AREA

13. When performing body contouring procedures using liposuction, it is important to have a concept of the "ideal" or "normal" aesthetically pleasing form for both males and females. This may differ according to personal tastes and with racial variations. Which one of the following is not a feature of the ideal female body contour?

A. A flat contour to the lower abdomen

The "ideal" female body form has a curvy silhouette, often described as an hourglass shape. It is wider at the shoulder and hip and narrower at the waist when viewed from the front (Fig. 98-3, *A*). This involves concavity below the ribcage and convexity over the hips and thighs. The convexity should continue over the proximal thighs and buttocks. In the lateral view, the abdomen should be concave in the epigastric area but slightly convex lower down in the periumbilical region. Since individual preferences vary, these must be discussed in detail with patients before surgery. Males have a more linear silhouette, with only limited convexity and concavity (Fig. 98-3, *B*). The flanks should taper from the lower ribs to the iliac crest. The abdomen should be flat in the periumbilical region.[1]

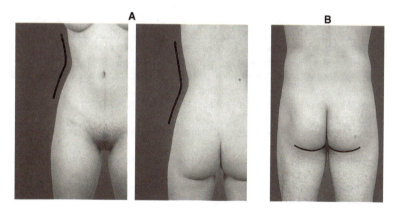

Fig. 98-3 A, An aesthetic female contour begins as a concavity at the flare of the lower ribcage that changes to a convexity over the hips and thighs. **B,** The male form has relative concavities above the pelvic area and convexities in the buttock area. The buttock crease is more angular and square than in females.

CLINICAL SCENARIO

14. A 34-year-old woman is seeking lower abdominal recontouring following pregnancy and weight loss. Her weight is stable within 30% of her ideal and she is otherwise fit and well. On examination, she has an excess of fat in the infraumbilical region and loose skin with striae. She has a Pfannenstiel scar and significant cellulite. **Which one of the following is correct?**
   C. She may be better served with an abdominoplasty.
   Understanding the limitations of liposuction is vital for practitioners and patients. Given the clinical features described, this woman may be best managed with an abdominoplasty rather than liposuction, as this will address both the skin and fat excesses. From a technical perspective, she is unlikely to obtain a good outcome following liposuction as her skin is thin and stretched, as evidenced by the striae. Removing the residual volume in this case will lead to an exaggerated residual skin excess. Liposuction is generally indicated in patients with fat excess but minimal skin excess. Patients should also be close to their ideal weight (within 30%). Therefore further weight loss is not required in this case. As discussed in question 2, cellulite probably represents a combination of fat hypertrophy within fibrous septae and skin laxity. It is not well treated with liposuction and it is important to inform patients of this preoperatively. It may be more effectively treated using skin-tightening procedures. Where mild skin-tightening effects are desired, then laser liposuction may be helpful, but suction-assisted liposuction is not beneficial.[8,9]

REFERENCES

1. Rohrich RJ, Smith PD, Marcantonio DR, et al. The zones of adherence: role in minimizing and preventing contour deformities in liposuction. Plast Reconstr Surg 107:1562-1569, 2001.
2. Rodriguez RL, Condé-Green A. Quantification of negative pressures generated by syringes of different calibers used for liposuction. Plast Reconstr Surg 130:383e-384e, 2012.
3. Hetter GP. The effect of low-dose epinephrine on the hematocrit drop following lipolysis. Aesthet Plast Surg 8:19-21, 1984.
4. Coleman WP III. The history of liposuction and fat transplantation in America. Dermatol Clin 17:723-727, 1999.
5. Gingrass MK, Shermak MA. The treatment of gynecomastia with ultrasound-assisted lipoplasty. Perspect Plast Surg 12:101-106, 1999.
6. Klein JA. Tumescent technique for regional anesthesia permits lidocaine doses of 35 mg/kg for liposuction. J Dermatol Surg Oncol 16:248-263, 1990.
7. Pace MM, Chatterjee A, Merrill DG, et al. Local anesthetics in liposuction: considerations for new practice advisory guidelines to improve patient safety. Plast Reconstr Surg 131:820e-826e, 2013.
8. Illouz YG. Study of subcutaneous fat. Aesthetic Plast Surg 14:165, 1990.
9. Lockwood TE. Superficial fascial system (SFS) of the trunk and extremities: a new concept. Plast Reconstr Surg 86:1009, 1991.

99. Brachioplasty

See *Essentials of Plastic Surgery*, second edition, pp. 1253-1263.

ANATOMY

1. Six months following brachioplasty a patient complains of continued pain around the elbow and paresthesia in the forearm. **What nerve is most likely to have been injured during the procedure?**
   A. Anterior brachial cutaneous nerve
   B. Ulnar nerve
   C. Musculocutaneous nerve
   D. Lateral antebrachial cutaneous nerve
   E. Medial antebrachial cutaneous nerve

2. **Where in the arm is most subcutaneous fat generally found?**
   A. Anterior
   B. Posterior
   C. Medial
   D. Lateral
   E. Distal

PATIENT EVALUATION

3. *For each of the following scenarios, select the best surgical option for each patient. (Each option may be used once, more than once, or not at all.)*
   A. A 28-year-old woman has achieved sustained weight loss after gastric banding. Her BMI has reduced from 39 to 28, but this has left her with significant skin redundancy in a number of areas. Examination shows scars from a belt lipectomy and medial thigh lift. She has minimal fat excess in the upper arms but has skin laxity passing onto the chest wall, with empty ptotic breasts.
   B. A 35-year-old woman has lost 14 pounds and currently has a BMI of 29. She is unhappy with the appearance of her arms which she feels still look fat. Examination shows she has good quality skin and soft tissues with moderate fat excess.
   C. A 50-year-old man has lost 40 pounds over the past 3 years by diet and exercise modification. Examination shows his BMI to be 34, with moderate fat excess and vertical skin excess along the length of the upper arm.

   Options:
   a. Liposuction only
   b. Liposuction and brachioplasty with vertical skin excision
   c. Liposuction and brachioplasty with horizontal skin excision
   d. Brachioplasty with horizontal skin excision only
   e. Brachioplasty with vertical skin excision only
   f. Brachioplasty with combined vertical and horizontal skin excision
   g. Minibrachioplasty only
   h. Extended brachioplasty with vertical and horizontal skin excision

4. **Which one of the following represents an absolute contraindication to brachioplasty?**
   A. Connective tissue disorders
   B. Diabetes mellitus
   C. Lymphedema
   D. Rheumatoid arthritis
   E. Raynaud's disease

PATIENT EDUCATION

5. **What is the main limitation of a standard brachioplasty procedure in terms of patient satisfaction when compared to many other commonly performed aesthetic procedures?**
   A. The pain incurred following the procedure
   B. The downtime following the procedure
   C. The visibility of the scars
   D. The residual contour deformity
   E. The functional outcome after surgery

6. A patient is seen in clinic having decided to undergo brachioplasty under your care. Since the last meeting she has heard about a minibrachioplasty technique and wishes to know how this differs from a standard brachioplasty. **What should you tell her?**
   A. Skin excision is usually avoided
   B. Liposuction is usually avoided
   C. The incision is usually limited to the axilla
   D. The incision is usually limited to the posterior arm
   E. It relies solely on fascial suspension

STANDARD BRACHIOPLASTY

7. **When marking a patient for a standard brachioplasty, which one of the following is correct?**
   A. The patient should face you with arms extended at the elbows and abducted 90 degrees at the shoulder.
   B. A dotted line should be placed in the bicipital groove from the axilla to the elbow to mark the lower incision.
   C. The amount of planned skin excision can be estimated using a pinch test so the upper incision can be marked.
   D. With experience, it may be beneficial to place the scar inferior/posterior to the bicipital groove.
   E. Placement of the scar more posteriorly will usually provide a less favorable scar quality.

8. You are performing simultaneous bilateral brachioplasties with your resident. You have decided that no liposuction is required and have jointly marked the patient preoperatively with a 3 by 20 cm ellipse. **Which one of the following is the most useful advice for you to give your resident?**
   A. Infiltration of a wetting solution will not offer any benefit in this case.
   B. He or she should begin with excision of the marked area as an ellipse.
   C. Some undermining may be required to facilitate wound closure.
   D. Two-layer closure should be performed with a short-acting monofilament suture.
   E. Wound closure should be staggered by partial closure as tissue is excised.

You are performing a brachioplasty and note you have cut through a medium-sized sensory nerve at the distal arm. There is segmental loss as a portion of the nerve has been excised with the redundant skin, which has already been discarded. **What should you do before continuing with the procedure?**
A. Do nothing with the nerve.
B. Remove a larger segment of nerve.
C. Repair the nerve with a nerve graft.
D. Cauterize the nerve end.
E. Cauterize the nerve end and bury it in muscle.

Answers

ANATOMY

1. Six months following brachioplasty a patient complains of continued pain around the elbow and paresthesia in the forearm. **What nerve is most likely to have been injured during the procedure?**
   ### E. Medial antebrachial cutaneous nerve
   Most nerves in the arm such as the median, radial, ulnar, and musculocutaneous nerve lie deep to the deep fascia and are not at risk of injury during brachioplasty. However, the cutaneous nerves of the arm and forearm lie superficial to the deep fascia and are therefore at risk of damage. The median antebrachial cutaneous nerve (MABC) (also known as the medial cutaneous nerve of the forearm) travels with the basilic vein and is most at risk of injury just proximal to the elbow, resulting in a painful neuroma, as in this scenario. The initial treatment of a neuroma is nonsurgical with massage, desensitization, physiotherapy, and analgesics. If the problem persists for more than 6 months as in this case, surgical intervention with resection of the neuroma and insertion of the ends into the triceps muscle may be beneficial.[1]

   The anterior brachial and lateral antebrachial cutaneous nerves are both superficial but should remain outside of the zone of dissection during brachioplasty. The lateral antebrachial cutaneous nerve is the continuation of the musculocutaneous nerve that supplies sensation to the lateral (radial) aspect of the forearm. The other nerve that is at risk during brachioplasty when close to the axilla is the intercostobrachial nerve.

2. **Where in the arm is most subcutaneous fat generally found?**
   ### B. Posterior
   Subcutaneous fat in the arms tends to collect posteriorly and inferiorly with very little medially. It also tends to be found more proximally than distally. Therefore when performing liposuction, the main target zone is the posterior arm with more subtle suctioning performed on the medial aspect, taking care not to overly thin the soft tissues such that 0.5 cm of subcutaneous fat is left in the skin and contour irregularities are avoided. The fat of the arm is supported by two fascial systems relevant to brachioplasty: the superficial system and the longitudinal system. The superficial system encases the fat circumferentially from the axilla to the elbow. The longitudinal fascial system begins at the clavicle and extends to the axillary fascia and superficial system. This is used in some techniques to support the arm tissues using permanent sutures to anchor the superficial system to the longitudinal fascia.[2] The skin is also thinner medially than it is posteriorly or laterally so there is less dermal support for scars, particularly when closed under tension.

PATIENT EVALUATION

3. **For each of the following scenarios, select the best surgical option for each patient. (Each option may be used once, more than once, or not at all).**

   A. *A 28-year-old woman has achieved sustained weight loss after gastric banding. Her BMI has reduced from 39 to 28, but this has left her with significant skin redundancy in a number of areas. Examination shows scars from a belt lipectomy and medial thigh lift. She has minimal fat excess in the upper arms but has vertical and horizontal skin laxity extending onto the chest wall, with empty ptotic breasts.*
   h. **Extended brachioplasty with vertical and horizontal skin excision.**
   This patient requires an extended brachioplasty as shown in Fig. 99-1. As can be seen in the figure, the excision pattern passes the full length of the arm to the axilla and onto the chest wall. It has both horizontal and vertical components.

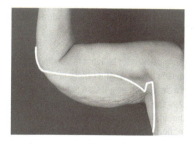

Fig. 99-1 Laxity in this patient extends onto the lateral chest wall and requires extended brachioplasty technique.

   B. *A 35-year-old woman has lost 14 pounds and currently has a BMI of 29. She is unhappy with the appearance of her arms which she feels still look fat. Examination shows she has good quality skin and soft tissues with moderate fat excess.*
   a. **Liposuction only**
   This patient requires liposuction only because there is fat excess without any current skin excess. As she is young and her skin quality is good, she should respond well to the liposuction with subsequent skin tightening over time.

   C. *A 50-year-old man has lost 40 pounds over the past 3 years by diet and exercise modification. Examination shows his BMI to be 34, with moderate fat excess and vertical skin excess along the length of the upper arm.*
   c. **Liposuction and brachioplasty with horizontal skin excision**
   This patient requires a standard brachioplasty with a horizontal incision placed in the brachial groove as shown in Fig. 99-2. As can be seen in the figure, the excision pattern passes the full length of the arm to the axilla, but without extension onto the chest wall or a vertical component into the axillary crease. He will also benefit from liposuction given the excess fat present, and this will allow slightly more skin to be resected. The remaining common

brachioplasty incision patterns are shown in Figs. 99-2, 99-3, and 99-5, *Essentials of Plastic Surgery,* second edition. An algorithm for treatment is also shown in Fig. 99-7, *Essentials of Plastic Surgery,* second edition.

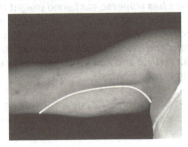

Fig. 99-2 This patient has isolated vertical skin redundancy that is treated with a horizontal excision along the brachial/bicipital groove.

When deciding on a surgical plan for patients requesting brachioplasty, a stepwise approach is helpful. The first step is to decide whether there is any fat excess. If there is, then liposuction may be useful, otherwise further weight loss may be advised. The next step is to see whether there is any skin excess and to note the anatomic location of this. When considering treatment for skin excess, it should be remembered that the resection is performed in the "opposite" vector from the direction of excess (i.e., vertical excess is removed through a horizontal [longitudinal] excision and horizontal excess is removed through a vertical [axillary] excision). These descriptors, vertical and horizontal, assume the patient is standing for the assessment with the shoulder abducted and elbow flexed to 90 degrees.

Therefore if the skin excess is horizontal, then a vertical scar in the axilla is used. If there is a vertical excess, then a longitudinal scar is used. If there is both horizontal and vertical excess, then a combination of horizontal and vertical scars is used. If the skin excess is restricted to the proximal arm only, then a short T-scar can be used. In patients with excess skin extending onto the chest wall such as may occur after massive weight loss, extension of the scar onto the chest wall may be indicated. This can be incorporated into a mastopexy/autoaugmentation if required (see Chapter 102).

4. **Which one of the following represents an absolute contraindication to brachioplasty?**
   C. Lymphedema
   Brachioplasty risks compromise to lymphatic flow from the upper limb and therefore should be avoided in patients who have chronic lymphedema, even if this is mild, as further interruption of lymphatic flow can be detrimental. Liposuction only in these patients may be beneficial as a treatment for their lymphedema, but compression garments will need to be worn long term (see Chapter 58).
   Other absolute contraindications to brachioplasty include reflex sympathetic dystrophy, smoking, and unrealistic patient expectations. Relative contraindications include symptomatic Raynaud's disease, connective tissue disorders, advanced rheumatoid arthritis, residual obesity, and diabetes mellitus.

PATIENT EDUCATION

5. What is the main limitation of a standard brachioplasty procedure in terms of patient satisfaction when compared to many other commonly performed aesthetic procedures?

C. The visibility of the scars

Brachioplasty is a good operation for recontouring the upper arms after weight loss in patients with excess skin ± fat, but the main limitation is that the scarring is extensive and visible. Furthermore, the scars can become stretched, as there will be some tension across the wound during closure and the medial skin is relatively thin. For this reason, it is vital that patients have a clear understanding of the scars preoperatively. Markings should be made on the patient to show them the site, orientation, and extent of the scars during their preoperative consultation. This should be documented in the medical record. Postoperative photos of other patients can also be useful to illustrate the scar pattern.

This procedure is not particularly painful for patients and the downtime is short. Early ambulation is advised postoperatively and most cases are performed as day cases.[3] The postoperative contour is usually good and patients tend to be satisfied with this. There is no functional loss following this surgery. In fact, it often helps function where larger skin volumes are resected.

6. A patient is seen in clinic having decided to undergo brachioplasty under your care. Since the last meeting she has heard about a minibrachioplasty technique and wishes to know how this differs from a standard brachioplasty. What should you tell her?

C. The incision is usually limited to the axilla

The main difference between a minibrachioplasty and a standard brachioplasty is the site and size of the excision. In a minibrachioplasty the incision is hidden in the axilla (Fig. 99-3). It still includes liposuction in the posteromedial upper arm where necessary. In some cases, a short dart extension onto the medial arm (not posterior) may be required, creating a T-shaped scar. Lockwood described a technique for anchoring the superficial fascia to the longitudinal fascial system (dense axillary and clavicopectoral fascia) in order to correct the laxity of the upper arm. However, this is not always performed and is not exclusive to a minibrachioplasty approach.

The minibrachioplasty is indicated in select patients only. They should have mild skin excess and mild to moderate fat excess. The most important step in successful minibrachioplasty is patient selection, and in the right patient it can be highly effective. However, patients who have more significant excess skin will benefit from a standard approach.

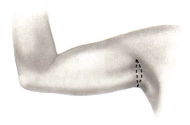

Fig. 99-3 Placement of the axillary incision for a minibrachioplasty.

STANDARD BRACHIOPLASTY

7. When marking a patient for a standard brachioplasty, which one of the following is correct?
   D. With experience, it may be beneficial to place the scar inferior/posterior to the bicipital groove.
   During marking for a brachioplasty, the patient should face you with their arms abducted 90 degrees at the shoulder and elbows flexed to 90 degrees as if flexing the biceps. A dotted line should be placed in the bicipital groove to help mark the planned scar. The upper incision should then be marked 1 cm above this, and the lower incision can then be estimated by pinching the skin (see Figs. 99-10 and 99-11, *Essentials of Plastic Surgery,* second edition). Placement of the scar posteriorly may provide a more favorable quality of scar but one that is more visible. A compromise between the two may be chosen, but should only be considered with experience of the procedure, as there is a risk of skin overresection. Vertical crosshatch markings are made to divide the incision into fifths and facilitate correct wound edge approximation.

8. You are performing simultaneous bilateral brachioplasties with your resident. You have decided that no liposuction is required and have jointly marked the patient preoperatively with a 3 by 20 cm ellipse. *Which one of the following is the most useful advice for you to give your resident?*
   E. Wound closure should be staggered by partial closure as tissue is excised.
   When undertaking a brachioplasty, the order of excision and closure must be modified from standard excisional and closure techniques. It is easy to overresect skin during this procedure, so a single upper incision is made first and the posterior skin flap is carefully elevated. Closure is tested before committing to the lower incision. The excision and closure are staged to close each part of the wound segmentally to minimize arm swelling that might otherwise prevent closure. A three-layer closure should be used without undermining. The superficial fascial system is closed with a long-lasting absorbable suture, and the skin can be closed with a shorter-acting one. Infiltration is useful to limit bleeding, regardless of whether liposuction is to be performed.

9. You are performing a brachioplasty and note you have cut through a medium-sized sensory nerve at the distal arm. There is segmental loss as a portion of the nerve has been excised with the redundant skin, which has already been discarded. *What should you do before continuing with the procedure?*
   E. Cauterize the nerve end and bury it in muscle.
   As discussed in question 1, the main problem with transection of a sensory nerve, such as the MABC during brachioplasty, is the risk of subsequent neuroma formation, leaving the patient with chronic pain in the upper limb. The loss of sensation tends to be much better tolerated than the neuroma symptoms. For this reason, when a sensory nerve is divided, it should either be repaired or managed such that a neuroma is unlikely to occur. By cauterizing the nerve and burying it in muscle the risk of neuroma formation will be reduced. Smaller nerve branches can just be cauterized. Use of a graft is not indicated, as the harvest will create a similar defect elsewhere anyway.

REFERENCES

1. Stahl S, Rosenberg N. Surgical treatment of painful neuroma in medial antebrachial cutaneous nerve. Ann Plast Surg 48:154-158, 2002.
2. Lockwood T. Brachioplasty with superficial fascial system suspension. Plast Reconstr Surg 96:912-920, 1995.
3. Aly AS, Capella JF. Staging, reoperation, and treatment of complications after body contouring in the massive-weight-loss patient. In Grotting J, ed. Reoperative Aesthetic and Reconstructive Surgery, ed 2. St Louis: Quality Medical Publishing, 2007.

100. Abdominoplasty

See *Essentials of Plastic Surgery*, second edition, pp. 1264-1278.

ANATOMY

1. **When elevating an abdominal skin flap during a standard abdominoplasty, which one of the following statements is correct?**
   A. The flap receives its blood supply from vessels in Huger's zone I.
   B. Striae present on the flap will normally be improved by this procedure.
   C. Sensory innervation from the lateral branches of intercostal nerves T10-12 is divided.
   D. If flap thinning is required, it should be performed in the subscarpal fat layer.
   E. Umbilical blood supply becomes dependent upon the ligamentum teres and median umbilical ligament.

2. **What is the clinical relevance of the arcuate line with respect to performing surgery on the anterior abdominal wall?**
   A. It represents the ideal anatomic position for the umbilicus.
   B. It marks the superior extent of abdominoplasty flap dissection.
   C. It represents the point at which rectus diastasis repair must be started.
   D. It marks the distinction between superficial and deep fat layers.
   E. It marks the point below which the posterior rectus sheath is absent.

PREOPERATIVE EVALUATION

3. **You are consenting a patient for abdominoplasty and find out that she has been smoking approximately 5 cigarettes per day since you met her in clinic to plan surgery 1 month ago. She previously denied smoking. How should you now proceed knowing this information?**
   A. Proceed with surgery as planned without further discussion.
   B. Start her on nicotine replacement therapy and proceed as planned.
   C. Check her blood and urine nicotine levels then proceed as planned.
   D. Proceed with surgery, explaining the increased risk of complications.
   E. Postpone surgery until smoking cessation is complete.

4. **When assessing a patient for an abdominoplasty, what is the key clinical relevance of a positive diver's test?**
   A. That there is an excess of lower abdominal fat
   B. That there is an excess of lower abdominal skin
   C. That there is rectus diastasis present
   D. That there is myofascial laxity present
   E. That there is a hernia present

5. **Which one of the following scars represents the most significant contraindication to standard abdominoplasty surgery?**
   A. McBurney (appendectomy)
   B. Kocher's (subcostal)
   C. Pfannenstiel (cesarian)
   D. Lower midline
   E. Periumbilical laparoscopic

INFORMED CONSENT

6. You are consenting a patient preoperatively to undergo a full abdominoplasty with rectus sheath plication. She has a moderate amount of skin and soft tissue excess and wants to know about the likely outcomes. **Which one of the following is least likely in her case?**
   A. A long transverse scar will curve from hip to hip but should be hidden in her underwear.
   B. Her umbilicus will need to be relocated, leaving a visible scar around it.
   C. She will need a short vertical scar given her current tissue laxity.
   D. Minor scar revision may be necessary after her original procedure.
   E. The rectus plication is likely to increase her recovery time.

7. A patient returns to the clinic after an initial consultation for an abdominoplasty where she was seen by your resident. She has since read through the information sheet describing the risks of surgery and wants to know why she was advised that she may have "dog-ears" after her surgery. She asks you to clarify exactly what this means. **Which one of the following would be correct to tell her about "dog-ears"?**
   A. They are the result of abnormal scarring at the wound edge.
   B. They can occur at any point along the transverse scar.
   C. They usually resolve spontaneously with massage and scar maturation.
   D. They normally occur secondary to surgical error.
   E. They are treated with liposuction or surgical excision.

8. A 46-year-old nurse is scheduled to undergo standard abdominoplasty surgery and wants to clarify some aspects of the surgical procedure and downtime. **Regarding the perioperative and postoperative periods surrounding her surgery, which one of the following statements is true?**
   A. It is standard practice to include concomitant liposuction to the central and upper abdomen.
   B. Her surgery would normally be performed under local anesthetic with sedation.
   C. She may be unable to stand up straight for several days following surgery.
   D. Two weeks off work will provide her with sufficient time to fully recover.
   E. She will be unable to use the gym for 9 months following surgery.

PROCEDURE SELECTION

9. For each of the following clinical scenarios, select the most appropriate surgical option from those listed. (Each option may be used once, more than once, or not at all.)

   A. A 44-year-old woman has a mild soft tissue and moderate skin excess involving the lower abdomen and back after major weight loss. She is clinically fit and well, has a stable weight for the past year, and is a nonsmoker.

   B. A fit and well 24-year-old woman has a moderate infraumbilical skin and soft tissue excess following pregnancy. Her skin quality is average, and she has multiple striae in the lower abdomen. She is generally slim, but this area seems unresponsive to diet and physical exercise.

   C. A 54-year-old woman has significant rectus diastasis following five pregnancies, all delivered vaginally. She is generally well and has a slim build, with moderate lower abdominal fat excess only. She is a nonsmoker and has not had any other surgical procedures.

   Options:
   a. Liposuction to the lower abdomen
   b. Standard abdominoplasty
   c. Endoscopic rectus plication with liposuction
   d. Miniabdominoplasty
   e. Fleur-de-lis abdominoplasty
   f. Lipoabdominoplasty (combined liposuction and abdominoplasty)
   g. Circumferential abdominoplasty

PERIOPERATIVE MANAGEMENT

10. Which one of the following is true of the perioperative management of patients undergoing abdominoplasty?
    A. The pubic area should be shaved the day before surgery.
    B. Intravenous antibiotics should be given 30 to 60 minutes before starting surgery.
    C. Intraoperative TED hose (stockings) are usually reserved for high-risk individuals.
    D. A single dose of low-molecular-weight heparin should be given on induction.
    E. Postoperative antibiotics should continue for 7 days after surgery.

SURGICAL PROCEDURE

11. What is the main benefit of leaving a layer of fat over the anterior superior iliac spine (ASIS) during abdominoplasty?
    A. A reduction in seroma rate
    B. A reduction in hematoma rate
    C. A better abdominal wall contour
    D. A reduced risk of nerve damage
    E. A reduced rate of fat necrosis

12. Which one of the following is correct when incorporating rectus plication into a standard abdominoplasty technique?
    A. The upper skin flap should be elevated widely to allow access for plication.
    B. Plication is best achieved using a heavy, permanent suture.
    C. Plication should begin 2 inches below the xiphisternum.
    D. Plication should be performed with a single layer of interrupted sutures.
    E. Plication negates the need for progressive tension sutures.

MINIABDOMINOPLASTY

13. You are discussing the relative merits of using a miniabdominoplasty with a patient. She is of slim build and has modest lower abdominal soft tissue excess. She has had a previous cesarian section and wants to minimize further scarring. Examination shows mild rectus diastasis. **Which one of the following is true of this procedure?**
    A. It involves a standard abdominoplasty transverse scar.
    B. It is mainly indicated for infraumbilical skin and fat excess.
    C. It is contraindicated in the presence of rectus diastasis.
    D. It should be avoided after cesarean section.
    E. The umbilicus is normally relocated level with the iliac crest.

PROGRESSIVE TENSION SUTURES

14. **Which one of the following is not a recognized benefit of using progressive tension sutures during closure of an abdominoplasty?**
    A. Reduced seroma formation
    B. Reduced hematoma formation
    C. Reduced operative time
    D. Improved scar appearance
    E. Reduced wound-edge necrosis

FLEUR-DE-LIS ABDOMINOPLASTY

15. **Which one of the following is the main advantage of using the fleur-de-lis abdominoplasty technique?**
    A. Postoperative scars are easier to conceal in underwear.
    B. Postoperative complications are less likely to occur.
    C. Rectus plication is avoided.
    D. Horizontal and vertical abdominal tissue excess is addressed.
    E. Anterior and lateral thigh soft tissue excess is addressed.

POSTOPERATIVE MANAGEMENT

16. You see a 44-year-old fit and healthy woman the morning after an abdominoplasty. She previously had two pregnancies by cesarean section and has undergone previous limb and breast surgery in the past, coping well with postoperative pain management. On this occasion she is really quite sore, despite having access to a morphine pump (patient controlled analgesia [PCA]) and background acetaminophen. She is wearing an external abdominal binder and lying with knees on a pillow. Her abdomen remains soft but tender and is otherwise unremarkable. Her CRP is elevated to 20 (normal range is <5) and her observations are normal. **What is the most likely explanation for her continued discomfort?**
    A. Abdominoplasty is generally a very painful procedure.
    B. She is not regularly using her morphine PCA.
    C. She is developing a postoperative infection.
    D. She has an intraperitoneal injury and developing peritonitis.
    E. She has undergone correctional surgery for rectus diastasis.

COMPLICATIONS

17. A patient who had a standard abdominoplasty surgery 6 months ago has called your secretary concerned about residual fullness to the epigastric region. She had a standard abdominoplasty approach with rectus plication, but no liposuction. **What is the most likely cause of the bulge in this area?**
    A. Inadequate flap dissection
    B. Inadequate fat excision
    C. Chronic seroma
    D. Solidified hematoma
    E. Postoperative weight gain

Answers

ANATOMY

1. **When elevating an abdominal skin flap during a standard abdominoplasty, which one of the following statements is correct?**
   D. If flap thinning is required, it should be performed in the subscarpal fat layer.
   Abdominal fat has two layers separated by a layer of superficial fascia. These layers have different vascular supplies. The overlying skin is reliant on blood supply through the superficial fat layer, whereas the deep fat vascularity is distinct from the skin. For this reason, superficial fat should be preserved when flap thinning is required.
   After raising a skin flap during an abdominoplasty, the blood supply arises from superolateral, which will correspond to Huger's zone III. Huger's zone I normally supplies the central area of the flap through the rectus abdominis muscles, but these perforating vessels are divided during flap elevation (Fig. 100-1).
   The normal sensory innervation to this part of the abdomen arises from T7-12 (ventral) intercostal nerves, which have anterior and lateral branches. The lateral branches are preserved during an abdominoplasty and travel within the superficial tissues anterior to the anterior axillary line. The anterior branches remain deep to the internal intercostal until they reach the rectus sheath. At this point they pass anteriorly through the sheath to supply overlying skin and will be divided during flap elevation. Patients probably will not have long-term sensory loss at this level because of sensory nerve arborization and reinnervation.
   The umbilicus normally receives its vascular supply through perforators from the deep inferior epigastric arteries (DIEA), the subdermal plexus, the medial umbilical ligament, and the ligamentum teres.[1] During an abdominoplasty the subdermal supply is divided, but the main perforators from the DIEA are still preserved. The blood supply would normally only rely on the medial umbilical ligament and ligamentum teres, if, for example, a bilateral DIEP flap had been performed. Striae are caused by thinning or absence of the dermis. Those present below the umbilicus will be excised during a standard abdominoplasty procedure. However, those above this line will remain and are likely to appear worse, as the flap will be stretched during wound closure.

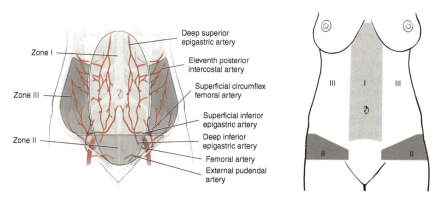

Fig. 100-1 Huger vascular zones of the abdominal wall.

2. **What is the clinical relevance of the arcuate line with respect to performing surgery on the anterior abdominal wall?**
   E. It marks the point below which the posterior rectus sheath is absent.

   The arcuate line is located halfway between the umbilicus and symphysis pubis. Above this line there are both anterior and posterior rectus sheaths. Below this line there is only an anterior rectus sheath present, therefore making this area of the abdomen more prone to weakness and herniation. It is particularly relevant when performing abdominal wall reconstruction and raising rectus abdominis flaps, as this area will need reinforcement if the anterior sheath is deficient.

   The ideal anatomic position for the umbilicus is the midline at the level of the iliac crest, although in less than 2% of patients is the umbilicus truly sited in the midline. Diastasis should be repaired from the xiphisternum down to the top of the symphysis in most cases. For this reason, the superior limit of dissection in an abdominoplasty is also the xiphisternum. Scarpa's fascia marks the junction between superficial and deep fat layers of the abdominal wall.

PREOPERATIVE EVALUATION

3. **You are consenting a patient for abdominoplasty and find out that she has been smoking approximately 5 cigarettes per day since you met her in clinic to plan surgery 1 month ago. She previously denied smoking. How should you now proceed knowing this information?**
   E. Postpone surgery until smoking cessation is complete.

   Abdominoplasty places a large stress on the abdominal wall flap vasculature and, accordingly, is not recommended in active smokers. During the preoperative consultation patients should be asked about their smoking status and advised of the increased risks of surgery while actively smoking. For example, wound healing complications in smokers are nearly 50% as compared to 15% in nonsmokers. Any plans for surgery should be postponed until smoking cessation has been successfully completed. Urine or blood tests can be used to assess nicotine levels and can help confirm whether patients have abstained from smoking. There remains debate regarding the effects of nicotine replacement therapy on wound healing; however, continuing with surgery in a patient who has recently stopped smoking and is on nicotine replacement therapy is still likely to carry a higher risk of postoperative complications. As discussed in Chapter 1, some of the effects of smoking are reversed after a month of cessation, but other factors take longer to reverse.

4. **When assessing a patient for an abdominoplasty, what is the key clinical relevance of a positive diver's test?**
   D. That there is myofascial laxity present

   Myofascial laxity of the anterior abdominal wall must be assessed before undertaking an abdominoplasty so that a plan to treat it can be made in advance of surgery. Laxity can be measured by the diver's test, a pinch test, and by assessment of rectus diastasis. The diver's test is performed with the patient standing and then flexing at the waist. Worsening of lower abdominal wall fullness indicates myofascial laxity is present (Fig. 100-2, *A* and *B*).

   The pinch test assesses abdominal fullness with the patient both relaxed and actively tensing the abdominal wall (Fig. 100-2, *C*). If the amount of fullness that can be pinched is significantly decreased by tensing the abdominal wall, then significant myofascial laxity is present. Midline rectus diastasis is assessed by asking the patient to raise their legs off the examination table while lying supine. This allows palpation of the rectus muscles in most patients. Examination of a hernia can also be undertaken at this time.

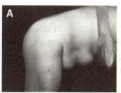 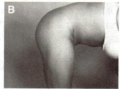 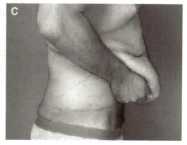

Fig. 100-2 **A** and **B,** Diver's test. **C,** Pinch test.

5. Which one of the following scars represents the most significant contraindication to standard abdominoplasty surgery?
   B. Kocher's (subcostal)
   Scars represent an alteration of the blood supply to the abdominal wall. Those in the subcostal area, such as a Kocher's for cholecystectomy, are of particular concern, as they interrupt the superolateral blood supply on which the abdominoplasty flap will be reliant. For this reason, a standard abdominoplasty is contraindicated in these patients. It may be more appropriate to perform a procedure that avoids undermining such as a fleur-de-lis procedure for patients with subcostal scars. The other scars would not usually present a problem for a standard abdominoplasty. The McBurney, Pfannenstiel, and lower midline scars could all be excised during the procedure. Periumbilical laparoscopic surgery can affect blood supply to the umbilicus and patients must be made aware of this; however, it does not represent a contraindication to surgery. Any of these scars may be associated with abdominal wall weakness and hernia formation. They can also distort the planes of dissection and make surgery more challenging.

INFORMED CONSENT

6. You are consenting a patient preoperatively to undergo a full abdominoplasty with rectus sheath plication. She has a moderate amount of skin and soft tissue excess and wants to know about the likely outcomes. *Which one of the following is least likely in her case?*
   C. She will need a short vertical scar given her current tissue laxity.
   This woman must be made aware of the extent of potential scarring that an abdominoplasty carries with it. She is unlikely to need a vertical component to the scar, but consent for this should be obtained in case she does not have sufficient laxity to fully remove the original periumbilical site. She must also be informed of the risk of umbilical necrosis and be made aware that the periumbilical scar will still be visible in a bikini or underwear. In most cases the transverse scar can be well hidden in underwear or swimwear, but a short vertical scar would not be. Minor revisional surgery may be required following an abdominoplasty and this is usually done 3 to 6 months after the original surgery. Rectus plication can increase recovery time, due to discomfort and decreased mobility.

7. A patient returns to the clinic after an initial consultation for an abdominoplasty where she was seen by your resident. She has since read through the information sheet describing the risks of surgery and wants to know why she was advised that she may have "dog-ears" after her surgery. She asks you to clarify exactly what this means. **Which one of the following would be correct to tell her about "dog-ears"?**
   E. **They are treated with liposuction or surgical excision**

   Dog-ears (also known as "standing cones") represent an excess of skin and subcutaneous fat at the end of a closed wound. Their formation is affected by wound geometry, and traditional thinking is that elliptical wounds with a length/width ratio of 3:1 or 4:1 (or maintaining closing angles of less than 30 degrees) can avoid dog-ear formation.[2] However, other factors may also be responsible such as tissue dynamics, surface contour, and surgical technique.

   Dog-ears may be present after abdominoplasty where there is lateral skin and fat excess not incorporated into the original excision pattern. The decision to exclude this area from the abdominoplasty is normally made to limit lateral scar length, so it is not a surgical error. In cases where there is lateral and posterior soft tissue excess, patients must be made aware that lateral fullness or dog-ears are likely to occur. Such patients may require belt lipectomy or liposuction to fully address these areas. Minimizing dog-ears during surgery is achieved by careful closure of the wound apex and serial halving or feeding in the shorter side of asymmetric wounds. Surgical removal of dog-ears will lengthen the original scar and a compromise must be reached between scar length and residual contour. Dog-ears do not usually resolve spontaneously unless they are very small. Massage to the scar will still be useful to help it soften.

8. A 46-year-old nurse is scheduled to undergo standard abdominoplasty surgery and wants to clarify some aspects of the surgical procedure and downtime. **Regarding the perioperative and postoperative periods surrounding her surgery, which one of the following statements is true?**
   C. **She may be unable to stand up straight for several days following surgery.**

   Following abdominoplasty, patients will have to initially mobilize slightly flexed at the hip due to the wound closure. They should be nursed with knees flexed on pillows and the hips also flexed. This takes tension off the wound repair during the early phase of healing. A standard abdominoplasty does not necessarily include liposuction, although it may do so. Many surgeons prefer to stage the liposuction, if it is required, following the initial surgery. It is used to target lateral fullness that is not addressed by the abdominoplasty technique. Therefore it is commonly directed at the flanks, rather than the central and upper abdomen which may risk flap viability, particularly if the suprascarpal fat is aspirated. The procedure is performed under general anesthetic with an overnight stay in the hospital. This patient has an active job with heavy manual lifting of patients. She will require more than a week off work, even if light duties are possible. She will need to avoid heavy abdominal exercise such as sit-ups or heavy weights in the immediate postoperative period, but she can resume lighter cardiovascular work after a few weeks. She will certainly be recovered enough to resume going to the gym after 9 months.

Chapter 100 ■ Abdominoplasty 859

PROCEDURE SELECTION

9. **For each of the following clinical scenarios, select the most appropriate surgical option from those listed. (Each option may be used once, more than once, or not at all.)**
   A. **A 44-year-old woman has a mild soft tissue and moderate skin excess involving the lower abdomen and back after major weight loss. She is clinically fit and well, has a stable weight for the past year, and is a nonsmoker.**
      g. Circumferential abdominoplasty
      This woman has an excess of skin and fat to both the anterior and posterior abdominal walls and therefore will not be served well with a standard abdominoplasty procedure. The best surgical procedure for this patient is a belt lipectomy, as this will address the circumferential tissue excess.
   B. **A fit and well 24-year-old woman has a moderate infraumbilical skin and soft tissue excess following pregnancy. Her skin quality is average, and she has multiple striae in the lower abdomen. She is generally slim, but this area seems unresponsive to diet and physical exercise.**
      d. Miniabdominoplasty
      This patient could benefit from a miniabdominoplasty procedure. It will target both the excess skin and fat, as well as remove some of the striae. It will, however, have a tendency to lower the umbilicus, and she must be counseled about this. She would not be a good candidate for liposuction, given her skin quality. A full abdominoplasty would be excessive.
   C. **A 54-year-old woman has significant rectus diastasis following five pregnancies, all delivered vaginally. She is generally well and has a slim build, with moderate lower abdominal fat excess only. She is a nonsmoker and has not had any other surgical procedures.**
      c. Endoscopic rectus plication with liposuction
      This woman has two main issues: excess lower abdominal fat and diastasis of the rectus. Since there is no skin excess, she could benefit from a minimal access procedure, such as liposuction and endoscopic rectus plication.

PERIOPERATIVE MANAGEMENT

10. **Which one of the following is true of the perioperative management of patients undergoing abdominoplasty?**
    B. Intravenous antibiotics should be given 30 to 60 minutes before starting surgery.
    Current guidelines from the Surgical Care Improvement Project (SCIP)[3] suggest that intravenous antibiotics are given 30 to 60 minutes before surgery begins. Cefazolin (Ancef) 1 g or clindamycin 900 mg are recommended, but institutions usually have their own individual guidelines based on local microbiological data. These are then given at regular intervals during surgery and continued for up to 24 hours. A full week's course is not required. The pubic area should not be shaved in advance, as skin damage can increase the risk of infection, but clipping is acceptable. TED hose (stockings) are recommended in all patients undergoing abdominoplasty, as it carries a high risk of thromboembolic events. In addition to TED hose, calf compression devices should also be used intraoperatively. Most patients should be considered for prophylactic low-molecular-weight heparin (e.g. Lovenox 40 mg) on the evening of surgery and for 7 days after.[4]

SURGICAL PROCEDURE

11. What is the main benefit of leaving a layer of fat over the anterior superior iliac spine (ASIS) during abdominoplasty?
D. A reduced risk of nerve damage

It is very important to leave a small amount of fat on the fascia overlying the ASIS, as this helps prevent injury to the lateral femoral cutaneous nerve. Damage to this nerve can lead to significant postoperative pain, numbness, and dysesthesia in the hip and lateral thigh region. There is no proven benefit on seroma development, or leaving this small area of fascia covered with fat, although in general leaving a thin layer of tissue overlying the rectus and external oblique fascia may help reduce seroma formation by preserving lymphatic channels. Quilting sutures may also reduce seroma formation following abdominoplasty. There is no reduction in hematoma rate secondary to leaving a layer of tissue over the fascia and there is no discernible difference on abdominal wall contour, as the layer preserved is very thin.

12. Which one of the following is correct when incorporating rectus plication into a standard abdominoplasty technique?
B. Plication is best achieved using a heavy permanent suture.

Choice of suture for repair of rectus diastasis is very important with regard to longevity of the repair and should be performed using a heavy, nonabsorbable suture. Recurrence of diastasis following rectus plication is much higher when an absorbable suture is used compared with a permanent suture.[5-8] When using an absorbable suture, there was a 40% recurrence rate by 5 years as confirmed by ultrasound imaging.[5] In contrast, a study conducted when a permanent suture material was used, found no diastasis recurrence observed at 5 to 7 years after surgery.

The findings were confirmed by CT imaging in this case.[6] The upper skin flap needs to be elevated up to the xiphisternum to allow access for rectus plication and a central area of undermining is adequate. Lateral undermining is unnecessary and reduces blood supply to the flap. Rectus plication must start just below the xiphisternum, otherwise a postoperative bulge may form and is apparent to the patient. There are different techniques of plication but a typical example would be to use a two-layer approach combining interrupted and then continuous sutures to reinforce the repair. The use of plication does not negate the use of progressive tension sutures, as these are used to advance and distribute tension of wound closure away from the suture line. They may also reduce hematoma and seroma formation.

MINIABDOMINOPLASTY

13. You are discussing the relative merits of using a miniabdominoplasty with a patient. She is of slim build and has modest lower abdominal soft tissue excess. She has had a previous cesarian section and wants to minimize further scarring. Examination shows mild rectus diastasis. Which one of the following is true of this procedure?
B. It is mainly indicated for infraumbilical skin and fat excess.

The miniabdominoplasty is a useful technique for correcting small to moderate fat and skin excesses in the infraumbilical region. The benefits over a full abdominoplasty are that it creates a shorter transverse scar and avoids the periumbilical scar completely (see Fig. 100-9, *Essentials of Plastic Surgery,* second edition). Rectus plication is still possible but access will require transection of the umbilicus at the level of deep fascia, and the small fascial weak point this leaves must be closed over to prevent a hernia. Any upper abdominal wall skin and fat excess is not addressed. Because the umbilicus is not dissected and relocated, the umbilicus may be artificially lowered on the abdominal wall and will not sit level with the iliac crest. Transection of the umbilical stalk at the deep fascia will remove the dominant blood supply to it, but there will be sufficient blood supply from the surrounding subdermal plexus.

PROGRESSIVE TENSION SUTURES

14. Which one of the following is not a recognized benefit of using progressive tension sutures during closure of an abdominoplasty?

C. Reduced operative time

Progressive tension sutures have many benefits but tend to increase, not decrease, surgical time. Progressive tension sutures involve placement of interrupted resorbable sutures between the muscular fascia and the underside of the abdominal flap. As the flap is advanced, progressive tension is exerted on each suture and thereby directed away from the incision. Decreased tension on the incision helps to prevent wound-edge necrosis and hypertrophic scars. The dead space underneath the flap is closed, thereby reducing hematoma and seroma formation. Pollock and Pollock[9,10] have shown extremely low rates of seroma formation when using this technique.

FLEUR-DE-LIS ABDOMINOPLASTY

15. Which one of the following is the main advantage of using the fleur-de-lis abdominoplasty technique?

D. Horizontal and vertical abdominal tissue excess is addressed.

The main advantage of the fleur-de-lis abdominoplasty is that it facilitates correction of combined horizontal and vertical soft tissue and skin excesses of the anterior abdominal wall. It is possible to achieve a good contour of the waistline with this technique at the expense of a long, vertical midline scar on the anterior abdomen. It is often a good choice in patients who may otherwise need a circumferential approach, such as a belt lipectomy, to address these areas. It can therefore avoid a posterior or very lateral scar for such patients. It is also well suited to patients who have previous scarring to the upper abdominal wall that may compromise the vascularity of a standard abdominoplasty skin flap. It is important that no flap undermining is performed during this procedure.

When performing a fleur-de-lis abdominoplasty, a standard lower abdominoplasty incision is made and the lower tissue ellipse is excised at the level of the umbilicus with no undermining of the flap above this point. The horizontal excess can be estimated at this stage by pinching the supraumbilical tissues together. A vertical elliptical excision can then be made from the umbilicus to the xiphisternum. It is important when performing this technique not to overestimate the amount of tissue that needs to be removed. It can also be difficult to avoid leaving epigastric fullness with this technique, particularly in massive-weight-loss patients. The benefits and risks should be fully discussed with the patient before surgery.

Postoperative complications are similar to a standard abdominoplasty. Rectus plication is generally required in patients undergoing fleur-de-lis abdominoplasty, as they tend to have been through significant fluctuations in body shape, such as multiple pregnancies or massive weight loss. This technique facilitates easy access to perform plication. The Lockwood high-lateral-tension technique addresses tissue excess on the thigh, but the fleur-de-lis does not.

POSTOPERATIVE MANAGEMENT

16. You see a 44-year-old fit and healthy woman the morning after an abdominoplasty. She previously had two pregnancies by cesarean section and has undergone previous limb and breast surgery in the past, coping well with postoperative pain management. On this occasion she is really quite sore, despite having access to a morphine pump (patient controlled analgesia [PCA]) and background acetaminophen. She is wearing an external abdominal binder and lying with knees on a pillow. Her abdomen remains soft but tender and is otherwise unremarkable. Her CRP is elevated to 20 (normal range is <5) and her observations are normal. **What is the most likely explanation for her continued discomfort?**

E. She has undergone correctional surgery for rectus diastasis.

Abdominoplasty is generally well tolerated by patients providing no adjunctive procedures have been performed. Even when given morphine PCAs many patients will use them minimally, yet remain comfortable. Correction of rectus diastasis can be very painful in the early postoperative period. This is the most likely explanation in this case. It is often well controlled by using continuous local anesthetic infusion catheters placed near to the rectus or within the sheath. It is too early for a postoperative soft tissue infection to be likely in a healthy patient and there would usually be evidence of swelling, cellulitis, or warmth to the abdomen if this were the case. CRP will be elevated as a result of surgery and does not by itself suggest infection. If peritonitis was present the patient would be acutely unwell and have guarding or a rigid abdomen. The possibility of a rectus sheath hematoma should also be considered.

COMPLICATIONS

17. A patient who had a standard abdominoplasty surgery 6 months ago and has called your secretary concerned about residual fullness to the epigastric region. She had a standard abdominoplasty approach with rectus plication, but no liposuction. **What is the most likely cause of the bulge in this area?**

A. Inadequate flap dissection

The patient in this scenario most likely has epigastric fullness because the rectus plication was not started high enough. Failure to elevate the flap up to the xiphisternum is the most likely cause in this case. A dog-ear can occur here following a fleur-de-lis abdominoplasty if there has been inadequate fat removal or if the skin flaps are particularly thick. Seromas can present late but are unlikely at this stage, and usually occur around the waist rather than superiorly as in this case. Postoperative weight gain can often be a reason for late changes in appearance and patient dissatisfaction following surgery, but fat gain affecting this area alone is not likely.

REFERENCES

1. Stokes RB, Whetzel TP, Sommerhaug E, et al. Arterial vascular anatomy of the umbilicus. Plast Reconstr Surg 102:761-764, 1998.
2. Weisberg NK, Nehal KS, Zide BM. Dog-ears: a review. Dermatol Surg 26:363-370, 2000.
3. Bratzler DW, Houck PM, Richards C, et al. Use of antimicrobial prophylaxis for major surgery: baseline results from the National Surgical Infection Prevention Project. Arch Surg. 140:174-182, 2005.
4. Buck DW, Mustoe TA. An evidence-based approach to abdominoplasty. Plast Reconstr Surg 126:2189-2195, 2010.

5. van Uchelen JH, Kon M, Werker PM. The long-term durability of plication of the anterior rectus sheath assessed by ultrasonography. Plast Reconstr Surg 107:1578-1584, 2001.
6. Nahas FX, Augusto SM, Ghelfond C. Should diastasis recti be corrected? Aesthetic Plast Surg 21:285-289, 1997.
7. Nahas FX, Ferreira LM, Mendes Jde A. An efficient way to correct recurrent rectus diastasis. Aesthetic Plast Surg 28:189-196, 2004.
8. Nahas FX, Ferreira LM, Augusto SM, et al. Long-term follow-up of correction of rectus diastasis. Plast Reconstr Surg 115:1736-1743, 2005.
9. Pollock H, Pollock T. Progressive tension sutures: a technique to reduce local complications in abdominoplasty. Plast Reconstr Surg 105:2583-2586, 2000.
10. Pollock T, Pollock H. Progressive tension sutures in abdominoplasty: a review of 597 consecutive cases. Aesthet Surg J 32:729-742, 2012.

101. Medial Thigh Lift

See *Essentials of Plastic Surgery*, second edition, pp. 1279-1284.

ANATOMY

1. **Which one of the following statements is correct regarding the anatomy of the thigh?**
   A. Thigh skin is of uniform thickness throughout.
   B. There are three distinct fat layers within the thigh.
   C. Colles' fascia lies within the superficial fat in the thigh.
   D. The femoral nerve runs adjacent to the femoral triangle to supply all thigh sensation.
   E. Colles' fascia anatomy is particularly relevant to thigh-lift techniques.

2. **What marks the medial border of the femoral triangle?**
   A. The medial border of the sartorius
   B. The medial border of the adductor longus
   C. The medial border of the adductor magnus
   D. The lateral border of the biceps femoris
   E. The lateral border of the gracilis

3. **When performing a medial thigh lift, what superficial muscle is particularly useful to guide location of the anatomic shelf of Colles' fascia used to suspend the thigh soft tissues?**
   A. Sartorius
   B. Gluteus maximus
   C. Adductor longus
   D. Vastus medialis
   E. Semitendinosus

PROCEDURE SELECTION

4. **For each of the following scenarios, select the next best step in surgical management. (Each option may be used once, more than once, or not at all.)**
   A. A 28-year-old woman has moderate skin laxity and subcutaneous fat extending from the distal third of her thigh up to the medial thigh crease.
   B. A 45-year-old woman has an excess of fat to both medial and lateral aspects of the thigh. Her skin quality is good and there is minimal skin excess.
   C. A 30-year-old woman has lost more than 40 pounds and has recently undergone a lower body lift. She has a small excess of subcutaneous fat in the medial thigh and skin laxity in the upper third.

   Options:
   a. Liposuction only
   b. Liposuction and horizontal skin excision
   c. Liposuction with horizontal and vertical skin excision
   d. Horizontal skin excision only
   e. Vertical skin excision only
   f. Combined horizontal and vertical skin excision

OPERATIVE TECHNIQUE

5. How should a patient be positioned when performing preoperative marking for a medial thigh lift?
A. Standing straight with feet placed together
B. Standing straight with knees placed slightly apart
C. Lying supine with legs straight and externally rotated
D. Lying supine in the frog-leg position
E. Lying prone with legs slightly apart

6. When marking a patient for a classic medial thigh lift to address a proximal one-third skin excess, which one of the following is correct?
A. A transverse incision should be marked 2 cm distal and parallel to the medial thigh crease.
B. A vertical incision should be marked along the anterior border of adductor longus.
C. A transverse incision should be marked parallel to the inguinal ligament on the anterior thigh.
D. A transverse incision should pass from the pubic tubercle to the buttock crease in the medial thigh crease.
E. The transverse skin resection is usually around 5 cm but should be estimated using a pinch test.

7. How should the patient be positioned on the operating table during a classic medial thigh lift?
A. Lateral with pillows between the legs
B. Supine with knees on pillows
C. Supine with legs elevated in stirrups
D. Supine in frog-leg position
E. Prone with hips flexed

8. During a medial thigh lift, why is it particularly important to preserve the soft tissue that lies between the mons pubis and femoral triangle?
A. To avoid nerve damage
B. To minimize vulval distortion
C. To reduce infection risk
D. To minimize risk of hypertrophic scarring
E. To minimize risk of lymphedema

MEDIAL THIGH LIFT IN MASSIVE-WEIGHT-LOSS PATIENTS

9. You are planning a medial thigh lift on a patient following a belt lipectomy after massive weight loss. On examination, the patient has type V lipodystrophy, with moderate residual fat excess in the medial thigh. The skin excess is very large and extends from the groin crease to the knee. Which one of the following is correct regarding the excisional component of the procedure?
A. It requires a full-length longitudinal incision in the medial thigh without a transverse component.
B. Anchoring the superficial fascia to Colles' fascia is not required in this case.
C. The patient should be placed supine on the operating table with stirrups to hold the ankles.
D. The long saphenous vein should be identified and carefully tied off to avoid bleeding risk.
E. Segmental excision and closure, as used for a brachioplasty, is not required in this case.

FASCIOFASCIAL SUSPENSION TECHNIQUE

10. The fasciofascial suspension technique for medial thigh lift uses a different fixation than a standard medial thigh lift. *What structures are used to suspend the thigh in this technique?*
    A. Superficial fascia and inguinal ligament
    B. Superficial fascia and Colles' fascia
    C. Adductor fascia and inguinal ligament
    D. Gracilis fascia and adductor fascia
    E. Gracilis fascia and inguinal ligament

Answers

ANATOMY

1. **Which one of the following statements is correct regarding the anatomy of the thigh?**
   E. Colles' fascia anatomy is particularly relevant to thigh-lift techniques.
   The superficial anatomy of the thigh is highly relevant to thigh-lift procedures, and knowledge and understanding of Colles' fascia is particularly important. Colles' fascia is a thick, strong fascial layer found deep to the subcutaneous fat of the thigh. It attaches to the ischiopubic rami of the bony pelvis, Scarpa's fascia of the abdominal wall, and the posterior border of the urogenital diaphragm. It has a particularly strong area at the junction of the perineum and medial thigh, where it defines the perineal thigh crease. The Colles' fascia is relevant to medial thigh lift as it is used to resuspend the elevated soft tissues. Thigh skin thickness differs according to anatomic location and is thinner medially than laterally. The medial skin also contains fewer hairs. The thigh has two distinct fat layers and between the two is a weak superficial fascial system also relevant to thigh-lift procedures. The femoral nerve travels in the femoral triangle (not adjacent to it) and provides some sensation to the thigh through its branches. The medial femoral cutaneous nerve supplies most of the medial thigh (L1-2). The proximal aspect of the medial thigh close to the groin crease is supplied by the ilioinguinal nerve (L1). The genitofemoral nerve (L1 component) supplies the skin over the femoral triangle. The lateral aspect of the thigh is supplied by the lateral cutaneous nerve of the thigh (L2-3) and this may be damaged during an abdominoplasty over the ASIS, as discussed in Chapter 100 (Fig. 101-1).

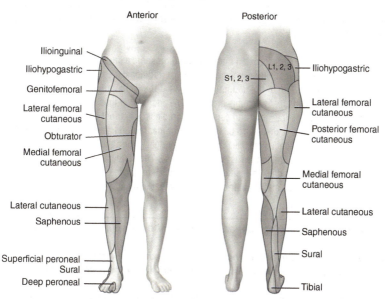

Fig. 101-1 Dermatomes of the lower limb.

868 Part VII ■ Aesthetic Surgery

2. **What marks the medial border of the femoral triangle?**
   B. **The medial border of the adductor longus**

   The femoral triangle is bounded by three structures: the medial border of the sartorius (laterally), the medial border of the adductor longus (medially), and the inguinal ligament superiorly (Fig. 101-2). The triangle contains the femoral vessels and nerve and lymphatic channels. It is relevant to a medial thigh lift, in that it should not be violated to avoid damage to these structures.

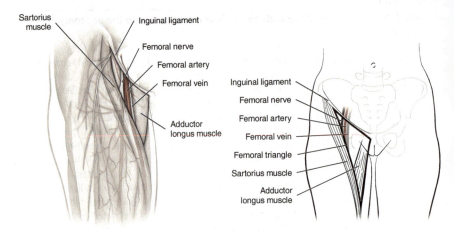

Fig. 101-2 Boundaries of the femoral triangle.

3. **When performing a medial thigh lift, what superficial muscle is particularly useful to guide location of the anatomic shelf of Colles' fascia used to suspend the thigh soft tissues?**
   C. **Adductor longus**

   The junction of the perineum and medial thigh represents a particularly strong area of Colles' fascia that is the site of fixation when performing a traditional medial thigh lift. This site is found by following the origin of the adductor muscles at the ischiopubic ramus and retracting the skin and superficial fat of the pubis medially. The adductor longus is the best guide to locating this area, as it lies superficial and can be palpated easily in most patients when their hips are externally rotated and knees flexed. The adductor magnus and gracilis origins are close to this area but deep to the longus muscle. The sartorius origin is the anterior superior iliac spine (ASIS) and therefore lies lateral to the medial thigh crease. The gluteus maximus lies posterior to the adductor insertion, as does the semitendinosus which originates from the ischial tuberosity. The vastus medialis is one of the quadriceps muscles that originates from the femur.

PROCEDURE SELECTION

4. **For each of the following scenarios, the next best step in surgical management is as follows:**
   A. *A 28-year-old woman has moderate skin laxity and subcutaneous fat extending from the distal third of her thigh up to the medial thigh crease.*
   C. **Liposuction with horizontal and vertical skin excision**

   The approach to medial thigh lift is both straightforward and logical. If there is excess fat then liposuction or further weight loss is required. If there is excess skin then resection is required. If

both fat and skin excess are present, a combination of each is required. If skin excess is confined to the upper third of the thigh, then a horizontal excision is performed, if skin excess affects the majority of the thigh then a vertical excision is performed. In some cases both horizontal and vertical excisions are combined to create a T-shaped excision.

If there are other areas that need to be addressed, such as the abdomen, back, and lateral thighs, then these are generally performed first. If there is severe fat excess, then the procedure is staged with liposuction first then skin resection is performed secondarily.

The patient in this scenario has moderate skin and fat excess for most of the thigh, so she will benefit from liposuction with horizontal and vertical skin resection.

B. A 45-year-old woman has an excess of fat to both medial and lateral aspects of the thigh. Her skin quality is good and there is minimal skin excess.
a. **Liposuction only**
The patient in this scenario has only fat excess without a need for skin resection. Assuming that her weight is stable, she is best managed with liposuction to target both medial and lateral thigh areas. As the skin is in good condition, it should tighten satisfactorily over time. It may be that laser-assisted liposuction is useful in this case to enhance skin tightening (see Chapter 98).

C. A 30-year-old woman has lost more than 40 pounds and has recently undergone a lower body lift. She has a small excess of subcutaneous fat in the medial thigh and skin laxity in the upper third.
b. **Liposuction and horizontal skin excision**
The patient in this scenario should be treated with liposuction to address the mild fat excess, then a horizontal skin resection should be performed (Table 101-1).

Table 101-1 *Classification and Surgical Recommendation*

Classification	Description	Treatment
Type I	Lipodystrophy with no sign of skin laxity	Liposuction alone
Type II	Lipodystrophy and skin laxity confined to the upper third of the thigh	Liposuction and a **horizontal skin** excision
Type III	Lipodystrophy and moderate skin laxity that extends **beyond the upper third of the thigh**	Liposuction, horizontal and vertical excision
Type IV	Skin laxity that extends the **length of the thigh**	A **longer vertical resection** than for type III
Type V	Severe medial thigh skin laxity with lipodystrophy	**Two stages:** First stage: Aggressive liposuction Second stage: Excisional medial thigh lift

OPERATIVE TECHNIQUE

5. *How should a patient be positioned when performing preoperative marking for a medial thigh lift?*
   B. **Standing with knees placed slightly apart**
   When marking a patient for a medial thigh lift it is important to perform this with them standing upright with knees apart. This should be performed in the presence of a chaperone of the same sex as the patient, given the intimate nature of the markings. It is important to do these markings with the patient standing, as it more reliably allows assessment of the location and extent of excess soft tissue.

6. **When marking a patient for a classic medial thigh lift to address a proximal one-third skin excess, which one of the following is correct?**
   E. The transverse skin resection is usually around 5 cm but should be estimated using a pinch test.
   When marking a patient for a medial thigh lift it is best to assess the amount of excess skin that can safely be removed by performing a pinch test. This is done by gently grasping the soft tissues and lifting them towards the thigh crease. The exact amount that can be taken is patient dependent but on average 5 to 7 cm is excised. A further 3 to 5 cm of lift is achieved secondary to anchoring of the skin flap to the Colles' fascia.
   As discussed in question 4, the approach to medial thigh lift will be guided by skin and soft tissue excess. A standard approach for the patient described involves a transverse incision placed in the medial thigh crease, passing from the pubic tubercle to the perineal thigh crease. It is not necessary to extend the incision all the way posterior to the buttock crease. A vertical extension is only required where skin laxity extends beyond the upper third of the thigh, and is therefore not required in this case (see Fig. 101-2, *Essentials of Plastic Surgery,* second edition). When performing a fasciofascial suspension technique the transverse incision may be placed parallel to the inguinal crease, but not in a classic thigh lift.

7. **How should the patient be positioned on the operating table during a classic medial thigh lift?**
   D. Supine in frog-leg position
   Patients undergoing classic medial thigh lift should be positioned supine in a frog-leg position. Stirrups were previously used but are no longer needed because the incision ends at the perineal crease without extension to the buttocks. A prone position is unnecessary for the same reason and is less favorable from an anesthetic perspective. Lateral positioning would entail changing position and redraping intraoperatively when moving from one side to the next.

8. **During a medial thigh lift, why is it particularly important to preserve the soft tissue that lies between the mons pubis and femoral triangle?**
   E. To minimize risk of lymphedema
   It is important to carefully preserve the soft tissue that lies between the mons pubis and femoral triangle to prevent damage to the lymphatics and subsequent lymphedema. Lymphedema is difficult to manage, and medial thigh lift carries a small risk of this and must be discussed during the preoperative consent process. The risk of nerve damage is low and the risk of infection is not affected. Hypertrophic scarring is not common at this site and a small volume resection of this soft tissue is unlikely to significantly distort the vulva.

MEDIAL THIGH LIFT IN MASSIVE-WEIGHT-LOSS PATIENTS

9. **You are planning a medial thigh lift on a patient following a belt lipectomy after massive weight loss. On examination, the patient has type V lipodystrophy, with moderate residual fat excess in the medial thigh. The skin excess is very large and extends from the groin crease to the knee. Which one of the following is correct regarding the excisional component of the procedure?**
   B. Anchoring the superficial fascia to Colles' fascia is not required in this case.
   This patient has a significant horizontal excess of skin, and this requires a longitudinal (vertical), elliptical excision pattern (see Fig. 101-4, *Essentials of Plastic Surgery,* second edition). The addition of a short transverse upper incision will likely be required to avoid formation of a dog-ear. Because the vector of lift is horizontal instead of vertical, it is not necessary to anchor the skin flap to Colles' fascia. Stirrups are not required in this case.

A similar approach to a brachioplasty should be adopted, where excision and closure are staged to minimize the effects of soft tissue swelling and the risk of overresection. The long saphenous vein should be identified and preserved. A compression garment should be used after surgery.

FASCIOFASCIAL SUSPENSION TECHNIQUE

10. The fasciofascial suspension technique for medial thigh lift uses a different fixation than a standard medial thigh lift. *What structures are used to suspend the thigh in this technique?*

    D. Gracilis fascia and adductor fascia

    The fasciofascial suspension technique was described by Candiani et al[1] as an alternative to a classic medial thigh lift. It employs a transverse skin excision with a vertical vector of pull. Instead of relying on anchoring of the Colles' fascia, the technique relies on the strength of overlap between the Gracilis and the adductor longus muscles. Instead of making an incision in the medial thigh crease, it is made 6 to 7 cm below the inguinal crease. The skin and fat are undermined down to the fascia of the adductor longus and gracilis muscles. The fascia between the two muscles is then overlapped and closed to support the lift and allow skin closure under minimal tension.

REFERENCE

1. Candiani P, Campiglio GL, Signorini M. Fascio-fascial suspension technique in medial thigh lifts. Aesthetic Plast Surg 19:137-140, 1995.

102. Body Contouring in the Massive-Weight-Loss Patient

See *Essentials of Plastic Surgery*, second edition, pp. 1285-1299.

BODY MASS INDEX

1. ***How is body mass index calculated?***
   A. Height (m) divided by weight (kg)^2
   B. Weight (kg) divided by height (m)^2
   C. Height (m) multiplied by weight (kg)^2
   D. Weight (kg) multiplied by height (m)^2
   E. Height (m)^2 divided by weight (kg)

2. A patient is seen in clinic before surgery. They are 1.72 meters tall and weigh 86 kg. ***How would you describe their current health status according to their calculated BMI?***
   A. Underweight
   B. Normal weight
   C. Overweight
   D. Morbidly obese
   E. Super obese

BARIATRIC SURGERY TECHNIQUES

3. A patient is seen in clinic having undergone gastric bypass surgery and subsequent major weight loss. ***Why is gastric bypass considered to be a better procedure than gastric banding?***
   A. The surgery is less invasive
   B. Nutritional supplements are not required
   C. It is more easily reversed
   D. It reduces small bowel food absorption
   E. The effects can be adjusted postoperatively

4. ***For each of the following scenarios, select the most likely bariatric surgery technique being described. (Each option may be used once, more than once, or not at all.)***
   A. This procedure is effective in helping patients achieve weight reduction of approximately 80% but risks them developing significant nutritional deficiencies. It may be combined with a duodenal switch.
   B. This represents the benchmark and most commonly performed bariatric procedure, providing resolution of type II diabetes in more than 90% of patients. It combines both restrictive and malabsorptive elements.
   C. This purely restrictive, reversible bariatric procedure is performed laparoscopically and helps achieve approximately 50% reduction in weight.

   Options:
   a. Biliopancreatic diversion (BPD)
   b. Adjustable gastric band
   c. Roux- en-Y gastric bypass
   d. Gastric sleeve
   e. Vertical band gastroplasty

Chapter 102 ■ Body Contouring in the Massive-Weight-Loss Patient

PRIORITIES IN WEIGHT-LOSS CONTOURING

5. When planning body contouring after massive weight loss, which one of the following areas is commonly targeted first?
   A. Breasts
   B. Trunk
   C. Neck and face
   D. Arms
   E. Medial thighs

TIMING OF BODY CONTOURING AFTER BARIATRIC SURGERY

6. A 30-year-old patient is seeking breast and trunk recontouring 9 months after undergoing gastric bypass. She has lost 22 kg (44 pounds), to move from a BMI of 40.5 to a BMI of 32. Her breasts and abdomen have significant skin excess. Her weight has been stable for 3 months. **Which one of the following is correct?**
   A. She is ready to proceed with an initial panniculectomy.
   B. She is ready to proceed with a breast reduction.
   C. Body contouring surgery should be postponed until her BMI is less than 25.
   D. Body contouring surgery should be postponed for an additional 3 months.
   E. Body contouring surgery should be postponed for an additional year.

FUNCTIONS OF A BELT LIPECTOMY

7. Which one of the following areas is not addressed with a belt lipectomy?
   A. Lower abdominal pannus
   B. Central buttock region
   C. Lateral and medial thighs
   D. Lower and midback rolls
   E. Waistline and mons pubis

BELT LIPECTOMY PROCEDURE

8. When marking a massive-weight-loss patient for a belt lipectomy, which one of the following is correct?
   A. Preoperative markings are best done on the day of surgery with the patient standing.
   B. Upper and lower anterior transverse markings are placed at the same level as for an abdominoplasty.
   C. Strict adherence to preoperative markings during surgery is essential for good outcomes.
   D. The patient must bend forward while the posterior vertical excess is marked to avoid overexcision.
   E. Posterior and lateral areas are most important to the final outcome, so warrant generous resection.

PERFORMING A BELT LIPECTOMY

9. Which of the following is correct when performing a belt lipectomy in a massive-weight-loss patient?
   A. Supine and prone positioning provides optimal access.
   B. Umbilical lengthening is usually required during a standard belt lipectomy.
   C. Liposuction to the lateral thigh should preserve the zones of adherence.
   D. Posterior skin flap elevation should be performed at the level of the lumbar fascia.
   E. Incisions should be sited to place postoperative scars below the pelvic brim.

BREAST SURGERY AFTER MASSIVE WEIGHT LOSS

10. *For each of the patients described, select the best surgical option for management of their breasts after major weight loss.*
    A. A patient has lost 98 pounds after gastric banding. Her breasts are flat and underfilled. She has notch-to-nipple distances of 29 cm on both sides and has a BMI of 26.
    B. A patient has lost 42 pounds with diet and exercise. Her BMI is now 23. Her breasts measure an A cup and she has notch-to-nipple distances of 22 cm.
    C. A patient has had body contouring surgery to the trunk after massive weight loss, but still has concerns regarding her breasts which are ptotic and empty. On examination, she has notch-to-nipple distances of 28 cm with grade III ptosis and a significant lateral soft tissue excess passing from the breast toward the axillae. Her BMI is 33.

Options:
a. Augmentation only
b. Mastopexy only
c. Reduction only
d. Augmentation-mastopexy
e. Autoaugmentation

COMPLICATIONS AFTER MASSIVE-WEIGHT-LOSS SURGERY

11. You are discussing the risks of surgery with a patient who has reduced their BMI from 40 to 30 after bariatric surgery. **What is the most frequent complication after major body contouring surgery?**
    A. Venous thromboembolism
    B. Skin necrosis
    C. Wound infection
    D. Hematoma
    E. Wound dehiscence

Answers

BODY MASS INDEX

1. *How is body mass index calculated?*
   B. Weight (kg) divided by height (m)^2
   Body mass index is a measurement of body fat based on weight and height. It is calculated using the following equation:
   - Weight in kg/Height (m)^2

   It is useful when assessing patients before and after massive-weight-loss surgery and can be used to subclassify the degree of obesity.

2. A patient is seen in clinic before surgery. They are 1.72 meters tall and weigh 86 kg. *How would you describe their current health status according to their calculated BMI?*
   C. Overweight
   This patient has a body mass index of 29 kg/m^2 based on their height and weight, using the calculation shown in explanation 1. The National Institute of Health (NIH) classification for BMI is as follows:
   - BMI <18.5–Underweight
   - BMI 18.5-25–Normal/healthy weight
   - BMI 25-29.9–Overweight
   - BMI 30-34.0–Obese
   - BMI 35-39.9–Severely obese
   - BMI >40–Morbidly obese
   - BMI >50–Super obese

   Most patients following massive weight loss will reach a plateau to remain with a BMI around 30. Some will be able to go further and achieve a BMI less than this, but most patients tend to remain slightly overweight. The relevance of BMI to body contouring surgery is that operative risks are markedly reduced once patients reduce their BMI to less than 30 or are close to their ideal body weight. They are also more likely to achieve good cosmetic outcomes after surgery. The patient described remains overweight at present.

BARIATRIC SURGERY TECHNIQUES

3. A patient is seen in clinic having undergone gastric bypass surgery and subsequent major weight loss. *Why is gastric bypass considered to be a better procedure than gastric banding?*
   D. It reduces small bowel food absorption.
   Techniques commonly used to achieve massive weight loss are either restrictive (such as gastric banding or sleeve) or both restrictive and malabsorptive, such as gastric bypass and biliopancreatic diversion (Fig. 102-1). Restrictive procedures simply reduce the size of the stomach such that patient's feel full sooner and reduce their food intake. Malabsorptive procedures bypass food through parts of the small intestine to reduce absorption. In general, procedures that are both restrictive and malabsorptive achieve more rapid and sustained weight loss at the expense of potentially causing nutritional deficiencies. The main benefit of the gastric

bypass procedure over gastric banding therefore is the fact that it reduces food intake and absorption of food.

Both procedures are performed laparoscopically and surgery is similarly invasive for both procedures, but is simpler in gastric banding. Nutritional supplements are required for patients following absorptive procedures. The gastric band procedure is reversible and more adjustable than gastric bypass, as the port can be inflated or deflated in clinic. In contrast, the gastric bypass requires surgical intervention to reverse or adjust.

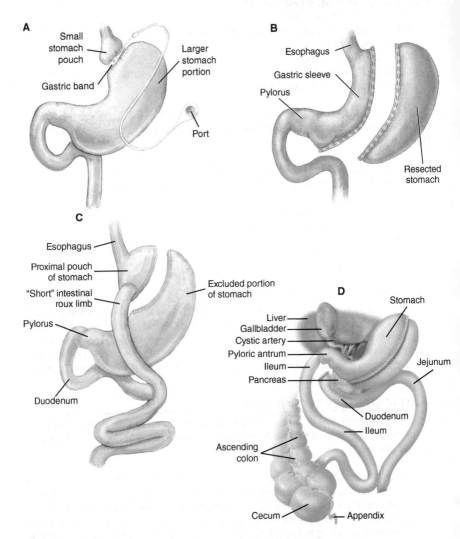

Fig. 102-1 Restrictive procedures for bariatric surgery. **A,** Laparoscopic adjustable gastric band. **B,** Sleeve gastrectomy. **C,** Roux-en-Y gastric bypass. **D,** Biliopancreatic diversion with duodenal switch.

4. **For each of the following scenarios, the best options are as follows:**
   A. **This procedure is effective in helping patients achieve weight reduction of approximately 80% but risks them developing significant nutritional deficiencies. It may be combined with a duodenal switch.**
   a. **Biliopancreatic diversion (BPD)**
      The biliopancreatic diversion procedure (BPD) involves removal of a part of the stomach to reduce its size by approximately 75%. The remaining stomach is then directly anastomosed to the lower portion of the small intestine. It is an effective procedure for achieving weight loss of 75% to 80% with good long-term maintenance. However, it may lead to significant nutritional deficiencies, such that patients require lifelong vitamin supplementation and experience foul smelling flatulence and loose stools.
   B. **This represents the benchmark and most commonly performed bariatric procedure, providing resolution of type II diabetes in more than 90% of patients. It combines both restrictive and malabsorptive elements.**
   c. **Roux-en-Y gastric bypass**
      The roux-en-Y gastric bypass is the current benchmark procedure for weight loss. It involves reducing the size of the stomach to create a pouch that is in continuity with the esophagus and intestine. Food consequently passes directly into the small intestine, while the stomach still releases gastric juices that also enter the small intestine and assist with digestion. This procedure means that food intake is restricted, as patients feel full rapidly. The absorption is less severely affected compared with other techniques such as the roux-en-Y (Fig. 102-1, *C*).
   C. **This purely restrictive, reversible bariatric procedure is performed laparoscopically and helps achieve approximately 50% reduction in weight.**
   b. **Adjustable gastric band**
      Gastric banding is usually performed laparoscopically and involves placement of an adjustable band around the top of the stomach. A separate port is connected to the band with silicone tubing and is sited in the subcutaneous tissues. This allows for adjustment of the band when required (Fig. 102-1, *A*).

PRIORITIES IN WEIGHT-LOSS CONTOURING

5. **When planning body contouring after massive weight loss, which one of the following areas is commonly targeted first?**
   B. **Trunk**
   The goals of surgery are to alleviate functional, aesthetic, and psychological impairments associated with skin redundancy. Often the functional component is most important, since this can limit the patient's ability to exercise fully. The order of treatment should therefore be patient specific, but in general, the trunk is treated first with a lower body lift or panniculectomy, because an overhanging abdominal pannus and trunk rolls can be quite restrictive. The breasts and arms would normally be targeted next, followed by the medial thighs, neck, and face.

TIMING OF BODY CONTOURING AFTER BARIATRIC SURGERY

6. A 30-year-old patient is seeking breast and trunk recontouring 9 months after undergoing gastric bypass. She has lost 22 kg (44 pounds), to move from a BMI of 40.5 to a BMI of 32. Her breast and abdomen have significant skin excess. Her weight has been stable for 3 months. **Which one of the following is correct?**
   D. **Body contouring surgery should be postponed for an additional 3 months.**
   It is too early to proceed with body contouring surgery at this stage because the patient has not reached a steady weight for sufficient time. Stability for 6 months is recommended

before proceeding with body contouring surgery. This usually corresponds to at least 12 to 18 months after gastric bypass. The benefits of delaying surgery include a reduction in the risk of perioperative complications, improved aesthetic outcomes, and better wound healing. Most patients following massive weight loss stabilize at a BMI of 30 to 35, and may benefit from an initial panniculectomy or breast reduction to assist further lifestyle changes such as diet or exercise. Although it may be optimal to wait until patients are less than BMI of 25, it is neither necessary nor realistic to wait until this time, as most patients' weight stabilizes around BMI 30.

FUNCTIONS OF A BELT LIPECTOMY

7. Which one of the following areas is not addressed with a belt lipectomy?
   C. Lateral and medial thighs

A belt lipectomy has the benefit of addressing multiple areas of trunk skin and soft tissue excess that are characteristic of the physique following massive weight loss. The circumferential excision pattern will address the anterior abdominal panniculus, the lateral excess, and the lower and midback folds. It cannot safely address the upper back fold, which is addressed during breast procedures. It also lifts the ptotic tissues from the buttocks, mons pubis, and lateral thighs. This improves the contour of these areas while improving the waistline. The medial thigh will need to be addressed separately (see Chapter 101, *Essentials of Plastic Surgery*, second edition).

BELT LIPECTOMY PROCEDURE

8. When marking a massive-weight-loss patient for a belt lipectomy, which one of the following is correct?
   D. The patient must bend forward while the posterior vertical excess is marked to avoid overexcision.

The preoperative markings can be done on the day of surgery, but it is preferable to do them the day before. This enables the surgeon to review photographs of the markings and make any necessary changes. It also increases time efficiency on the day of surgery. The markings will be made with the patient standing for some parts and supine with hips slightly flexed for others (see Fig. 102-4, *Essentials of Plastic Surgery*, second edition). The key aspect when marking is to ensure that sufficient excess will be removed anteriorly and laterally, where the patient can most easily see the result. It is important to ensure the posterior excision is not overdone, because this will lead to tension at the point of closure.

In massive-weight-loss patients, the anterior horizontal markings will differ from those for a standard abdominoplasty. The lower incision should be lower to correct mons pubis ptosis. The upper incision may be higher than the abdominoplasty level because of the presence of excess tissue. It will continue away from the midline, oriented horizontally, and will not taper back toward the lower incision. Preoperative markings must be used as a guide and may require adjustment in the operating room.

PERFORMING A BELT LIPECTOMY

9. Which of the following is correct when performing a belt lipectomy in a massive-weight-loss patient?
   E. Incisions should be sited to place postoperative scars below the pelvic brim.

Scars should be placed to minimize their appearance in most undergarments and swimwear, and this can be achieved by designing them to lie below the pelvic brim. Patients undergoing belt lipectomy will need to be positioned in supine, prone, and lateral decubitus positions to achieve adequate access. Umbilical lengthening is not required; however, an umbilicoplasty (shortening) is required regardless of the contouring technique used, because the umbilical stalk will have become stretched and elongated during the period of excess weight gain and will not shrink with weight loss. Liposuction to the lateral thighs should be performed with release of the zones of adherence, in this case to facilitate lateral thigh elevation. The anterior resection is made at the level of the deep fascia, as per a standard abdominoplasty, but posteriorly the resection is limited to the level of superficial fascia, as this minimizes seroma formation. In addition, the level at which the posterior inferior flap is raised can affect buttock projection. In massive-weight-loss patients the buttocks are usually underprojected, so it is wise to elevate the posterior flap at the level of the superficial fascia to maximize the soft tissue volume maintained in this region.[1]

BREAST SURGERY AFTER MASSIVE WEIGHT LOSS

10. *For each of the patients described, select the best surgical option for management of their breasts after major weight loss.*
    A. *A patient has lost 98 pounds after gastric banding. Her breasts are flat and underfilled. She has notch-to-nipple distances of 29 cm on both sides and has a BMI of 26.*
       d. **Augmentation-mastopexy**
          The patient in this scenario needs additional volume for her breasts, but is likely to be fairly slim following her weight loss. She is unlikely to have sufficient autologous tissue to augment her breasts and will therefore need prosthetic augmentation. Her notch-to-nipple distances are large and should be reduced. This requires skin excision in the form of a mastopexy. The best procedure for this patient is therefore a combined augmentation-mastopexy.
    B. *A patient has lost 42 pounds with diet and exercise. Her BMI is now 23. Her breasts measure an A cup and she has notch-to-nipple distances of 22 cm.*
       a. **Augmentation only**
          The patient in this scenario has a modest weight loss and is slim. Her breasts are not ptotic but are just underfilled. She should have an augmentation procedure only.
    C. *A patient has had body contouring surgery to the trunk after massive weight loss, but still has concerns regarding her breasts which are ptotic and empty. On examination, she has notch-to-nipple distances of 28 cm with grade III ptosis and a significant lateral soft tissue excess passing from the breast toward the axillae. Her BMI is 33.*
       e. **Autoaugmentation**
          The patient in this scenario requires additional breast volume and an uplift procedure with skin resection. She remains obese and has excess lateral tissue in the upper trunk which can be used to autoaugment her breasts (see Fig. 102-6, *Essentials of Plastic Surgery,* second edition).

COMPLICATIONS AFTER MASSIVE-WEIGHT-LOSS SURGERY

11. You are discussing the risks of surgery with a patient who has reduced their BMI from 40 to 30 after bariatric surgery. *What is the most frequent complication after major body contouring surgery?*
    E. **Wound dehiscence**
       There are a number of common complications that can occur in patients undergoing body contouring in massive-weight-loss surgery and many of these relate to the wounds themselves. The most common complication is wound dehiscence (22% to 30%), and this may be due to

excess tension across the wounds and the extent of the wounds. Most of the time this is self-limiting and will heal with prolonged wound care. Other complications include wound infection (1% to 7%) and skin necrosis (6% to 10%). The latter will obviously contribute to wound dehiscence. Patients are also at risk of venous thromboembolism (1%) and this is affected by BMI and procedure type. Prophylaxis is recommended with low-molecular-weight heparin shortly after surgery and continued for 7 days. Calf-compression garments should be used intraoperatively. Hematomas occur in 1% to 5% of cases following body contouring surgery and are most often seen in the early phase.

REFERENCE

1. Aly AS, Cram AE. Body lift: belt lipectomy. In Nahai F, ed. The Art of Aesthetic Surgery: Principles & Techniques, ed 2. St Louis: Quality Medical Publishing, 2011.

Credits

Chapter 7
Box 7-1 Data from Cendales LC, Kanitakis J, Schneeberger S, et al. The Banff 2007 working classification of skin-containing composite tissue allograft pathology. Am J Transplant 8:1396-1400, 2008.

Chapter 15
Tables 15-1 and 15-2 Data from Coit D, Andtbacka R, Anker C, et al. NCCN Guidelines: Clinical Practice Guidelines in Oncology: Melanoma Version 2.2013.

Chapter 32
Fig. 32-1 through 32-3 From Marcus JR, Erdmann D, Rodriguez ED, eds. Essentials of Craniomaxillofacial Trauma. St Louis: CRC Press, 2012.

Chapter 33
Box 33-1 Data from Edge SB, Byrd DR, Compton CC, et al, eds. American Joint Committee on Cancer Staging Handbook, ed 7. New York: Springer, 2010.

Chapter 36
Fig. 36-1 From Zenn MR, Jones G, eds. Reconstructive Surgery: Anatomy, Technique, and Clinical Applications. St Louis: CRC Press, 2012.

Fig. 36-2 From Jackson IT. Local Flaps in Head and Neck Reconstruction. St Louis: CRC Press, 2007.

Chapter 37
Fig. 37-1 From Zide BM. Deformities of the lips and cheeks. In McCarthy JR, ed. Plastic Surgery. Philadelphia: WB Saunders, 1990.

Chapter 39
Fig. 39-1 From Zenn MR, Jones G, eds. Reconstructive Surgery: Anatomy, Technique, and Clinical Applications. St Louis: CRC Press, 2012.

Fig. 39-2 From Jackson IT. Local Flaps in Head and Neck Reconstruction. St Louis: CRC Press, 2007.

Chapter 40
Fig. 40-1 From Zenn MR, Jones G, eds. Reconstructive Surgery: Anatomy, Technique, and Clinical Applications. St Louis: CRC Press, 2012.

Chapter 46
Fig. 46-1 Data from Kirwan L. Augmentation of the ptotic breast: simultaneous periareolar mastopexy/breast augmentation. Aesthet Surg J 19:34-39, 1999.

Chapter 48
Fig. 48-1 From Hall-Findley EJ. Aesthetic Breast Surgery: Concepts & Techniques. St Louis: CRC Press, 2011.

Chapter 54
Fig. 54-1 Data from Cordeiro PG, Pusic AL, Disa JJ. A classification system and reconstructive algorithm for acquired vaginal defects. Plast Reconstr Surg 110:1058, 2002.

Chapter 59
Fig. 59-3 From Rosenwasser M, Miyasajsa K, Strauch R. The RASL procedure: reduction and association of the scaphoid and lunate using the Herbert screw. Tech Hand U Extrem Surg 1:263-272, 1997.

Chapter 61
Table 61-1 Data from Swanson AB. A classification for congenital limb malformations. J Hand Surg Am 1:8-22, 1976.

Chapter 65
Fig. 65-3 From Rizzo M. Hand Surgery. New York: Springer, 2001. With kind permission from Springer Science and Business Media.

Chapter 67
Fig. 67-2 Modified from Green DP, Hotchkiss RN, Pederson WC, eds. Green's Operative Hand Surgery, ed 4. Philadelphia: Churchill Livingstone, 1999.

Chapter 73
Fig. 73-1 Data from Sebastin SJ, Chung KC. A systematic review of the outcomes of replantation of distal digital amputation. Plast Reconstr Surg 128:723-737, 2011.

Chapter 76
Fig. 76-1 From Zenn MR, Jones G, eds. Reconstructive Surgery: Anatomy, Technique, and Clinical Applications. St Louis: CRC Press, 2012.

Chapter 80
Fig. 80-1 From Brandt KE, Mackinnon SE. Microsugical repair of peripheral nerves and nerve grafts. In Aston JS, Beasley RW, Thorne CHM, eds. Grabb and Smith's Plastic Surgery, ed 6. Philadelphia: Lippincott, 1997; http://www.lww.com/Product/9781451109559.

Table 80-1 Data from Gutowski KA. Hand II: Peripheral nerve and tendon transfers. Sel Read Plast Surg 9:1-19, 2003.

Chapter 85
Table 85-1 Data from Eaton RG, Glickel SZ. Trapeziometacarpal arthritis: staging as a rationale for treatment. Hand Clin 3:455-471, 1987.

Chapter 87
Fig. 87-1 Data from Bashour M. History and current concepts in the analysis of facial attractiveness. Plast Reconstr Surg 118:741-756, 2006.

Figs. 87-2 through 87-6 From Gunter JP, Rohrich RJ, Adams WP Jr. Dallas Rhinoplasty: Nasal Surgery by the Masters. St Louis: CRC Press, 2002.

Chapter 88
Fig. 88-1 Data from Carruthers J, Fagien S, Matarasso SL; Botox Consensus Group. Consensus recommendations on the use of botulinum toxin type a in facial aesthetics. Plast Reconstr Surg 114(Suppl 6):S1-S22, 2004.

Chapter 90
Fig. 90-1 From Norwood OT. Male pattern baldness: classification and incidence. South Med J 68:1359-1365, 1975.

Chapter 91
Fig. 91-1 and 91-2 Data from Carruthers J, Fagien S, Matarasso SL: Botox Consensus Group. Consensus recommendations on the use of botulinum toxin type a in facial aesthetics. Plast Reconstr Surg 114(Suppl 6):S1-S22, 2004.

Fig. 91-3 From Nahai F, ed. The Art of Aesthetic Surgery: Principles & Techniques, ed 2. St Louis: CRC Press, 2011.

Chapter 93
Fig. 93-1 From McCord CD Jr, Codner MA. Eyelid & Periorbital Surgery. St Louis: CRC Press, 2008.

Fig. 93-2 From Marsh J, Perlyn C. Decision Making in Plastic Surgery. St Louis: CRC Press, 2010.

Chapter 97
Fig. 97-1 From Gunter JP, Rohrich RJ, Adams WP Jr. Dallas Rhinoplasty: Nasal Surgery by the Masters. St Louis: CRC Press, 2002.

Chapter 100
Fig. 100-1 Data from Huger WE Jr. The anatomic rationale for abdominal lipectomy. Am Surg 45:612-617, 1979.

Chapter 102
Fig. 102-1 From Aly A. Body Contouring After Massive Weight Loss. St Louis: CRC Press, 2006.

Index

A

Abbé flap, 316, 317, 318
Abdominal wall, anterior, anatomy of, 430
Abdominal wall reconstruction, 70, 430-434
Abdominoplasty, 98, 839, 855-862
Abductor digiti minimi tendon transfer, 585
Abductor pollicis brevis, 489
Ablative resurfacing; *see also* Laser therapy
  Er:YAG laser in, 82-83, 731
  target chromophore in, 80
Acellular dermal matrix (ADM), 67, 69
  in abdominal wall reconstruction, 432, 433
  in breast reconstruction, 407
Acetazolamide, 779
Achilles tendon exposure repair, 68
Acinic cell carcinoma, 270
Acoustic neuroma, 341
Actinic damage, 730
Actinic keratosis, 127
Action potentials, in local anesthesia, 88
Adductor longus, 868
Adductor pollicis, 495
Adenoid cystic carcinoma, 271
Adenoidectomy, velopharyngeal dysfunction and, 209
Adipocytes, 743
Adolescents, gynecomastia in, 395
Advanced Trauma and Life Support (ATLS), in burn patients, 134
Advancement flaps, 31
Adventitia, in microvascular manipulation, 59
Affricates, 209
Afrin, 204
Age, and burn prognosis, 132
Aging
  facial, 797
  photoaging, 717, 730

Airway
  in Pierre Robin sequence, 202
  in Treacher Collins syndrome, 181
Alar contour graft, 290
Alar-facial angle, in cleft lip, 192
Alar rim deformities, 822
Alar spreader graft, 290, 291, 820
Albumin levels, 15
Alexandrite, 82
Allen's test, 621
Allergies, local anesthetic, 89
AlloDerm, 17, 67
Allografts
  defined, 51
  materials for, 67-68
  rejection of, 52
  vascularized composite, 52, 54
Alloplastic materials, 70, 431-432
Alloplasts, 66
Alopecia, 751, 753-754
Alopecia areata, 753
Alpha-hydroxy acid peels (AHA), 735
Alveolar bone graft, 66
Amblyopia, 784
American Society of Anesthesiologists (ASA) patient classification, 88
Amides, 89
Amputation
  complications following, 592
  digital, 591, 597-598
  forearm, 592
  hand, 606-609
  preservation after, 598-599
  ray, 591-592
  wrist, 592
Anastomosis
  end-to-side, 59, 60
  microvascular
    backwalling of, 59
    clamp pressure in, 58
    size discrepancy in, 59
Androgenic alopecia, 753; *see also* Male pattern baldness
Anesthesia; *see also* Local anesthesia
  ASA patient classification, 88
  techniques, 92

Aneurysm
  traumatic, 708
  ulnar artery, 642-643, 680
  upper limb, 708
Animal bites, 671
Ankle-brachial pressure test, 16
Anotia, 216
Anterior chest wall muscles, 359-360
Anterior ethmoid nerve, 818
Anterior interosseous syndrome, 640-641
Anterior rectus sheath, 430
Anterior tibial nerve, 631-632
Anterolateral thigh flap (ALT), 29, 37-38
  in cheek reconstruction, 301
  in head and neck cancer reconstruction, 334-335
Antia-Buch flap, 309
Antibiotics
  in abdominoplasty, 859
  in bite wounds, 228
  in burn patients, 136-137
Anticoagulants, in microsurgery, 61
Antihelix, 722
Apert syndrome, 174-175, 203
Apligraf, 17, 68, 69
Aponeurotic layer, of scalp, 275
Appositional growth, of cranium, 170
Arcade of Frohse, 638
Arch bars, 259-260
Arcuate line, 430, 856
Arm flap, lateral, 29
Artefill, 737
Arterial emboli, 708
Arterial insufficiency, 470, 601
Arteriovenous malformation (AVM), 144, 709-710
Arthritis; *see also* Rheumatoid arthritis (RA)
  degenerative, in scaphoid fracture, 512
  osteoarthritis, 696, 700-703
  psoriatic, 696
  septic, 671
Arthroscopy, of wrist, 518

883

884　Index

Asian eyelids, 776
Aspirin, 33
Atasoy flaps, 547, 619
Augmentation-mastopexy, 380-381
Aural atresia, 215-216
Auricular appendages, 182
Auriculotemporal nerve, 165, 222, 798
Autografts; see also Bone grafts; Skin graft
　advantages of, 66
　bone, 69, 70
　defined, 51
Axillary nodes, 360

B

Backwalling, of microvascular anastomosis, 59
Baker classification, 367
Ballistic trauma, in face transplantation, 349
Banff grading, 52-53, 352
Bannayan-Zonana syndrome, 143
Bariatric surgery, 875-877
Barrel distortion, 97
Basal cell carcinoma (BCC), 116-119
Battle's sign, 243
Baux score, 132
Becker's nevus, 149
Bell flap, 412, 413
Bell's palsy, 342, 343, 817-818
Bell's phenomenon, 777
Belotero Balance, 738
Belt lipectomy, 878-879
Bier block, 92
Bilateral sagittal split osteotomy (BSSO), 260
Biliopancreatic diversion, 876, 877
Biobrane, 17, 68
Biofilms, 672
Biomaterials, principles of, 66
Bite wounds, 228, 308, 565, 576, 670-671
Bleomycin, for hemangioma, 141
Blepharochalasis, 776
Blepharophimosis syndrome, 783
Blepharoplasty
　anatomy in, 773-775
　complications after, 779
　lacrimal glandulopexy in, 777
　negative vector globe position in, 776-777
　preoperative assessment in, 776
　techniques, 778-779

Blepharoptosis, 783-788
Blindness, face transplantation and, 350
Blood loss, in burn excision, 135-136
Blood sugar, abdominal wall reconstruction and, 431
Body contouring, 838, 839, 877-880; see also Abdominoplasty
Body mass index (BMI), 875
Body views, 98
Bone anchors
　in central slip injuries, 577-578
　in flexor tendon repair, 564
Bone autografts, 69
Bone biopsy, 448
Bone grafts
　cortical versus cancellous, 69
　in mandibular reconstruction, 323
　in thumb reconstruction, 614
Bone lesions, benign, 679
Bone substitutes, synthetic, 70
Bony orbit anatomy, 238
Boot strap distribution, 461
Botulinum toxin
　in brachial plexus birth palsy, 652-653
　in facial rejuvenation, 736, 738, 762
　for glabellar rhytids, 761-762
　for migraines, 164-165
Bowen's disease, 126
Brachial plexus
　anatomy, 648
　assessment of injury to, 650
　electrophysiologic testing in, 651
　Erb's point, injury at, 648-649
　grading muscle power in injury to, 650-651
　mechanism of injury in, 650
　obstetric injury to, 649
　peripheral nerve branches from, 648
Brachial plexus birth palsy, 652-653
Brachioplasty, 844-848
Brachydactyly, 503
Braden scale, 446
Branchial arches, 155-156
Branchial grooves, 156
Branchial pouches, 157
Branchial sinus tracts, 156
Brava system, 746
BRCA genes, 402

Breast aesthetics, 360-361, 386
Breast anatomy, 358-359
Breast augmentation, 365-369; see also Augmentation-mastopexy
Breast cancer
　lymphedema in, 477
　in males, 396
　risk factors, 402
　staging, 403
　statistics, 402
Breast conservation therapy, 403
Breast development, 358
Breast embryology, 358
Breast hypertrophy, 387
Breast innervation, 359
Breast lymphatics, 360
Breast ptosis, 373-377
Breast reconstruction
　expanders in, 45, 47
　fat grafting in, 743-744
　implant-based, 404
　photography in, 99
　after weight loss, 879
Breast reduction, 60, 386-390
Breast rejuvenation, 380-381
Breast vasculature, 359
Brent technique, 217
Breslow thickness (BT), in melanoma, 121
Brow aesthetics, 763-764
Brow anatomy, 761-763
Brow lift
　botulinum toxin in, 761-762
　endoscopic, 765-766
　facial palsy and, 344
　postoperative complications after, 766-767
　sentinel vein in, 763
　surgical approaches to, 765-767
Buccal block, 258
Buccal branch, 798
Buccinator, 341
Buddy taping, 543
Buerger's disease, 711
Bupivacaine, 89-90, 91
Burn center, 133
Burns
　acute management of, 133-134
　Advanced Trauma and Life Support approach in, 134
　autologous skin grafts in, 66-67
　blistering in, 132
　blood loss in excision of, 135-136

Index

chemical, 134
degrees of, 107, 132
dressing of, 68
electrical, 133
extent estimation in, 135
histology in, 132
nutritional support with, 136
operative management of, 135-136
prognosis in severe, 132
resuscitation in, 134
sepsis with, 137
skin substitutes in, 17, 68
topical antimicrobials in, 136-137
zones in, 132
Burow's triangle, 30-31
Byrd classification, 456

C

Café au lait spots, 148
Calcium channel blockers, 33
Calvarial reconstruction, 70, 277
Cam effect, of metacarpophalangeal joint, 540
Camitz procedure, 585
Camptodactyly, 504, 505
Candida albicans, 673
Canthal elevation, 181-182
Canthoplasty, 345
Cantilever graft, 290
Capillary malformation, 81
Capitate fracture, 513
Caprosyn, 24
Capsular contracture, 367
Capsulopalpebral fascia, 774
Carotid bifurcation, 265
Carotid-cavernous fistula, traumatic, 241
Carpal bone fractures, 512-513
Carpal boss, 680
Carpal instability, 516, 517, 518
Carpal tunnel syndrome (CTS), 489, 496, 585, 639-640, 695
Carpometacarpal joint, in osteoarthritis, 701-702
Cartilage, hyaline, 108
Cartilage autografts, 70
Casting, contact, 468
Cat bites, 671
Cauliflower ear, 308
Central blocks, 92
Central retinal artery occlusion, 241
Central slip injuries, 577-578

Cephalic vein, in breast reconstruction, 406
Cerebrospinal fluid leak, in facial trauma, 241-242
Cervical branch, 798-799
Cervical plexus, 307
Cervical sinus, 156
Cervicofacial flap reconstruction, 300, 301
C flap, 194
Champy system, 248
Charles procedure, 476
Cheek reconstruction, 299-303
Chemical peels, 734-736
Chemotherapy, wound healing and, 11
Chest wall anatomy, 422
Chest wall deformity, in ear reconstruction, 218
Chest wall reconstruction, 423-426
Chin, 827-829
Chondrodermatitis nodularis helicis (CDNH), 308-309
Chondrosarcoma, 680
Chongchet technique, 224-225
Chromophores
 in facial rejuvenation, 731
 target, 80
Chronologic aging, 730-731
Circumflex scapular artery, 623
Cisplatin, in melanoma, 123-124
Cleft, craniofacial, 180-182;
 see also Distraction osteogenesis (DO)
Cleft hand, 506
Cleft lip
 alar-facial angle in, 192
 anatomy, 191
 demographics of, 191
 familial recurrence of, 192
 lip adhesion for, 193
 risk, 201
 timing of repair of, 193
 tip rhinoplasty in, 193
 types of repair of, 194
 whistle tip deformity in, 195
Cleft nasal deformity, 192
Cleft palate
 bifid uvula in, 201
 demographics of, 201
 environmental risk factors in, 203
 familial recurrence of, 192
 feeding of infants with, 193
 fistulas after repair of, 205

isolated, 202, 210
risk, 201, 202, 203
speech in, 210
submucous, 200-201
subtypes, 202
surgical repair of, 203-205
syndromic, 203
Cleland's ligament, 485, 684
Cleveland Clinic FACES scoring system, 350, 351
Clinodactyly, 505, 507
Closed reduction, of hand fractures, 530-531
Clostridium perfringens, 672
Cobblestone ectasia, 143
Coleman technique, in fat processing, 745
Collagen
 in aging, 730-731
 in negative pressure wound therapy, 74
 subtypes, in skin, 6-7, 108
 in wound healing, 7
Collagenase injection, for Dupuytren's disease, 685
Colles' fascia, 867
Colles' fracture, 522, 523
Colobomas, 180
Compartment syndromes
 in anterior compartment of lower leg, 628
 delayed presentation of, 630
 fasciotomy in, 629-630, 630-631
 in foot, 632-633
 in forearm, 628-629
 in lower extremity reconstruction, 460
 pressure in, 628
 six Ps in, 629
Complete decongestive therapy, 476
Component separation, in abdominal wall reconstruction, 432-433
Composite conchal bowl graft, 293
Composite grafting, in fingertip, 550
Composite mesh, in abdominal wall reconstruction, 70
Compression bandaging, 461
Computer-aided design, in mandibular reconstruction, 325
Conchoscaphal angle, 223

886 Index

Congenital unilateral lower lip palsy (CULLP), 343
Consent
 in abdominoplasty, 857
 for photography, 99
Constriction band syndrome, 506
Contact casting, 468
Contact inhibition, 8
Cooper's ligaments, 358-359, 374
Coronal synostosis, 172, 173
Corrugator supercilii, 342, 761
Cortical ring sign, 516
Counseling, patient, in breast augmentation, 368-369
C-Qur, 70
Cranial growth and development, 170
Cranial nerve foramina, 254
Cranial nerve relations, 254-255
Cranial sutures, 170, 171-172
Craniofacial embryology, 180
Craniosynostoses, 171-174
Creatinine phosphokinase (CPK), in compartment syndrome, 630
Creep, tissue, 44
Cricopharyngeal myotomy, 271
Cross-finger flap, 612
Cross-hatching, in fat graft injection, 746
Cross-linking, in acellular dermal matrix, 67
Croton oil, 735
Crouzon syndrome, 174, 203
Cryotherapy, for basal cell carcinoma, 118
Cubital tunnel syndrome, 643
Cultured epidermal autografts (CEA), 66-67
Curreri formula, 136
Cutis hyperelastica, 108
Cutis laxa, 9, 108
C-V flap, 414-415

D

Dacarbazine, in melanoma, 123-124
Daclizumab, 53
Dakin's solution, 449
"Dancing breasts," 366
Darrach procedure, 695
Darwin's tubercle, 225
Debridement
 of chronic wound, 10
 of diabetic foot ulcers, 469
 permanent tattooing and, 228
 of pressure sores, 449

Deep circumflex iliac artery flap, 323-324
Deep inferior epigastric artery perforator flap (DIEP), 29, 33-34, 38-39, 324, 433
Deep space abscess, in hand, 669-670
Deep temporal fascia, 795
Deformational plagiocephaly, 173-174
Degenerative arthritis, 512
Dellon's modification, 548
Deltopectoral flap, 302
Dental show, 800-801
Dental terminology, 256
Dentoalveolar fractures, 242
Depressor labii inferioris, 342
Depressor septi nasi, 818
de Quervain's tenosynovitis, 496
Dermagraft, 68
Dermis, 106-107
Dermoid cyst, 677
Dexon, 23, 24
Dextran, 32-33
Diabetic foot ulcers, 466-470
Diabetic patients
 epinephrine in local anesthesia in, 91
 wound healing and, 15
Digastric muscles, 155, 808
Digastric transfer, in facial nerve injury, 346
Digital amputation, 591, 597-598
Digital extensor tendon anatomy, 574-575
Digital replantation, 58, 597-601
Distal interphalangeal (DIP) joint, osteoarthritis in, 703
Distraction osteogenesis (DO), 186-187
Diver's test, 856
Diver's view, 98
Dog bite, 308, 671
Dog-ears, 858
Donor, transplantation, 54
Doppler ultrasound
 implantable, in buried free flap monitoring, 60
 in perforator flap design, 39
Dorsal intercalated segment instability (DISI), 516
Dorsal metacarpal artery flap, 551
Dorsal scapular nerve, 648
Double crush syndrome, 658
Drains, in breast reduction, 390
Dual plane breast implant placement, 366

Duane's syndrome, 783
Duodenal switch, 876
Dupuytren's disease, 683-686

E

Ear
 aesthetics, 222-223, 308
 anatomy, 307
 cauliflower, 308
 in facial analysis, 722-723
 height, 308
 innervation to, 222
 keloid scarring to, 308-309
 in microtia, 215-218
 normal, 222
 prominent, 223-225
 replantation, 310-311
 squamous cell carcinoma in, 119
 vascularity of, 222
Ear lobule, in facial analysis, 720
Ear reconstruction, 182, 216-218, 309-311
Ecchymosis, in mandibular fracture, 247
Eccrine sweat glands, 106
Ectoderm, 155
Ectropion, 776-777
Ehlers-Danlos syndrome, 108
Eikenella, 228
Eklund view, 368
Elasticity, of sutures, 21
Elbow, ulnar nerve compression at, 642
Elbow soft tissue coverage, 622
Eloesser flap, 423
Emboli, arterial, 708
Embolization, of arteriovenous malformation, 144
Embryology, 155
 breast, 358
 craniofacial, 180
 genitourinary, 438
 of lymphatic system, 474
 of microtia, 215
 of palate, 200
EMLA, 92
Encapsulation, with silicone, 71
Encephaloceles, 180
Enchondroma, 679
Endoderm, 155
Endoneurium, 657
End-to-side anastomosis, 59, 60
Epicel, 67
Epidermal growth factor, in wound healing, 8
Epidermal layers, 107

Epinephrine
  in diabetic patients, 91
  disadvantages of, 90-91
  in liposuction, 834, 836
Epineural repair, 661
Epispadias, 441
Epitendinous suture, 563
Epithelialization, 8
Eponychium, 556
Erb-Duchenne palsy, 651-652
Erb's point, 648-649
Eruption sequence, 256
Erythroplakia, 126-127
Erythroplasia of Queyrat, 126
Esters, 89
Estlander flap, 316, 317
Etanercept, 694
Ethmoid fractures, 237-238
Evoked potentials, 651
Expanders
  advantages of, 45
  in breast reconstruction, 45, 47
  in cheek reconstruction, 300
  complications with, 47
  crescentic, 45
  in fat grafting, 746
  in leg, 47
  in nasal reconstruction, 46
  permanent, in breast
    reconstruction, 45
  planning with, 45
  puncture of, 47
  in scalp reconstruction, 277
  silicone elastomer shell in, 44
  skin blanching and, 45-46
  soft tissue and, 44
  subtypes of, 44
  tissue availability after use
    of, 46
  in tuberous breast deformity,
    375
Extensor anatomy, 573
Extensor carpi radialis tendon,
  573
Extensor carpi ulnaris tendon, 573
Extensor compartments, 573-574
Extensor digiti communis, 486,
  495
Extensor digiti communis tendon,
  578
Extensor indicis proprius, 486
Extensor indicis proprius tendon,
  in pollicization, 614
Extensor pollicis brevis tendon,
  573
Extensor pollicis longus tendon,
  573, 614

Extensor tenolysis, 579
External oblique aponeurosis, 430
Eyebrow; see Brow
Eyelashes, in lymphedema, 475
Eyelid
  anatomy, 282, 773-775
  Asian, 776
  blood supply, 283
  in facial analysis, 721
  fat compartments of, 775
  gold weight insertion in, 344
  muscles, 773
  ptosis, 783-784
  reconstruction, 283-284
  retractors, 282
  shortening procedure, 345
Eye width, 721

F

Face lift
  complications, 801-802
  deep temporal fascia in, 795
  facial palsy and, 800
  hematoma in, 801-802
  incision placement in, 799
  minimal access cranial
    suspension, 799-800
  motor deficits after, 798-799
  photography for, 97
  sensory deficits after, 798
  smoking and, 801
  stigmata of, 802
  superficial muscular
    aponeurotic system in,
    794, 795, 799
  techniques, 799-800
Face transplantation, 52, 349-352
Facial aging, 797
Facial analysis
  brow in, 763-764
  ear in, 722-723
  Fibonacci ratio in, 717-718
  frontal view in, 719-720
  lateral view in, 720
  nose in, 721-722
  skin quality in, 717
  upper eyelid in, 721
Facial artery myomucosal flap
  (FAMM), 300, 301
Facial canons, 718-719
Facial ductal anatomy, 229-230
Facial expression muscles, 156
Facial fat compartments, 796
Facial implants alloplastic, 70
Facial ligaments, 796, 797
Facial musculature, 341-342
Facial nerve anatomy, 340-341

Facial nerve function grading, 343
Facial nerve graft, 345
Facial nerve palsy, 340
Facial proportions, 721
Facial rejuvenation; see also
  Face lift
  botulinum toxin in, 736, 738
  chemical peels in, 734-736
  chromophores in, 731
  face lift in, 787-802
  fillers in, 737-739
  fractional photothermolysis in,
    731, 732
  intense pulsed light in, 734
  laser therapy in, 82-83,
    731-734
Facial skeletal trauma, 236-243
Facial soft tissue layers, 794-795
Facial soft tissue trauma, 228-230
Facial wrinkles, acellular dermal
  matrix for, 69
Fasanella-Servat procedure,
  786-787
Fascicular repair, 661
Fasciofascial suspension, 871
Fasciotomy
  in compartment syndrome,
    629-630, 630-631
  in Dupuytren's disease, 686
  in electrical burns, 133
  leg, 630-631
Fat grafting
  benefits of, 744
  in breast reconstruction,
    743-744
  fat necrosis in, 747
  harvesting in, 744-745
  indications for, 743-744
  injection in, 746
  postoperative care for, 746-747
  principles of, 743
  processing in, 745-746
Feeding, in cleft palate, 193
Femoral triangle, 868
Fetal sexual differentiation, 438
Fetal tissue, wound healing in, 6
Fibonacci ratio, 717-718
Fibroblast
  neonatal, in skin substitutes, 68
  in wound healing, 6, 7-8
Fibroproliferative phase, in wound
  healing, 6
Fibrous encapsulation, with
  silicone, 44
Fibular fracture, 456
Fibular osseocutaneous flap, 323
"Fight bite," 576, 670-671

Filariasis, 474
Fillers, 737-739
Finasteride, 754
Fingertip
 abnormalities, 677-678
 anatomy, 547
 homodigital flaps for, 547-549, 619-620
 regional flaps for, 549
Finkelstein's test, 496
First dorsal metacarpal artery perforator flap, 548
First web space, in thumb reconstruction, 613-614
Fishtail flap, 414
Fistula, palatal, 205
Fitzpatrick classification, 717, 730
Flaps
 arterial versus venous occlusion in, 33-34
 blood supply to, 29
 clinical observation of, 34
 delay, 32
 failure of, 60-61
 heparin and, 32-33
 monitoring of, 33-34, 60
 muscle, classification of, 30
 pharmacologic influences on survival of, 32-33
 surface temperature of, 33-34
 vasoconstrictor for, 32
Flash, in photography, 96
Flexion creases, incisions crossing, 668
Flexor carpi ulnaris flap, 622
Flexor digitorum profundus, 495
Flexor digitorum profundus tendon, 562, 564
Flexor digitorum superficialis, 488, 640
Flexor hallucis flap, 458-459
Flexor pollicis longus, 488, 562, 628-629
Flexor pollicis longus tendon, 567
Flexor tendon repair, 563-567
Flexor tenosynovitis, 670
Flip-flap technique, 441
Fluid resuscitation, in liposuction, 838
Focal length, 96
Follicular unit extraction, 755
Fontanelles, closure of, 170
Foot compartment syndrome, 632-633
Foot ulcers, 466-470
Foramen ovale, 254

Forearm amputation, 592
Forearm compartments, 628-629
Forehead anatomy, 761-763
Forehead rhytids, 762
Foucher flap, 551
Fournier's gangrene, 442
Fractional photothermolysis, 731, 732
Fractures
 capitate, 513
 carpal bone, 512-513
 comminuted, 529
 ethmoid, 237-238
 facial, 236-243
 fibular, 456
 frontal sinus, 236-237
 hamate, 512
 healing of, 530
 hook of hamate, 513
 lunate, 513
 mandibular, 246-249
 maxillary, 239-240, 242
 metacarpal, 530-531, 531-532
 nasal, 238
 orbital, 239
 panfacial, 240
 phalangeal, 533-535
 radius, distal, 522-524, 578
 scaphoid, 511-512
 temporal bone, 240, 243
 terminology, 529
 tibial
  end-to-side anastomosis in, 60
  Gustilo classification for, 455
  reduction and stabilization of, 456-457
 trapezoid, 513
 zygomatic, 243
 zygomaticomaxillary complex, 239
Frankfort plane, 97
Frank's technique, 439
Free anterolateral thigh flap, 301
Free flap breast reconstruction, 406
Free flap failure, 60-61
Free flap monitoring, 60
Free jejunum flap, 334
Free tissue transfer, 58-59
Free toe transfer, in thumb reconstruction, 612-613, 614-615
Fricatives, 209
Fricke flap, 284

Froment-Rauber anastomosis, 658
Frontal bone fracture, 236
Frontal sinus fractures, 236-237
Frontal view, 719-720
Frontalis muscle, 761, 762
Frontalis suspension, 787
Frontonasal prominence, 157-158, 180
Frontotemporal flap, 292
Full-thickness skin graft, in hand, 619
Furlow flaps, 547
Furlow's double-opposing technique, 203
Furnas technique, 223, 224-225

G

Galeal sheath, 761
Gamekeeper's thumb, 541-542
Ganglion cysts, 677
Gangrene, 442, 672
Gas gangrene, 672
Gastric banding, 875, 876, 877
Gastric bypass, 875, 877
Genioplasty, 827-829
Genitourinary embryology, 438
Giant cell nevus, 147, 148
Giant cell tumor, of tendon sheath, 677
Gibson's principle, 224-225
Gigantomastia, 387
Gillies strut technique, 290
Glabellar flap, 293
Glabellar rhytids, 761-762
Glabrous graft, 619
Glandular ptosis, 373
Glomus tumors, 710, 711
Glucose levels, wound healing and, 15
Glycolide suture, 24
Goldenhar's syndrome, 182
Gore-Tex, 70
Gorlin's syndrome, 116-117, 126
Gracilis muscle flap, 440, 459, 623
Grafts; see Bone grafts; Fat grafting; Skin graft
Grayson's ligament, 485
Great auricular nerve, 222, 798
Greater occipital nerve, 163-164, 165-166
Greater palatine artery, 200
Great toe transfer, in thumb reconstruction, 615
Groin flap, 29, 624

Groin flap, in fingertip
  reconstruction, 551
Ground substance, 107
Group fascicular repair, 61
Growth factors, in wound healing,
  7-8
Gustilo classification, 449
Guyon's canal, 642-643
Gynecomastia, 395-397

H

Hair anatomy, 751
Hair density, 754
Hair growth, 751
Hair removal, in laser therapy,
  80, 82
Hair transplantation, 755-757
Hall-Findlay technique, 375
Halo nevus, 148
Hamate fracture, 512
Hand; see also Rheumatoid
    arthritis (RA)
  amputation, 606-609
  arterial supply to, 488-489
  autoimmune diseases affecting,
    696
  cleft, 506
  clinical joint evaluation in, 540
  deep fascial spaces in, 485-486
  Dupuytren's disease in,
    683-686
  embryology, 502
  extrinsic extensors in, 486-487
  extrinsic flexors in, 488
  flap reconstruction of, 621-622
  infections, 668-673
  innervation of, 489-490
  intrinsic muscles of, 574
  motor function examination
    in, 495
  range of motion of, 494
  retinacular system in, 485
  skin grafts on, 619
  vascular disorders of, 708-711
Hand transplantation, 606-609
Harlequin deformity, 173
Harvesting
  of fat grafts, 744-745
  in hair transplantation, 755
Head, development of, 157
Head and neck cancer
  examination in, 265
  human papillomavirus in,
    331-332
  minimally invasive surgery
    for, 333

referred otalgia in, 331
  tumor staging in, 266-269
  tumor types in, 265
Health Insurance Portability
    and Accountability Act
    (HIPAA), 99
Hearing, in microtia, 215-216
Helical rim, in prominent ear, 223
Helix tumors, 307-308
Hemangiomas, 141-142, 709
Hematoma
  in breast reduction, 390
  in face lift, 801-802
Hemifacial spasm, 343
Hemi-tongue flap, 300-301
Heparin, 32-33, 61, 708
Hepatitis A, hand transplantation
    and, 606
Hering's law, 787
Hernia grading, 430-431
Hernia repair, 433
High-pressure injection injuries,
    672
Hirudin, 33
Hitselberger's sign, 341
Homodigital flaps, 547-549,
    619-620
Hook-nail deformity, 558
Hook of hamate fracture, 513
House-Brackmann scale, 343
Human bite wound, 565
Human leukocyte antigen (HLA)
    molecules, 51
Human papilloma virus (HPV)
  in head and neck cancer,
    331-332
  squamous cell carcinoma
    and, 116
Hutchinson freckle, 121
Hutchinson-Gilford syndrome,
    108-109
Hyaline cartilage, 108
Hyaluronic acid (HA)
  in facial rejuvenation, 737, 739
  in ground substance, 107
Hyaluronidase, in skin graft donor
    site anesthesia, 90
Hydrofluoric acid burn, 134
Hynes pharyngoplasty, 211
Hyoid, 182, 330
Hyperacusis, 343
Hypermastia, 387
Hypernasality, in velopharyngeal
    dysfunction, 209
Hyponychium, 556
Hypopharyngeal anatomy, 331

Hypopharyngeal cancer, 332, 333
Hypopharyngeal reconstruction,
    334
Hypospadias, 440-441
Hypothenar hammer syndrome,
    710

I

Ibuprofen, in fracture healing, 530
Iliac crest free flap, 323-324
Immobilization, in diabetic foot,
    468
Immune suppression
  in hand transplantation, 608
  squamous cell carcinoma
    and, 119
Immune system, acquired, 51
Immunosuppression, 53-54
Implantable Doppler, 61
Implants, synthetic, 66, 70
Inclusion dermoid cyst, 677
Infants, hemangiomas in, 141
Infection
  hand, 668-673
  odontogenic, 259
  parapharyngeal space, 259
Inferior alveolar nerve block, 258
Inferior pole scoring, 375
Infiltration, in breast reduction,
    389
Inflammation
  suture materials and, 21
  in wound healing, 6
Informed consent, 857
Inframammary fold, 360, 365,
    374, 386
Inframammary fold wedge
    excision, 376
Infraorbital nerve block, 258
Injection, of fat grafts, 746
Injection injuries, 672
Integra, 68, 69
Intense pulsed light (IPL), 734
Intercanthal distance, 721
Intercostobrachial nerve, 361
Interior turbinate, 819
Internal intercostal muscles, 422
Internal mammary artery, 422
Internal maxillary artery, 236
Interphalangeal joint, in
    Dupuytren's disease, 685
Intracranial pressure (ICP)
  in Apert syndrome, 175
  in craniosynostoses, 171
  diagnosis of raised, 171
Intravelar veloplasty, 203

Inverted nipples, 415
Inverted-T breast reduction, 388-389
Ipilimumab, in melanoma, 125
Ischial tuberosity, pressure sore on, 446
Isograft, 51
Isotretinoin, in laser skin resurfacing, 83
Ivermectin, in secondary lymphedema, 478

J

Jahss maneuver, 530-531
Jessner's solution, 735
Joint fusion, in brachial plexus injury, 652
Joker's lines, 802
Jowls, 796
Jugular foramen, 254-255
Juncturae tendinum, 487
Juvéderm, 738
Juvenile virginal hypertrophy of breast, 387

K

Kanavel's signs, 670
Kaplan's line, 488-489
Karapandzic flap, 317, 318
Karnofsky stability score, 350, 351
Kasabach-Merritt syndrome, 142
Keloid, in lobule of ear, 308
Keloid scarring, 11-12, 308-309
Keratinocyte, 105
Keratoacanthoma, 126
Kienbock's disease, 513
Klinefelter's syndrome, 395
Klippel-Trenaunay syndrome, 143
Knee, soft tissue defects in, 459-460
Kocher's scars, 856
Krause end bulbs, 106
Kutler V-Y advancement, 547

L

Labyrinthine segment, of facial nerve, 340, 341
Lacrimal glandulopexy, 777
Lactiferous ducts, 358
Lagophthalmos, 784, 786
Lambdoid synostosis, 173
Lamella, in eyelid anatomy, 282
Landsmeer's ligament, 684
Langerhans cell, 105

Laryngeal muscles, 156
Laryngopharyngectomy, reconstruction after, 334-335
Laser-assisted liposuction, 837
Laser resurfacing, 731-734
Laser therapy
  alexandrite, 82
  carbon dioxide, 732, 733
  Er-YAG, 732, 733
  in facial rejuvenation, 82-83, 731-734
  for facial rhytids, 733-734
  in hair loss, 754
  hair removal in, 80, 82
  in hypertrophic scars, 82
  IPL, 82
  KTP, 80-81
  laser selection in, 80-81
  Nd:YAG, 81, 731
  pulsed dye, 82
  Q-switched Nd:YAG, 81
  safety with, 84
  skin resurfacing in, 83
  target chromophores in, 80
  vascular lesions in, 81
  wavelengths in, 83-84
Lassus technique, 375
Lateral arm flap, 623
Lateral canthoplasty, 778
Lateral circumflex femoral artery perforator flap, 39-40
Lateral crural strut graft, 291
Lateral nasal artery, 818
Lateral pedicle, in breast reduction, 388
Lateral sweep, 802
Lateral territory, of scalp, 275
Lateral view, 97, 99, 720
Latissimus dorsi flap, 99, 302, 405
Leddy type II tendon injury, 563
Leeches, 33
LeFort I fracture, 242
LeFort II fracture, 242
LeFort III fracture, 242
LeFort I osteotomy, 260
Leg; see also Lower limb
  compartments, 631-632
  fasciotomy, 630-631
  tissue expansion in, 47
Lejour technique, 375
Lesser occipital nerve, 798
Leukoplakia, 126-127
Levator advancement, 785-786
Levator anguli oris, 341

Levator aponeurosis advancement, 787
Levator dehiscence, 784-785
Levator labii alaeque nasi, 817-818
Levator palpebrae superioris, 774
Levator veli palatini, 156
Levobupivacaine, 89-90
Leydig cells, 438
L flap, 194
Lidocaine, 89, 92, 836
Lignocaine, 836
Linburg's anomaly, 565
Linguine sign, 368
Lip
  aging, 800-801
  anatomy, 315
  lower, 157
  reconstruction, 316-318
  upper, anatomy of, 191
Liposuction
  in abdominoplasty, 858
  in brachioplasty, 845-846
  cannula diameter in, 835-836
  fluid resuscitation in, 838
  in gynecomastia, 396
  history of, 834
  in lymphedema, 476
  in neck, 809
  in thigh lift, 868-869
  wetting solutions in, 836
Littler flap, 620
Local anesthesia
  action of, 88
  additives in, 90
  allergies, 89
  as amides, 89
  cardiotoxicity in, 91
  in diabetic patients, 91
  epinephrine in, 90-91
  as esters, 89
  safe dose selection of, 89
  in skin graft donor site, 90
  sodium bicarbonate in, 90
  techniques, 92
  topical, 92
  toxicity with, 91
Love's sign, 710
Lower lid pinch blepharoplasty, 778
Lower limb; see also Foot; Leg
  embryology, 502
  reconstruction, 458-461
Lower limb replantation, 599
Lumbrical plus, 550
Lumbricals, 574
Lunate dislocation, 517

Lunate fracture, 513
Lung cancer, 54
Lymphatic drainage, of breast, 360
Lymphatic malformations, 144
Lymphaticovenular bypass anastomoses, 476
Lymphatic physiology, 474
Lymphedema, 474-478, 846
Lymphedema tarda, 475
Lymphocytes, in wound healing, 6
Lymphoscintigraphy, 476

M

Macrodactyly, 503, 506
Macrophage, in wound healing, 6
Mafenide acetate, 136-137
Maffucci's syndrome, 141
Maggots, 469
Magnetic resonance angiography (MRA), 15-16, 210
Magnetic resonance imaging (MRI), in osteomyelitis, 448
Major histocompatibility complex (MHC) antigens, 51
Málaga technique, 439
Malar fat pad, 796
Male pattern baldness, 752-753, 754
Mallet deformities, 576-577, 578
Malocclusion, 257, 827
Mammography, 396
Mandible, 156
  anatomy, 246
  fracture, 246-249
  in panfacial fractures, 240
Mandibular distraction, 187
Mandibular ligament, 796
Mandibular nerve injury, 346
Mandibular prominence, 157-158
Mandibular reconstruction
  bone graft in, 323
  collapse in, 322
  computer-aided design in, 325
  soft tissue flaps for, 322-323
  vascularized bone flaps in, 322, 323-324
Mandibular reconstruction plates, 322
Mandibulocutaneous ligament, 808
Mannerfelt lesion, 694
Mannitol, 779
Marcus Gunn syndrome, 783
Marginal mandibular nerve, 807-808
Margination, 8

Marin-Amat syndrome, 783
Marionette lines, 796
Marlex, 70
Masseteric ligament, 796, 797
Mastectomy, 404
Mastication muscles, 156
Mastopexy, 373-377, 380-381
Maxilla, 156
Maxillary artery, 200
Maxillary fractures, 239-240, 242
Maxillary prominence, 157-158
Mayer-Rokitansky-Küster-Hauser syndrome, 438
Medial antebrachial cutaneous nerve, 844
Medial cord, 649
Medial femoral circumflex artery, 623
Medial gastrocnemius flap, 459
Median nerve
  in carpal tunnel syndrome, 639-640
  dysfunction, 638
  palsy, 585
  repair, 662
Medpor, 70
Meggitt-Wagner system, 467
Meissner's corpuscle, 105-106
Melanin, 80, 105
Melanoma
  acral-lentiginous, 120
  advanced, 125
  amelanotic, 126
  Breslow thickness in, 121
  cisplatin in, 123-124
  dacarbazine in, 123-124
  de novo development of, 121
  excision margins in, 124
  ipilimumab in, 125
  lifelong follow-up for, 125
  lymph node dissection in, 123
  in nail bed, 678
  nodular, 121
  nonsurgical management of, 123-124, 125
  prognosis, 121
  sentinel lymph node biopsy in, 123-124
  staging, 121-123
  subtypes, 120
  superficial spreading, 120
  surgical management of, 123
  vemurafenib in, 125
Melanonychia, 120
Melkersson-Rosenthal syndrome, 342
Meloschisis, 180

Men
  breast cancer in, 396
  gynecomastia in, 395-397
Mentalis, 341, 827
Mental nerve, 827
Merkel cell, 105
Merkel cell tumors, 127
Mersilene, 70
Mesoderm, 155
Mesoneurium, 657
Metacarpal fractures, 530-531, 531-532
Metacarpophalangeal (MP) joint, 540-542, 693, 695, 703
Metalloproteases, 10
Methicillin-resistant *Staphylococcus aureus* (MRSA), 469
Methylmethacrylate, 70
Methylparaben, 89
Metopic suture, 172
Metopic synostosis, 172
M flap, 194
Microneural repair, 61
Microsurgical anticoagulant, 61
Microsurgical sutures, 25
Microtia, 215-216
Microvascular clamps, 58
Midline forehead flap, 291
Migraine headaches, 162-166
Milk ridge, 358
Millard cleft lip repair, 194
Millard gull-wing flap, 290
Millard's hinged septal flap, 290
Miniabdominoplasty, 860-861
Minibrachioplasty, 847
Minimal access cranial suspension (MACS-lift), 799-800
Minoxidil, 754
Moberg flap, 547, 548, 613
Möbius syndrome, 343
Modified Manchester cleft lip repair, 194
Modified radical nodal dissections (MRND), 269
Mohs surgery, 118-119
Mongolian spot, 148
Monitoring, free flap, 60
Monocryl, 23, 24
Montgomery's glands, 358-359
Motor evoked potentials, 651
Mucoperichondrial flap, 292-293
Mucous cyst, 677, 678
Müller's muscle, 282, 775
Muscle denervation, 659
Muscle power grading, 650-651

892　Index

Muscles
　anterior chest wall, 359-360
　facial, 341-342
　hand, 574
　respiration, 422-423
Mustarde technique, 223, 224-225
Mycobacterium spp., 673
Mycophenolate mofetil (MMF), 608
Myelination, 658
Myocutaneous advancement flaps, 283
Myofibroblast, in wound healing, 8
Myoglobinuria, in burn, 133

N

Nagata technique, 217
Nail bed injury, 556-558
Nail growth, 556-557
Nasal alae, 158
Nasal base, in facial analysis, 720
Nasal fractures, 238
Nasal innervation, 289
Nasal lining reconstruction, 289
Nasal packing, in facial injury, 236
Nasal prominences, 158
Nasal reconstruction; *see also* Rhinoplasty
　cartilage grafting in, 70
　tissue expansion in, 46
Nasal root, in deformational plagiocephaly, 173-174
Nasal septum, 158
Nasal substitution, 210
Nasal tip
　in cleft lip, 193
　grafts, 821
　projection in facial analysis, 722
　rotation, in facial analysis, 721
Nasal valve, 819
Nasal vasculature, 289
Nasofrontal duct, 236
Nasolabial angle, 720, 721
Nasolabial folds, 797, 800
Nasoorbital ethmoid fractures, 237-238
Nasopalatine nerve block, 258
Nasopharyngeal anatomy, 330
Nasopharyngeal carcinoma, 331, 332, 333
Neck; *see also* Head and neck cancer
　development of, 157
　dissections, 269-270
　levels, 265
　nerves in, 807-808
Neck lift, 808-811

Needles, 22
Negative pressure wound therapy (NPWT)
　collagen in, 74
　contact layers in, 74
　contraindications to, 75
　in directly closed ankle wound, 75
　foam pore size in, 74
　granulation tissue production in, 16
　intermittent pressure mode in, 75
　macrostrain in, 74
　polyurethane foam in, 74
　pressures in, 75
　silver-coated sponge dressings in, 75
　in venous ulcers, 76
　wound odor in, 75
Nerve anatomy, 657-658
Nerve block, 92, 165, 258
Nerve compression, 639
Nerve degeneration, 658
Nerve gap, 661
Nerve grafts, 662
Nerve injury classification, 660
Nerve repair, primary, 661
Nerve root injury, 649
Nerve transfer, in brachial plexus injury, 652
Neurofibromatosis type 1 (NF1), 783-784
Neurotropism, 659
Neurovascular island flap, 620
Neutrophils, in soft tissue injury, 6
Nevus, congenital, 45, 46, 147-149
Nevus of Ito, 149
Nevus of Jadassohn, 126
Nevus of Ota, 149
Nevus spilus, 149
Nicotine replacement, 10-11
Nifedipine, 708-709
Nipple aesthetics, 360-361
Nipple-areolar complex (NAC), 365, 373, 388, 389-390
Nipple inversion, 415
Nipple positioning, 411
Nipple projection, 414
Nipple reconstruction, 411, 412-415
Nonabsorbable sutures, 21, 24
Norwood classification, 752-753
Nose
　anatomy, 817-819
　in facial analysis, 721-722

Notch-to-nipple distance, 386
Notta's node, 507
Nutrition, preoperative assessment of, 15
Nutritional support, of burn patients, 136
Nylon suture, 24, 25

O

Obstetric brachial plexus injury, 649
Odontogenic infections, 259
Odor, wound, 75
Omental flap, in chest wall reconstruction, 423, 425
Omohyoid, in neck levels, 265
Optic foramen, 254
Optic neuropathy, traumatic, 241
Oral-ocular clefts, 180
Orbicularis oculi, 282, 762, 774
Orbicularis oris, 315
Orbital apex syndrome, 241
Orbital fat, 775
Orbital fractures, 239
Orbital rhytids, 762
Orbit anatomy, 238
Orcel, 68
Oropharyngeal anatomy, 330
Oropharyngeal cancer, 331-332, 335
Orticochea flaps, 276
Orticochea pharyngoplasty, 211
Osler-Weber-Rendu disease, 143
Osteoarthritis, 696, 700-703
Osteoid osteoma, 680
Osteoinduction, 69
Osteomyelitis, 448, 460
Otalgia, referred, in head and neck cancer, 1070
Outcomes, photography and, 96
Oxygen supply, wound healing and, 10
Oxyhemoglobin, as target chromophore, 80
Oxymetazoline, 204

P

PABA, 89
Pacinian corpuscles, 105-106
Paget's disease, 415
Palate; *see also* Cleft palate
　embryology of, 200
　hard, 200
　primary, 158
　secondary, 157, 200
　soft, 200
Palatoplasty, 193

Panel reactive antibody test, 54, 351
Panfacial fractures, 240
Papaverine, in replantation, 600-601
Papillary cystadenoma lymphomatosum, 271
Paramedian forehead flap, 283-284, 292-293
Parascapular flap, 623
Parietex, 70
Parkes-Weber syndrome, 143
Parkland formula, 134
Parona's space, 485-486, 669-670
Paronychia, 556, 669
Parotid gland tumors, 270
Parotidomasseteric fascia, 794
Pasteurella multocida, 673
Patient classification, for anesthesia, 88
Patient counseling, in breast augmentation, 368-369
Pectoralis major, 360, 361, 404
Pectoralis major flap
 in cheek reconstruction, 302, 303
 in mandibular reconstruction, 322-323
Pectoralis major turnover, 424
Pectoralis minor, 359, 425
Pectus carinatum, 426
Pectus excavatum, 426
Pediatric patients
 facial palsy in, 343
Pedicle designs, in breast reduction, 387-388
Pedicled island flap, 548-549
Peels, 734-736
Perforating artery, in ear, 307
Perforator flaps, 29
 anatomy of, 37
 classification of, 37
 handheld Doppler in, 39
 plane of dissection in, 39
 raising, 38-39
Periareolar techniques
 in breast augmentation, 366
 in breast reduction, 388
 in mastopexy, 376
Perineurial repair, 61
Perineurium, 657
Perioral wounds, 229
Peripheral arterial disease, 15-16
Permacol, 67
Permanence, of implants, 66

Peyronie's disease, 441-442
Pfeiffer syndrome, 175
PHACE syndrome, 141
Phalangeal fractures, 533-535
Pharyngeal anatomy, 330
Pharyngeal arches, 155-156
Pharyngeal flap, 211
Pharyngeal grooves, 156
Pharyngeal pouches, 157
Pharyngeal reconstruction, 60
Phenol injury, 134
Phenol peels, 735-736
Philtral column, 191
Philtrum, 157
Photoaging, 717, 730
Photodynamic therapy (PFT), for basal cell carcinoma, 117-118
Photography
 in abdominoplasty, 98
 benefits of, 96
 in breast reconstruction, 99
 consent for, 99
 in face lift, 97
 focal length in, 96
 in rhinoplasty, 98
 standardized, 96
Pierre Robin sequence, 202, 211
Pigeon chest, 426
Pitanguy's point, 386
Platysma, 807
Platysma-auricular ligament, 808
Platysma sling, 810
Pleomorphic adenomas, 270, 271
Plosives, 209
Plummer-Vinson syndrome, 332
Pogonion, 259
Poland's syndrome, 361, 424, 425
Poliglecaprone, 23, 24
Pollicization, 614
Polybutester suture, 24
Polydactyly, 505, 507-508
Polydioxanone, 24
Polyester suture, 23, 24
Polyethylene glycol, 134
Polyglycolic acid, in abdominal wall reconstruction, 431
Polyglyconate, 24
Polyglytone, 24, 25
Poly-L-lactic acid (PLLA), 738
Polymastia, 358
Polypropylene suture, 24, 25
Polythelia, 358
Porion, 259
Port-wine stains, 81, 143
Posterior auricular artery, 307

Posterior interosseous artery (PIA), 622
Posterior interosseous flap, 622
Posterior interosseous nerve palsy, 490
Posterior interosseous syndrome, 643
Posterior pharyngeal wall augmentation, 211
Pouce flottant, 507
Power-assisted liposuction (PAL), 837
Prednisolone, 53-54
Preservation, of amputated digits, 598-599
Pressure sores, 446-449
Prilocaine, in EMLA, 92
Proceed, 70
Progeria, 108-109
Progressive tension sutures, 861
Pronator syndrome, 640
Propranolol, for hemangioma, 141
Proximal interphalangeal (PIP) joint
 in digital amputation, 591
 injury, 542-543
 osteoarthritis, 703
Pseudomonas, in pressure sores, 449
Pseudoxanthoma elasticum, 108
Psoriatic arthritis, 696
Ptosis, eyelid
 acquired, 784
 congenital, 783-784
Pulley system, flexor tendon, 562
Punching injuries, 530, 576
Pyogenic granuloma, 126
Pyrocarbon hemiarthroplasty, 702

Q

Quaba flap, 548

R

Radial forearm flap, 38, 318, 621
Radial nerve
 compression, 638, 641
 neurapraxia, 497
 palsy, 586
 repair, tendon transfer in, 585
 in Wartenberg's syndrome, 641-642
Radial tunnel syndrome, 641
Radiation therapy, for basal cell carcinoma, 118
Radiesse, 737

Index

Radiocarpal joint, in rheumatoid arthritis, 692
Radius fracture, distal, 522-524, 578
Radix graft, 820
Railroad scar, 25
Random pattern nasolabial flap, 301
Range of motion, in and wrist, 494
Ray amputation, 591-592
Raynaud's disease, 708-709
Raynaud's phenomenon, 708-709
Reconstructive ladder concept, 16
Rectus abdominis flap, 440
Rectus abdominis muscle, 360
Rectus abdominis myocutaneous flap, 424
Rectus diastasis, 862
Rectus plication, 860
Red line, 191
Red-line sign, 600
Regional anesthesia, 92
Remodeling phase, of wound healing, 7
Replantation, digital, 597-601
Resection arthroplasty, 469
Respiration muscles, 422-423
Restylane, 737
Resuscitation, burn, 134
Retinacular system of hand, 485
Reverse cross-finger flap, 551, 620
Reverse lateral arm flap, 623
Reverse radial forearm flap, 621
Revision surgery
 in augmentation-mastopexy, 381
 in fingertip amputation, 550
Rheumatoid arthritis (RA)
 common procedures in, 694-695
 Darrach procedure in, 695
 deformities in, 692
 diagnosis of, 691
 Mannerfelt lesion in, 694
 medications, surgical considerations with, 694
 metacarpophalangeal joint in, 693, 695
 pathophysiology of, 691
 Sauve-Kapandji procedure in, 695
 swan neck deformity in, 692-693
 tendon transfer in, 584-585, 588
 thumb deformity in, 693-694
 unsalvageable joints in, 695-696

Rhinophyma, 294
Rhinoplasty, 98, 820-824
Rhomboid flap, 302
Rhytids
 laser therapy for, 733-734
 lateral orbital, 762
 transverse forehead, 762
 vertical glabellar, 761-762
Riche-Cannieu anastomosis, 490, 658
Riedel's plane, 828
Rieger's dorsal nasal flap, 290
Right pectoralis major turnover, 424
Right vertical rectus abdominis myocutaneous flap, 424
Riley-Smith syndrome, 143
Rives-Stoppa procedure, 434
Robert's view, 700
Rosacea, 81
Rose-Thompson cleft lip repair, 194
Rotation flaps, 30-31
Roux-en-Y gastric bypass, 877
Ruffini ending, 106

S

Saethre-Chotzen syndrome, 175
Safe dosing, of local anesthetics, 89
Safety, in laser therapy, 84
Sagittal suture, 170
Sagittal synostosis, 172
Salivary gland tumors, 270, 271
Salivary pharyngeal bypass tube, 334-335
Salter-Harris classification, 529
Scalp anatomy, 275-276
Scalp defect, expanders with, 46
Scalp reconstruction, 276-278
Scalp wounds, 229, 230
Scaphocephaly, 172
Scaphoid, 490, 511
Scaphoid fractures, 511-512
Scapholunate ligament, 517, 677
Scapular flap, 623
Scapular osseocutaneous flaps, 324
Scarring
 in abdominoplasty, 857
 in brachioplasty, 847, 848
 hypertrophic, 11, 82
 keloid, 11-12
 laser therapy in, 82
 railroad, 25
Scleral show, 776-777
Scroll area, 819

Sculptra, 737, 738
Sebaceous nevus, 149
Seborrheic keratoses, 126
Secondary palate, 200
Sensation, abnormal, 660
Sentinel lymph node biopsy (SLNB), in melanoma, 123-124
Sentinel vein, 763
Sepramesh, 70
Sepsis, in burn patients, 137
Septal mucoperichondrial flaps, 289
Septal pivot flap, 290
Septic arthritis, 671
Septocutaneous perforators, 37-38
Serratus anterior flap, 624
Serratus anterior muscle, 359, 422-423
Serum inhibition, 67
Sexual differentiation, fetal, 438
S flap, 414
Shiffman classification, 717
Shprintzen's syndrome, 203
Silicone, fibrous encapsulation with, 71
Silicone elastomer shell, 44
Silk suture, 24
Silver-containing agents, in burn patients, 137
Simonart's band, 191
Simvastatin, gynecomastia and, 395
Singapore flap, 440
Skate flap, 412
Skin
 antigenicity of, 52
 cellular content of, 105
 collagen subtypes in, 6-7, 108
 dermal appendages in, 106
 layers, 107
 sensory receptors of, 105-106
 viscoelastic properties of, 44
Skin cancer, 54; *see also* Basal cell carcinoma (BCC); Melanoma; Squamous cell carcinoma (SCC)
Skin graft
 autologous, 66-67
 donor site anesthesia, 90
 in hand, 619
 on hand, 619
 loss of contact inhibition in, 8
 in lower limb reconstruction, 459

Index

Skin quality, in facial analysis, 717
Skin resurfacing, in laser therapy, 83
Skin substitutes, 17, 68
Sleep apnea, in velopharyngeal insufficiency, 211
Sleeve gastrectomy, 876
Smoking, 58, 331, 801, 856
Snodgrass technique, 440
Sodium bicarbonate, in local anesthetics, 90
Soft tissue
 injury, neutrophils in, 6
 substitutes, 68
 in tissue expansion, 44
Soft tissue sarcoma, 678-679
Soft triangle reconstruction, 293
Somatosensory evoked potentials (SSEPs), 651
Souquet flap, 547
Space of Poirier, 491, 517
Spasticity, tendon transfer and, 584-585
Spider nevus, 80-81
Spinal accessory nerve, 266, 798
Spinal block, 92
Spitz nevus, 148
Splinting
 for carpal tunnel syndrome, 639-640
 in central slip injuries, 577
 in extensor tendon injury, 579
 in flexor tendon repair, 566
 of hand injuries, 530, 542
 in mallet deformities, 576-577
Split-thickness skin graft, 67
 in hand, 619
 in lower limb reconstruction, 459
Sporothrix schenckii, 673
Spreader graft, 820, 822
Squamous cell carcinoma (SCC), 54
 deaths from, 119
 in ear, 119
 excision margins in, 120
 in head and neck, 265
 human papillomavirus and, 116
 in lower limb, 470
 lymph node dissection in, 120
 metastatic, in parotid gland, 342
 recurrence of, 119-120
 risk factors for, 119
 treatment of, 120
 verrucous, 119-120

Squint, 784
Staged tubed pedicle flap, 310
Staging, of head and neck cancers, 266-269
Stahl's ear, 225
Standing cones, 858
Stapedius, 155
Staphylococcus aureus, in capsular contracture, 367
Staphylococcus epidermidis, 367
Staples, in scalp wounds, 229
Star flap, 412, 413
Steel suture, 24, 25
Stemmer sign, 477
Stensen's duct, 229-230
Sterile matrix, 556-557
Sternal defects, 423
Sternocleidomastoid, 422, 808, 809
Sternotomy defects, 424
Steroid injections, in osteoarthritis, 701-702
Stewart-Treves syndrome, 477
Stickler syndrome, 203
Strabismus, 784
Stratum basale, 107
Stratum corneum, 107
Stratum granulosum, 107
Stratum spinosum, 107
Strauss-Bacon stability score, 350
Streeter's syndrome, 502
Streptococcus, in bite wounds, 228
Streptococcus pyogenes, 367
Streptococcus viridans, 367
Streptokinase, 33
Sturge-Weber syndrome, 143
Sauve-Kapandji procedure, 695
Submandibular transposition flap, 301
Submental artery flap, 300
Submucous cleft palate, 200-201
Suborbital zone, 299
Subscapular nerve, 648
Suction-assisted lipectomy, in lymphedema, 476
Suction lipectomy, in breast reduction, 387
Sumatriptan, 162
Sunderland classification, 660
Sunnybrook facial nerve function grading, 343, 344
Superciliary brow lift, 344
Superficial circumflex iliac artery, 624

Superficial inferior epigastric vein (SIEV) anastomosis, in deep inferior epigastric perforator flap, 38-39
Superficial muscular aponeurotic system (SMAS), 794, 795, 799
Superficial palmar arch, 488-489
Superficial temporal artery, 222, 307, 310
Superior labial artery, 289
Superior orbital fissure, 254
Superior orbital fissure syndrome, 241
Superior pedicle, in breast reduction, 387-388
Supraorbital nerve, 766-767
 in migraines, 163
 in scalp anatomy, 275-276
Suprascapular nerve, 648
Sural nerve, 662
SurgiMend, 17
Suture materials, 21-25
Swallowing, 332-333
Swan neck deformities, 579, 587, 692-693
Sweat glands, 106
Swing flap, 309-310
Swinging door flap, 822-823
Sympathetic ophthalmia, 243
Syndactyly, 174-175, 502, 504
Synkinesis, in face transplantation, 349-350
Synovium, in rheumatoid arthritis, 691
Systemic lupus erythematosus, 696

T

Tacrolimus, 53, 608
Tanner classification, of breast development, 358
Tarsal fixation techniques, 778-779
Tarsal plate, 282
Tarsoligamentous complex, 774-775
Tarsus, 282
Tattooing, in soft tissue trauma, 228
Tattoo removal, 80, 81, 82
Tear-trough deformity, 796
Teeth
 in mandibular fracture, 247
 primary, 254-255
 secondary, 254-255

Telangiectasia, 81
Telecanthus, 784
Temporal bone fractures, 240, 243
Temporal forehead flap, 284
Temporomastoid flap, 292
Tendon, exposed, defect repair with, 68
Tendon nutrition, 563
Tendon transfers
 in combined nerve palsy, 587
 contraindications after, 587
 donor muscle in, 584
 indications for, 584
 in median nerve palsy, 585
 principles of, 584
 in radial nerve palsy, 586
 in rheumatoid arthritis, 584-585, 588
 spasticity and, 584-585
 in ulnar nerve palsy, 586
Tenolysis, after digital replantation, 601
Tensile strength, in healed wounds, 7
Tensor fascia lata flap, 30
Tensor veli palatini, 155, 156, 200
Tessier clefts, 180-181
Testosterone, in male pattern baldness, 752
Tetanus, 228
Thenar flap, 549, 620
Thigh anatomy, 867
Thigh lift, medial, 867-871
Thoracic outlet syndrome, 709, 711
Thoracodorsal artery, 624
Thoracoplasty, 423
Thromboxane A_2, 32
Thumb
 in anterior interosseous syndrome, 640-641
 duplication, 503, 507
 local flaps for, 620
 mallet deformity of, 578
 metacarpophalangeal joint injury in, 541-542
 osteoarthritis in, 700, 701-702
 in rheumatoid arthritis, 693-694
 stiff replanted versus alternative reconstruction, 612
 tip injury, 551
Thumb reconstruction, 612-615
Thyroid gland, development of, 157
Tibial blood supply, 457

Tibial fracture
 end-to-end anastomosis in, 60
 fibular fracture with, 456
 Gustilo classification for, 455
 reduction and stabilization of, 456-457
 soft tissue reconstruction in, 456-457
TIFF photo format, 96
TiMesh, 70
Tinel's sign, 496
Tissue creep, in scalp wounds, 276
Tissue expansion; *see* Expanders
Tissue plasminogen activator, 33
Tongue base, in oropharyngeal defects, 335
Transaxillary approach, in breast augmentation, 366
Transcyte, 17, 68, 69
Transforming growth factor beta, in wound healing, 7-8
Transplantation
 candidates for, 54
 face, 52, 349-352
 hair, 755-757
 hand, 606-609
Transplant rejection, 51, 52, 351, 352
Transplant tissue types, 51
Transverse rectus abdominis flap, 60
Transverse rectus abdominis myocutaneous (TRAM) flap, 405-407
Transverse upper gracilis (TUG) flap, 623
Trapeziectomy, 702
Trapezius flap, 302
Trapezoid fracture, 513
Trauma
 as face transplantation indication, 349
 facial skeletal, 236-243
 facial soft tissue, 228-230
Traumatic alopecia, 754
Traumatic aneurysm, 708
Traumatic optic neuropathy (TON), 241
Treacher Collins syndrome, 181-182
Trichloroacetic acid peels, 735
Trigeminal nerve
 in ear innervation, 307
 foramina, 254
 in migraines, 162

Trigger finger, 694, 695
Trigger thumb, 502, 507
Trigonocephaly, 172
Triptans, 162
Tuberous breast deformity, 374-375
Tubular incised plate (TIP), 440, 441
Tunica albuginea, 441-442
Turning, for pressure sore prevention, 448
Turribrachycephaly, 174
Tutopatch, 69
TWIST gene mutation, 175
Two-point discrimination, 660
Two-stage Wise pattern augmentation-mastopexy, 376
Tympanic segment, of facial nerve, 340, 341
Tyndall effect, 739

U

Ulcer
 foot, 466-470
 pressure, 446-449
 vascular, 16, 76
Ulnar artery aneurysm, 642-643, 680
Ulnar collateral ligament injury, 541
Ulnar nerve compression, 497
 at elbow, 642
 in Guyon's canal, 642-643
Ulnar nerve palsy, 586, 638
Ulnar nerve repair, 662
Ulnar nerve transection, 61
Ultrasound-assisted liposuction (UAL), 396, 837
Umbrella graft, 821
Upper limb; *see also* Hand; Wrist
 aneurysm, 708
 brachioplasty in, 844-848
 compression syndromes, 643
 innervation of, 489-490
Urine output, in burn patients, 133
Urokinase, 33
Uvula, bifid, 201

V

Vaginal agenesis, 439
Vaginal defects, 438
Vaginal reconstruction, 440
Vaginal wall defects, 439
Vagus nerve, 222, 331
Valleculae, 330

Vancomycin-resistant *Enterococcus* (VRE), 469
Van der Woude syndrome, 203
Vascular disorders, of hand and wrist, 708-711
Vascular endothelial growth factor (VEGF), in wound healing, 7-8
Vascularized bone flaps, 322, 323-324
Vascularized composite allografts (VCAs), 52, 54
 in face transplantation, 350
 in hand transplantation, 608
Vascular lesions, in laser therapy, 81
Vascular malformations, 142-143
Vasoconstriction, in wound healing, 6
Vasodilation, in wound healing, 6
Vastus lateralis, in lateral circumflex femoral artery perforator flap, 39-40
Veau-Wardill-Kilner pushback palatoplasty, 203-204
Vecchietti procedure, 439
Velocardiofacial syndrome, 203, 210
Velopharyngeal dysfunction
 adenoidectomy and, 209
 evaluation in, 210
 hypernasality in, 209
 speech assessment in, 209-210
 terminology with, 209
 treatment of, 211-212
Velopharyngeal incompetence, 209
Vemurafenib, in melanoma, 125
Venkataswamy flap, 551
Venous flaps, 30
Venous insufficiency, foot lesions in, 470
Venous malformations, 144
Venous thromboembolism (VTE), 58
Venous thrombosis, 711
Venous ulcers, negative pressure wound therapy in, 76
Vermilion, 191, 195, 315
Vermilion defect repair, 316
Vertical scar mastopexy, 376, 381
V flap, 414-415
Vicryl sutures, 21, 24
Videofluoroscopy
 in swallowing assessment, 332-333

 in velopharyngeal dysfunction, 210
Vinculae, 575
Viscoelasticity, of skin, 44
Vitamin A, wound healing and, 9-10
Volar abscess, 669-670
Volar advancement flaps, 613
Volar compartment, 628-629
Volar plate, 542
Volcano sign, 171
Vomer flaps, 204
von Hippel-Lindau disease, 142
von Langenbeck palatoplasty, 204

W

Warfarin, 708
Wartenberg's syndrome, 641-642, 643
Warthin's tumor, 271
Washio flap, 292
Waterfall deformity, 368
Wavelengths, in laser resurfacing, 731
Web space, in thumb reconstruction, 613-614
Weight loss
 bariatric surgery for, 875-877
 body contouring after, 877-880
 breast reconstruction after, 879
 mastopexy after, 377
 thigh lift after, 870-871
Werner's syndrome, 108
Whistle tip deformity, 195
White roll, 191, 315
Whites
 alopecia in, 751
 malocclusion in, 827
Whitnall's ligament, 774
Wise pattern autoaugmentation-mastopexy, 377
Wood-Smith technique, 223-224
Wound dehiscence, 879-880
Wound healing
 blood glucose and, 15
 cell types in, 6, 8
 chemotherapy and, 11
 collagen in, 7
 in cutis laxa, 9
 cutis laxa and, 108
 debridement and, 10
 edge apposition in, 8-9
 epidermal growth factor in, 8
 factors affecting, 9-11
 in fetal tissue, 6
 fibroblast in, 6, 7-8

 growth factors in, 7-8
 lymphocytes in, 6
 macrophage in, 6
 myofibroblast in, 8
 neutrophil in, 6
 nicotine and, 10-11
 oxygen supply and, 10
 phases of, 6
 reconstructive ladder concept in, 16
 remodeling phase of, 7
 tensile strength and, 7
 transforming growth factor beta in, 7-8
 types of, 8-9
 vascular endothelial growth factor in, 7-8
 vitamin A and, 9-10
Wrist
 bones, 490-491
 ligaments, 517
 range of movement in, 494
 ulnar deviation of, 496
 vascular disorders of, 708-711
Wrist amputation, 592
Wrist arthroscopy, 518
Wrist splinting, for carpal tunnel syndrome, 639-640
Wuchereria bancrofti, 474
Würinger's septum, 359

X

Xenograft, 51, 66

Z

Zinc oxide, 294
Zone of inflammation, 132
Zone of necrosis, 132
Zone of polarizing activity (ZPA), 502
Zone of stasis, 132
Zones of adherence, 834, 835
Z-plasty
 angles in, 31
 double-opposing, 31-32
 in ear reconstruction, 310
Zygomatic fracture, 243
Zygomatic ligament, 796, 797
Zygomaticocutaneous ligament, 796
Zygomaticomaxillary complex fractures, 239
Zygomaticotemporal nerve, 165
Zygomaticus major, 342